Systemic Lupus Erythematosus: Pathogenesis, Diagnosis and Treatment

Systemic Lupus Erythematosus: Pathogenesis, Diagnosis and Treatment

Guest Editor

Matteo Piga

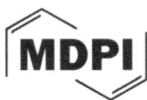

Basel • Beijing • Wuhan • Barcelona • Belgrade • Novi Sad • Cluj • Manchester

Guest Editor
Matteo Piga
University of Cagliari
Cagliari
Italy

Editorial Office
MDPI AG
Grosspeteranlage 5
4052 Basel, Switzerland

This is a reprint of the Special Issue, published open access by the journal *Journal of Clinical Medicine* (ISSN 2077-0383), freely accessible at: https://www.mdpi.com/journal/jcm/special_issues/Erythematosus_Treatment.

For citation purposes, cite each article independently as indicated on the article page online and as indicated below:

Lastname, A.A.; Lastname, B.B. Article Title. *Journal Name* **Year**, *Volume Number*, Page Range.

ISBN 978-3-7258-2869-2 (Hbk)
ISBN 978-3-7258-2870-8 (PDF)
https://doi.org/10.3390/books978-3-7258-2870-8

© 2024 by the authors. Articles in this book are Open Access and distributed under the Creative Commons Attribution (CC BY) license. The book as a whole is distributed by MDPI under the terms and conditions of the Creative Commons Attribution-NonCommercial-NoDerivs (CC BY-NC-ND) license (https://creativecommons.org/licenses/by-nc-nd/4.0/).

Contents

About the Editor ix

Alvaro Gomez, Sofia Soukka, Petter Johansson, Emil Åkerström, Sharzad Emamikia, Yvonne Enman, et al.
Use of Antimalarial Agents Is Associated with Favourable Physical Functioning in Patients with Systemic Lupus Erythematosus
Reprinted from: *J. Clin. Med.* **2020**, *9*, 1813, https://doi.org/10.3390/jcm9061813 1

Muna Saleh, Christopher Sjöwall, Helena Strevens, Andreas Jönsen, Anders A. Bengtsson and Michele Compagno
Adverse Pregnancy Outcomes after Multi-Professional Follow-Up of Women with Systemic Lupus Erythematosus: An Observational Study from a Single Centre in Sweden
Reprinted from: *J. Clin. Med.* **2020**, *9*, 2598, https://doi.org/10.3390/jcm9082598 18

Sabrina Porta, Alvaro Danza, Maira Arias Saavedra, Adriana Carlomagno, María Cecilia Goizueta, Florencia Vivero and Guillermo Ruiz-Irastorza
Glucocorticoids in *Systemic Lupus Erythematosus*. Ten Questions and Some Issues
Reprinted from: *J. Clin. Med.* **2020**, *9*, 2709, https://doi.org/10.3390/jcm9092709 32

Elena Monzón Manzano, Ihosvany Fernández-Bello, Raúl Justo Sanz, Ángel Robles Marhuenda, Francisco Javier López-Longo, Paula Acuña, et al.
Insights into the Procoagulant Profile of Patients with Systemic Lupus Erythematosus without Antiphospholipid Antibodies
Reprinted from: *J. Clin. Med.* **2020**, *9*, 3297, https://doi.org/10.3390/jcm9103297 45

Tomoyuki Asano, Naoki Matsuoka, Yuya Fujita, Haruki Matsumoto, Jumpei Temmoku, Makiko Yashiro-Furuya, et al.
Serum Levels of T Cell Immunoglobulin and Mucin-Domain Containing Molecule 3 in Patients with Systemic Lupus Erythematosus
Reprinted from: *J. Clin. Med.* **2020**, *9*, 3563, https://doi.org/10.3390/jcm9113563 62

Matteo Piga and Laurent Arnaud
The Main Challenges in Systemic Lupus Erythematosus: Where Do We Stand?
Reprinted from: *J. Clin. Med.* **2021**, *10*, 243, https://doi.org/10.3390/jcm10020243 71

Farah Tamirou and Frédéric A. Houssiau
Management of Lupus Nephritis
Reprinted from: *J. Clin. Med.* **2021**, *10*, 670, https://doi.org/10.3390/jcm10040670 83

Kennedy C. Ukadike and Tomas Mustelin
Implications of Endogenous Retroelements in the Etiopathogenesis of Systemic Lupus Erythematosus
Reprinted from: *J. Clin. Med.* **2021**, *10*, 856, https://doi.org/10.3390/jcm10040856 94

Irini Gergianaki, Panagiotis Garantziotis, Christina Adamichou, Ioannis Saridakis, Georgios Spyrou, Prodromos Sidiropoulos and George Bertsias
High Comorbidity Burden in Patients with SLE: Data from the Community-Based Lupus Registry of Crete
Reprinted from: *J. Clin. Med.* **2021**, *10*, 998, https://doi.org/10.3390/jcm10050998 112

Berta Magallares, David Lobo-Prat, Ivan Castellví, Patricia Moya, Ignasi Gich, Laura Martinez-Martinez, et al.
Assessment of EULAR/ACR-2019, SLICC-2012 and ACR-1997 Classification Criteria in SLE with Longstanding Disease
Reprinted from: *J. Clin. Med.* **2021**, *10*, 2377, https://doi.org/10.3390/jcm10112377 . . . . **128**

Yen-Fu Chen, Ao-Ho Hsieh, Lian-Chin Wang, Kuang-Hui Yu and Chang-Fu Kuo
Cytomegalovirus-Associated Autoantibody against TAF9 Protein in Patients with Systemic Lupus Erythematosus
Reprinted from: *J. Clin. Med.* **2021**, *10*, 3722, https://doi.org/10.3390/jcm10163722 . . . . **137**

Renen Taub, Danny Horesh, Noa Rubin, Ittai Glick, Orit Reem, Gitit Shriqui and Nancy Agmon-Levin
Mindfulness-Based Stress Reduction for Systemic Lupus Erythematosus: A Mixed-Methods Pilot Randomized Controlled Trial of an Adapted Protocol
Reprinted from: *J. Clin. Med.* **2021**, *10*, 4450, https://doi.org/10.3390/jcm10194450 . . . . **146**

Tsu-Yi Hsieh, Yi-Ching Lin, Wei-Ting Hung, Yi-Ming Chen, Mei-Chin Wen, Hsin-Hua Chen, et al.
Change of Renal Gallium Uptake Correlated with Change of Inflammation Activity in Renal Pathology in Lupus Nephritis Patients
Reprinted from: *J. Clin. Med.* **2021**, *10*, 4654, https://doi.org/10.3390/jcm10204654 . . . . **164**

Katarzyna Pawlak-Buś, Wiktor Schmidt and Piotr Leszczyński
Lack of Association between Serum Interleukin-23 and Interleukin-27 Levels and Disease Activity in Patients with Active Systemic Lupus Erythematosus
Reprinted from: *J. Clin. Med.* **2021**, *10*, 4788, https://doi.org/10.3390/jcm10204788 . . . . **180**

Nesreen M. Ismail, Eman A. Toraih, Mai H. S. Mohammad, Eida M. Alshammari and Manal S. Fawzy
Association of microRNA-34a rs2666433 (A/G) Variant with Systemic Lupus Erythematosus in Female Patients: A Case-Control Study
Reprinted from: *J. Clin. Med.* **2021**, *10*, 5095, https://doi.org/10.3390/jcm10215095 . . . . **194**

Ioannis Parodis and Paul Studenic
Patient-Reported Outcomes in Systemic Lupus Erythematosus. Can Lupus Patients Take the Driver's Seat in Their Disease Monitoring?
Reprinted from: *J. Clin. Med.* **2022**, *11*, 340, https://doi.org/10.3390/jcm11020340 . . . . **209**

Marlene Plüß, Silvia Piantoni, Chris Wincup and Peter Korsten
Rapid Response of Refractory Systemic Lupus Erythematosus Skin Manifestations to Anifrolumab—A Case-Based Review of Clinical Trial Data Suggesting a Domain-Based Therapeutic Approach
Reprinted from: *J. Clin. Med.* **2022**, *11*, 3449, https://doi.org/10.3390/jcm11123449 . . . . **216**

Minhui Wang, Ziqian Wang, Shangzhu Zhang, Yang Wu, Li Zhang, Jiuliang Zhao, et al.
Progress in the Pathogenesis and Treatment of Neuropsychiatric Systemic Lupus Erythematosus
Reprinted from: *J. Clin. Med.* **2022**, *11*, 4955, https://doi.org/10.3390/jcm11174955 . . . . **225**

Eleni Kapsia, Smaragdi Marinaki, Ioannis Michelakis, George Liapis, Petros P. Sfikakis, John Boletis and Maria G. Tektonidou
Predictors of Early Response, Flares, and Long-Term Adverse Renal Outcomes in Proliferative Lupus Nephritis: A 100-Month Median Follow-Up of an Inception Cohort
Reprinted from: *J. Clin. Med.* **2022**, *11*, 5017, https://doi.org/10.3390/jcm11175017 . . . . **241**

Miguel Marín-Rosales, Claudia Azucena Palafox-Sánchez, Ramón Antonio Franco-Topete,
Francisco Josué Carrillo-Ballesteros, Alvaro Cruz, Diana Celeste Salazar-Camarena, et al.
Renal Tissue Expression of BAFF and BAFF Receptors Is Associated with Proliferative Lupus Nephritis
Reprinted from: J. Clin. Med. 2023, 12, 71, https://doi.org/10.3390/jcm12010071 256

Fernanda Isadora Corona-Meraz, Mónica Vázquez-Del Mercado, Flavio Sandoval-García,
Jesus-Aureliano Robles-De Anda, Alvaro-Jovanny Tovar-Cuevas,
Roberto-Carlos Rosales-Gómez, et al.
Biomarkers in Systemic Lupus Erythematosus along with Metabolic Syndrome
Reprinted from: J. Clin. Med. 2024, 13, 1988, https://doi.org/10.3390/jcm13071988 267

Mohamed H. Omer, Areez Shafqat, Omar Ahmad, Juzer Nadri, Khaled AlKattan and
Ahmed Yaqinuddin
Urinary Biomarkers for Lupus Nephritis: A Systems Biology Approach
Reprinted from: J. Clin. Med. 2024, 13, 2339, https://doi.org/10.3390/jcm13082339 282

Joanna Kosałka-Węgiel, Radosław Dziedzic, Andżelika Siwiec-Koźlik,
Magdalena Spałkowska, Mamert Milewski, Anita Wach, et al.
Comparison of Clinical and Laboratory Characteristics in Lupus Nephritis vs. Non-Lupus
Nephritis Patients—A Comprehensive Retrospective Analysis Based on 921 Patients
Reprinted from: J. Clin. Med. 2024, 13, 4486, https://doi.org/10.3390/jcm13154486 298

Noemí Espinoza-García, Diana Celeste Salazar-Camarena, Miguel Marín-Rosales,
María Paulina Reyes-Mata, María Guadalupe Ramírez-Dueñas,
José Francisco Muñoz-Valle, et al.
High Interleukin 21 Levels in Patients with Systemic Lupus Erythematosus: Association with
Clinical Variables and rs2221903 Polymorphism
Reprinted from: J. Clin. Med. 2024, 13, 4512, https://doi.org/10.3390/jcm13154512 316

María Recio-Barbero, Janire Cabezas-Garduño, Jimena Varona, Guillermo Ruiz-Irastorza,
Igor Horrillo, J. Javier Meana, et al.
Clinical Predictors of Mood Disorders and Prevalence of Neuropsychiatric Symptoms in
Patients with Systemic Lupus Erythematosus
Reprinted from: J. Clin. Med. 2024, 13, 5423, https://doi.org/10.3390/jcm13185423 331

About the Editor

Matteo Piga

Matteo Piga is an Associate Professor of Rheumatology at the University of Cagliari (Italy). He completed his rheumatology qualification in 2007 at the University of Cagliari. From 2007 to 2008, he worked at the Louise Coote Lupus Unit at St. Thomas's Hospital in London, UK, as a Research Fellow. Professor Piga is mainly interested in Systemic Lupus Erythematosus in both clinical and scientific aspects. He is dedicated to caring for and treating patients in a longitudinal lupus clinic. His current research focuses on immunogenetics, epidemiology, developing biomarkers and tools for assessing SLE disease activity and organ damage, and implementing digital health for diagnosing and monitoring the disease.

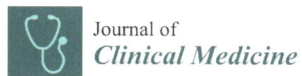

Article

Use of Antimalarial Agents Is Associated with Favourable Physical Functioning in Patients with Systemic Lupus Erythematosus

Alvaro Gomez [1,2], Sofia Soukka [1,2], Petter Johansson [1,2], Emil Åkerström [1,2], Sharzad Emamikia [1,2], Yvonne Enman [1,2], Katerina Chatzidionysiou [1,2] and Ioannis Parodis [1,2,*]

[1] Division of Rheumatology, Department of Medicine Solna, Karolinska Institutet, 171 76 Stockholm, Sweden; alvaro.gomez.gonzalez@ki.se (A.G.); sofia.soukka@gmail.com (S.S.); petter.johansson@stud.ki.se (P.J.); emil.akerstrom@stud.ki.se (E.Å.); sharzad.emamikia@ki.se (S.E.); yvonne.enman@ki.se (Y.E.); aikaterini.chatzidionysiou@ki.se (K.C.)
[2] Rheumatology, Karolinska University Hospital, 171 76 Stockholm, Sweden
* Correspondence: ioannis.parodis@ki.se; Tel.: +46-72-232-1322

Received: 14 May 2020; Accepted: 8 June 2020; Published: 10 June 2020

Abstract: Impaired health-related quality of life (HRQoL) is a major problem in patients with systemic lupus erythematosus (SLE). Antimalarial agents (AMA) are the cornerstone of SLE therapy, but data on their impact on HRQoL are scarce. We investigated this impact using baseline data from the BLISS-52 (NCT00424476) and BLISS-76 (NCT00410384) trials (n = 1684). HRQoL was self-reported using the Medical Outcomes Study short-form 36 (SF-36), functional assessment of chronic illness therapy (FACIT)-Fatigue and 3-level EuroQoL 5-Dimension (EQ-5D) questionnaires. Patients on AMA (n = 1098/1684) performed better with regard to SF-36 physical component summary, physical functioning, role physical, bodily pain, FACIT-Fatigue, EQ-5D utility index and EQ-5D visual analogue scale scores. The difference in SF-36 physical functioning (mean ± standard deviation (SD): 61.1 ± 24.9 versus 55.0 ± 26.5; $p < 0.001$) exceeded the minimal clinically important difference (≥5.0). This association remained significant after adjustment for potential confounding factors in linear regression models (standardised coefficient, β = 0.07; p = 0.002). Greater proportions of AMA users than non-users reported no problems in the mobility, self-care, usual activities and anxiety/depression EQ-5D dimensions. AMA use was particularly associated with favourable HRQoL in physical aspects among patients with active mucocutaneous and musculoskeletal disease, and mental aspects among patients with active renal SLE. These results provide support in motivating adherence to AMA therapy. Exploration of causality in the relationship between AMA use and favourable HRQoL in SLE has merit.

Keywords: systemic lupus erythematosus; health-related quality of life; antimalarial agents; treatment; patient-reported outcomes; health perceptions; medication adherence

---

1. Introduction

Systemic lupus erythematosus (SLE) is a chronic inflammatory multisystem disease that commonly affects women during their reproductive life span. It is characterised by relapses and periods of remission, and permanent organ damage may accrue during the course of the disease [1]. SLE negatively affects the patients' health-related quality of life (HRQoL), not only because it causes pain and physical dysfunction, but also because it is associated with end-organ damage, several comorbidities and medication-related adverse events [2]. Certain disease characteristics signify particular propensity for HRQoL diminutions, i.e., early disease onset, and cutaneous, musculoskeletal and renal involvement [3,4].

Treatment of SLE includes broad immunosuppressants or immunomodulatory agents, aiming for remission or low disease activity state [5,6]. Antimalarial agents (AMA) are considered the cornerstone of SLE therapy and are recommended for all patients with SLE, unless contraindicated [7]. Administration of AMA reduces the probability of disease relapses and contributes to long-term remission, reduces the rate of organ damage accrual, increases patient survival, and is associated with protective effects against complications and comorbidities, e.g., cardiovascular disease and impairment of the renal function [8–10].

The concept of the patients' perspective as an integral part of the clinical evaluation gains increasing acknowledgment within the SLE researcher community, and HRQoL outcomes are nowadays commonly used in drug trials [11]. This has to be seen as a paradigm shift, knowing that the patients' perspective historically has rather been neglected in clinical practice. However, data on the impact of AMA on HRQoL among SLE patients are scarce and conflicting, with some studies reporting beneficial effects [12,13] while other investigations show no impact [14].

Our aim in the present study was to determine the impact of AMA on self-reported physical and mental HRQoL in a large SLE population from two phase III clinical trials.

2. Experimental Section

2.1. Study Design and Population

We conducted a post-hoc analysis of data from two multicentre, double-blinded placebo-controlled phase III trials of belimumab, i.e., BLISS-52 [15] and BLISS-76 [16], which comprised 865 and 819 participants, respectively. The two trials included SLE patients of 18 years of age and above, classified having SLE according to the American College of Rheumatology revised criteria [17]. All patients in the trials were seropositive, defined as having an ANA titre of ≥1:80 and/or anti-double stranded (ds)DNA antibody level ≥ 30 IU/mL, and had an active SLE disease defined as a Safety of Estrogens in Lupus National Assessment-Systemic Lupus Erythematosus Disease Activity Index (SELENA-SLEDAI) [18] score of 6 or more.

All patients recruited were also on a stable background treatment comprising glucocorticoids, AMA and/or immunosuppressants, or, in the majority of the cases, combinations thereof (termed standard of care therapy), for at least one month prior to treatment initiation.

For the purpose of the present study, we utilised baseline data only in a cross-sectional manner, i.e., data obtained prior to exposure to belimumab or placebo. The almost identical trial designs facilitated utilisation of pooled data from both trials. Data were made available by GlaxoSmithKline (Uxbridge, UK) through the Clinical Study Data Request (CSDR) consortium.

The patients' rights, privacy and safety were protected in compliance with the ethical principles of the Declaration of Helsinki. Written informed consent was obtained from all study participants prior to enrolment in the BLISS-52 and BLISS-76 trial programmes. The study protocols from all participating centres were reviewed and approved by regional ethics review boards, and the study protocol for this post-hoc analysis was reviewed and approved by the regional ethics review board in Stockholm, Sweden (reference number 2019-05498).

2.2. Evaluation of HRQoL

Patient-reported data of HRQoL were registered using generic instruments, i.e., the medical outcome study (MOS) short form-36 (SF-36) questionnaire [19], the functional assessment of chronic illness therapy (FACIT)-Fatigue scale [20] and the 3-level EuroQoL research foundation 5-dimension (EQ-5D) health survey [21].

The MOS SF-36 is one of the most common generic questionnaires used for assessment of HRQoL in patients with different health conditions, as well as in the general population [19]. It contains 36 questions, analysis of which results in eight subscales representing different HRQoL aspects, i.e., physical functioning (PF), role physical (RP), bodily pain (BP), general health (GH), social functioning (SF), vitality (VT), role emotional (RE) and mental health (MH). The response from SF-36 was scored using the SF-36v2 manual [22], yielding subscale scores from 0 to 100. Next, the SF-36 subscales were computed according to a three-step procedure, including Z-score transformation and weighting based on the general US population to generate two summary measures, i.e., the physical component summary (PCS) and the mental component summary (MCS). Although all subscales are weighted in the derivation of both PCS and MCS, PF, RP, BP and GH are referred to as the physical aspects, and SF, VT, RE and MH are referred to as the mental aspects of SF-36. In terms of interpretation, high scores in SF-36 component summaries and subscales are considered a favourable perception of HRQoL and low scores are interpreted as poor HRQoL.

The FACIT-Fatigue scale is an instrument that includes 13 items and is designed to assess the level of fatigue over the preceding seven days. The scores generated have a span from 0 (maximal fatigue) to 52 (minimal fatigue), with scores < 30 representing severe fatigue.

The 3-level EQ-5D health survey consists of two distinct sections, i.e., a visual analogue scale (VAS), measuring patients' health perception from 0 (worst health status) to 100 (best health status), and a descriptive system, consisting of a questionnaire that comprises five dimensions, i.e., self-care, mobility, usual activities, pain/discomfort and anxiety/depression. Each dimension is scored by the respondent, with possible answers being no problems (level 1), some/moderate problems (level 2), or extreme/major problems (level 3). Responses to these five questions are next summarised into a utility index score. In the present study, EQ-5D utility index scores were calculated based on the valuation of EQ-5D health states from a general US population sample [23]. In terms of interpretation, higher utility index scores represent a better HRQoL. "Full-health state" was defined as statement of no problems in all five dimensions [24].

Apart from numerical and statistical differences, we endorsed the concept of minimal clinically important differences (MCIDs), and registered fulfilment of MCIDs in comparisons between AMA users and non-users. Based on previous literature, we set the MCID for SF-36 PCS and MCS scores to ≥2.5 points and for SF-36 subscales to ≥5.0 points [25], for FACIT-Fatigue scores to ≥4 points [26], for EQ-5D utility index scores to ≥0.040 points, used for scores calculated using the US valuation algorithm [27], and for EQ-5D VAS scores to ≥10 points [28]. For MCIDs that in previous studies were meant for evaluation of changes of the HRQoL between different time points, with different benchmarks for improvement and worsening, we considered the greatest benchmark as the MCID for the respective HRQoL item in the cross-sectional design of the present study.

2.3. Evaluation of Disease Activity and Organ Damage

In the BLISS trials, SLE disease activity was measured using the SELENA-SLEDAI [18] and the classic British Isles Lupus Assessment Group Index (BILAG) [29] indices. Organ damage was assessed using the Systemic Lupus International Collaborating Clinics/American College of Rheumatology Damage Index (SDI) [30].

2.4. Patient Subgroups based on Organ-Specific Activity

For patient subgroup analyses, we evaluated associations between use of AMA and patient perceptions of HRQoL in study participants with active mucocutaneous, musculoskeletal and renal disease, herein defined as BILAG A or B in the respective domain.

2.5. Statistical Analysis

Data are presented as numbers (percentage) or means ± standard deviation (SD). Comparisons of continuous data between AMA users and non-users were conducted using the Mann-Whitney U test. The Pearson's chi-square test was used to investigate contingent associations between binomial variables. Subsequently, linear regression analysis was carried out for comparisons yielding clinically important differences in order to adjust for potential confounding factors, selected based on previous literature [12,31–33]. Covariates included age, sex, ethnicity, SELENA-SLEDAI scores, SLE disease duration, SDI scores, prednisone (or equivalent) dose and use of immunosuppressants. Multivariable linear regression models included items that showed statistically significant associations in preceding univariable analysis. p-values < 0.05 were considered statistically significant. Statistical analyses were performed using the IBM SPSS software version 25 (IBM Corp., Armonk, NY, USA). GraphPad Prism 7 (GraphPad Software Inc., La Jolla, CA, USA) was used for the construction of graphs.

3. Results

3.1. Patient Characteristics

Of 1684 SLE patients recruited to the BLISS trials, 1098 patients were on AMA at the baseline evaluation (65.2%), and 94.1% were women. Demographics and SLE disease characteristics for the entire study population are presented in Table 1, and include AMA compounds and dose, as well as comparisons between AMA users and non-users. In Supplementary Materials Table S1, we present patient characteristics in the BLISS-52 and BLISS-76 trials separately.

Table 1. Demographic characteristics and clinical data of antimalarial agents (AMA) users versus non-users.

Patient Characteristics	Pooled BLISS	AMA Use +	AMA Use −	p Value
Number of Patients	1684	1098	586	
Demographic Characteristics				
Age (years)	37.8 (11.5)	36.8 (11.4)	39.6 (11.5)	**<0.001**
Female sex	1585 (94.1%)	1033 (94.1%)	552 (94.2%)	0.922
Ethnicity				
Asian	353 (21.0%)	243 (22.1%)	110 (18.8%)	0.107
Black/African American	146 (8.7%)	98 (8.9%)	48 (8.2%)	0.610
Indigenous American	374 (22.2%)	254 (23.1%)	120 (20.5%)	0.212
White/Caucasian	798 (47.4%)	491 (44.7%)	307 (52.4%)	**0.003**
Clinical Data				
SELENA-SLEDAI score	9.7 (3.8)	9.6 (3.6)	10.0 (4.0)	0.145
SLE disease duration (years)	6.4 (6.3)	6.1 (6.2)	7.0 (6.6)	**0.007**
SDI score	0.78 (1.24)	0.69 (1.15)	0.95 (1.37)	**<0.001**
SDI score = 0	977 (58.1%)	673 (61.3%)	304 (52.0%)	**<0.001**
Glucocorticoid use	1453 (86.3%)	929 (84.6%)	524 (89.4%)	**0.006**
Prednisone eq. dose (mg/day)	10.8 (8.7)	10.1 (8.5)	12.1 (8.8)	**<0.001**
AMA use	1098 (64.8%)	1098 (100%)	N/A	N/A
Hydroxychloroquine	836 (49.6%)	836 (76.1%)	N/A	N/A
Chloroquine	265 (15.7%)	265 (24.1%)	N/A	N/A
Other antimalarial agents *	5 (0.3%)	5 (0.5%)	N/A	N/A
Hydroxychloroquine eq. dose (mg/day)	219.6 (183.5)	336.2 (111.0)	N/A	N/A
Immunosuppressants	816 (48.5%)	476 (43.4%)	340 (58.0%)	**<0.001**
Azathioprine	389 (23.1%)	221 (20.1%)	168 (28.7%)	**<0.001**
Methotrexate	231 (13.7%)	144 (13.1%)	87 (14.8%)	0.325
Mycophenolic acid	189 (11.2%)	104 (9.5%)	85 (14.5%)	**0.002**

Data are presented as numbers (percentage) or means (standard deviation). Statistically significant p-values are indicated in bold. * Mepacrine, mepacrine hydrochloride, quinine sulphate. AMA: antimalarial agents; SELENA-SLEDAI: Safety of Estrogens in Lupus National Assessment Systemic Lupus Erythematosus Disease Activity Index; SDI: Systemic Lupus International Collaborating Clinics (SLICC)/American College of Rheumatology (ACR) Damage Index. N/A: not applicable.

Patients receiving AMA were younger than patients who were not on AMA, whereas no difference was seen in sex distributions. The groups had a similar composition of races/ethnic origins, with an overall greater representation of white/Caucasian patients, followed by indigenous American, Asian and black/African American patients. SELENA-SLEDAI scores did not differ between the AMA groups (9.6 ± 3.6 versus 10.0 ± 4.0; $p = 0.145$). AMA users (0.69 ± 1.15) had lower SDI scores compared with AMA non-users (0.95 ± 1.37; $p < 0.001$), and a shorter disease duration (6.1 ± 6.2 versus 7.0 ± 6.6 years; $p = 0.007$).

Fewer patients were on corticosteroids within the AMA group (84.6%) compared with AMA non-users (89.4%; $p = 0.006$), and AMA users had lower average prednisone equivalent doses (10.1 ± 8.5 versus 12.1 ± 8.8 mg/day; $p < 0.001$). Use of immunosuppressants was less frequent in AMA users (43.4%) compared with non-users (58.0%; $p < 0.001$).

3.2. MOS SF-36

As delineated in Figure 1, SLE patients who received AMA reported higher SF-36 PCS (39.6 ± 9.5 versus 38.1 ± 9.9; $p = 0.001$), physical functioning (61.1 ± 24.9 versus 55.0 ± 26.5; $p < 0.001$), role physical (53.2 ± 26.9 versus 50.3 ± 27.7; $p = 0.036$) and bodily pain (49.5 ± 23.8 versus 47.1 ± 25.3; $p = 0.016$) scores compared with patients who did not. Notably, only the difference in the physical functioning subscale was greater than the corresponding MCID. There were no differences between the AMA groups with regard to SF-36 MCS scores or SF-36 subscales scores representing the mental compartment.

3.3. FACIT-Fatigue

Patients who received AMA (30.5 ± 11.8) reported better FACIT-Fatigue scores compared with patients who did not (29.3 ± 11.9; $p = 0.046$), yielding, however, no greater difference than the MCID (Figure 1).

3.4. EQ-5D

Patients in the AMA group reported higher EQ-5D VAS scores (64.6 ± 19.4) compared with patients who did not receive AMA (61.7 ± 18.6; $p < 0.001$), but the difference was not clinically important (<MCID; Figure 1). Accordingly, AMA users reported better EQ-5D utility index scores (0.747 ± 0.185) than AMA non-users (0.720 ± 0.192; $p = 0.004$), but the difference did not reach the MCID. We next analysed the different dimensions of the questionnaire separately: we used the Pearson's chi-square test to compare AMA groups in relation to patients reporting no problems versus moderate or major problems. In this analysis, a higher proportion of patients reporting no problems was seen among AMA users versus non-users with regard to mobility (60.0% versus 52.6%; odds ratio, OR: 1.35; 95% confidence interval, CI: 1.10–1.66; $p = 0.004$), self-care (82.9% versus 78.1%; OR: 1.35; 95% CI: 1.05–1.74; $p = 0.020$), usual activities (46.5% versus 37.8%; OR: 1.43; 95% CI: 1.16–1.76; $p = 0.001$) and anxiety/depression (47.6% versus 41.4%; OR: 1.29; 95% CI: 1.05–1.58; $p = 0.015$), but not pain/discomfort (20.5% versus 18.9%; OR: 1.11; 95% CI: 0.86–1.43; $p = 0.444$) (Figure 2). Finally, the proportion of patients experiencing "full-health state" was higher within AMA users (14.1% versus 10.3%; OR: 1.44; 95% CI: 1.04–1.97; $p = 0.026$; Figure 1).

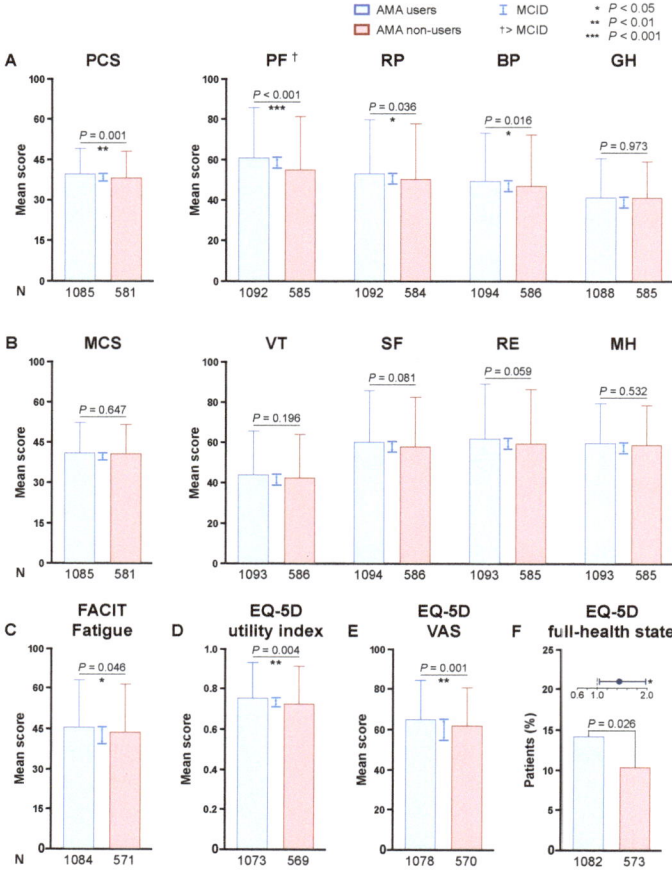

Figure 1. Comparisons of HRQoL between AMA users and non-users. This figure illustrates comparisons of HRQoL perceptions between patients with SLE who received AMA and patients with SLE who did not. Heights of the boxes represent mean HRQoL item scores (**A**–**E**) or percentage of patients (**F**), and whiskers indicate standard deviations. Vertical bidirectional arrows indicate MCIDs. The forest plot in panel F illustrates the odds ratio (circle) and 95% confidence interval (whiskers) of the corresponding comparison. Actual number of observations is indicated below the bars. Asterisks indicate statistically significant associations. AMA: antimalarial agents; SLE: systemic lupus erythematosus; HRQoL: health-related quality of life; FACIT-Fatigue: functional assessment of chronic illness therapy-Fatigue; EQ-5D: EuroQol research foundation 5-dimension; VAS: visual analogue scale; MCID: minimal clinically important difference.

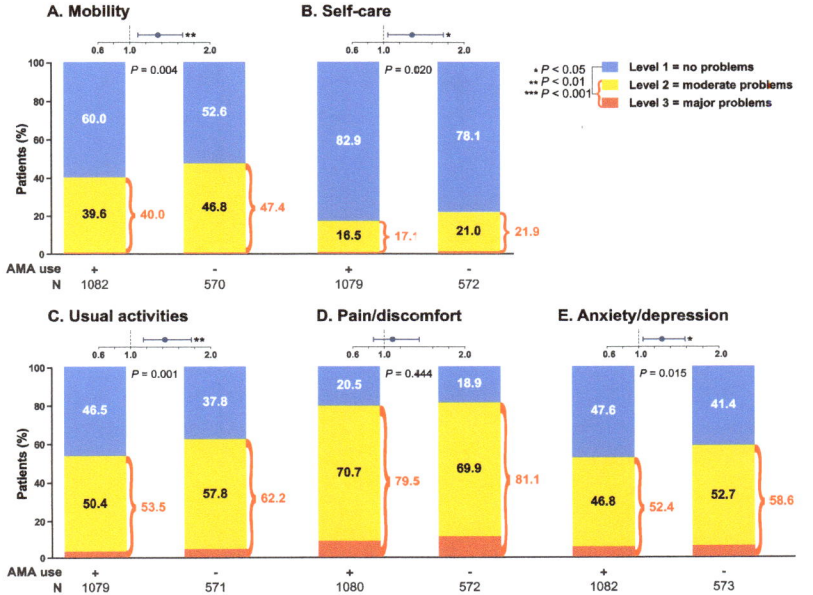

Figure 2. Response to EQ-5D dimensions in AMA users versus non-users. This figure illustrates comparisons between the response of patients with SLE who received AMA and the response of patients who did not receive AMA to the five different dimensions of the EQ-5D questionnaire, i.e., mobility (**A**), self-care (**B**), usual activities (**C**), pain/discomfort (**D**) and anxiety/depression (**E**). Proportions of patients reporting each one of the three levels (no problems, moderate problems, major problems) are indicated by colour-coded sections (blue, yellow, red) within the bars. *p*-values are derived from Pearson's chi-square tests and signify comparisons of level 1 responders between AMA users and non-users. The forest plots illustrate the odds ratio (circles) and 95% confidence interval (whiskers) of the corresponding comparison. Actual number of observations is indicated below the bars. Asterisks indicate statistically significant associations. AMA: antimalarial agents.

3.5. Associations with SF-36 Physical Functioning

We next selected HRQoL aspects where the difference between AMA users and non-users exceeded the corresponding MCID, i.e., the SF-36 PF subscale, for further evaluation in relation to demographical and disease-associated factors with confounding potentiality, employing linear regression analysis.

In multivariable analysis, use of AMA was associated with higher SF-36 PF scores (standardised coefficient, $\beta = 0.07$; $p = 0.002$), independently of the other factors analysed (Figure 3). In the same model, Asian ancestry was also associated with a healthier perception of SF-36 PF ($\beta = 0.08$; $p = 0.002$), whereas African American origin ($\beta = -0.07$; $p = 0.004$), high SELENA-SLEDAI scores ($\beta = -0.11$; $p < 0.001$) and high SDI scores ($\beta = -0.11$; $p < 0.001$) were associated with lower SF-36 PF scores.

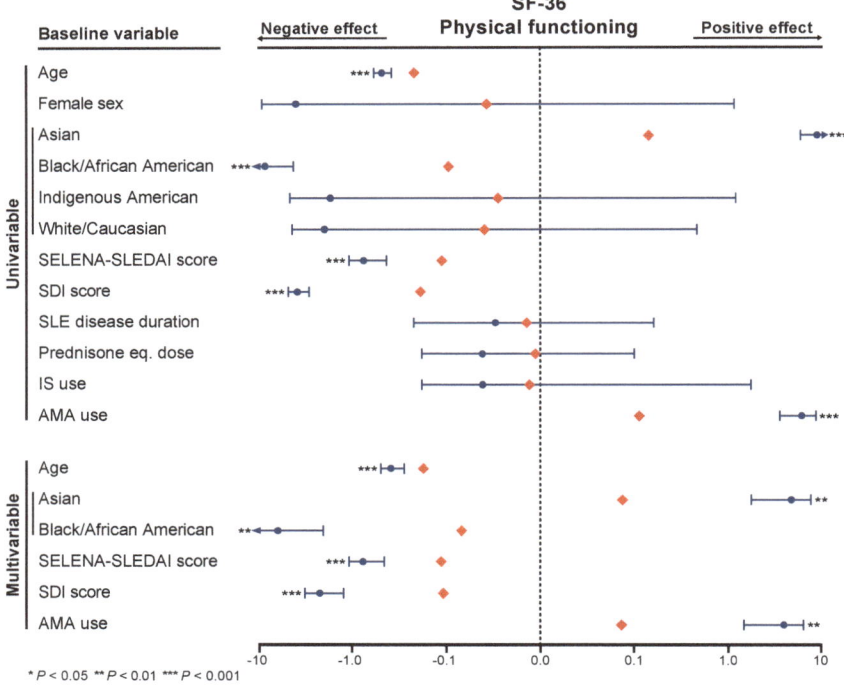

Figure 3. Association between AMA use and SF-36 physical functioning. The forest plots illustrate results from linear regression analysis, employed to investigate the association between AMA use (covariate) and SF-36 physical functioning (outcome), in relation to demographical and disease-specific factors. Factors showing statistically significant associations in univariable analysis were next included in a multivariable model. The dark blue circles represent the un-standardised coefficients, and the whiskers represent the 95% confidence intervals. The red diamonds represent the standardised coefficients. Asterisks indicate statistically significant associations. SF-36: short-form 36; PF: physical functioning; SLE: systemic lupus erythematosus; SELENA-SLEDAI: Safety of Estrogens in Lupus National Assessment SLE Disease Activity Index; SDI: Systemic Lupus International Collaborating Clinics/American College of Rheumatology Damage Index; IS: immunosuppressive; AMA: antimalarial agents.

3.6. Stratification into Subgroups Based on Organ-Specific Activity

We next studied the impact of AMA use on HRQoL in SLE patients with active (BILAG A or B) mucocutaneous, musculoskeletal and renal disease. Similar to the findings in the total study population, patients with active mucocutaneous SLE who received AMA reported higher scores than patients who did not receive AMA in the SF-36 PCS and three of four physical subscales, i.e., PF, RP and BP, as well as SF from the mental compartment of SF-36; however, only the difference in the PF subscale was clinically important (Table 2). Among patients with active musculoskeletal manifestations, AMA users reported higher SF-36 PF scores (55.34 ± 24.10) than AMA non-users (49.98 ± 26.06; $p = 0.002$), and this difference exceeded the MCID (Table 3). Distributions of scores did not differ between the AMA groups in any other SF-36 subscale or component summaries (p = not significant, ns for all). Among patients with active renal SLE, AMA users reported higher scores than patients who did not receive AMA, exceeding the MCID in the SF-36 BP from the physical compartment, and the SF and RE subscales from the mental compartment, but none of these differences reached statistical significance (Table 4).

Table 2. Comparisons of HRQoL between AMA users and non-users in patients with active mucocutaneous disease.

HRQoL Items		AMA Users		AMA Non-Users		p Value	MCID
Number of Patients		638		353			
SF-36							
Physical component summary		39.63	(9.31)	37.82	(9.76)	**0.006**	No
Mental component summary		40.60	(11.44)	40.02	(10.82)	0.448	No
Physical functioning		61.46	(24.71)	54.16	(26.58)	**<0.001**	**Yes**
Role physical		52.51	(26.59)	49.00	(27.52)	**0.033**	No
Bodily pain		48.81	(22.71)	46.17	(24.82)	**0.038**	No
General health		41.40	(19.22)	40.98	(18.09)	0.763	No
Vitality		43.86	(21.34)	41.91	(21.33)	0.175	No
Social functioning		60.63	(25.14)	57.01	(25.01)	**0.043**	No
Role emotional		61.13	(27.44)	58.96	(27.07)	0.165	No
Mental health		59.20	(20.19)	57.60	(19.31)	0.245	No
FACIT-Fatigue							
Score		30.32	(11.74)	28.87	(12.09)	0.077	No
EQ-5D							
Utility index		0.747	(0.173)	0.716	(0.189)	**0.003**	No
VAS		65.10	(19.27)	60.53	(18.99)	**<0.001**	No
EQ-5D Dimensions							
Mobility	L 1	377	(60.2%)	169	(49.4%)		
	L 2	249	(39.8%)	172	(50.3%)	**0.001**	N/A
	L 3	0	(0%)	1	(0.3%)		
Self-care	L 1	518	(82.9%)	261	(75.9%)		
	L 2	103	(16.5%)	78	(22.7%)	**0.009**	N/A
	L 3	4	(0.6%)	5	(1.5%)		
Usual activities	L 1	281	(44.9%)	118	(34.3%)		
	L 2	331	(52.9%)	213	(61.9%)	**0.001**	N/A
	L 3	14	(2.2%)	13	(3.8%)		
Pain or discomfort	L 1	116	(18.6%)	58	(16.9%)		
	L 2	460	(73.6%)	248	(72.1%)	0.510	N/A
	L 3	49	(7.8%)	38	(11.0%)		
Anxiety or depression	L 1	295	(47.1%)	132	(38.4%)		
	L 2	295	(47.1%)	196	(57.0%)	**0.009**	N/A
	L 3	36	(5.8%)	16	(4.7%)		
Full-health state		77	(12.3%)	34	(9.9%)	0.262	N/A

Data are presented as means (standard deviation (SD)) or numbers (percentage). In comparisons of SF-36, FACIT-Fatigue, EQ-5D utility index and EQ-5D VAS scores, p-values are derived from Mann-Whitney U tests. In comparisons of EQ-5D dimensions, p-values are derived from Pearson's chi-square tests and signify comparisons between AMA groups in relation to patients reporting no problems (level 1) versus moderate or major problems (level 2 and level 3 combined). Statistically significant p-values and differences exceeding the MCID are indicated in bold. AMA: antimalarial agents; MCID: minimal clinically important difference; SF-36: Short Form-36; FACIT: Functional Assessment of Chronic Illness Therapy; EQ-5D: EuroQol 5 Dimensions; VAS: visual analogue scale; L: level; N/A: not applicable.

Table 3. Comparisons of HRQoL between AMA users and non-users in patients with active musculoskeletal disease.

HRQoL Items		AMA Users		AMA Non-Users		*p* Value	MCID
Number of Patients		363		372			
SF-36							
Physical component summary		37.18	(9.12)	35.95	(8.99)	**0.042**	No
Mental component summary		40.22	(11.39)	40.08	(11.58)	0.903	No
Physical functioning		55.34	(24.10)	49.98	(26.06)	**0.002**	Yes
Role physical		48.87	(25.78)	46.27	(25.87)	0.131	No
Bodily pain		43.26	(21.24)	40.96	(22.31)	0.053	No
General health		38.89	(18.83)	39.94	(17.45)	0.298	No
Vitality		40.16	(21.53)	39.45	(21.05)	0.584	No
Social functioning		56.91	(25.85)	55.01	(24.47)	0.361	No
Role emotional		59.33	(27.46)	57.40	(27.77)	0.207	No
Mental health		58.54	(19.68)	57.80	(20.50)	0.654	No
FACIT-Fatigue							
Score		28.37	(11.93)	27.22	(11.96)	0.167	No
EQ-5D							
Utility index		0.706	(0.182)	0.684	(0.195)	0.080	No
VAS		61.76	(19.91)	59.21	(18.28)	**0.042**	No
EQ-5D Dimensions							
Mobility	L 1	318	(50.5%)	157	(43.9%)		
	L 2	311	(49.4%)	200	(55.9%)	**0.045**	N/A
	L 3	1	(0.2%)	1	(0.3%)		
Self-care	L 1	491	(78.2%)	258	(71.9%)		
	L 2	132	(21.0%)	98	(27.3%)	**0.026**	N/A
	L 3	5	(0.8%)	3	(0.8%)		
Usual activities	L 1	230	(36.7%)	111	(31.0%)		
	L 2	374	(59.6%)	224	(62.6%)	0.072	N/A
	L 3	23	(3.7%)	23	(6.4%)		
Pain or discomfort	L 1	66	(10.5%)	31	(8.6%)		
	L 2	489	(77.7%)	276	(76.9%)	0.345	N/A
	L 3	74	(11.8%)	52	(14.5%)		
Anxiety or depression	L 1	261	(41.4%)	147	(40.8%)		
	L 2	326	(51.7%)	188	(52.2%)	0.855	N/A
	L 3	43	(6.8%)	25	(6.9%)		
Full-health state		43	(6.8%)	20	(5.6%)	0.431	N/A

Data are presented as means (SD) or numbers (percentage). In comparisons of SF-36, FACIT-Fatigue, EQ-5D utility index and EQ-5D VAS scores, *p*-values are derived from Mann-Whitney *U* tests. In comparisons of EQ-5D dimensions, *p*-values are derived from Pearson's chi-square tests and signify comparisons between AMA groups in relation to patients reporting no problems (level 1) versus moderate or major problems (level 2 and level 3 combined). Statistically significant *p*-values and differences exceeding the MCID are indicated in bold. AMA: antimalarial agents; MCID: minimal clinically important difference; SF-36: Short Form-36; FACIT: Functional Assessment of Chronic Illness Therapy; EQ-5D: EuroQol 5 Dimensions; VAS: visual analogue scale; L: level; N/A: not applicable.

Table 4. Comparisons of HRQoL between AMA users and non-users in patients with active renal disease.

HRQoL Items		AMA Users		AMA Non-Users		p Value	MCID
Number of Patients		112		67			
SF-36							
Physical component summary		40.70	(9.88)	39.39	(11.87)	0.471	No
Mental component summary		41.44	(10.89)	39.54	(11.42)	0.288	No
Physical functioning		60.69	(26.23)	57.93	(28.50)	0.547	No
Role physical		56.10	(28.05)	52.33	(31.74)	0.503	No
Bodily pain		54.42	(26.78)	49.28	(31.18)	0.149	**Yes**
General health		43.19	(20.16)	40.34	(19.56)	0.309	No
Vitality		46.27	(22.28)	44.40	(24.19)	0.516	No
Social functioning		62.39	(25.14)	56.90	(26.68)	0.138	**Yes**
Role emotional		63.58	(25.69)	57.90	(27.58)	0.183	**Yes**
Mental health		59.99	(19.73)	57.87	(19.89)	0.545	No
FACIT-Fatigue							
Score		32.19	(11.64)	30.03	(13.11)	0.357	No
EQ-5D							
Utility index		0.768	(0.206)	0.733	(0.221)	0.286	No
VAS		65.61	(21.59)	59.86	(19.48)	**0.041**	No
EQ-5D Dimensions							
Mobility	L 1	69	(63.9%)	35	(53.0%)	0.156	N/A
	L 2	39	(36.1%)	31	(47.0%)		
	L 3	0	(0%)	0	(0%)		
Self-care	L 1	84	(78.5%)	54	(81.8%)	0.598	N/A
	L 2	22	(20.6%)	12	(18.2%)		
	L 3	1	(0.9%)	0	(0%)		
Usual activities	L 1	52	(48.6%)	30	(45.5%)	0.688	N/A
	L 2	54	(50.5%)	32	(48.5%)		
	L 3	1	(0.9%)	4	(6.1%)		
Pain or discomfort	L 1	33	(30.8%)	22	(33.3%)	0.732	N/A
	L 2	63	(58.9%)	35	(53.0%)		
	L 3	11	(10.3%)	9	(13.6%)		
Anxiety or depression	L 1	59	(54.6%)	23	(34.8%)	**0.011**	N/A
	L 2	45	(41.7%)	37	(56.1%)		
	L 3	4	(3.7%)	6	(9.1%)		
Full-health state		27	(25.0%)	13	(19.7%)	0.420	N/A

Data are presented as means (SD) or numbers (percentage). In comparisons of SF-36, FACIT-Fatigue, EQ-5D utility index and EQ-5D VAS scores, p-values are derived from Mann-Whitney U tests. In comparisons of EQ-5D dimensions, p-values are derived from Pearson's chi-square tests and signify comparisons between AMA groups in relation to patients reporting no problems (level 1) versus moderate or major problems (level 2 and level 3 combined). Statistically significant p-values and differences exceeding the MCID are indicated in bold. AMA: antimalarial agents; MCID: minimal clinically important difference; SF-36: Short Form-36; FACIT: Functional Assessment of Chronic Illness Therapy; EQ-5D: EuroQol 5 Dimensions; VAS: visual analogue scale; L: level; N/A: not applicable.

FACIT-Fatigue scores did not differ between AMA groups in any of the three subgroups studied. Among patients with mucocutaneous BILAG A or B, AMA users reported lower EQ-5D VAS (65.10 ± 19.27 versus 60.53 ± 18.99; $p < 0.001$) and utility index (0.747 ± 0.173 versus 0.716 ± 0.189; $p = 0.003$) scores compared with AMA non-users. These differences did not reach the level of MCID (Table 2). Among subjects with active musculoskeletal (Table 3) and renal (Table 4) disease, EQ-5D utility index scores did not differ between the AMA groups ($p = $ ns for all), and the differences in EQ-5D VAS scores did not reach the level of MCID.

Notably, a higher proportion of AMA users versus non-users reported no problems within the mobility (60.2% versus 49.4%; OR: 1.55; 95% CI: 1.12–2.02; $p = 0.001$), self-care (82.9% versus

75.9%; OR: 1.54; 95% CI: 1.12–2.13; $p = 0.009$), usual activities (44.9% versus 34.3%; OR: 1.56; 95% CI: 1.19–2.05; $p = 0.001$) and anxiety/depression (47.1% versus 38.4%; OR: 1.43; 95% CI: 1.10–1.87; $p = 0.009$) EQ-5D dimensions among patients with active mucocutaneous disease, and within mobility (50.5% versus 43.9%; OR: 1.31; 95% CI: 1.01–1.69; $p = 0.45$) and self-care (78.2% versus 71.9%; OR: 1.40; 95% CI: 1.04–1.89; $p = 0.026$) among patients with active musculoskeletal disease. By contrast, in the active renal subgroup, proportions differed only in the anxiety/depression dimension (54.6% versus 34.8%; OR: 2.25; 95% CI: 1.20–4.24; $p = 0.011$).

4. Discussion

In the present post-hoc analysis of the BLISS-52 and BLISS-76 trials, we demonstrated that patients with active SLE receiving AMA reported better physical functioning than patients who were not on AMA. This association was clinically important, and independent of age, ethnic origin, disease activity and organ damage accrual. Furthermore, AMA users reported more favourable perceptions of mobility, ability to carry out self-care and usual activities, and level of anxiety or depression. Notably, a greater proportion of patients among AMA users experienced a full-health state, defined as no problems in all dimensions of the EQ-5D questionnaire.

In patients with SLE, AMA have been coupled with numerous beneficial effects, including reductions in disease activity, organ damage accrual and flare rates, as well as prolonged patient survival [8–10]. Mechanisms involved in the immunomodulatory effects of AMA include an altered peptide processing in antigen-presenting cells, reduced B cell activity and altered binding of anti-phospholipid antibody-β_2-glycoprotein I complexes to phospholipid bilayers [34,35]. In the present study, we confirmed that SLE patients using AMA had accrued less organ damage and were on lower prednisone doses compared with patients not treated with AMA. Importantly, our study was not designed to address causality, and these observations could be explained, at least partly, by the fact that AMA users were younger and had a shorter SLE disease duration at the time of assessment. The rather low proportion of patients on AMA treatment (65%) signifies that the need for increased awareness of the favourable effects of AMA and for alignment with current recommendations [7] remains.

With regard to HRQoL, data on the impact of AMA have been scarce and conflicting. In one study comprising 277 SLE patients from Peru, past and current use of AMA was associated with a better perception of physical health, burden to others and body image [13], as assessed using the LupusQoL, an SLE-specific questionnaire for self-reported HRQoL [36]. In a Swedish cohort of 69 SLE patients with active disease, selected for treatment with biological agents, i.e., belimumab or rituximab, patients receiving AMA performed better in social functioning and mental health [12], based on self-reports using the SF-36 health survey [19]. By contrast, in a post-hoc analysis of the PLUS trial, a trial of hydroxychloroquine that comprised 166 SLE patients with low and stable disease activity, hydroxychloroquine concentrations were not associated with scores in any of the SF-36 component summaries or subscales, either at baseline or at month 7 [14]. Discrepancies in the different cohorts may be due to different disease phenotypes among the study participants. For example, patients selected for biological therapy in the aforementioned Swedish study had a more active disease, with an overrepresentation of active renal SLE, as opposed to the quiescent SLE cohort of the PLUS trial. Another explanation could be traced to the different instruments used to evaluate HRQoL. While generic indices provide information that has the advantage of being directly comparable with that of the general population and other disorders, disease-specific indices are expected to be more sensitive to change and perform better in discriminating across distinct subgroups of patients [37]. In this respect, the sole use of generic instruments in the present study may have contributed to omission of important disease-associated and disease-specific attributes that potentially influence the inventories and could be better captured by SLE-specific HRQoL questionnaires, such as the LupusQoL [36].

The BLISS populations included in this post-hoc analysis consisted of SLE patients with active disease despite standard of care treatment, with a high prevalence of mucocutaneous and musculoskeletal involvement. In the total study population, use of AMA was associated with better

HRQoL perceptions in physical aspects of the SF-36, but the differences between AMA groups were moderate and only that in the physical functioning subscale exceeded the threshold of minimal clinically important difference. In the same fashion, the observed statistically significant difference in FACIT-Fatigue scores favouring the use of AMA was not clinically important. Lastly, differences in favour of AMA were also observed in the EQ-5D dimensions of mobility, self-care and usual activities. Although no MCIDs have to date been validated for the EQ-5D dimensions, patients using AMA had a 1.4-fold increased chance to report no problems in each one of the three aforementioned dimensions. It should be mentioned that factors such as concomitant medications, especially glucocorticoids, and SLE disease activity, as well as common comorbid conditions with immense impact on levels of pain and fatigue, such as fibromyalgia, may have influenced our findings. Comparisons yielding clinically important differences in HRQoL perception in AMA users versus non-users qualified for further exploration of independence and confounding potentiality. Importantly, glucocorticoid doses and use of immunosuppressants were not found to impact physical functioning, and the favourable impact of AMA use on physical functioning was independent of the negative impact of age, disease activity and organ damage in multivariable linear regression analysis.

Patients with SLE and mucocutaneous or musculoskeletal involvement suffer from a higher degree of HRQoL diminutions than SLE patients with other manifestations, especially regarding physical aspects [4]. When we herein analysed these subgroups of patients independently, AMA use was associated with more favourable perceptions in physical aspects of HRQoL, including SF-36 physical functioning and EQ-5D mobility, self-care and usual activities. Furthermore, patients with active mucocutaneous manifestations who received AMA also reported a better health profile in the anxiety or depression EQ-5D dimension compared with patients who did not. These findings further support current treatment recommendations, which advocate that patients with mucocutaneous and musculoskeletal involvement might particularly benefit from treatment with AMA. Currently, AMA remain the first-line systemic therapy for cutaneous SLE [7,38], and are considered an effective option for the management of lupus polyarthritis [35].

An observation of particular interest was that, in contrast to the entire study population and the subgroups of active mucocutaneous and musculoskeletal SLE, patients with active renal disease benefited from AMA regarding perceptions of mental HRQoL. These differences were found to be clinically important with respect to SF-36 social functioning and role emotional, and yielded a 2.3-fold increased chance to report no problems in the EQ-5D anxiety or depression dimension. These observations are in line with the aforementioned Swedish study of SLE patients, in which lupus nephritis was the most frequent clinical phenotype, showing that AMA users reported better scores than non-users in SF-36 social functioning and mental health [12]. The lack of statistical significance in some of the differences in mental HRQoL aspects in the present study may be due to the fact that patients with severe active lupus nephritis were, as per study protocol, excluded from the BLISS trials, resulting in a relatively low number of patients in the renal subgroup analysis, and, reasonably, a rather moderate renal activity in these patients. Further investigation of the impact of AMA on HRQoL in renal SLE is merited.

Despite the widely known benefits of AMA on SLE disease activity and course, non-adherence remains a major problem [14,39,40]. Costedoat-Chalumeau et al. found that the most common reasons for AMA treatment discontinuation by patient initiative included the perception of AMA not being an effective treatment and apprehension about potential side-effects [41]. This may be partially explained by the fact that the long-term benefits of AMA, which constitute a main reason for prescription, do not have a direct impact on SLE patients' perception of health status. Indeed, while AMA prescription by physicians is predominantly steered by evidence with regard to both organ-specific and long-term benefits, the latter including atheroprotective effects and reduced flare rates [1,6], patients' principal concerns have been shown to be related to their ability to perform physical and usual activities, as well as the degree of fatigue and pain [42]. In recent years, including patient-reported outcomes in shared therapeutic decision-making between physician and patient has received increasing embracement in all medical fields [43]. In this regard, our findings contribute with further evidence on the beneficial effects of AMA on SLE patients' HRQoL and may provide support to motivate adherence to AMA therapy.

The cross-sectional design of our study constituted a major limitation. For example, it limited us from exploring a potential causality in the relationship between AMA use and HRQoL benefits. Furthermore, no quantification of blood AMA concentrations was attempted in the BLISS trials. Thus, medication non-adherence may have resulted in unintentional inaccuracies in our findings, which therefore have to be interpreted with caution. Information about comorbid conditions with confounding potentiality, such as fibromyalgia, was not available. Finally, patients with severe active lupus nephritis and neuropsychiatric SLE were excluded from the BLISS trials, and the conclusions of this study should therefore not be extrapolated to these patient subgroups. Nonetheless, the strengths of this investigation included the large study population, the diversity of patients enrolled from 32 different countries, the variety of instruments utilised to evaluate HRQoL and the extensive availability of homogeneous data in the BLISS-52 and BLISS-76 trials that allowed us to pool the two cohorts and adjust for multiple factors. To our knowledge, to date, this is the largest analysis of AMA use in relation to HRQoL in patients with SLE.

5. Conclusions

In the present cohort of 1684 patients with active SLE, mainly comprising patients with active mucocutaneous and musculoskeletal disease, we observed a clinically important benefit of AMA use with respect to physical functioning. Importantly, this effect was not impacted by patients' age, ethnic origin, SLE disease activity or organ damage accrual. A particular benefit of AMA use on mental aspects of HRQoL was observed in the subgroup of patients with active renal disease. Results from this investigation provide further support in motivating adherence to AMA therapy. Exploration of a potential causality in the relationship between AMA use and favourable HRQoL in people living with SLE has merit.

Supplementary Materials: The following are available online at http://www.mdpi.com/2077-0383/9/6/1813/s1, Table S1: Characteristics of AMA users versus non-users in BLISS-52 and BLISS-76.

Author Contributions: A.G., S.S. and I.P. were responsible for conceptualisation, design, and coordination of the project; A.G., S.S., P.J., E.Å., S.E. and I.P. were responsible for acquisition of data and for the statistical analysis; Y.E. contributed as a patient research partner; A.G., S.S., Y.E., K.C. and I.P. contributed to the interpretation of the results; A.G., S.S., Y.E. and I.P. drafted the manuscript. All authors read and critically revised the manuscript for intellectual content, approved its final version prior to submission, and agree to be accountable for all aspects of the work. All authors have read and agreed to the published version of the manuscript.

Funding: This work was supported by the GlaxoSmithKline Investigator-Sponsored Studies (ISS) programme and grants or stipends from the Swedish Rheumatism Association (R-932236), Professor Nanna Svartz Foundation (2019-00290), Ulla and Roland Gustafsson Foundation (2019-12), Swedish Society of Rheumatology, Eli Lilly and Company, Region Stockholm and Karolinska Institutet.

Acknowledgments: The authors would like to thank GlaxoSmithKline (Uxbridge, UK) for sharing the data from the BLISS-52 (NCT00424476) and BLISS-76 (NCT00410384) trials through the Clinical Study Data Request (CSDR) consortium, as well as all participating patients.

Conflicts of Interest: I.P. has received research funding from GlaxoSmithKline, and honoraria/stipends from GlaxoSmithKline, Novartis and Eli Lilly and Company. The other authors declare no conflict of interest. The funders had no role in the design of the study; in the analyses or interpretation of data; in the writing of the manuscript, or in the decision to publish the results.

References

1. Kaul, A.; Gordon, C.; Crow, M.K.; Touma, Z.; Urowitz, M.B.; van Vollenhoven, R.; Ruiz-Irastorza, G.; Hughes, G. Systemic lupus erythematosus. *Nat. Rev. Dis. Prim.* **2016**, *2*, 16039. [CrossRef]
2. Waldheim, E.; Elkan, A.-C.; Pettersson, S.; Vollenhoven, R.V.; Bergman, S.; Frostegård, J.; Henriksson, E.W. Health-related quality of life, fatigue and mood in patients with SLE and high levels of pain compared to controls and patients with low levels of pain. *Lupus* **2013**, *22*, 1118–1127. [CrossRef] [PubMed]
3. Jolly, M.; Toloza, S.; Goker, B.; Clarke, A.E.; Navarra, S.V.; Wallace, D.; Weisman, M.; Mok, C.C. Disease-specific quality of life in patients with lupus nephritis. *Lupus* **2018**, *27*, 257–264. [CrossRef]
4. Bjork, M.; Dahlstrom, O.; Wettero, J.; Sjowall, C. Quality of life and acquired organ damage are intimately related to activity limitations in patients with systemic lupus erythematosus. *BMC Musculoskelet. Disord.* **2015**, *16*, 188. [CrossRef] [PubMed]
5. Van Vollenhoven, R.; Voskuyl, A.; Bertsias, G.; Aranow, C.; Aringer, M.; Arnaud, L.; Askanase, A.; Balazova, P.; Bonfa, E.; Bootsma, H.; et al. A framework for remission in SLE: Consensus findings from a large international task force on definitions of remission in SLE (DORIS). *Ann. Rheum. Dis.* **2017**, *76*, 554–561. [CrossRef]
6. Durcan, L.; O'Dwyer, T.; Petri, M. Management strategies and future directions for systemic lupus erythematosus in adults. *Lancet* **2019**, *393*, 2332–2343. [CrossRef]
7. Fanouriakis, A.; Kostopoulou, M.; Alunno, A.; Aringer, M.; Bajema, I.; Boletis, J.N.; Cervera, R.; Doria, A.; Gordon, C.; Govoni, M.; et al. 2019 update of the EULAR recommendations for the management of systemic lupus erythematosus. *Ann. Rheum. Dis.* **2019**, *78*, 736–745. [CrossRef]
8. Ruiz-Irastorza, G.; Egurbide, M.-V.; Pijoan, J.-I.; Garmendia, M.; Villar, I.; Martinez-Berriotxoa, A.; Erdozain, J.-G.; Aguirre, C. Effect of antimalarials on thrombosis and survival in patients with systemic lupus erythematosus. *Lupus* **2006**, *15*, 577–583. [CrossRef]
9. Petri, M. Hydroxychloroquine use in the Baltimore Lupus Cohort: Effects on lipids, glucose and thrombosis. *Lupus* **1996**, *5*, 16–22. [CrossRef]
10. Alarcón, G.S.; McGwin, G.; Bertoli, A.M.; Fessler, B.J.; Calvo-Alén, J.; Bastian, H.M.; Vilá, L.M.; Reveille, J.D. Effect of hydroxychloroquine on the survival of patients with systemic lupus erythematosus: Data from LUMINA, a multiethnic US cohort (LUMINA L). *Ann. Rheum. Dis.* **2007**, *66*, 1168–1172. [CrossRef]
11. Annapureddy, N.; Devilliers, H.; Jolly, M. Patient-reported outcomes in lupus clinical trials with biologics. *Lupus* **2016**, *25*, 1111–1121. [CrossRef] [PubMed]
12. Parodis, I.; Lopez Benavides, A.H.; Zickert, A.; Pettersson, S.; Moller, S.; Welin Henriksson, E.; Voss, A.; Gunnarsson, I. The Impact of Belimumab and Rituximab on Health-Related Quality of Life in Patients With Systemic Lupus Erythematosus. *Arthritis Care Res.* **2019**, *71*, 811–821. [CrossRef] [PubMed]
13. Elera-Fitzcarrald, C.; Alva, M.; Gamboa-Cardenas, R.; Mora-Trujillo, C.S.; Zevallos, F.; García-Poma, A.; Medina, M.; Rodriguez-Bellido, Z.; Perich-Campos, R.A.; Pastor-Asurza, C.A.; et al. Factors associated with health-related quality of life in Peruvian patients with systemic lupus erythematosus. *Lupus* **2018**, *27*, 913–919. [CrossRef] [PubMed]
14. Jolly, M.; Galicier, L.; Aumaître, O.; Francès, C.; Le Guern, V.; Lioté, F.; Smail, A.; Limal, N.; Perard, L.; Desmurs-Clavel, H.; et al. Quality of life in systemic lupus erythematosus: Description in a cohort of French patients and association with blood hydroxychloroquine levels. *Lupus* **2016**, *25*, 735–740. [CrossRef]
15. Navarra, S.V.; Guzmán, R.M.; Gallacher, A.E.; Hall, S.; Levy, R.A.; Jimenez, R.E.; Li, E.K.M.; Thomas, M.; Kim, H.-Y.; León, M.G.; et al. Efficacy and safety of belimumab in patients with active systemic lupus erythematosus: A randomised, placebo-controlled, phase 3 trial. *Lancet* **2011**, *377*, 721–731. [CrossRef]
16. Furie, R.; Petri, M.; Zamani, O.; Cervera, R.; Wallace, D.J.; Tegzova, D.; Sanchez-Guerrero, J.; Schwarting, A.; Merrill, J.T.; Chatham, W.W.; et al. A phase III, randomized, placebo-controlled study of belimumab, a monoclonal antibody that inhibits B lymphocyte stimulator, in patients with systemic lupus erythematosus. *Arthritis Rheumat.* **2011**, *63*, 3918–3930. [CrossRef]
17. Hochberg, M.C. Updating the American college of rheumatology revised criteria for the classification of systemic lupus erythematosus. *Arthritis Rheumat.* **1997**, *40*, 1725. [CrossRef]
18. Petri, M.; Kim, M.Y.; Kalunian, K.C.; Grossman, J.; Hahn, B.H.; Sammaritano, L.R.; Lockshin, M.; Merrill, J.T.; Belmont, H.M.; Askanase, A.D.; et al. Combined Oral Contraceptives in Women with Systemic Lupus Erythematosus. *N. Engl. J. Med.* **2005**, *353*, 2550–2558. [CrossRef]

19. Ware, J.; Sherbourne, C. The MOS 36-item short-form health survey (SF-36). I. Conceptual framework and item selection. *Med. Care* **1992**, *30*, 473–483. [CrossRef]
20. Webster, K.; Cella, D.; Yost, K. The Functional Assessment of Chronic Illness Therapy (FACIT) Measurement System: Properties, applications, and interpretation. *Health Qual. Life Outcomes* **2003**, *1*, 79. [CrossRef]
21. EuroQol—A new facility for the measurement of health-related quality of life. *Health Policy* **1990**, *16*, 199–208. [CrossRef]
22. Ware, J.E.J. SF-36 Health Survey Update. *Spine* **2000**, *25*, 3130–3139. [CrossRef] [PubMed]
23. Shaw, J.W.; Johnson, J.A.; Coons, S.J. US Valuation of the EQ-5D Health States: Development and Testing of the D1 Valuation Model. *Med. Care* **2005**, *43*, 203–220. [CrossRef] [PubMed]
24. EuroQol Research Foundation. EQ-5D-3L User Guide. 2018. Available online: https://euroqol.org/publications/user-guides (accessed on 9 June 2020).
25. Strand, V.; Crawford, B. Improvement in health-related quality of life in patients with SLE following sustained reductions in anti-dsDNA antibodies. *Expert Rev. Pharmacoecon. Outcomes Res.* **2005**, *5*, 317–326. [CrossRef]
26. Strand, V.; Levy, R.A.; Cervera, R.; Petri, M.A.; Birch, H.; Freimuth, W.W.; Zhong, Z.J.; Clarke, A.E. Improvements in health-related quality of life with belimumab, a B-lymphocyte stimulator-specific inhibitor, in patients with autoantibody-positive systemic lupus erythematosus from the randomised controlled BLISS trials. *Ann. Rheum. Dis.* **2014**, *73*, 838–844. [CrossRef] [PubMed]
27. Coretti, S.; Ruggeri, M.; McNamee, P. The minimum clinically important difference for EQ-5D index: A critical review. *Expert Rev. Pharmacoecon. Outcomes Res.* **2014**, *14*, 221–233. [CrossRef]
28. Bangert, E.; Wakani, L.; Merchant, M.; Strand, V.; Touma, Z. Impact of belimumab on patient-reported outcomes in systemic lupus erythematosus: Review of clinical studies. *Patient Relat. Outcome Meas.* **2019**, *10*, 1. [CrossRef]
29. Hay, E.M.; Bacon, P.A.; Gordon, C.; Isenberg, D.A.; Maddison, P.; Snaith, M.L.; Symmons, D.P.M.; Viner, N.; Zoma, A. The BILAG index: A reliable and valid instrument for measuring clinical disease activity in systemic lupus erythematosus. *QJM Int. J. Med.* **1993**, *86*, 447–458. [CrossRef]
30. Gladman, D.; Ginzler, E.; Goldsmith, C.; Fortin, P.; Liang, M.; Sanchez-Guerrero, J.; Urowitz, M.; Bacon, P.; Bombardieri, S.; Hanly, J.; et al. The development and initial validation of the systemic lupus international collaborating clinics/American college of rheumatology damage index for systemic lupus erythematosus. *Arthritis Rheumat.* **1996**, *39*, 363–369. [CrossRef]
31. Azizoddin, D.R.; Gandhi, N.; Weinberg, S.; Sengupta, M.; Nicassio, P.M.; Jolly, M. Fatigue in systemic lupus: The role of disease activity and its correlates. *Lupus* **2019**, *28*, 163–173. [CrossRef]
32. Tamayo, T.; Fischer-Betz, R.; Beer, S.; Winkler-Rohlfing, B.; Schneider, M. Factors influencing the health related quality of life in patients with systemic lupus erythematosus: Long-term results (2001–2005) of patients in the German Lupus Erythematosus Self-Help Organization (LULA Study). *Lupus* **2010**, *19*, 1606–1613. [CrossRef] [PubMed]
33. Alarcon, G.S.; McGwin, G., Jr.; Uribe, A.; Friedman, A.W.; Roseman, J.M.; Fessler, B.J.; Bastian, H.M.; Baethge, B.A.; Vila, L.M.; Reveille, J.D. Systemic lupus erythematosus in a multiethnic lupus cohort (LUMINA). XVII. Predictors of self-reported health-related quality of life early in the disease course. *Arthritis Care Res.* **2004**, *51*, 465–474. [CrossRef] [PubMed]
34. Rand, J.H.; Wu, X.X.; Quinn, A.S.; Chen, P.P.; Hathcock, J.J.; Taatjes, D.J. Hydroxychloroquine directly reduces the binding of antiphospholipid antibody-beta2-glycoprotein I complexes to phospholipid bilayers. *Blood* **2008**, *112*, 1687–1695. [CrossRef] [PubMed]
35. Lee, S.J.; Silverman, E.; Bargman, J.M. The role of antimalarial agents in the treatment of SLE and lupus nephritis. *Nat. Rev. Nephrol.* **2011**, *7*, 718–729. [CrossRef]
36. McElhone, K.; Abbott, J.; Shelmerdine, J.; Bruce, I.N.; Ahmad, Y.; Gordon, C.; Peers, K.; Isenberg, D.; Ferenkeh-Koroma, A.; Griffiths, B.; et al. Development and validation of a disease-specific health-related quality of life measure, the LupusQol, for adults with systemic lupus erythematosus. *Arthritis Care Res.* **2007**, *57*, 972–979. [CrossRef]
37. Yazdany, J. Health-related quality of life measurement in adult systemic lupus erythematosus: Lupus Quality of Life (LupusQoL), Systemic Lupus Erythematosus-Specific Quality of Life Questionnaire (SLEQOL), and Systemic Lupus Erythematosus Quality of Life Questionnaire (L-QoL). *Arthritis Care Res.* **2011**, *63* (Suppl. 11), S413–S419. [CrossRef]

38. Kuhn, A.; Ruland, V.; Bonsmann, G. Cutaneous lupus erythematosus: Update of therapeutic options part I. *J. Am. Acad. Dermatol.* **2011**, *65*, e179–e193. [CrossRef]
39. Iudici, M.; Pantano, I.; Fasano, S.; Pierro, L.; Charlier, B.; Pingeon, M.; Dal Piaz, F.; Filippelli, A.; Izzo, V. Health status and concomitant prescription of immunosuppressants are risk factors for hydroxychloroquine non-adherence in systemic lupus patients with prolonged inactive disease. *Lupus* **2018**, *27*, 265–272. [CrossRef]
40. Chehab, G.; Sauer, G.M.; Richter, J.G.; Brinks, R.; Willers, R.; Fischer-Betz, R.; Winkler-Rohlfing, B.; Schneider, M. Medical adherence in patients with systemic lupus erythematosus in Germany: Predictors and reasons for non-adherence—A cross-sectional analysis of the LuLa-cohort. *Lupus* **2018**, *27*, 1652–1660. [CrossRef]
41. Costedoat-Chalumeau, N.; Amoura, Z.; Hulot, J.S.; Aymard, G.; Leroux, G.; Marra, D.; Lechat, P.; Piette, J.C. Very low blood hydroxychloroquine concentration as an objective marker of poor adherence to treatment of systemic lupus erythematosus. *Ann. Rheum. Dis.* **2007**, *66*, 821–824. [CrossRef]
42. Golder, V.; Ooi, J.J.Y.; Antony, A.S.; Ko, T.; Morton, S.; Kandane-Rathnayake, R.; Morand, E.F.; Hoi, A.Y. Discordance of patient and physician health status concerns in systemic lupus erythematosus. *Lupus* **2018**, *27*, 501–506. [CrossRef] [PubMed]
43. Anker, S.D.; Agewall, S.; Borggrefe, M.; Calvert, M.; Jaime Caro, J.; Cowie, M.R.; Ford, I.; Paty, J.A.; Riley, J.P.; Swedberg, K.; et al. The importance of patient-reported outcomes: A call for their comprehensive integration in cardiovascular clinical trials. *Eur. Heart J.* **2014**, *35*, 2001–2009. [CrossRef] [PubMed]

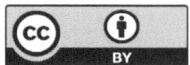

© 2020 by the authors. Licensee MDPI, Basel, Switzerland. This article is an open access article distributed under the terms and conditions of the Creative Commons Attribution (CC BY) license (http://creativecommons.org/licenses/by/4.0/).

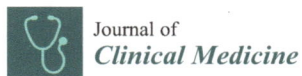

Article

Adverse Pregnancy Outcomes after Multi-Professional Follow-Up of Women with Systemic Lupus Erythematosus: An Observational Study from a Single Centre in Sweden

Muna Saleh [1,*], Christopher Sjöwall [1], Helena Strevens [2], Andreas Jönsen [3], Anders A. Bengtsson [3] and Michele Compagno [3]

1. Department of Biomedical and Clinical Sciences, Division of Inflammation and Infection, Linköping University, SE-581 85 Linköping, Sweden; christopher.sjowall@liu.se
2. Department of Clinical Sciences Lund, Department of Obstetrics and Gynaecology, Lund University, SE-222 42 Lund, Sweden; helena.strevens@med.lu.se
3. Department of Clinical Sciences Lund, Rheumatology, Lund University, SE-222 42 Lund, Sweden; andreas.jonsen@med.lu.se (A.J.); anders.bengtsson@med.lu.se (A.A.B.); michele.compagno@med.lu.se (M.C.)
* Correspondence: muna.saleh@liu.se

Received: 7 June 2020; Accepted: 7 August 2020; Published: 11 August 2020

Abstract: While the management of pregnant patients with systemic lupus erythematosus (SLE) has improved over the last decades, the risk of maternal, foetal, and neonatal complications is still substantial. We evaluated the occurrence of adverse pregnancy outcomes (APO) occurring in 2002–2018 among patients with SLE from the catchment area of the Department of Rheumatology in Lund, Sweden. Longitudinal clinical and laboratory data were collected and analysed. Results were stratified according to the sequence of conception. We investigated a total of 59 pregnancies in 28 patients. Prior lupus nephritis was the clinical feature that, in a multivariable regression analysis, displayed the strongest association with APO overall (OR 6.0, $p = 0.02$). SLE combined with antiphospholipid syndrome (APS) was associated with the risk of miscarriage (OR 3.3, $p = 0.04$). The positivity of multiple antiphospholipid antibodies (aPL) was associated with APO overall (OR 3.3, $p = 0.05$). IgG anti-cardiolipin during pregnancy resulted in a higher risk of preterm delivery (OR 6.8, $p = 0.03$). Hypocomplementaemia was associated with several APO, but only in the first pregnancies. We conclude that, despite the close follow-up provided, a majority of pregnancies resulted in ≥1 APO, but a few of them were severe. Our study confirms the importance of previous lupus nephritis as a main risk factor for APO in patients with SLE.

Keywords: SLE; pregnancy; conception; adverse pregnancy outcomes; maternal and foetal complications; Lupus nephritis; antiphospholipid syndrome; risk factors

1. Introduction

Systemic lupus erythematosus (SLE) is a systemic autoimmune disease that often affects fertile women. Adverse pregnancy outcomes (APO), commonly grouped into maternal and foetal/neonatal complications, occur in the obstetric general population. Pregnant SLE patients are at increased risk of both maternal and foetal/neonatal APO [1,2]. In the past, patients with SLE have been advised and warned from getting pregnant and giving birth, due to the high risk of severe complications for both the mother and the offspring. In recent times, modern treatment strategies and established preventive measures have led to less risk of APO, but there is more to be done to keep the risk as low as in the obstetric population.

Maternal APO observed in SLE include increased disease activity, pre-eclampsia, eclampsia and Haemolysis, Elevated Liver enzymes and Low Platelet count (HELLP) syndrome, as well as obstetrical complications, such as preterm labour, unplanned Caesarean delivery, and conditions related to pre-eclampsia [3–5]. Foetal and neonatal complications frequently associated with SLE are miscarriage, stillbirth, intrauterine growth restriction (IUGR), neonatal lupus erythematosus (NLE), congenital heart block, and prematurity [6–8]. Moreover, women with SLE are at increased risk of foetal loss around the 10th gestational week, particularly in the presence of active SLE, active lupus nephritis (LN), or concomitant antiphospholipid syndrome (APS) [9]. However, a decline in the risk of foetal loss in SLE has been reported over the last decades [9–12]. Up to 30% of pregnancies in SLE patients are complicated by IUGR and small-for-gestational-age (SGA) newborns, compared to approximately 10% of pregnancies in the general obstetric population [13,14]. Lower birth weight at any gestational age is also more prevalent among the offspring of SLE patients [15]. Pre-eclampsia is one of the most frequent maternal APO in SLE, occurring in 16% to 30%, compared with 5% of pregnancies in the general obstetric population [16,17]. Poorly controlled SLE, a history of LN, low levels of complement proteins, and thrombocytopenia have been identified as risk factors for pre-eclampsia in SLE [16,18,19]. The role played by the antiphospholipid antibodies (aPL) in the occurrence of pre-eclampsia is still controversial [16,19]. Active SLE, previous LN, presence of APS or aPL, and thrombocytopenia have been suggested as predictors, as well as putative risk factors of other APO [16,20–22], but studies are needed to evaluate this further.

The study aimed to contribute to the field of knowledge with a report of real-world longitudinal data from one single tertiary referral rheumatology centre in southern Sweden, where a multi-professional follow-up of pregnant SLE patients has been carried out since 2002. In particular, we aimed to assess the occurrence of APO in our cohort and how some established and putative SLE-related risk factors may predict the pregnancy outcomes.

2. Methods

2.1. Patients and Clinical Follow-Up

In patients affected by SLE, from the catchment area of Skåne University Hospital, Sweden, we investigated the outcome of all the pregnancies occurred between 2002 and 2018. Each included patient fulfilled the 1997 American College of Rheumatology (ACR) and/or the 2012 Systemic Lupus International Collaborating Clinics (SLICC) classification criteria [23,24] and was regularly followed at the Department of Rheumatology, since the time-point of diagnosis. All patients had consented to join a prospective follow-up program, intending to improve care of SLE patients and to identify clinical and laboratory features that could be used as a marker or a predictor of complications and exacerbations of the disease. Patients were followed longitudinally with scheduled visits every 60 ± 20 days and extra visits in case of disease flares. An extensive set of clinical and laboratory variables were registered in a database tailored for the study. Serum samples were collected regularly, also before and after the date of clinical assessment.

Whenever pregnant, the patients underwent multi-professional follow-up, with recurrent visits at the local antenatal clinic, often in presence of one of the health professionals responsible for the regular follow-up at the rheumatology department. After informed consent from the pregnant patients, we gathered the relevant clinical features and laboratory data already recorded in the local SLE database, to define the clinical phenotype of each patient [25], as well as the data recorded during each and every gestation that occurred during the study period, including the medical records from obstetrics and neonatal units concerning all the maternal and perinatal outcomes. Concomitant APS, meeting the Sydney classification criteria [26], was accounted for only if APS had been recognized before conception.

Disease activity and acquired organ damage were assessed using the SLEDAI-2000 (SLEDAI-2K) [27] and the SLICC/ACR damage index (SDI) [28], respectively. A SLEDAI-2K score of ≥4 was recorded as "active SLE". To the purpose of this study, we gathered the SLEDAI-2K scores determined at 6-months before conception, at each trimester, and at 6-months post-pregnancy, as well as the SDI scores determined at 1 year before conception and at 1 year after termination of each gestation.

To account for systematic bias, we analysed all the first pregnancies occurring after the diagnosis of SLE apart from the remaining pregnancies. Women who had been pregnant up to 12 months before the time-point of SLE diagnosis were not suitable for the "first pregnancy group" but for the "subsequent pregnancy" group. Identical statistical analyses were employed separately in these two subgroups, as well as in the pooled data of all pregnancies.

2.2. APO

We collected data concerning the following maternal complications, documented during the investigated pregnancies: gestational hypertension, pre-eclampsia (or eclampsia or HELLP syndrome), preterm delivery (<37th gestational week), and gestational diabetes.

We assessed the occurrence of the following foetal/neonatal complications: foetal loss, defined as early miscarriage (occurring before 10th week of gestation), or late miscarriage (occurring between the 10th and 24th week of gestation), or intrauterine foetal death (IUFD) (occurring at >24th gestational weeks); stillbirth; IUGR (a foetus not reaching its target weight based on sonographic estimated foetal weight); SGA newborns (weight and length at birth below 10th percentile for gestational age); low birth weight (LBW-below 2500 gram, regardless of gestational age); congenital heart block and NLE.

2.3. Risk Factors

We investigated the role of SLE-related clinical and immunological features as putative risk factors for the development of APO. The following clinical features were assessed and gathered as binary variables (yes/no): concomitant APS (recognized before the time of conception) and history of LN (documented by renal biopsy). In addition, acknowledged risk factors for APO in the general obstetric population were studied, such as smoking habits (tobacco smoking; ever or current), obesity (body mass index >30) and age ≥35 years at the time of conception [29].

The following immunological findings were gathered as binary variables (yes/no) and grouped as "ever present", "present 1-year before conception" and "present during pregnancy": presence of anti-dsDNA, anti-Ro/SSA, anti-La/SSB, anti-cardiolipin (aCL, IgG isotype), anti-β2-glycoprotein-I (anti-β2GPI, IgG isotype), lupus anticoagulant (LA) test and hypocomplementaemia (decreased levels of complement proteins: C3 and/or C4 and/or C1q).

The assessments were made at the local clinical immunology laboratory, according to the validated assays and methods in current use at the time of evaluation.

2.4. Statistics

Statistical analyses were performed with SPSS Statistics, version 25.0 (IBM, Armonk, NY, USA) and GraphPad Prism, version 6.07 (GraphPad Software, La Jolla, CA, USA). Median values were calculated for continuous variables. Other variables were presented as binary categorical variables, apart from the SLEDAI-2K and SDI scores, collected as continuous variables and presented (mean ± SD) in a Box-whisker plots graph. To handle with repeated measurements during each gestation and with data collected from recurrent gestations in the same patient, we used Generalized Estimating Equation (GEE) to assess the association between potential risk factors and outcomes (APO). A p-value of <0.05 was considered significant. Potential risk factors for developing any APO in each studied pregnancy were examined also by logistic regression analysis (univariate and multivariable). All the significant associations in the univariate model were included in the multivariable analysis. No corrections for multiple comparisons were made, but by reporting the exact p-values, we enable this by any preferred method [30].

2.5. Ethical Considerations

Oral and written informed consent was obtained from all participants. The study protocol was approved by the regional ethics board in Lund (Dnr: LU 378–02).

3. Results

Twenty-eight patients affected by SLE experienced 1–5 gestations each during the study period. We totally investigated 59 pregnancies, whereof 26 were categorised as "1st pregnancies". The remaining 2 patients had had ≥1 gestation before the onset of SLE; therefore, only their subsequent pregnancies were recorded. Twenty-one patients accounted for the 33 "subsequent pregnancies". Overall, 61 embryos were conceived, being 2 out of the 59 gestations multiple (3.4%) with twins.

All recorded demographic data, clinical manifestations, immunological features, and pharmacological therapy concerning the included patients are summarized in Tables 1 and 2.

Table 1. Characteristics and descriptive data of the studied pregnancies ($n = 59$) in included patients ($n = 28$).

Variable	Value	Range or Percent (%)
Caucasian race/ethnicity, n/total	27/28	96.4%
Age at SLE diagnosis, median (years)	20.5	10–33
Age at time of conception, median (years)	31	22–41
Disease duration at time of conception, median (years)	10	0–25
BMI at time of conception, median (kg/m^2)	23.5	19–33
Ever smoked tobacco before conception, n/total	10/48	20.8%
Ever treated with antihypertensives, n/total	12/59	20.3%
Diabetes mellitus, n/total	0/59	0%
Pregnancies with prior APS, n/total	19/59	32.2%
2012 SLICC criteria [23]	**In 28 patients (%)**	**In 59 pregnancies (%)**
Acute cutaneous lupus, n (%)	17 (60.7)	34 (57.6)
Chronic cutaneous lupus, n (%)	4 (14.3)	6 (10.2)
Oral ulcers, n (%)	7 (25)	12 (20.3)
Non-scarring alopecia, n (%)	8 (28.6)	10 (16.9)
Synovitis, n (%)	27 (96.4)	58 (98.3)
Serositis, n (%)	9 (32.1)	16 (27.1)
Renal, n (%)	15 (53.6)	36 (61.0)
Neurologic, n (%)	6 (21.4)	13 (22.0)
Haemolytic anaemia, n (%)	3 (10.7)	7 (11.9)
Leukopenia, n (%)	18 (64.3)	41 (69.5)
Lymphopenia, n (%)	25 (89.3)	54 (91.5)
Thrombocytopenia, n (%)	11 (39.3)	20 (33.9)
ANA, n (%)	28 (100)	59 (100)
Anti-Sm antibody, n (%)	5 (17.9)	13 (22.0)
Anti-dsDNA antibody, n (%)	17 (60.7)	35 (59.3)
Antiphospholipid antibodies *, (%) n	17 (60.7)	38 (64.4)
Low complement, n (%)	25 (89.3)	40 (67.8)
Positive direct Coombs' test in the absence of haemolytic anaemia, n (%)	5 (17.9)	10 (16.9)

* With or without APS diagnosis; ANA, antinuclear antibodies; APS, antiphospholipid syndrome; BMI, Body Mass index.

Table 2. Pharmacotherapy and immunological features in the study population.

Pharmacotherapy	Ever Documented Total (n = 59)	Up to 1 Year before Pregnancy			During Pregnancy		
		Total (n = 59)	FP (n = 26)	SP (n = 33)	Total (n = 59)	FP (n = 26)	SP (n = 33)
<15 mg prednisolone		28	14	14	30	14	16
≥15 mg prednisolone		2	2	0	9	5	4
Antimalarials	50	47	21	26	44	20	24
Azathioprine	41	31	14	17	31	14	17
Mycophenolate mofetil	19	1	1	0	0	0	0
Cyclophosphamide	15	0	0	0	0	0	0
Cyclosporine	6	0	0	0	0	0	0
Tacrolimus	3	0	0	0	0	0	0
Protein A *	3	0	0	0	0	0	0
Intravenous immunoglobulin	4	0	0	0	1	1	0
Biologics	0	0	0	0	0	0	0
Methotrexate	2	0	0	0	0	0	0
Warfarin	10	7	3	4	0	0	0
LMWH	17	1	1	0	17	6	11
Acetylsalicylic acid	18	16	7	9	34	12	22
Immunological data							
Anti-dsDNA, n/total (%)	35/59 (59.3)	12/55 (21.8)			17/51 (33.3)		
Anti-Ro/SSA, n/total (%)	14/59 (23.7)	12/53 (22.6)			13/51 (25.5)		
Anti-La/SSB, n/total (%)	13/59 (22.0)	10/53 (18.9)			12/51 (23.5)		
Anti-cardiolipin, n/total (%)	38/59 (64.4)	12/54 (22.2)			5/51 (9.8)		
Anti-β2-GPI, n/total (%)	15/59 (25.4)	8/52 (15.4)			9/51 (17.6)		
LA test, n/total (%)	16/54 (29.6)	4/22 (18.2)			5/41 (12.2)		
Low C3, n/total (%)	40/59 (67.8)	22/53 (41.5)			20/51 (39.2)		
Low C4, n/total (%)	38/59 (64.4)	24/53 (45.3)			21/51 (41.2)		
Low C1q, n/total (%)	35/53 (66.0)	12/53 (22.6)			26/51 (51.0)		

* Immune-adsorption Staphylococcal protein A; aCL, anti-cardiolipin antibody; anti-β2-GPI, anti-β2-glycoprotein I antibody; FP, first pregnancy after SLE diagnosis; IVIG, intravenous immunoglobulin; LA, lupus anticoagulant test; LMVH, low molecular-weight heparin; SP, subsequent pregnancy.

3.1. APO

At least 1 APO complicated 33 pregnancies (56%) in 18 patients (64%). A total of 44 gestations (75%) ended with delivery, whereof 8 (18%) were preterm. No post-term deliveries were recorded. As shown in Table 3, pre-eclampsia (25%), preterm deliveries (18%), and Caesarean Section (30%) were the most common maternal APO.

Regarding foetal/neonatal adverse outcomes, we observed 13 cases (22%) of early foetal loss, but no cases of late miscarriage, IUFD, or stillbirth. Restricted foetal growth (IUGR and/or, SGA, and/or LBW) was recorded in 13 pregnancies (30%). One case (1.7%) of NLE and no congenital heart block was observed.

Among the 26 "1st pregnancies", 22 (85%) ended with delivery and 4 with early miscarriage. A total of 11 of these 22 deliveries (50%) were complicated with ≥1 APO. The 33 "subsequent pregnancies" resulted in 22 (66%) deliveries, 9 (27%) early miscarriage and 2 (6%) induced abortions.

Seven deliveries (32%) were complicated with ≥1 APO. Further details concerning types of APO observed are summarized in Table 3. The incidence of APO over time decreased around 10%, despite about 2/3 of the investigated pregnancies were recorded during the period 2010–2018, as illustrated in Table 4.

Table 3. Maternal and foetal adverse pregnancy outcomes (divided by pregnancy number in the case of early outcome, or by number of deliveries in the case of late outcome).

	APO in All Pregnancies ($n = 59$)	APO in FP ($n = 26$)	APO in S ($n = 33$)
Maternal APO			
Pre-eclampsia, n/total (%)	11/44 (25)	6/22 (27)	5/22 (23)
Eclampsia, n/total (%)	0/44 (0)	0/22 (0)	0/22 (0)
HELLP syndrome, n/total (%)	1/44 (2)	1/22 (5)	0/22 (0)
Preterm deliveries (<37th gestational week), n/total (%)	8/44 (18)	4/22 (18)	4/22 (18)
Gestational hypertension, n/total (%)	2/44 (5)	2/22 (10)	0/22 (0)
Gestational diabetes, n/total (%)	1/44 (2)	0/22 (0)	1/22 (5)
Caesarean delivery, n/total (%)	13/44 (30)	7/22 (32)	5/22 (23)
Foetal/Neonatal APO			
Miscarriage <10 weeks, n/total (%)	13/59 (22)	4/26 (15)	9/33 (27)
Miscarriage ≥10 weeks, n/total (%)	0/59 (0)	0/26 (0)	0/33 (0)
Induced abortion	2/59 (3)	0/26 (0)	2/33 (6)
IUFD >24 weeks, n/total (%)	0/44 (0)	0/22 (0)	0/22 (0)
Stillbirths, n/total (%)	0/44 (0)	0/22 (0)	0/22 (0)
Prematurity, n/total (%)	10/44 * (23)	5/22 (23)	5/22 (23)
Restricted foetal growth, n/total	13/44 (30)	8/22 (36)	5/22 (23)
IUGR, n/total (%)	5/44 (11)	3/22 (14)	2/22 (9)
SGA, n/total (%)	1/44 (2)	1/22 (0.5)	0/22 (0)
LBW, n/total (%)	10/44# (23)	6/22 (27)	4/22 (18)
Congenital heart block, n/total (%)	0/44 (0)	0/22 (0)	0/22 (0)
Neonatal lupus erythematosus, n/total (%)	1/44 (2)	1/22 (0.5)	0/22 (0)

* Birth before 37th week of gestation (2 multiple gestations with twins). # 2 cases already diagnosed with IUGR and 1 case also diagnosed with SGA. These gestations resulted in 15 newborns (2 multiple gestations with twins). FP, first pregnancy after SLE diagnosis; IUFD, intrauterine foetal death; IUGR, intrauterine growth restriction; LBW, low birth weight; SGA, small for gestational age; SP, subsequent pregnancies.

Table 4. Incidence of adverse pregnancy outcomes (APO) grouped according to the decade of occurrence. Observe that one pregnancy may have been complicated by >1 APO.

Year Interval	Gestations/Patients		Total APO n (%)	Pregnancies with APO ($n = 33$)		Pre-Eclampsia/ HELLP ($n = 12$)		Miscarriage (<10 weeks) ($n = 13$)		Preterm Delivery ($n = 8$)		Restricted Foetal Growth * ($n = 13$)	
Sequence of conception	FP	SP		FP	SP	FP	SP	FP	SP	FP	SP	FP	SP
2002–2009	11/11	9/5	12 (60%)	6	6	1	1	2	4	2	2	3	2
2010–2018	15/15	24/16	21 (54%)	9	12	6	4	2	5	2	2	5	3
Total	26/26	33/21		15	18	7	5	4	9	4	4	8	5

* IUGR (intra-uterine growth restriction) and/or SGA (small-for-gestational-age) newborns and/or LBW (low birth weight). FP, first pregnancy after SLE diagnosis; SP, subsequent pregnancies.

3.2. Risk Factors

The analysis of all the 59 gestations showed that APS diagnosed before the time of conception in SLE patients may enhance the risk (OR 3.3, $p = 0.04$) of early miscarriage. Furthermore, the presence of aPL was associated with increased risk (OR 3.3, $p = 0.05$) of any APO. In particular, the presence of aCL during pregnancy resulted in a higher risk (OR 6.8, $p = 0.03$) of preterm delivery, regardless of APS. A history of LN was associated with increased risk of any APO (OR 5.9, $p = 0.005$), particularly any kind of restricted foetal growth (OR 16.6, $p = 0.01$).

At first pregnancy after the onset of SLE, the detection of aCL during the gestation was associated with an increased risk of preterm delivery (OR 32.0, $p = 0.03$). Restricted foetal growth was associated with presence of different immunological features and clinical manifestations, such as low levels of C3 (OR 13.0, $p = 0.04$) and C4 (OR 20.0, $p = 0.02$) up to 1-year before conception, as well as presence of aPL during pregnancy (OR 17.3, $p = 0.03$), concomitant APS diagnosis (OR 13.0, $p = 0.04$) and previous LN (OR 12.6, $p = 0.04$). In addition, increased risk of pre-eclampsia/HELLP was associated with low C4 levels detected up to 1-year before conception (OR 12.5, $p = 0.04$).

In the subgroup of 33 subsequent pregnancies, a positive aCL test ≤1-year before the time of conception (OR 3.8, $p = 0.01$), concomitant APS diagnosis (OR 4.9, $p = 0.02$) and a history of LN (OR 5.7, $p = 0.04$) indicated higher risk of miscarriage. Ever documented presence of aPL (OR 11.3, $p = 0.04$) and previous LN (OR 12.0, $p = 0.01$) were also associated with increased risk for any APO. In contrast, ever documented low C3 levels (OR 0.05, $p = 0.03$) showed an inverse association with pre-eclampsia/HELLP. The associations between risk factors and APO are summarized in Table 5 and are further detailed in Supplementary Materials (Tables S1–S3).

Table 5. Associations between investigated risk factors and the APO reaching statistical significance at any time-point among all included pregnancies (59 conceptions, whereof 44 led to delivery). p-values, odds ratios, and 95% confidence intervals are given.

Risk Factor		Total APO ($n = 33$)	Pre-Eclampsia and HELLP ($n = 12$)	Miscarriage (<10 Weeks) ($n = 13$)	Preterm Delivery ($n = 8$)	Restricted Foetal Growth * ($n = 13$)
	Denominators	$n = 59$	$n = 44$	$n = 59$	$n = 44$	$n = 44$
aCL	Ever	0.40 (OR 1.7, CI 0.5–5.7)	0.51 (OR 1.8, CI 0.3–9.5)	0.08 (OR 3.9, CI 0.9–17.2)	0.31 (OR 2.7, CI 0.4–18.3)	0.83 (OR 0.8, CI 0.2–3.9)
	≤1-year before	0.74 (OR 0.8, CI 0.3–2.6)	0.33 (OR 0.3, CI 0.03–3.1)	0.47 (OR 1.4, CI 0.6–3.7)	0.12 (OR 4.8, CI 0.7–35.0)	0.61 (OR 1.5, CI 0.3–7.1)
	During pregnancy	0.46 (OR 1.6, CI 0.4–6.1)	N.E.	N.T.	**0.03 (OR = 6.8, CI 1.2–39.4)**	0.19 (OR 2.9, CI 0.6–14.1)
≥1 pos. aCL, anti-β2-GPI or LA test	Ever	**0.05 (OR 3.3, CI 1.0–11.11)**	0.17 (OR 3.4, CI 0.6–19.6)	0.20 (OR 2.7, CI 0.6–11.8)	0.59 (OR 1.7, CI 0.2–11.8)	0.36 (OR 2.1, CI 0.4–10.2)
	≤1-year before	0.73 (OR 0.8, CI 0.3–2.6)	0.57 (OR 0.6, CI 0.1–3.3)	0.87 (OR 1.1, CI 0.4–3.1)	0.23 (OR 3.4, CI 0.5–24.5)	0.97 (OR 1.0, CI 0.2–5.3)
	During pregnancy	0.25 (OR 1.9, CI 0.7–5.5)	0.73 (OR 0.7, CI 0.1–6.4)	N.T.	0.72 (OR 1.4, CI 0.2–8.8)	0.26 (OR 2.1, CI 0.6–7.5)
APS before pregnancy		0.12 (OR 3.1, CI 0.8–12.7)	0.28 (OR 2.6, CI 0.5–13.9)	**0.04 (OR = 3.3, CI 1.1–10.2)**	0.22 (OR 3.5, CI 0.5–26.2)	0.13 (OR 3.6, CI 0.7–18.5)
Previous LN		**0.005 (OR = 5.9, CI 1.7–20.8)**	0.06 (OR 5.7, CI 0.9–34.6)	0.20 (OR 2.6, CI 0.6–10.7)	0.10 (OR 7.0, CI 0.7–71.5)	**0.01 (OR = 16.6, CI 1.8–156.5)**

* IUGR, (intra-uterine growth restriction) and/or; SGA (small-for-gestational-age) newborns and/or; LBW, (low birth weight). Yellow background indicates statistical significance. aCL, anti-cardiolipin antibody; anti-β2-GPI, anti-β2-glycoprotein I antibody; APS, antiphospholipid syndrome; CI, 95% confidence intervals; LA, lupus anticoagulant test; LN, lupus nephritis; N.E.; not estimated (used for calculations with division by zero); N.T., not tested; OR, odds ratio.

Next, we performed a multivariable logistic regression analysis, emphasizing that previous LN was the only significant risk factor in our study population for the occurrence of any APO (OR 6.0, $p = 0.02$), particularly in the subsequent pregnancy group (OR 25.7, $p = 0.02$). In the subgroup of 26 first pregnancies, none of the investigated risk factors showed any significant associations with maternal or foetal APO in the univariate model.

3.3. Damage Accrual and Disease Activity

SDI and SLEDAI-2K were determined at each visit, to assess accrual of organ damage and disease activity, respectively. No major changes in SDI score were found before and after each pregnancy, regardless of the number of pregnancies and the occurrence of APO (Figure 1). Moreover, a modest increase in disease activity during the last two trimesters and the near period post-delivery was observed. Active SLE (SLEDAI-2K score of ≥4) was found in around 30% during the period before conception and during the 1st trimester of each gestation. The rate of pregnant patients with active SLE increased up to 49% and 43% during the 2nd and the 3rd trimester of gestation, respectively. We documented, at last, active SLE in 51% of the investigated pregnancies during the six months following the termination of the gestations (Figure 1).

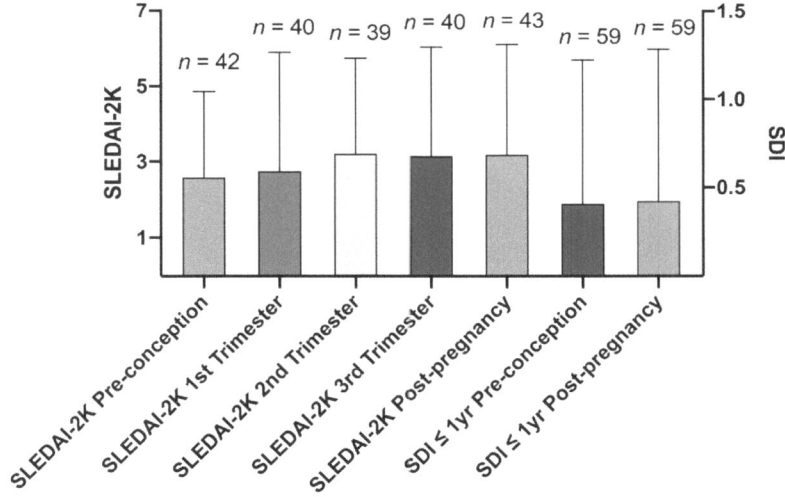

Figure 1. SLEDAI-2K scores illustrated during each trimester as well as 6 months pre-conception and 6 months post-pregnancy; and SLICC/ACR damage index (SDI) up to 1 year pre-conception and 1 year post-pregnancy (termination of pregnancy). Data show mean ± standard deviations.

4. Discussion

This is the first Swedish study that describes the occurrence of APO in a well-defined population of patients affected by SLE, undergoing regular multi-professional check-ups throughout pregnancy, at one single university centre. In previous studies, this kind of regular follow-up has been suggested to facilitate a positive outcome of pregnancy in patients with SLE, particularly those with a history of LN and concomitant APS or with the presence of aPL [9,15,20]. Despite progress in the management of pregnancies in SLE patients during the last decades [2,13], our data indicate that SLE is still associated with high risks of maternal and foetal complications. While pre-eclampsia occurs in 2–8% of pregnancies in the general obstetric population and is seldom complicated by eclampsia and the HELLP syndrome, pre-eclampsia occurred in >20% of the pregnancies investigated in the present study, which is comparable to the results reported in previous investigations [3,16,31].

Early foetal loss and preterm deliveries were also more common than usually observed in the general population [3,6,9,32]. Late foetal loss, stillbirth, and congenital heart defects are generally less prevalent [33]. The absence of these APO in our experience could simply be due to the limited number of pregnancies investigated, though the regular multi-professional follow-up may have contributed to fewer major foetal/neonatal APO in the later phase of pregnancies. IUGR occurs in about 10–30% among pregnant women with SLE, as compared to approximately 10% in the general obstetric population [4,13,15]. Around 30% of gestations in our study resulted in restricted foetal growth, such as IUGR and SGA or LBW. Among the risk factors assessed in this study, a history of LN, diagnosis of APS, and the presence of one or more aPL were associated with major APO.

Nevertheless, the results of the present investigation may suggest a trend towards a lower incidence of APO in SLE patients during the last years (54%), as compared with the incidence recorded between 2002 and 2009 (60%). We speculate that the accurate use of effective and safe drugs, as well as the implementation of a multi-professional follow-up program, has contributed to achieving a lower rate of APO among patients with SLE, despite the growing number of recorded gestations in our centre.

Renal involvement in SLE has previously been reported as a risk factor for developing several APO, mainly foetal loss, preterm delivery, restricted foetal growth, and pre-eclampsia [13,14,34,35]. Previous LN among our patients showed a significant association with the development of any APO, in particular with restricted foetal growth, as confirmed by the assessment in a multivariable regression model (Table 6). However, none had active LN at the time of conception or up to 6 months before conception. One patient developed LN during the 2nd trimester of pregnancy and needed to terminate the gestation at the 20th week.

Table 6. Logistic regression analysis with associations between risk factors and development of any APO.

Risk Factors	Univariate			Multivariable		
	OR	CI	p-Value	OR	CI	p-Value
APO in all pregnancies (n = 59)						
Previous LN	5.9	1.9–18.8	0.002	6.0	1.3–27.9	0.02
≥1 pos. aCL, anti-β2-GPI or LA test (ever)	3.3	1.0–10.7	0.05	2.8	0.6–13.9	0.20
≥1 pos. aCL, anti-β2-GPI or LA test (≤1-year before)	0.8	0.2–2.8	0.75	0.12	0.01–1.3	0.09
≥1 pos. aCL, anti-β2-GPI or LA test (during pregnancy)	1.9	0.5–6.6	0.32	2.6	0.2–30.4	0.45
APO in subsequent pregnancies (n = 33)						
Previous LN	12.0	2.0–72.4	0.007	25.7	1.8–362.3	0.02
≥1 pos. aCL, anti-β2-GPI or LA test (ever)	11.3	1.2–109.3	0.04	15.3	0.71–329.9	0.08
≥pos. aCL, anti-β2-GPI or LA test (≤1-year before)	1.3	0.26–5.9	0.78	0.3	0.008–11.6	0.52
≥pos. aCL, anti-β2-GPI or LA test (during pregnancy)	1.3	0.26–5.9	0.78	0.3	0.008–11.6	0.52

aCL, anti-cardiolipin antibody; anti-β2-GPI, anti-β2-glycoprotein I antibody; CI, 95% confidence intervals; LA, lupus anticoagulant test; LN, lupus nephritis; OR, odds ratios.

Concomitant APS and the presence of aPL have already been reported as potential risk factors for the development of APO [20,21,36,37], and this was confirmed herein. We could confirm that abnormal levels of aCL during pregnancy indeed were associated with the occurrence of preterm delivery, as previously described [38,39]. Worth noting is that, in our population, APS appeared to be a significant risk factor for APO, despite that the diagnosis was already known since before the time of conception and the treatment was ongoing.

The results of our investigation show that hypocomplementaemia, or activation of the complement system, during the first pregnancy after the presumptive onset of SLE, may have a pathological role in the occurrence of some APO, such as pre-eclampsia and restricted foetal growth (Table S2). This is consistent with previous investigations that indicate the activation of the classical pathway of the complement system, and hypocomplementaemia overall, as variables associated with a significant risk of APO. In particular, a higher occurrence of foetal loss, IUGR, and pre-eclampsia have been observed, especially when concomitant APS or aPL [18,40–45] are present. Moreover, the activation of the complement system has been demonstrated to be of importance regarding the risk of pre-eclampsia and IUGR, even in women without autoimmune diseases [46,47].

On the other hand, any decreased level of C3 ever documented in our patients showed an inverse association with the occurrence of pre-eclampsia/HELLP syndrome during the subsequent pregnancies. These results were unexpected and should be interpreted with caution. However, it may reflect the tailored interventions usually undertaken to minimize the risk of APO in patients with a history of hypocomplementaemia [48]. In line with this, the use of antimalarials, low-molecular-weight heparin, and acetylsalicylic acid increased during subsequent pregnancies, in comparison with first pregnancies (Table 2), which might have contributed to reducing the risk of APO.

Many reports have emphasized the importance of low disease activity in women with SLE at the time of conception and throughout the entire pregnancy period, to minimize the risk of APO [49–51]. Kwok et al., concluded that a SLEDAI score of ≥ 4 during the 6 months before conception predicts adverse maternal outcomes, while a disease flare during pregnancy rather predicts adverse foetal outcomes [51]. Similar conclusions have been drawn in other studies [49–52]. In our study population, SLEDAI-2K scores were generally low 6 months prior to conception and during the 1st trimester. The mean values of SLEDAI-2K were slightly higher during the latter part of the investigated pregnancies, as well as during 6 months post-partum, as shown in Figure 1, consistent with other investigations [53,54]. No significant increase of organ damage was recorded among our cases, which also was observed in a recently published study, suggesting that pregnancies before and after the diagnosis of SLE may not be significant predictors of irreversible damage [55]. Effects of other general risk factors for APO (i.e., smoking, ≥ 35 years of age at the time of conception, or obesity) did not fall out significant. However, the general risk factors among the included women were uncommon. Subsequently, firm conclusions regarding this cannot be drawn based on our data.

Some limitations should be acknowledged. Firstly, we could not investigate the effect of medication on the major APO. Moreover, the small number of studied pregnancies in a limited number of patients from one single centre may have led to uncertain results, and conclusions could thus be difficult to generalize to a broader population of SLE patients. Finally, one must also consider the risk of observation and treatment bias; patients so closely followed might run the risk of being delivered at the first signs of a developing APO, such as pre-eclampsia or restricted foetal growth, thereby increasing the number of abnormal parameters observed but limiting the number of serious APO. On the other hand, a major strength is the Swedish healthcare system, which is public, tax-funded, and offers universal access. This significantly reduces the risk of selection bias and ensures a very high coverage of cases, especially at a tertiary referral centre, offering high-specialized health-care services with longstanding experience of SLE care [25]. A clear advantage of a single centre study in comparison with a multi-centre study is the homogeneity in both care and management over time in this patient group. For this reason, though small in size, this study provides reliable data concerning appropriate management of these women.

5. Conclusions

To conclude, the results of the present investigation highlight the risks of APO in SLE. No new predictors could be identified in this study. Nonetheless, our data indicate the importance of planning pregnancy and organizing a multi-professional follow-up during pregnancy, with regular visits, to minimize the prevalence of APO and/or the consequences of APO. The early detection of unfavourable conditions may help to step up surveillance and to provide the patients with the best treatment to prevent and avoid serious adverse outcomes.

The sequence of conception may play an important role in the risk stratification and prevention. We confirm the importance of some clinical phenotypes (e.g., previous LN, APS) and immunological factors (e.g., aPL, hypocomplementaemia) as risk factors for the occurrence of APO. Larger multicentre studies would be needed to identify further reliable predictors of APO and to investigate the actual impact of pharmacological treatments.

Supplementary Materials: The following are available online at http://www.mdpi.com/2077-0383/9/8/2598/s1. Supplementary Table S1: Associations between all investigated risk factors and the most frequent APO among all included pregnancies (59 conceptions, whereof 44 led to delivery); Table S2: Associations between all investigated risk factors and the most frequent APO among 1st pregnancies (26 conceptions, whereof 22 led to delivery); Table S3: Associations between all investigated risk factors and the most frequent APO among subsequent pregnancies, not defined as 1st pregnancy after SLE diagnosis (33 conceptions, whereof 22 led to delivery).

Author Contributions: Conceptualization, M.S., A.J., A.A.B. and M.C.; data collection, M.S., A.J., A.A.B. and M.C.; formal analysis, M.S., C.S., A.J., A.A.B., H.S. and M.C.; investigation, M.S., C.S., A.J., A.A.B., H.S. and M.C.; writing—original draft preparation, M.S., C.S. and M.C.; writing—review and editing, M.S., C.S., A.J., A.A.B., H.S. and M.C.; visualization, M.S., C.S. and M.C.; supervision, C.S., H.S. and M.C.; funding, C.S., A.J. and A.A.B. All authors have read and agreed to the published version of the manuscript.

Funding: This study was funded by grants from the Swedish Rheumatism Association, the Region Östergötland (ALF grants), the King Gustaf V's 80-year Anniversary Foundation, the King Gustaf V and Queen Victoria's Freemasons Foundation, the Swedish Research Council, Alfred Österlund's Foundation, the Anna-Greta Crafoord Foundation, the Greta and Johan Kock's Foundation, the Skåne University Hospital and the Medical Faculty of Lund University.

Acknowledgments: Sofia Pihl, Specialist physician in obstetrics and gynaecology, Linköping University Hospital, and Rheumatology Thomas Skogh, Linköping University, for kindly reviewing the manuscript. Jan-Åke Nilsson, Lund, and Lars Valter, Linköping, for advice on statistical analyses.

Conflicts of Interest: The authors declare no conflict of interest.

References

1. Nili, F.; McLeod, L.; O'Connell, C.; Sutton, E.; McMillan, D. Maternal and neonatal outcomes in pregnancies complicated by systemic lupus erythematosus: A population-based study. *J. Obstet. Gynaecol. Can.* **2013**, *35*, 323–328. [CrossRef]
2. Molokhia, M.; Maconochie, N.; Patrick, A.L.; Doyle, P. Cross-sectional analysis of adverse outcomes in 1029 pregnancies of Afro-Caribbean women in Trinidad with and without systemic lupus erythematosus. *Arthritis Res. Ther.* **2007**, *9*, R124. [CrossRef] [PubMed]
3. Clowse, M.E.; Jamison, M.; Myers, E.; James, A.H. A national study of the complications of lupus in pregnancy. *Am. J. Obstet. Gynecol.* **2008**, *199*, 127.e1. [CrossRef] [PubMed]
4. Clowse, M.E. Lupus activity in pregnancy. *Rheum. Dis. Clin. N. Am.* **2007**, *33*, 237–252. [CrossRef] [PubMed]
5. Arkema, E.V.; Palmsten, K.; Sjöwall, C.; Svenungsson, E.; Salmon, J.E.; Simard, J.F. What to Expect When Expecting With Systemic Lupus Erythematosus (SLE): A Population-Based Study of Maternal and Fetal Outcomes in SLE and Pre-SLE. *Arthritis Care Res.* **2016**, *68*, 988–994. [CrossRef] [PubMed]
6. Petri, M.; Allbritton, J. Fetal outcome of lupus pregnancy: A retrospective case-control study of the Hopkins Lupus Cohort. *J. Rheumatol.* **1993**, *20*, 650–656. [CrossRef]
7. Zhan, Z.; Yang, Y.; Zhan, Y.; Chen, D.; Liang, L.; Yang, X. Fetal outcomes and associated factors of adverse outcomes of pregnancy in southern Chinese women with systemic lupus erythematosus. *PLoS ONE* **2017**, *12*, e0176457. [CrossRef]
8. Vanoni, F.; Lava, S.A.G.; Fossali, E.F.; Cavalli, R.; Simonetti, G.D.; Bianchetti, M.G.; Bozzini, M.A.; Agostoni, C.; Milani, G.P. Neonatal Systemic Lupus Erythematosus Syndrome: A Comprehensive Review. *Clin. Rev. Allergy Immunol.* **2017**, *53*, 469–476. [CrossRef]
9. Carvalheiras, G.; Vita, P.; Marta, S.; Trovão, R.; Farinha, F.; Braga, J.; Rocha, G.; Almeida, I.; Marinho, A.; Mendonça, T.; et al. Pregnancy and systemic lupus erythematosus: Review of clinical features and outcome of 51 pregnancies at a single institution. *Clin. Rev. Allergy Immunol.* **2010**, *38*, 302–306. [CrossRef]
10. Wang, X.; Chen, C.; Wang, L.; Chen, D.; Guang, W.; French, J. Conception, early pregnancy loss, and time to clinical pregnancy: A population-based prospective study. *Fertil. Steril.* **2003**, *79*, 577–584. [CrossRef]
11. Wilcox, A.J.; Weinberg, C.R.; O'Connor, J.F.; Baird, D.D.; Schlatterer, J.P.; Canfield, R.E.; Armstrong, E.G.; Nisula, B.C. Incidence of early loss of pregnancy. *N. Engl. J. Med.* **1988**, *319*, 189–194. [CrossRef] [PubMed]
12. Clark, C.A.; Spitzer, K.A.; Laskin, C.A. Decrease in pregnancy loss rates in patients with systemic lupus erythematosus over a 40-year period. *J. Rheumatol.* **2005**, *32*, 1709–1712. [PubMed]

13. Smyth, A.; Oliveira, G.H.; Lahr, B.D.; Bailey, K.R.; Norby, S.M.; Garovic, V.D. A systematic review and meta-analysis of pregnancy outcomes in patients with systemic lupus erythematosus and lupus nephritis. *Clin. J. Am. Soc. Nephrol. CJASN* **2010**, *5*, 2060–2068. [CrossRef] [PubMed]
14. Saavedra, M.A.; Cruz-Reyes, C.; Vera-Lastra, O.; Romero, G.T.; Cruz-Cruz, P.; Arias-Flores, R.; Jara, L.J. Impact of previous lupus nephritis on maternal and fetal outcomes during pregnancy. *Clin. Rheumatol.* **2012**, *31*, 813–819. [CrossRef] [PubMed]
15. Yasmeen, S.; Wilkins, E.E.; Field, N.T.; Sheikh, R.A.; Gilbert, W.M. Pregnancy outcomes in women with systemic lupus erythematosus. *J. Matern. Fetal Med.* **2001**, *10*, 91–96. [CrossRef] [PubMed]
16. Chakravarty, E.F.; Colón, I.; Langen, E.S.; Nix, D.A.; El-Sayed, Y.Y.; Genovese, M.C.; Druzin, M.L. Factors that predict prematurity and preeclampsia in pregnancies that are complicated by systemic lupus erythematosus. *Am. J. Obstet. Gynecol.* **2005**, *192*, 1897–1904. [CrossRef]
17. Bramham, K.; Hunt, B.J.; Bewley, S.; Germain, S.; Calatayud, I.; Khamashta, M.A.; Nelson-Piercy, C. Pregnancy outcomes in systemic lupus erythematosus with and without previous nephritis. *J. Rheumatol.* **2011**, *38*, 1906–1913. [CrossRef]
18. Salmon, J.E.; Heuser, C.; Triebwasser, M.; Liszewski, M.K.; Kavanagh, D.; Roumenina, L.; Branch, D.W.; Goodship, T.; Fremeaux-Bacchi, V.; Atkinson, J.P. Mutations in complement regulatory proteins predispose to preeclampsia: A genetic analysis of the PROMISSE cohort. *PLoS Med.* **2011**, *8*, e1001013. [CrossRef]
19. Gibbins, K.J.; Ware Branch, D. Pre-eclampsia as a manifestation of antiphospholipid syndrome: Assessing the current status. *Lupus* **2014**, *23*, 1229–1231. [CrossRef]
20. Buyon, J.P.; Kim, M.Y.; Guerra, M.M.; Laskin, C.A.; Petri, M.; Lockshin, M.D.; Sammaritano, L.; Branch, D.W.; Porter, T.F.; Sawitzke, A.; et al. Predictors of Pregnancy Outcomes in Patients With Lupus: A Cohort Study. *Ann. Intern. Med.* **2015**, *163*, 153–163. [CrossRef]
21. Borella, E.; Lojacono, A.; Gatto, M.; Andreoli, L.; Taglietti, M.; Iaccarino, L.; Casiglia, E.; Punzi, L.; Tincani, A.; Doria, A.; et al. Predictors of maternal and fetal complications in SLE patients: A prospective study. *Immunol. Res.* **2014**, *60*, 170–176. [CrossRef] [PubMed]
22. Cortes-Hernandez, J.; Ordi-Ros, J.; Paredes, F.; Casellas, M.; Castillo, F.; Vilardell-Tarres, M. Clinical predictors of fetal and maternal outcome in systemic lupus erythematosus: A prospective study of 103 pregnancies. *Rheumatology* **2002**, *41*, 643–650. [CrossRef] [PubMed]
23. Petri, M.; Orbai, A.M.; Alarcón, G.S.; Gordon, C.; Merrill, J.T.; Fortin, P.R.; Bruce, I.N.; Isenberg, D.; Wallace, D.J.; Nived, O.; et al. Derivation and validation of the Systemic Lupus International Collaborating Clinics classification criteria for systemic lupus erythematosus. *Arthritis Rheum.* **2012**, *64*, 2677–2686. [CrossRef] [PubMed]
24. Hochberg, M.C. Updating the American College of Rheumatology revised criteria for the classification of systemic lupus erythematosus. *Arthritis Rheum* **1997**, *40*, 1725. [CrossRef]
25. Ingvarsson, R.F.; Bengtsson, A.A.; Jönsen, A. Variations in the epidemiology of systemic lupus erythematosus in southern Sweden. *Lupus* **2016**, *25*, 772–780. [CrossRef]
26. Miyakis, S.; Lockshin, M.D.; Atsumi, T.; Branch, D.W.; Brey, R.L.; Cervera, R.H.W.M.; Derksen, R.H.W.M.; De Groot, P.G.; Koike, T.; Meroni, P.L.; et al. International consensus statement on an update of the classification criteria for definite antiphospholipid syndrome (APS). *J. Thromb. Haemost. JTH* **2006**, *4*, 295–306. [CrossRef]
27. Gladman, D.D.; Ibanez, D.; Urowitz, M.B. Systemic lupus erythematosus disease activity index 2000. *J. Rheumatol.* **2002**, *29*, 288–291.
28. Gladman, D.; Ginzler, E.; Goldsmith, C.; Fortin, P.; Liang, M.; Sanchez-Guerrero, J.; Urowitz, M.; Bacon, P.; Bombardieri, S.; Hanly, J.; et al. The development and initial validation of the Systemic Lupus International Collaborating Clinics/American College of Rheumatology damage index for systemic lupus erythematosus. *Arthritis Rheum.* **1996**, *39*, 363–369. [CrossRef]
29. Cnattingius, S.; Lambe, M. Trends in smoking and overweight during pregnancy: Prevalence, risks of pregnancy complications, and adverse pregnancy outcomes. *Semin. Perinatol.* **2002**, *26*, 286–295. [CrossRef]
30. Proschan, M.A.; Waclawiw, M.A. Practical guidelines for multiplicity adjustment in clinical trials. *Control. Clin. Trials* **2000**, *21*, 527–539. [CrossRef]
31. Abalos, E.; Cuesta, C.; Grosso, A.L.; Chou, D.; Say, L. Global and regional estimates of preeclampsia and eclampsia: A systematic review. *Eur. J. Obstet. Gynecol. Reprod. Biol.* **2013**, *170*, 1–7. [CrossRef] [PubMed]

32. Georgiou, P.E.; Politi, E.N.; Katsimbri, P.; Sakka, V.; Drosos, A.A. Outcome of lupus pregnancy: A controlled study. *Rheumatology* **2000**, *39*, 1014–1019. [CrossRef] [PubMed]
33. Lateef, A.; Petri, M. Systemic Lupus Erythematosus and Pregnancy. *Rheum. Dis. Clin. N. Am.* **2017**, *43*, 215–226. [CrossRef] [PubMed]
34. Gladman, D.D.; Tandon, A.; Ibanez, D.; Urowitz, M.B. The effect of lupus nephritis on pregnancy outcome and fetal and maternal complications. *J. Rheumatol.* **2010**, *37*, 754–758. [CrossRef]
35. Wagner, S.J.; Craici, I.; Reed, D.; Norby, S.; Bailey, K.; Wiste, H.J.; Wood, C.M.; Moder, K.G.; Liang, K.P.; Liang, K.V.; et al. Maternal and foetal outcomes in pregnant patients with active lupus nephritis. *Lupus* **2009**, *18*, 342–347. [CrossRef]
36. Lateef, A.; Petri, M. Managing lupus patients during pregnancy. *Best Pract. Res. Clin. Rheumatol.* **2013**, *27*, 435–447. [CrossRef]
37. Chighizola, C.B.; Andreoli, L.; de Jesus, G.R.; Banzato, A.; Pons-Estel, G.J.; Erkan, D. The association between antiphospholipid antibodies and pregnancy morbidity, stroke, myocardial infarction, and deep vein thrombosis: A critical review of the literature. *Lupus* **2015**, *24*, 980–984. [CrossRef]
38. Yamada, H.; Atsumi, T.; Kobashi, G.; Ota, C.; Kato, E.H.; Tsuruga, N.; Ohta, K.; Yasuda, S.; Koike, T.; Minakami, H. Antiphospholipid antibodies increase the risk of pregnancy-induced hypertension and adverse pregnancy outcomes. *J. Reprod. Immunol.* **2009**, *79*, 188–195. [CrossRef]
39. Clark, C.A.; Spitzer, K.A.; Nadler, J.N.; Laskin, C.A. Preterm deliveries in women with systemic lupus erythematosus. *J. Rheumatol.* **2003**, *30*, 2127–2132.
40. Kim, M.Y.; Guerra, M.M.; Kaplowitz, E.; Laskin, C.A.; Petri, M.; Branch, D.W.; Lockshin, M.D.; Sammaritano, L.R.; Merrill, J.T.; Porter, T.F.; et al. Complement activation predicts adverse pregnancy outcome in patients with systemic lupus erythematosus and/or antiphospholipid antibodies. *Ann. Rheum. Dis.* **2018**, *77*, 549–555. [CrossRef]
41. Girardi, G.; Berman, J.; Redecha, P.; Spruce, L.; Thurman, J.M.; Kraus, D.; Hollmann, T.J.; Casali, P.; Caroll, M.C.; Wetsel, R.A.; et al. Complement C5a receptors and neutrophils mediate fetal injury in the antiphospholipid syndrome. *J. Clin. Investig.* **2003**, *112*, 1644–1654. [CrossRef] [PubMed]
42. Wang, W.; Irani, R.A.; Zhang, Y.; Ramin, S.M.; Blackwell, S.C.; Tao, L.; Kellems, R.E.; Xia, Y. Autoantibody-mediated complement C3a receptor activation contributes to the pathogenesis of preeclampsia. *Hypertension (Dallas Tex 1979)* **2012**, *60*, 712–721. [CrossRef] [PubMed]
43. Holers, V.M.; Girardi, G.; Mo, L.; Guthridge, J.M.; Molina, H.; Pierangeli, S.S.; Espinola, R.; Xiaowei, L.E.; Mao, D.; Vialpando, C.G.; et al. Complement C3 activation is required for antiphospholipid antibody-induced fetal loss. *J. Exp. Med.* **2002**, *195*, 211–220. [CrossRef] [PubMed]
44. Carolis, S.; Botta, A.; Santucci, S.; Salvi, S.; Moresi, S.; Di Pasquo, E.; Del Sordo, G.; Martino, C. Complementemia and obstetric outcome in pregnancy with antiphospholipid syndrome. *Lupus* **2012**, *21*, 776–778. [CrossRef]
45. Reggia, R.; Ziglioli, T.; Andreoli, L.; Bellisai, F.; Iuliano, A.; Gerosa, M.; Ramoni, V.; Tani, C.; Brucato, A.; Galeazzi, M.; et al. Primary anti-phospholipid syndrome: Any role for serum complement levels in predicting pregnancy complications? *Rheumatology* **2012**, *51*, 2186–2890. [CrossRef]
46. Penning, M.; Chua, J.S.; Van Kooten, C.; Zandbergen, M.; Buurma, A.; Schutte, J.; Bruijn, J.A.; Khankin, E.V.; Bloemenkamp, K.; Karumanchi, S.A.; et al. Classical Complement Pathway Activation in the Kidneys of Women with Preeclampsia. *Hypertension (Dallas Tex 1979)* **2015**, *66*, 117–125. [CrossRef]
47. Buurma, A.; Cohen, D.; Veraar, K.; Schonkeren, D.; Claas, F.H.; Bruijn, J.A.; Bloemenkamp, K.W.; Baelde, H.J. Preeclampsia is characterized by placental complement dysregulation. *Hypertension (Dallas Tex 1979)* **2012**, *60*, 1332–1337. [CrossRef]
48. Andreoli, L.; Bertsias, G.K.; Agmon-Levin, N.; Brown, S.; Cervera, R.; Costedoat-Chalumeau, N.; Doria, A.; Fischer-Betz, R.; Forger, F.; Moraes-Fontes, M.F.; et al. EULAR recommendations for women's health and the management of family planning, assisted reproduction, pregnancy and menopause in patients with systemic lupus erythematosus and/or antiphospholipid syndrome. *Ann. Rheum. Dis.* **2017**, *76*, 476–485. [CrossRef]
49. Clowse, M.E.; Magder, L.S.; Witter, F.; Petri, M. The impact of increased lupus activity on obstetric outcomes. *Arthritis Rheum.* **2005**, *52*, 514–521. [CrossRef]
50. Yang, H.; Liu, H.; Xu, D.; Zhao, L.; Wang, Q.; Leng, X.; Zheng, W.; Zhang, F.; Tang, F.; Zhang, X. Pregnancy-related systemic lupus erythematosus: Clinical features, outcome and risk factors of disease flares—a case control study. *PLoS ONE* **2014**, *9*, e104375. [CrossRef]

51. Kwok, L.W.; Tam, L.S.; Zhu, T.; Leung, Y.Y.; Li, E. Predictors of maternal and fetal outcomes in pregnancies of patients with systemic lupus erythematosus. *Lupus* **2011**, *20*, 829–836. [CrossRef] [PubMed]
52. Davis-Porada, J.; Kim, M.Y.; Guerra, M.M.; Laskin, C.A.; Petri, M.; Lockshin, M.D.; Sammaritano, L.R.; Branch, D.W.; Sawitzke, A.; Merrill, J.T.; et al. Low frequency of flares during pregnancy and post-partum in stable lupus patients. *Arthritis Res. Ther.* **2020**, *22*, 52. [CrossRef] [PubMed]
53. Ruiz-Irastorza, G.; Lima, F.; Alves, J.; Khamashta, M.A.; Simpson, J.; Hughes, G.R.V.; Buchanan, N.M.M. Increased rate of lupus flare during pregnancy and the puerperium: A prospective study of 78 pregnancies. *Br. J. Rheumatol.* **1996**, *35*, 133–138. [CrossRef]
54. Eudy, A.M.; Siega-Riz, A.M.; Engel, S.M.; Franceschini, N.; Howard, A.G.; Clowse, M.E.; Petri, M. Effect of pregnancy on disease flares in patients with systemic lupus erythematosus. *Ann. Rheum. Dis.* **2018**, *77*, 855–860. [CrossRef] [PubMed]
55. Morishita, M.; Sada, K.E.; Ohashi, K.; Miyawaki, Y.; Asano, Y.; Hayashi, K.; Asano, S.H.; Yamamura, Y.; Watanabe, H.; Narazaki, M.; et al. Damage accrual related to pregnancies before and after diagnosis of systemic lupus erythematosus: A cross-sectional and nested case-control analysis from a lupus registry. *Lupus* **2020**, *29*, 176–181. [CrossRef] [PubMed]

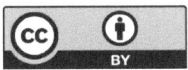

© 2020 by the authors. Licensee MDPI, Basel, Switzerland. This article is an open access article distributed under the terms and conditions of the Creative Commons Attribution (CC BY) license (http://creativecommons.org/licenses/by/4.0/).

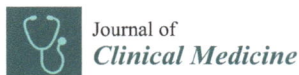

Review

Glucocorticoids in *Systemic Lupus Erythematosus*. Ten Questions and Some Issues

Sabrina Porta [1], Alvaro Danza [2], Maira Arias Saavedra [1], Adriana Carlomagno [2], María Cecilia Goizueta [3], Florencia Vivero [4] and Guillermo Ruiz-Irastorza [5,6,*]

[1] Rheumatology Department, Hospital JM Ramos Mejía, Buenos Aires 1221, Argentina; psachu@gmail.com (S.P.); mairaariassaavedra@gmail.com (M.A.S.)
[2] Department of Internal Medicine, Faculty of Medicine, Universidad de la República, Montevideo 11000, Uruguay; alvarodanza@gmail.com (A.D.); adrianacarlomagno@gmail.com (A.C.)
[3] Autoimmune Disease Unit, Sanatorio 9 de Julio, Tucumán T4000, Argentina; cecigoizueta@yahoo.com.ar
[4] Autoimmune Disease Unit, Hospital Privado de Comunidad, Mar del Plata B7600, Argentina; florenciavivero82@gmail.com
[5] Autoimmune Diseases Research Unit, BioCruces Bizkaia Health Research Institute, Cruces Univeristy Hospital, 48903 Bizkaia, Spain
[6] University of the Basque Country, 48940 Leioa, Spain
* Correspondence: r.irastorza@outlook.es

Received: 9 July 2020; Accepted: 17 August 2020; Published: 21 August 2020

Abstract: Since the discovery of glucocorticoids (GCs), their important anti-inflammatory effect, rapid mechanism of action, low cost, and accessibility have made them one of the mainstays of treatment for *Systemic lupus erythematosus* (SLE). Although their use has allowed controlling the disease and reducing acute mortality in severe conditions, the implementation of a scheme based on high doses for long periods has inevitably been accompanied by an increase in adverse effects and infections, including long-term damage. The objective of this review is to answer some important questions that may arise from its use in daily clinical practice, and to propose a paradigm based on the use of methylprednisolone pulses followed by medium-low doses and a rapid decrease of prednisone.

Keywords: systemic lupus erythematosus; SLE; prednisone; methylprednisolone; glucocorticoids; mortality; prognosis; damage

1. Introduction

Systemic lupus erythematosus (SLE) is a complex disease characterized by autoimmunity, inflammation, and a variable degree of organ damage, which depends on the number and severity of flares but also on the treatments received. The management of SLE is often challenging. Most guidelines refer to "standard of care" as a combination of hydroxychloroquine, glucocorticoids (GCs), and, sometimes, an immunosuppressive agent. Such therapy often achieves disease remission, but too many times at the cost of a large degree of damage accrual.

Irreversible organ damage is not only very frequent in SLE, but also particularly relevant considering that most patients are young or middle-aged women. According to a growing amount of scientific evidence, irreversible damage, as well as other serious side effects, such as infections, are strongly associated with the use of GCs [1–3]. Indeed, the recently updated EULAR guidelines highlight the need to prevent organ damage and to optimize pharmacological strategies in order to improve health-related quality of life and to achieve long-term patient survival [4].

The purpose of this review is to answer ten daily clinical practice questions by updating the current evidence about the optimal doses of GCs in several scenarios, based on pharmacological and clinical evidence, as well as to offer our point of view regarding the "standard of care" of GC use.

1.1. What Is the Main Mechanism of Action of GCs?

The first mechanism of action of GCs is to interfere with the genomic transcription of inflammatory molecules. This process starts by means of GCs binding the cytosolic-GC receptor (cGR). The GC-cGR complex is translocated into the nucleus where it modulates gene expression. This is called the genomic pathway [5,6]. The first effect generated by the GC-cGR complex within the nucleus is transrepression, consisting of the inhibition of those genes which promote cytokine and other protein synthesis involved in the inflammatory process, with the resulting anti-inflammatory effect. As the intranuclear concentration of GCs increases, a second process named transactivation starts. Although this mechanism stimulates the transcription of some inhibitory genes, it mainly mediates the activation of gluconeogenesis, insulin resistance, skin atrophy, and the inhibition of bone formation, all well-known adverse effects of GCs [7–9].

The use of low doses of prednisone (≤7.5 mg/day) is associated with a progressive saturation up to 50% of the cGR. At medium doses (>7.5 mg/day to 30 mg/day of prednisone), the receptor becomes progressively saturated from 50 to close to 100%, keeping a less lineal relation with the daily dose. It is estimated that the almost complete saturation of cGR occurs at approximately 30–40 mg/day of prednisone. At higher doses, up to 100 mg/day, the predominant effect is transactivation, and therefore the occurrence of unwanted effects with no major increase in anti-inflammatory actions [10–12]. This pharmacodynamic behavior is the basis of the new GC dosage schemes [12].

1.2. What Is the Non-Genomic Way and How Does It Get Activated?

A second mechanism of action of GCs, the non-genomic pathway, acts by modulating inflammatory and immune cells by three molecular mechanisms independent from nuclear interactions. First, the GC-cGR complex directly blocks the activation of phospholipase A2 and thus the production of arachidonic acid by a transcription-independent mechanism. Second, the activation of the membrane-bound GR (mGR) leads to the reduction of lymphocyte activity via the p38 MAP kinase. Third, nonspecific interactions with the cellular membranes of immune cells result in the inhibition of ATP production and thus decrease cell activity [13]. In addition, mGR activation also modifies gene expression, so priming the immune cells for the upcoming genomic effects [13]. These non-genomic mechanisms are characterized by a rapid onset of action (less than 15 min) because they do not need time for translation to the nucleus and modulation of gene transcription.

The activation of the non-genomic pathway starts at doses >100 mg/day of prednisone or equivalent. This pathway is especially sensitive to methylprednisolone (MP) and dexamethasone, which have non-genomic effects up to five times more potent than genomic ones [8].

Non-genomic effects are responsible for the efficacy of pulse therapy with GCs at doses over 125 mg of MP [14]. Work by the group of Buttgeterit et al. has shown the relative anti-inflammatory potency of different GCs by the non-genomic method, based on the effects on respiration, protein synthesis, and Na+−K+-ATPase and Ca2+−ATPase in concanavalin A-stimulated rat thymocytes [15]. MP and dexamethasone show the highest non-genomic-mediated potency (Table 1). The potency of treatment with MP also allows a faster tapering of oral prednisone and therefore, a reduction in the cumulative dose of GC [14,16,17]. A summary of the genomic and non-genomic GC effects is shown in Table 2.

Table 1. Anti-inflammatory potency exerted by genomic/non-genomic ways of the different glucocorticoids [15,18].

Glucocorticoid	Anti-Inflammatory Effect (Genomic Way)	Anti-Inflammatory Effect (Non-Genomic Way)
Cortisol/hydrocortisone	1	Low
Prednisone/prednisolone	4	4
Methylprednisolone	5	10–15
Dexamethasone	20–30	20
Betamethasone	20–30	<4

Table 2. Summary of the mechanisms of action of glucocorticoids.

	Genomic Pathway	Non-Genomic Pathway
Cells targeted	All the organism	Inflammatory cells
Mechanism of action	Genomic modulation	Membrane receptor and intracellular inflammatory pathways
Start of action	~4 to 6 h	~15 min
Saturation dose of the immunosuppressive – anti-inflammatory effects	~100% at 30 to 40 mg/day of prednisone-equivalent	Unknown
Minimum effective dose	2.5 to 5 mg/day of prednisone-equivalent	Over 100 mg of prednisone-equivalent
Maximum effective doses that minimize adverse effects	30 to 40 mg/day of prednisone-equivalent (for trans-repression)	500/day mg of methylprednisolone
Damage accrual with cumulative doses	Proven	Not proven
Glucocorticoids acting by this way	All	Mainly methylprednisolone and dexamethasone

1.3. Should High Doses of Prednisonse Be Still Considered the Standard Starting Dose?

The "classical" standard 1 mg/kg/day prednisone dose is not supported by either basic pharmacology or clinical evidence (Figure 1) [19,20]. It is unlikely that anti-inflammatory effects increase significantly after prednisone doses have reached 30–40 mg/day, since such doses already result in a saturation of almost 100% of the genomic pathway [12,19]. Recent data suggest that higher initial doses of prednisone are associated with higher cumulative doses [21] with the well proven result of increasing damage accrual [1,22–25].

Instead, the combination of MP pulses followed by doses of prednisone up to 30 mg/day, depending on severity, is more effective, more rapid, and safer than the use of the "classical" 1 mg/kg/day (Figure 2). Several studies support this view. A European multicenter randomized, controlled study compared standard dose (1 mg/kg/day, $n = 42$) and reduced dose prednisone groups (0.5 mg/kg/day; $n = 39$), both associated with mycophenolic acid, during the induction phase of class III-IV lupus nephritis (LN). The complete remission rates at week 24 were similar for both groups, with fewer infections in the reduced prednisone dose group [26].

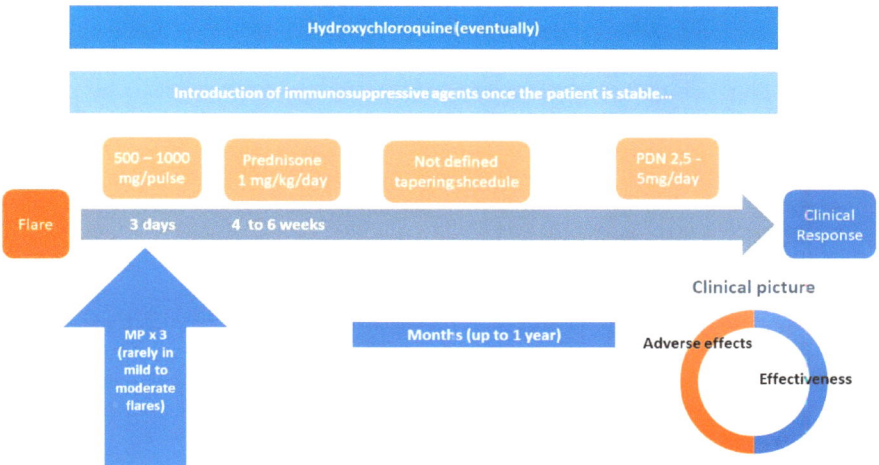

Figure 1. The "classical paradigm" in SLE therapy. Note: PDN: prednisone; MP: methylprednisolone pulses; proportions showed in "clinical picture" are merely illustrative.

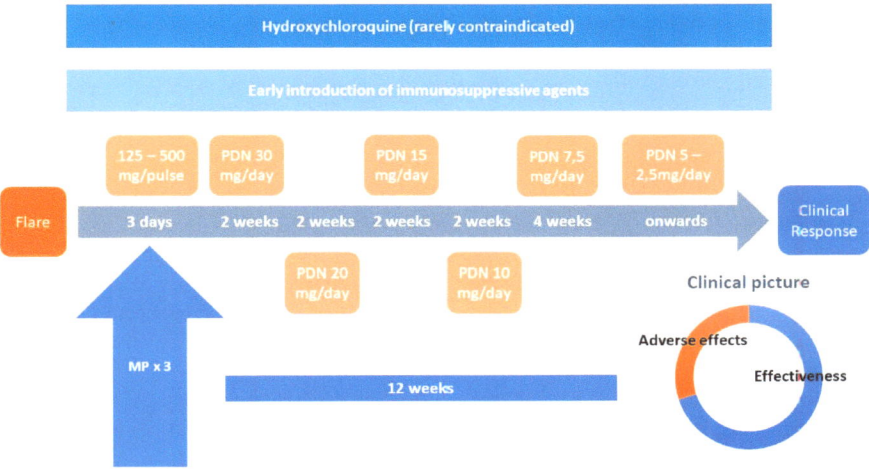

Figure 2. The "new paradigm" in SLE therapy. Note: PDN: prednisone; MP: methylprednisolone pulses; proportions showed in "clinical picture" are merely illustrative.

In an observational study of patients with class III-IV-V LN from the *Lupus-Cruces* (CC; $n = 29$) and the *Lupus-Bordeaux* cohorts (BC; $n = 44$), the number of pulses of MP per patient (9.3 vs. 2.3), but not the cumulative dose, and the proportion of patients on hydroxychloroquine (100% vs. 63%) were higher in the CC. The maximum doses of prednisone (21 vs. 42 mg/day), the number of weeks until 5 mg/day (12 vs. 22), and the mean doses at six months (8.3 vs. 21 mg/day) were all lower in the CC. Complete renal remission rates were significantly higher in the CC at six (69% vs. 30) and 12 months (86% vs. 43%) [27]. Of note, the number (not the total dose) of MP pulses was the only independent therapeutic predictor of achieving complete remission and of reducing GCs-related side effects [27].

The AURA–LV was a 48-week randomized clinical trial comparing the efficacy in the treatment of LN of two doses of voclosporin or placebo added to mycophenolate mofetil. All patients received a maximum initial dose of 25 mg/day of prednisone with tapering to 5 mg in 8 weeks and to 2.5 mg in 12 weeks. Remission rates at 48 weeks were 49.45% and 39.8% in both voclosporin groups [28]. Even patients in the control arm of the AURA trial had remission rates higher than those in previous studies such as ALMS [29] and LUNAR [30,31].

The "Rituxilup" schedule, which consisted of rituximab and MP, followed by maintenance treatment with mycophenolate mofetil and no oral steroids, resulted in 72% of patients with LN class III, IV, or V eventually achieving complete remission within a median period of 36 weeks [32].

In patients presenting with an SLEDAI score ≥6 (those with severe LN excluded), initial therapy with doses of prednisone ≤30 mg/day resulted in a similar decrease in SLEDAI scores at one year and reduced damage at five years compared with initial doses >30 mg/day. It must be noted that, in order to reduce prednisone doses, hydroxychloroquine was used in 100% vs. 33% of patients and MP pulses in 34% vs. 10%, respectively [1].

Thus, current evidence, based on large observational cohorts and a few clinical trials, supports the idea that low-medium initial doses of prednisone (i.e., ≤30 mg/day) are at least as effective as high-dose schemes and with a better safety profile [31,33]. MP pulses offer additional potency and allow the use of lower doses of prednisone. Of note, no studies of similar quality have ever shown the superiority of high-dose prednisone regimes.

1.4. Are 1000 mg MP Pulses More Effective than Lower Doses?

In a study from 1987 including 21 patients with active SLE with severe manifestations refractory to other treatments, patients were either treated with intravenous MP 100 mg/day or 1000 mg/day for three days. The study did not find significant differences between the two groups [34]. In addition, a retrospective study by Badsha et al., 2002 reported that 1500 mg of MP given throughout three days were equally effective in controlling the disease and associated with fewer serious infections than 3000 to 5000 mg in the same period [35]. The same authors carried out a prospective study comparing the use of 500 mg/day of methylprednisolone for three days with a historical cohort given higher doses and obtained the same results [36].

In the *Lupus-Cruces* cohort, the use of intravenous MP pulses, in all cases between 125 and 500 mg/day for three consecutive days, were not associated with long-term damage accrual [17]. In the previously mentioned study of patients with class III-IV-V LN from the CC and the BC, the number of intravenous MP pulses, rather than the total dose, was an independent predictor of complete response and of reduced GC-related toxicity. CC patients were treated with three consecutive 250–500 mg intravenous pulses and then with additional 125 mg pulses every two weeks before each intravenous dose of cyclophosphamide [27].

In 2018, Danza et al. compared the efficacy and rates of infections among patients with several autoimmune conditions, including SLE, treated with MP pulses, for a total dose over three days ≤1500 mg, <1500 to ≤3000 mg and >3000 mg [19]. No differences among the different doses were seen in patients achieving complete response, partial response, or no response. No patients in the ≤1500 mg group suffered infections, vs. 9.1% in the high dose group.

1.5. Should Pulses of MP Be Reserved for Life Threatening Flares?

It is well assumed that MP pulses, due to their higher potency and faster mechanism of action compared to oral prednisone, are indicated in those patients with severe manifestations of SLE in whom a rapid effect is necessary [4,14]. However, they might not be limited to this clinical scenario. The rapidity and potency of action make MP pulses at doses 125–250 mg/day for three days is ideal to deal with many moderate lupus flares, like arthritis, skin rashes, and pericarditis, and also for recurrent or non-responding mild flares. Thus, MP pulses may contribute to avoid high-dose prednisone and to promote a faster tapering, reducing the cumulative GC dose and thus the short and long-term side effects of oral prednisone [4,33].

1.6. Can GC-Related Damage Be Avoided without Reducing Efficacy?

There are several factors that contribute to organ damage accrual in patients with SLE. Among them, the role of GCs has proven fundamental. In 2003, Gladman et al. categorized damage as definite, probable and not related to GCs [3] and found that the latter increased over disease course, being the most frequent in latter stages of SLE. Joo et al. have also found that patients with LN have more damage associated than non-associated to GCs [37]. In the Hopkins cohort, GC-related irreversible damage has been shown to depend on the cumulative dose of prednisone [38]. Compared to patients who did not receive prednisone, the risk of accruing damage increased 1.2 times if they had received a cumulative dose of 180 mg per month, and twice for a cumulative dose >540 mg per month [23]. On the other hand, the use of MP pulses has not been associated with damage accrual in large series [17,38].

A possible reason explaining this is the different toxicity associated with the activation of the genomic (increasing toxicity in parallel with activation) and the non-genomic ways (free of genomic transactivation-related toxicity). Therefore, the use of MP pulses (activating non-genomic mechanisms), rather than prednisone doses >30 mg/day (fully activating the genomic way), for inducing rapid remission, followed by maintenance doses of prednisone ≤5 mg/day (activating less than 25% of the genomic way) may be a good approach to minimize GC-related side effects. In addition, hydroxychloroquine helps spare prednisone and, by itself, also prevents damage accrual [39]. Ruiz-Arruza et al found that the use of this treatment scheme achieved the same efficacy, with no increase in SLE-related damage and less global, cardiovascular and GC-related damage [33].

Whilst the eventual discontinuation of GC is the ultimate goal, a recent monocentric, 12-month, superiority, open label, randomized controlled trial compared the efficacy to prevent flares of maintenance versus withdrawal of 5 mg/day prednisone in patients with clinically quiescent SLE. The study found that maintenance therapy with 5 mg/day of prednisone prevents relapses, with no worsening of damage and no GC toxicity observed during the follow-up period [40]. Therefore, long-term therapy with low-dose GC may be necessary in a number of patients with SLE. This could contrast with the results of the aforementioned Rituxilup study [32], in which no oral GCs were used during the induction phase in patients with LN. However, the clinical setting (maintenance and induction) is different, and no data were given regarding how many patients in this study eventually needed GCs for other manifestations of SLE.

1.7. How Can the Risk of Infections Be Reduced during GC Treatment?

Infections represent one of the most important causes of morbidity and mortality in patients with SLE [41]. The factors predisposing lupus patients to infection are not only disease activity and the malfunction of the immune system, but also the use of immunosuppressive drugs, particularly GCs [41,42]. GCs suppress the production of inflammatory cytokines, the microbicidal activity of activated macrophages, the adhesion of neutrophils to endothelial cells, the release of lysosomal enzymes, the respiratory burst, and the chemotaxis. In addition, they cause marked lymphopenia in all lymphocyte subpopulations, inhibit the activation of T cells and have immunosuppressive effects on the maturation and function of dendritic cells, responsible for triggering the adaptive immune response [43]. Although these effects increase with the dose and the duration of treatment, the risk of infection is already high at maintained doses of 7.5 mg/day. Indeed, the chance of suffering a severe infection increases by 12% for each mg/day of prednisone [2].

According to the data obtained from the Spanish Registry of *Systemic Lupus Erythematosus* (RELES), 6.4% of patients had a documented episode of major infection during the first year of follow-up and 5.67% during the second. Mean prednisone doses >30 mg/day during the first month and >7.5 mg/day during the first year independently predicted major infections within the first and the second year of follow-up, respectively [44]. Regarding MP pulses, the use of 1000 mg/day for three days has been associated with an increase in infections compared with 500 mg/day [35].

A number of prophylactic measures, such as the administration of vaccines, can be recommended in SLE, and the use of hydroxychloroquine is also protective against infections [45]. However, a retrospective, new-user study including 3030 SLE patients found that the rate of severe infections in patients on prednisone >15 mg/day was high and not influenced by antimalarials use [22]. Thus, the use of maintenance doses of prednisone not exceeding 5 mg/day with pulses of 500 mg of MP instead of 1000 mg is probably a good way to reduce the infectious complications in lupus patients.

1.8. How Should GC Therapy Be Managed during Pregnancy?

Since the therapeutic possibilities are lower in pregnant women, GCs are one of main therapeutic resources during gestation in case of lupus flares [46]. Indeed, their potent anti-inflammatory effect seems not to be accompanied by any significant teratogenicity.

The choice of GC will depend on whether our goal is to treat the mother or the fetus. According to the most recent EULAR and BSR guidelines, in the first case, the use of non-fluorinated GCs such as prednisone or MP will be of choice, while in the second case, the treatment will be with fluorinated GCs, such as betamethasone or dexamethasone [46,47]. This is due to the presence of the placental 11-beta dehydrogenase enzyme that converts non-fluorinated GCs into relatively inactive forms, with less than 10% of the drug reaching the fetal circulation [48].

The adverse effects observed are similar to those occurring outside pregnancy, however, hypertension, preeclampsia, insulin resistance, infections and premature rupture of membranes represent additional serious problems during gestation. For this reason, prednisone is recommended at doses not exceeding 20 mg/day for the treatment of severe manifestations of the disease, and 7.5 mg/day for minor manifestations, with rapid tapering in both cases to maintenance doses ≤5 mg/day. If necessary, in moderate-severe flares, intravenous pulses of MP 125–500 mg can be safely used [49].

During the lactation, the amount of prednisone found in breast milk is very low, although it is advisable to delay breastfeeding until four hours after taking doses greater than 50 mg/day (which are not recommended, anyhow) [46].

In women undergoing corticotherapy during pregnancy or lactation, adequate supplementation with calcium 1000 mg/day and vitamin D 800 IU/day is recommended for the prevention of GC-induced osteoporosis [50].

1.9. What Are the Current Recommendations?

The current recommendations are, once a SLE flare is diagnosed, to achieve remission or low disease activity as soon as possible, and then prevent new flares [4,51,52]. An intensification of the immunosuppressive regimen is universally recommended for this purpose. Although there is no universal agreement regarding the definition of low dose of GCs, most authors accept doses ≤7.5–5 mg/day of prednisone or equivalent [52,53]. Since no consensus about tapering has been established, such doses can be reached within variable periods ranging from four weeks to up to 12 months.

Table 3 shows how starting doses of GCs vary among the different guidelines, from 0.3 to 2 mg/kg/day for patients with severe, renal or extra-renal involvement [51,52,54–56], or whenever the administration of MP pulses during induction therapy is not possible [54]. Even though the recent 2019 EULAR recommendations do not provide a specific tapering scheme, they recommend avoiding an initial dose of 1 mg/kg/day of prednisone and highlight the importance of using early MP pulses and immunosuppressants in order to spare oral GCs [4], with some significant recommendations: in cases of mild to moderate disease, start with prednisone doses ≤0.5 mg/kg/day, with "gradual tapering"; in cases of severe or organ-threatening disease, MP pulses (250–1000 mg/day) for 1–3 days are suggested, followed by prednisone 0.5–0.7 mg/kg/day "with tapering" [4]. Recommended MP doses vary from 250 mg/day to 1000 mg/day for 3 days when a flare is diagnosed [54]. Again, there is no agreement on its use during induction, often being reserved for severely active patients who do not achieve a sufficient response after initial high doses of prednisone [54,55].

Table 3. Recommended doses of glucocorticoids in recent lupus guidelines.

Guideline	Methodology	Clinical Setting	Pulses Recommended?	Dose of Prednisone Recommended?	Tapering Scheme?	Maintenance Dose?
ACR (2012) [54]	Opinions of highly-qualified experts.	LN III-IV	YES. 500–1000 mg/day methyl-prednisolone for 1–3 days	YES. 0.5–1 mg/kg/day or 1 mg/kg/day if crescents seen	NO. Only "a few weeks"	NO Only "to lowest effective dose"
		LN V	NO	YES. 0.5 mg/kg/day	NO. Maintain initial dose by for 6 months	
EULAR/ERA-EDTA (2012) [55]	A modified Delphi method was used to compile questions, elicit expert opinions and reach consensus	LN III-IV	YES. 500–750 mg/day methyl-prednisolone for 1–3 days	YES. 0.5 mg/kg/day	YES. Maintain initial dose by 4 weeks, reducing to ≤10 mg/day by 4–6 months.	YES. ≤10 mg/day
		LN II	NO	YES. If proteinuria >1 g/24 h: 0.25–0.5 mg/kg/day		
BSR (2018) [51]	Evidence-based guidelines, supplemented as necessary with expert opinion and consensus agreement.	Mild activity flare	NO	YES. ≤20 mg/day	NO. Only maintain initial dose by 1–2 weeks	YES. ≤7.5 mg/day
		Moderate activity flare	YES. ≤250 mg/day methyl-prednisolone for 1–3 days	YES. ≤0.5 mg/kg/day	NO	YES. ≤7.5 mg/day
		Severe activity flare:	YES 500 mg/day methyl-prednisolone for 1–3 days	YES. ≤0.75–1 mg/kg/day or ≤0.5 mg/kg/day with pulses	NO	YES. ≤7.5 mg/day
EULAR (2019) [4]	Delphi method, to form questions, elicit expert opinions and reach consensus.	Mild-moderate flare	NO	YES. ≤0.5 mg/kg/day	NO. Only gradual tapering	YES. ≤7.5 mg/day
		Severe/organ-threatening disease:	YES. "Consider" 250–1000 mg/day methyl-prednisolone for 1–3 days	YES. 0.5–0.7 mg/kg/day	NO. Only "gradual tapering"	YES. ≤7.5 mg/day.
GLADEL/PANLAR (2019) [52]	GRADE	LN	NO	YES. 1–2 mg/kg/ maximum 60 mg/day	NO. "Regardless of manifestations of disease, should prescribed at the lowest doses and for the shortest period of weather"	YES. ≤7.5 mg/day.
		Diffuse alveolar haemorrhage	YES	NO		
EULAR/ERA-EDTA (2020) [56]	Delphi methodology. Task Force voted on their level of agreement with the formed statements.	LN III-IV	YES. Total dose 500–2500 mg, depending on disease severity.	YES. 0.3–0.5 mg/kg/day	YES. 0.3–0.5 mg/kg/day for up to 4 weeks. Tapered to ≤7.5 mg/day by 3 to 6 months. Gradual withdrawal of treatment (glucocorticoids first, then immunosuppressive)	YES. ≤7.5 mg/day
		LN V		YES. 20 mg/day	YES. Tapered to ≤5 mg/day by 3 months	YES. ≤5 mg/day

ACR: American College of Rheumatology. EULAR: European League Against Rheumatism. ERA-EDTA: European Renal Association-European Dialysis and Transplant Association. BSR: British Society of Rheumatology. LN: Lupus nephritis. GLADEL: Grupo Latino-Americano de Estudio del Lupus. PANLAR: Liga Panamericana de Asociaciones de Reumatología.

1.10. What Is our Proposed "Standard of Care" for GC Use?

We advocate for a new paradigm in the use of GCs in SLE. The old, vague expression "the shortest time and at the lowest dose possible" is not enough, since many doctors feel that a rapid decrease in the dose of prednisone can precipitate a flare or a situation of adrenal insufficiency (Figure 1). Nowadays, there is enough evidence to support the use of doses of prednisone ≤30 mg/day in most severe flares, equally effective than higher doses, with a much better safety profile, both in the short and in the long term. MP pulses should not be limited life-threatening situations since they contribute to rapid disease control while sparing oral GCs. Pulses can be used in a wide range of doses, from 125 mg to 500 mg, depending on the severity of flares (Figures 2 and 3). Using this scheme, along with hydroxychloroquine and early immunosuppressive therapy, it is possible to accomplish a quick tapering of prednisone, and therefore to achieve maintenance doses ≤5 mg/day within a maximum period of 12 weeks [57,58].

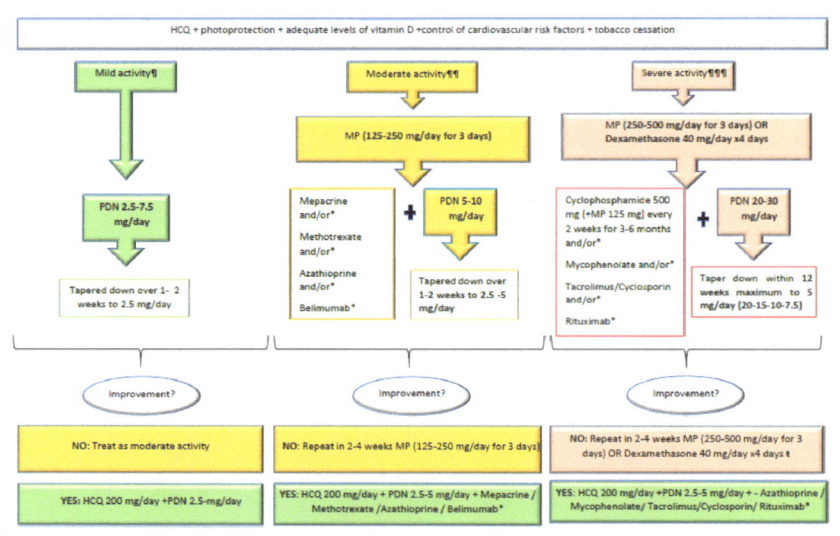

Figure 3. The Lupus-Cruces protocol for the treatment of SLE according to severity. Note: HCQ: hydroxychloroquine; PDN: prednisone; MP: methylprednisolone pulses; ¶ Polyarthralgia, small joint monooligoarthritis, limited skin lesions; ¶¶ Polyarthritis, moderate thrombocytopenia (20,000–50,000/mm^3), haemolytic anaemia with a low rate of haemolysis, widespread skin lupus lesions, non-severe pericardial effusion/pericarditis, pleural effusion; ¶¶¶ Lupus nephritis, pneumonitis, severe thrombocytopenia (<20,000/mm^3), haemolytic anaemia with a high rate of haemolysis, severe pericardial effusion, refractory pleural effusion, severe neuropsychiatric manifestations; * depending on specific organ involvement.

2. Conclusions

- Glucocorticoids may act by genomic and non-genomic pathways. The second way is faster and non-related to chronic damage.
- The classic glucocorticoid dose of 1 mg/kg/day is not evidence-supported and has a well-known range of serious adverse effects
- Recruiting the non-genomic pathway by methylprednisolone pulses followed by a reduced dose scheme of prednisone may avoid adverse effect and chronic damage
- Immunosuppressive agents should be early introduced in the treatment of moderate-severe SLE to spare glucocorticoids

- Prednisone maintenance doses ≤5 mg/day should be ideally achieved in no more than 12 weeks.
- Hydroxychloroquine is mandatory in SLE treatment, except in the exceptional cases with contraindications.

Author Contributions: Conceptualization, S.P., A.D., and G.R.-I.; comprehensive literature review, S.P., A.D., M.A.S., A.C., M.C.G., F.V., and G.R.-I.; writing—original draft preparation, S.P., A.D., M.A.S., A.C., M.C.G., and F.V.; writing—review and editing, S.P., A.D., and G.R.-I.; supervision, G.R.-I. All authors have read and agreed to the published version of the manuscript.

Funding: This research received no external funding.

Conflicts of Interest: The authors declare no conflict of interest.

References

1. Ruiz-Arruza, I.; Barbosa, C.; Ugarte, A.; Ruiz-Irastorza, G. Comparison of high versus low-medium prednisone doses for the treatment of systemic lupus erythematosus patients with high activity at diagnosis. *Autoimmun. Rev.* **2015**, *14*, 875–879. [CrossRef] [PubMed]
2. Ruiz-Irastorza, G.; Olivares, N.; Ruiz-Arruza, I.; Martinez-Berriotxoa, A.; Egurbide, M.V.; Aguirre, C. Predictors of major infections in systemic lupus erythematosus. *Arthritis Res. Ther.* **2009**, *11*, R109. [CrossRef] [PubMed]
3. Gladman, D.D.; Urowitz, M.B.; Rahman, P.; Ibanez, D.; Tam, L.S. Accrual of organ damage over time in patients with systemic lupus erythematosus. *J. Rheumatol.* **2003**, *30*, 1955–1959. [PubMed]
4. Fanouriakis, A.; Kostopoulou, M.; Alunno, A.; Aringer, M.; Bajema, I.; Boletis, J.N.; Cervera, R.; Doria, A.; Gordon, C.; Govoni, M.; et al. 2019 update of the EULAR recommendations for the management of systemic lupus erythematosus. *Ann. Rheum. Dis.* **2019**, *78*, 736–745. [CrossRef]
5. Buttgereit, F.; Wehling, M.; Burmester, G.R. A new hypothesis of modular glucocorticoid actions: Steroid treatment of rheumatic diseases revisited. *Arthritis Rheum.* **1998**, *41*, 761–767. [CrossRef]
6. Kleiman, A.; Tuckermann, J.P. Glucocorticoid receptor action in beneficial and side effects of steroid therapy: Lessons from conditional knockout mice. *Mol. Cell. Endocrinol.* **2007**, *275*, 98–108. [CrossRef]
7. Buttgereit, F.; Straub, R.H.; Wehling, M.; Burmester, G.R. Glucocorticoids in the treatment of rheumatic diseases: An update on the mechanisms of action. *Arthritis Rheum.* **2004**, *50*, 3408–3417. [CrossRef]
8. Buttgereit, F.; Burmester, G.R.; Lipworth, B.J. Optimised glucocorticoid therapy: The sharpening of an old spear. *Lancet* **2005**, *365*, 801–803. [CrossRef]
9. Ruiz-Irastorza, G.; Danza, A.; Khamashta, M. Glucocorticoid use and abuse in SLE. *Rheumatology* **2012**, *51*, 1145–1153. [CrossRef]
10. Bijlsma, J.W.; Saag, K.G.; Buttgereit, F.; da Silva, J.A. Developments in glucocorticoid therapy. *Rheum. Dis. Clin. N. Am.* **2005**, *31*, 1–17. [CrossRef]
11. Buttgereit, F.; Saag, K.G.; Cutolo, M.; da Silva, J.A.; Bijlsma, J.W. The molecular basis for the effectiveness, toxicity, and resistance to glucocorticoids: Focus on the treatment of rheumatoid arthritis. *Scand. J. Rheumatol.* **2005**, *34*, 14–21. [CrossRef] [PubMed]
12. Buttgereit, F.; da Silva, J.A.; Boers, M.; Burmester, G.R.; Cutolo, M.; Jacobs, J.; Kirwan, J.; Kohler, L.; Van Riel, P.; Vischer, T.; et al. Standardised nomenclature for glucocorticoid dosages and glucocorticoid treatment regimens: Current questions and tentative answers in rheumatology. *Ann. Rheum. Dis.* **2002**, *61*, 718–722. [CrossRef] [PubMed]
13. Strehl, C.; Buttgereit, F. Unraveling the functions of the membrane-bound glucocorticoid receptors: First clues on origin and functional activity. *Ann. N. Y. Acad. Sci.* **2014**, *1318*, 1–6. [CrossRef] [PubMed]
14. Badsha, H.; Edwards, C.J. Intravenous pulses of methylprednisolone for systemic lupus erythematosus. *Semin. Arthritis Rheum.* **2003**, *32*, 370–377. [CrossRef]
15. Schmid, D.; Burmester, G.R.; Tripmacher, R.; Kuhnke, A.; Buttgereit, F. Bioenergetics of human peripheral blood mononuclear cell metabolism in quiescent, activated, and glucocorticoid-treated states. *Biosci. Rep.* **2000**, *20*, 289–302. [CrossRef] [PubMed]
16. Parker, B.J.; Bruce, I.N. High dose methylprednisolone therapy for the treatment of severe systemic lupus erythematosus. *Lupus* **2007**, *16*, 387–393. [CrossRef]

17. Ruiz-Arruza, I.; Ugarte, A.; Cabezas-Rodriguez, I.; Medina, J.A.; Moran, M.A.; Ruiz-Irastorza, G. Glucocorticoids and irreversible damage in patients with systemic lupus erythematosus. *Rheumatology* **2014**, *53*, 1470–1476. [CrossRef]
18. Buttgereit, F.; Brand, M.D.; Burmester, G.R. Equivalent doses and relative drug potencies for non-genomic glucocorticoid effects: a novel glucocorticoid hierarchy. *Biochem. Pharmacol.* **1999**, *58*, 363–368. [CrossRef]
19. Danza, A.; Borgia, I.; Narvaez, J.I.; Baccelli, A.; Amigo, C.; Rebella, M.; Dominguez, V. Intravenous pulses of methylprednisolone to treat flares of immune-mediated diseases: How much, how long? *Lupus* **2018**, *27*, 1177–1184. [CrossRef]
20. Ugarte, A.; Danza, A.; Ruiz-Irastorza, G. Glucocorticoids and antimalarials in systemic lupus erythematosus: An update and future directions. *Curr. Opin. Rheumatol.* **2018**, *30*, 482–489. [CrossRef]
21. Ruiz-Irastorza, G.; Garcia, M.; Espinosa, G.; Caminal, L.; Mitjavila, F.; González-León, R.; Sopeña, B.; Canora, J.; Villalba, M.V.; Rodríguez-Carballeira, M.; et al. First month prednisone dose predicts prednisone burden during the following 11 months: An observational study from the RELES cohort. *Lupus Sci. Med.* **2016**, *3*, e000153. [CrossRef] [PubMed]
22. Tarr, T.; Papp, G.; Nagy, N.; Cserep, E.; Zeher, M. Chronic high-dose glucocorticoid therapy triggers the development of chronic organ damage and worsens disease outcome in systemic lupus erythematosus. *Clin. Rheumatol.* **2017**, *36*, 327–333. [CrossRef] [PubMed]
23. Thamer, M.; Hernan, M.A.; Zhang, Y.; Cotter, D.; Petri, M. Prednisone, lupus activity, and permanent organ damage. *J. Rheumatol.* **2009**, *36*, 560–564. [CrossRef] [PubMed]
24. Ruiz-Irastorza, G.; Danza, A.; Khamashta, M. Treatment of systemic lupus erythematosus: Myths, certainties and doubts. *Med. Clin.* **2013**, *141*, 533–542. [CrossRef]
25. Little, J.; Parker, B.; Lunt, M.; Hanly, J.G.; Urowitz, M.B.; Clarke, A.E.; Romero-Diaz, J.; Gordon, C.; Bae, S.C.; Bernatsky, S.; et al. Glucocorticoid use and factors associated with variability in this use in the systemic lupus international collaborating clinics inception cohort. *Rheumatology* **2018**, *57*, 677–687. [CrossRef]
26. Zeher, M.; Doria, A.; Lan, J.; Aroca, G.; Jayne, D.; Boletis, I.; Hiepe, F.; Prestele, H.; Bernhardt, P.; Amoura, Z. Efficacy and safety of enteric-coated mycophenolate sodium in combination with two glucocorticoid regimens for the treatment of active lupus nephritis. *Lupus* **2011**, *20*, 1484–1493. [CrossRef]
27. Ruiz-Irastorza, G.; Ugarte, A.; Saint-Pastou Terrier, C.; Lazaro, E.; Iza, A.; Couzi, L.; Saenz, R.; Richez, C.; Porta, S.; Blanco, P. Repeated pulses of methyl-prednisolone with reduced doses of prednisone improve the outcome of class III, IV and V lupus nephritis: An observational comparative study of the Lupus-Cruces and lupus-Bordeaux cohorts. *Autoimmun. Rev.* **2017**, *16*, 826–832. [CrossRef]
28. Sin, F.E.; Isenberg, D. An evaluation of voclosporin for the treatment of lupus nephritis. *Expert Opin. Pharmacother.* **2018**, *19*, 1613–1621. [CrossRef]
29. Appel, G.B.; Contreras, G.; Dooley, M.A.; Ginzler, E.M.; Isenberg, D.; Jayne, D.; Li, L.S.; Mysler, E.; Sánchez-Guerrero, J.; Solomons, N.; et al. Mycophenolate mofetil versus cyclophosphamide for induction treatment of lupus nephritis. *J. Am. Soc. Nephrol.* **2009**, *20*, 1103–1112. [CrossRef]
30. Rovin, B.H.; Furie, R.; Latinis, K.; Looney, R.J.; Fervenza, F.C.; Sanchez-Guerrero, J.; Maciuca, R.; Zhang, D.; Garg, J.P.; Brunetta, P.; et al. Efficacy and safety of rituximab in patients with active proliferative lupus nephritis: The Lupus Nephritis Assessment with Rituximab study. *Arthritis Rheum.* **2012**, *64*, 1215–1226. [CrossRef]
31. Lightstone, L.; Doria, A.; Wilson, H.; Ward, F.L.; Larosa, M.; Bargman, J.M. Can we manage lupus nephritis without chronic corticosteroids administration? *Autoimmun. Rev.* **2018**, *17*, 4–10. [CrossRef] [PubMed]
32. Condon, M.B.; Ashby, D.; Pepper, R.J.; Cook, H.T.; Levy, J.B.; Griffith, M.; Cairns, T.D.; Lightstone, L. Prospective observational single-centre cohort study to evaluate the effectiveness of treating lupus nephritis with rituximab and mycophenolate mofetil but no oral steroids. *Ann. Rheum. Dis.* **2013**, *72*, 1280–1286. [CrossRef]
33. Ruiz-Arruza, I.; Lozano, J.; Cabezas-Rodriguez, I.; Medina, J.A.; Ugarte, A.; Erdozain, J.G.; Ruiz-Irastorza, G. Restrictive use of oral glucocorticoids in systemic lupus erythematosus and prevention of damage without worsening long-term disease control: An observational study. *Arthritis Care Res.* **2018**, *70*, 582–591. [CrossRef] [PubMed]
34. Edwards, J.C.; Snaith, M.L.; Isenberg, D.A. A double blind controlled trial of methylprednisolone infusions in systemic lupus erythematosus using individualised outcome assessment. *Ann. Rheum. Dis.* **1987**, *46*, 773–776. [CrossRef] [PubMed]

35. Badsha, H.; Kong, K.O.; Lian, T.Y.; Chan, S.P.; Edwards, C.J.; Chng, H.H. Low-dose pulse methylprednisolone for systemic lupus erythematosus flares is efficacious and has a decreased risk of infectious complications. *Lupus* **2002**, *11*, 508–513. [CrossRef]
36. Kong, K.O.; Badsha, H.; Lian, T.Y.; Edwards, C.J.; Chng, H.H. Low-dose pulse methylprednisolone is an effective therapy for severe SLE flares. *Lupus* **2004**, *13*, 212–213. [CrossRef]
37. Joo, Y.B.; Won, S.; Choi, C.B.; Bae, S.C. Lupus nephritis is associated with more corticosteroid-associated organ damage but less corticosteroid non-associated organ damage. *Lupus* **2017**, *26*, 598–605. [CrossRef]
38. Zonana-Nacach, A.; Barr, S.G.; Magder, L.S.; Petri, M. Damage in systemic lupus erythematosus and its association with corticosteroids. *Arthritis Rheum.* **2000**, *43*, 1801–1808. [CrossRef]
39. Pakchotanon, R.; Gladman, D.D.; Su, J.; Urowitz, M.B. More consistent antimalarial intake in first 5 years of disease is associated with better prognosis in patients with systemic lupus erythematosus. *J. Rheumatol.* **2018**, *45*, 90–94. [CrossRef]
40. Mathian, A.; Pha, M.; Haroche, J.; Cohen-Aubart, F.; Hié, M.; Pineton de Chambrun, M.; Boutin, T.H.D.; Miyara, M.; Gorochov, G.; Yssel, H.; et al. Withdrawal of low-dose prednisone in SLE patients with a clinically quiescent disease for more than 1 year: a randomised clinical trial. *Ann. Rheum. Dis.* **2020**, *79*, 339–346. [CrossRef]
41. Danza, A.; Ruiz-Irastorza, G. Infection risk in systemic lupus erythematosus patients: Susceptibility factors and preventive strategies. *Lupus* **2013**, *22*, 1286–1294. [CrossRef]
42. Duffy, K.N.; Duffy, C.M.; Gladman, D.D. Infection and disease activity in systemic lupus erythematosus: a review of hospitalized patients. *J. Rheumatol.* **1991**, *18*, 1180–1184.
43. Youssef, J.; Novosad, S.A.; Winthrop, K.L. Infection risk and safety of corticosteroid use. *Rheum. Dis. Clin. N. Am.*. [CrossRef]
44. Gonzalez-Echavarri, C.; Capdevila, O.; Espinosa, G.; Suarez, S.; Marin-Ballve, A.; Gonzalez-Leon, R.; Rodriguez-Carballeira, M.; Fonseca-Aizpuru, E.; Pinilla, B.; Pallares, L.; et al. Infections in newly diagnosed Spanish patients with systemic lupus erythematosus: Data from the RELES cohort. *Lupus* **2018**, *27*, 2253–2261. [CrossRef]
45. Rua-Figueroa, I.; Lopez-Longo, J.; Galindo-Izquierdo, M.; Calvo-Alen, J.; Del Campo, V.; Olive-Marques, A.; Perez-Vicente, S.; Fernandez-Nebro, A.; Andres, M.; Erausquin, C.; et al. Incidence, associated factors and clinical impact of severe infections in a large, multicentric cohort of patients with systemic lupus erythematosus. *Semin. Arthritis Rheum.* **2017**, *47*, 38–45. [CrossRef]
46. Götestam Skorpen, C.; Hoeltzenbein, M.; Tincani, A.; Fischer-Betz, R.; Elefant, E.; Chambers, C.; da Silva, J.; Nelson-Piercy, C.; Cetin, I.; Costedoat-Chalumeau. N.; et al. The EULAR points to consider for use of antirheumatic drugs before pregnancy, and during pregnancy and lactation. *Ann. Rheum. Dis.* **2016**, *75*, 795–810. [CrossRef]
47. Flint, J.; Panchal, S.; Hurrell, A.; van de Venne, M.; Gayed, M.; Schreiber, K.; Arthanari, S.; Cunningham, J.; Flanders, L.; Moore, L.; et al. BSR and BHPR guideline on prescribing drugs in pregnancy and breastfeeding-Part I: Standard and biologic disease modifying anti-rheumatic drugs and corticosteroids. *Rheumatology* **1693**. [CrossRef]
48. Diederich, S.; Eigendorff, E.; Burkhardt, P.; Quinkler, M.; Bumke-Vogt, C.; Rochel, M.; Seidelmann, D.; Esperling, P.; Oelkers, W.; Bahr, V. 11beta-hydroxysteroid dehydrogenase types 1 and 2: An important pharmacokinetic determinant for the activity of synthetic mineralo- and glucocorticoids. *J. Clin. Endocrinol. Metab.* **2002**, *87*, 5695–5701. [CrossRef] [PubMed]
49. Rodríguez Almaraz, E.; Sáez-Comet, L.; Casellas, M.; Delgado, P.; Ugarte, A.; Vela-Casasempere, P.; Martínez Sánchez, N.; Galindo-Izquierdo, M.; Espinosa, G.; Marco, B.; et al. Pregnancy control in patients with systemic lupus erythematosus/antiphospholipid syndrome: Part 2: Pregnancy follow-up. *Reumatol. Clin.* **2019**. [CrossRef]
50. Ruiz-Irastorza, G.; Khamashta, M.A.; Nelson-Piercy, C.; Hughes, G.R. Lupus pregnancy: Is heparin a risk factor for osteoporosis? *Lupus* **2001**, *10*, 597–600. [CrossRef] [PubMed]
51. Gordon, C.; Amissah-Arthur, M.B.; Gayed, M.; Brown, S.; Bruce, I.N.; D'Cruz, D.; Empson, B.; Griffiths, B.; Jayne, D.; Khamashta, M.; et al. The British Society for Rheumatology guideline for the management of systemic lupus erythematosus in adults. *Rheumatology* **2018**, *57*, e1–e45. [CrossRef] [PubMed]

52. Pons-Estel, B.A.; Bonfa, E.; Soriano, E.R.; Cardiel, M.H.; Izcovich, A.; Popoff, F.; Criniti, J.M.; Vasquez, G.; Massardo, L.; Duarte, M.; et al. First Latin American clinical practice guidelines for the treatment of systemic lupus erythematosus: Latin American Group for the Study of Lupus (GLADEL, Grupo Latino Americano de Estudio del Lupus)-Pan-American League of Associations of Rheumatology (PANLAR). *Ann. Rheum. Dis.* **2018**, *77*, 1549–1557. [CrossRef] [PubMed]
53. Ruiz-Irastorza, G.; Espinosa, G.; Frutos, M.A.; Jimenez Alonso, J.; Praga, M.; Pallares, L.; Rivera, F.; Robles Marhuenda, A.; Segarra, A.; Quereda, C. Diagnosis and treatment of lupus nephritis. *Rev. Clin. Esp.* **2012**, *212*, 147.e1–147.e30. [CrossRef]
54. Hahn, B.H.; McMahon, M.A.; Wilkinson, A.; Wallace, W.D.; Daikh, D.I.; Fitzgerald, J.D.; Karpouzas, G.A.; Merrill, J.T.; Wallace, D.J.; Yazdany, J.; et al. American College of Rheumatology guidelines for screening, treatment, and management of lupus nephritis. *Arthritis Care Res.* **2012**, *64*, 797–808. [CrossRef] [PubMed]
55. Bertsias, G.K.; Tektonidou, M.; Amoura, Z.; Aringer, M.; Bajema, I.; Berden, J.H.; Boletis, J.; Cervera, R.; Dörner, T.; Doria, A.; et al. Joint European League Against Rheumatism and European Renal Association-European Dialysis and Transplant Association (EULAR/ERA-EDTA) recommendations for the management of adult and paediatric lupus nephritis. *Ann. Rheum. Dis.* **2012**, *71*, 1771–1782. [CrossRef]
56. Fanouriakis, A.; Kostopoulou, M.; Cheema, K.; Anders, H.J.; Aringer, M.; Bajema, I.; Boletis, J.; Frangou, E.; Houssiau, F.A.; Hollis, J.; et al. 2019 Update of the Joint European League Against Rheumatism and European Renal Association-European Dialysis and Transplant Association (EULAR/ERA-EDTA) recommendations for the management of lupus nephritis. *Ann. Rheum. Dis.* **2020**. [CrossRef]
57. Ruiz-Irastorza, G.; Ugarte, A.; Ruiz-Arruza, I.; Khamashta, M. Seventy years after Hench's Nobel prize: Revisiting the use of glucocorticoids in systemic lupus erythematosus. *Lupus* **2020**. [CrossRef]
58. Ruiz-Irastorza, G.; Ugarte, A.; Ruiz-Arruza, I.; Erdozain, J.G.; Gonzalez-Echavarri, C.; Martin-Cascon, M.; Soto, A.; Ferreiro, M.; Espinosa, G. Autoinmunes. Mobile Application Version 1.05. Osakidetza. 2019. Available online: https://play.google.com/store/apps/details?id=com.ionicframework.apautoinmun; https://apps.apple.com/es/app/autoinmunes/id1344571564 (accessed on 1 July 2020).

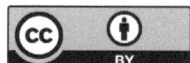

© 2020 by the authors. Licensee MDPI, Basel, Switzerland. This article is an open access article distributed under the terms and conditions of the Creative Commons Attribution (CC BY) license (http://creativecommons.org/licenses/by/4.0/).

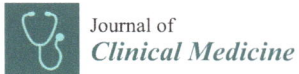 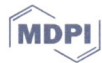

Article

Insights into the Procoagulant Profile of Patients with Systemic Lupus Erythematosus without Antiphospholipid Antibodies

Elena Monzón Manzano [1,†], Ihosvany Fernández-Bello [1,†,‡], Raúl Justo Sanz [1,‡], Ángel Robles Marhuenda [2], Francisco Javier López-Longo [3], Paula Acuña [1], María Teresa Álvarez Román [1], Víctor Jiménez Yuste [1,4] and Nora V. Butta [1,*]

1. Hematology Unit, University Hospital La Paz-Idipaz, Paseo de la Castellana 231, 28046 Madrid, Spain; elenamonzonmanzano@hotmail.com (E.M.M.); ihosvanyf@yahoo.es (I.F.-B.); rauljustosanz@gmail.com (R.J.S.); paulaacbu@gmail.com (P.A.); talvarezroman@gmail.com (M.T.Á.R.); vjyuste@gmail.com (V.J.Y.)
2. Internal Medicine Unit, Hospital Universitario La Paz-IdiPAZ, 28046 Madrid, Spain; aroblesmarhuenda@gmail.com
3. Rheumatology Unit, University Hospital Gregorio Marañón, 28007 Madrid, Spain; hemostasia.hulp@gmail.com
4. Faculty of Medicine, Universidad Autónoma de Madrid, 28029 Madrid, Spain
* Correspondence: nora.butta@salud.madrid.org; Tel.: +34-91-727-0000 (ext. 42258)
† E.M.M. and I.F.-B. contributed equally to the manuscript.
‡ At present, I.F.-B. is employee at NovoNordiskEspaña and R.J.S. is employee at Takeda FarmacéuticaEspaña SA.

Received: 15 September 2020; Accepted: 11 October 2020; Published: 14 October 2020

Abstract: We aimed to identify the key players in the prothrombotic profile of patients with systemic lupus erythematosus (SLE) not mediated by antiphospholipid antibodies, as well as the potential utility of global coagulation tests to characterize hemostasis in these patients. Patients with SLE without antiphospholipid antibodies and without signs of thrombosis were included. The kinetics of clot formation were determined by ROTEM®. Platelet activation markers were determined by flow cytometry. Thrombin generation associated with Neutrophil Extracellular Traps (NETs) and microparticles (MPs) was measured by calibrated automated thrombogram (CAT). The plasma levels of PAI-1 were also determined. ROTEM® showed a procoagulant profile in SLE patients. SLE patients had activated platelets and more leukocyte/platelet aggregates at basal conditions. The plasma PAI-1 and platelet aggregates correlated with several ROTEM® parameters. The thrombin generation associated with the tissue factor (TF) content of MPs and with NETs was increased. Our results suggest the utility of global tests for studying hemostasis in SLE patients because they detect their procoagulant profile, despite having had neither antiphospholipid antibodies nor any previous thrombotic event. A global appraisal of hemostasis should, if possible, be incorporated into clinical practice to detect the risk of a thrombotic event in patients with SLE and to consequently act to prevent its occurrence.

Keywords: systemic lupus erythematosus; thromboelastometry; thrombin generation; neutrophil extracellular traps

1. Introduction

Systemic lupus erythematosus (SLE) is a potentially fatal multiorgan inflammatory immune-mediated disease that primarily affects females. The disease is characterized by the production of antibodies against various tissues, which triggers a wide variety of cutaneous and systemic manifestations that in many cases become serious, compromising the patient's life. Thrombosis contributes to substantial morbidity and mortality in patients with SLE due to a complex interplay between traditional risk factors and the dysregulation of autoimmunity. Up to 15% of patients with SLE have had myocardial infarction [1], and approximately 20–30% of deaths in patients with SLE are due to cardiovascular disease (CVD) [2,3]. Conflicting data on the mechanisms involved in the increase in risk and in the prediction of CVD complicate prevention of its occurrence.

The duration of the disease correlates with the degree of cardiovascular involvement [4], suggesting that chronic exposure to immune system dysregulation contributes to the development of CDV in these patients. The proposed predictors of cardiovascular events in this population are dyslipidemia, hypertension, a family medical history of coronary artery disease (CAD), and smoking. In addition, although the presence of antiphospholipid and anticardiolipin antibodies and lupus anticoagulant is correlated with the occurrence of cardiovascular events, 40% of SLE thrombosis cases are autoantibody-negative [5,6], suggesting the involvement of other factors. Thus, we aim to identify the key players in the prothrombotic profile of patients with SLE not mediated by antiphospholipid antibodies.

Recently, there has been growing interest in the use of global coagulation tests to evaluate hypercoagulable states [7,8]. Among them, rotational thromboelastometry (ROTEM®), a viscoelastometric clotting test that measures the kinetics of clot formation and fibrinolysis, and calibrated automated thrombogram (CAT), a thrombin generation test that quantifies thrombin generation, are the most widely used. Given that hemostasis is the consequence of the relationship between various cells, coagulation factors, and plasma components, we considered that these tests would be a good approach to evaluate the hypercoagulable condition in SLE. Therefore, we investigated the potential utility of ROTEM® and CAT in the characterization of the procoagulant state in SLE not mediated by antiphospholipid antibodies, giving a new insight into the relationship between different factors involved in this pathology.

2. Materials and Methods

2.1. Participants and Study Design

This study was approved by the ethics committees of two hospitals: Gregorio Marañón University Hospital (Code 324/14) and La Paz University Hospital (Code PI-3293). All the included patients had been diagnosed with SLE according to the American College of Rheumatology (ACR) criteria for SLE [9]. The global disease activity was measured with the Systemic Lupus Erythematosus Activity Index 2000 (SLEDAI-2K).

Exclusion criteria were infection with hepatitis C virus or human immunodeficiency virus; alcohol abuse or addiction; oral contraceptive intake or hormonal therapy (excepting steroids as an immunosuppressive treatment for SLE); patients with antiphospholipid antibodies (lupus anticoagulant, anti-β2-GPI, and anticardiolipin antibodies); a history of acute myocardial infarction, angina, or CAD; diabetes, hyperlipemia, or uncontrolled arterial hypertension; overweight defined by a body mass index ≥ 30 kg/m^2; smoking in the 12 months before our study; pregnancy in the previous 3 months prior to the study; or cancer.

Patients older than 18 years who fulfilled 4 or more ACR criteria, with a titer of antinuclear antibodies ≥1:80 and/or anti-double-stranded DNA antibody (anti-dsDNA antibody) levels ≥ 30 UI/mL, with a stable standard SLE therapy for the last 30 days, and who signed written informed consent were included in this study.

2.2. Collection and Preparation of Samples

Human peripheral blood samples were collected in tubes containing 3.2% trisodium citrate (BD Vacutainer, Madrid, Spain). Platelet-rich plasma (PRP) was prepared within 60 min of blood collection by centrifugation (150 g for 20 min at 23 °C). To obtain platelet-poor plasma (PPP), the PRP was centrifuged twice at 23 °C, first at 1500 g for 15 min and then at 13,000 g for 2 min.

Acid-citrate-dextrose (1:10) was added to the top two-third volumes of PRP and centrifuged at 650 g for 10 min at 23 °C to obtain washed platelets. The pellet was then resuspended in an equal volume of 4-(2-hydroxyethyl)-1-piperazineethanesulfonic acid (HEPES) buffer (10 mM of HEPES, 145 mM of NaCl, 5 mM of KCl, and 1 mM of $MgSO_4$, pH 7.4).

For serum preparation, peripheral blood was collected in serum tubes (BD Vacutainer, Plymouth, UK) and separated by centrifuging clotted blood (2500 g for 15 min at 23 °C).

Plasma and serum aliquots were stored at −80 °C until analysis.

2.3. Cell Count and Biochemical Parameters

The blood cell count was performed using a Coulter AcT Diff cell counter (Beckman Coulter, Madrid, Spain). The plasminogen activator inhibitor type 1 (PAI-1) (Invitrogen, Vienna, Austria) levels were determined in serum or plasma according to the manufacturer's instructions and measured in a Multiskan FC microplate photometer (ThermoScientific, Madrid, Spain).

The cell-free DNA (cfDNA) was determined in PPP by the Quant-iT™ PicoGreen dsDNA assay (Thermo Fisher Scientific, Waltham, MA, USA) according to the manufacturer's instructions.

C-reactive protein (CRP), serum complement C3 and C4, erythrocyte sedimentation rate (ESR), creatinine, 24-hproteinuria, and anti-DNA titer were only determined in the SLE groups.

2.4. Rotational Thromboelastometry

The kinetics of clot formation and fibrinolysis were assessed by rotational thromboelastometry (ROTEM®, Pentapharm, Munich, Germany) with the recalcification of whole blood (NATEM® test).

The following parameters were recorded: clotting time (CT) (time from the start of clot formation until an amplitude of 2 mm, in seconds); alpha angle (α) (the slope of the tangent line to the clotting curve through the 20 mm amplitude that reflects the rate of fibrin polymerization, in degrees); the clot firmness X min after CT; the maximal clot firmness (MCF, in mm); and clot lysis as the percentage of clot lysed after 60 min.

2.5. Analysis of Platelet Activation and Platelet Receptors

PRP was diluted 1:5 with HEPES buffer and incubated with either buffer, 100 µmol/L of thrombin receptor-activating peptide (TRAP)-6 (Bachem, Switzerland), or 10 µmol/L of adenosine diphosphate (ADP, Sigma, Madrid, Spain) at room temperature (RT). Later, fluorescein-isothiocyanate (FITC)-PAC1 (BD, Madrid, Spain), a monoclonal antibody (mAb) that recognizes only the activated conformation of fibrinogen receptor, FITC-anti P-selectin mAb (BD Pharmingen, San Diego, CA, USA), or FITC anti-CD63 mAb (BD, Madrid, Spain) were added and incubated for 15 min at RT. To determine the platelet receptors, diluted PRP was incubated with phycoerythrin (PE) anti-CD41 mAb (Biocytex, Marseille, France) or FITC anti-CD61mAb (BD, Madrid, Spain)—which recognized, respectively, the αIIb and β3 subunits of fibrinogen receptor—or it was incubated with FITC anti-CD42a mAb (BD, Madrid, Spain) or anti-CD42b mAb (BD Pharmingen, San Diego, CA, USA), against, respectively, the GPIX and GPIbα subunits of von Willebrand factor (vWF) receptor. These samples were analyzed using a FACScan flow cytometer (BD Biosciences, Madrid, Spain) after being diluted in 1:6 HEPES buffer.

2.6. Determination of Platelet-Leukocyte Aggregates

To determine the platelet-leukocyte aggregates, whole blood was diluted 1:10 in HEPES buffer and coincubated with FITC anti-CD45 mAb (BD Pharmingen, San Diego, CA, USA), PE anti-CD41 mAb, and 50 µM of TRAP or 40 µM of ADP for 15 min at RT in the dark. Platelet-leukocyte aggregates were defined as leukocytes positive for CD41.

2.7. Determination of Phosphatidylserine Exposure on Platelet Surface and Caspase Activity

The surface exposure of phosphatidylserine (PS) in washed platelets was assessed by measuring the binding of (FITC)-labeled Annexin V (BD Pharmingen, San Diego, CA, USA). Washed platelets were resuspended in annexinV binding buffer (10 mM of HEPES, 10 mM of NaOH, 140 mM of NaCl, 2.5 mM of $CaCl_2$, pH 7.4) and labeled with FITC-annexinV. After incubation for 15 min at RT in the dark, the samples were analyzed by flow cytometry.

To analyze the caspase-3, -7, -8, and -9 activity, PRP was diluted 10-fold with isotonic HEPES buffer containing 2 mM of $CaCl_2$ and 2 mM of Gly-Pro-Arg-Pro acetate (Sigma Aldrich, Madrid, Spain) to prevent fibrin formation, and either FAM-DEVD-FMK, FAM-LETD-FMK, or FAM-LEHD-FMK (Millipore, Madrid, Spain). The samples were analyzed by flow cytometry.

2.8. Calibrated Automated Thrombogram

The procoagulant activity of MPs associated with their content of either tissue factor (TF) or PS was determined, respectively, with MP reagent (4 µM of phospholipids) or PRP reagent (1 pM of recombinant human TF) by calibrated automated thrombogram (CAT). All CAT reagents were from Diagnostica Stago (Madrid, Spain). The thrombin generation was determined with a Fluoroskan FL instrument (ThermoLabsystems, Helsinki, Finland) under the control of Thrombinoscope software, version 3.6 (Thrombinoscope BV, Maastricht, Holand), filtered for excitation at 390 nm and emission at 460 nm.

The following parameters were determined: lagtime (LT) (time from the start of the assay until 10 nM of thrombin is formed, in min), time to peak (ttPeak) (time required to reach the maximum thrombin concentration, in min), peak height (Peak) (maximum thrombin concentration reached, in nM), and endogenous thrombin potential (ETP) (the total amount of thrombin generated over time, in nMxmin).

2.9. Neutrophil Isolation and Generation of Neutrophil Extracellular Traps

Neutrophils were isolated from 10 mL of whole blood from controls and from patients with SLE using a Percoll gradient centrifuged at 500 g for 25 min at 5 °C. The isolated neutrophils (2.5×10^6 cells/mL) were incubated with and without 100 nM of phorbol 12-myristate 13-acetate (PMA) (Sigma-Aldrich, Madrid, Spain) for 45 min at 37 °C in Roswell Park Memorial Institute (RPMI)-1640 medium (Invitrogen, Madrid, Spain). Later, the samples were centrifuged at 5000 g for 3 min and resuspended in PRP from healthy controls. The Neutrophil Extracellular Traps (NETs) formation was verified by fluorescence microscopy.

2.10. Assessment of Neutrophil Extracellular Trap Generation by Fluorescence Microscopy

Neutrophils were seeded on 12 mm cover glasses pretreated with poly-L-lysine (Sigma-Aldrich, Sweden) in 24-well plates in 500 µL of RPMI-1640 medium with and without 100 nM of PMA, for 45 min at 37 °C. The samples were fixed with a final concentration of 2% paraformaldehyde for 15 min at RT. Then, the preparations were blocked, adding 2% bovine serum albumin–phosphate-buffered saline for 45 min at RT and incubated first with a 1:300 dilution of rabbit anti-human myeloperoxidase (Dako, Madrid, Spain) and then with Alexa Fluor 488 goat anti-rabbit IgG (Invitrogen, Madrid, Spain) for 45 min at RT in dark. Finally, the samples were embedded in mounting medium with 4′,6-diamidino-2-phenylindole (Vector Laboratories, Burlingame, CA, USA) and kept at 4 °C in the dark until visualization with fluorescence microscopy using the Nikon Eclipse 90i microscope.

2.11. Thrombin Generation Associated with Neutrophil Extracellular Traps

Blood from healthy controls was drawn in 2 tubes with citrate as an anticoagulant (Vacutainer, Madrid, Spain) and in 2 tubes with citrate plus 50 µg/µL of corn trypsin inhibitor (CTI) (Cell Systems Biotechnologie, Troisdorf, Germany) to inhibit activated factor XII (FXII). One of each kind of tube was centrifuged to obtain PRP, and the others were centrifuged for PPP. PRP either with or without CTI was adjusted to 1×10^5 platelets/µL with the corresponding PPP. Neutrophils were isolated from healthy controls and from patients with SLE from citrated blood, as described above. Neutrophils were added to wells at a final concentration of 2.5×10^5 cells to 40 µL aliquots of PRP from healthy controls, with and without CTI, to perform CAT experiments after incubation for 30 min at 37 °C with either buffer or 100 nM of PMA without the addition of any trigger.

2.12. Statistical Analysis

The Shapiro–Wilk test was used to assess the distribution of the data, and the results were expressed as mean ± SD or median (p25–p75) depending on the distribution. The differences between the 2 groups were assessed using the 2-tailed unpaired Student's t-test or the non-parametric Mann–Whitney U-test, as appropriate. The correlation analysis was performed using Pearson's or Spearman's test. The GraphPad Prism 5 software (GraphPad Software version 5.03, GraphPad Software, San Diego, CA, USA) was used for all the statistical analyses, and significance was set at $p \leq 0.05$.

3. Results

3.1. Experimental Results

3.1.1. Features of the Patients with SLE

The study was performed on 32 patients with SLE treated at the Rheumatology Unit of the Gregorio Marañón University Hospital and at the Internal Medicine Unit of La Paz University Hospital, with a median age of 41.9 ± 12.9 years, who were recruited after signing informed consent. Eighty-eight sex- and age-matched healthy controls, with a mean age of 38.3 ± 11.6 years, were recruited as controls at the Blood Donation Center of La Paz University Hospital. The study was performed between January 2017 and October 2019. None of the patients had a history or signs or symptoms of thrombosis at inclusion.

A summary of the clinical and demographic data of the patients with SLE is shown in Table 1.

Table 1. Features of the patients with Systemic lupus erythematosus (SLE).

Patient	Disease Duration (Years)	Age (Years)	Medication at the Time of the Study	Concomitant Diseases	SLEDAI-2K
1	23	44	No treatment		12
2	21	50	Omeprazole, mycophenolate mofetil, prednisone, calcifediol	Autoimmune thrombocytopenia	6
3	9	35	Tramadol, levothyroxine, prednisone, rituximab	Sjogren's syndrome, Graves-Basedow disease, autoimmune hepatitis, fibromyalgia	3
4	18	35	Ramipril, phenelzine, abatacept, immunoglobulins		4
5	26	32	No treatment	Raynaud's phenomenon, endometriosis,	1
6	19	31	No treatment	Photosensitivity, inflammatory arthralgias, lymphopenia	5
7	13	49	Ferrous sulfate, omeprazole, prednisone, belimumab, azathioprine	Sjogren's syndrome	4

Table 1. *Cont.*

Patient	Disease Duration (Years)	Age (Years)	Medication at the Time of the Study	Concomitant Diseases	SLEDAI-2K
8	19	35	Quetiapine, duloxetine, omeprazole, diazepam, hydroxychloroquine, azathioprine, pregabalin, prednisone, tramadol, ferrous sulfate, calcifediol, rituximab		2
9	27	57	Prednisone, azathioprine, belimumab, rituximab		14
10	12	46	Calcifediol		2
11	4	45	Clobetasol propionate, trazodone, calcipotriol, diazepam, hydroxychloroquine, calcifediol, pregabalin, metamizole, omeprazole, almotriptan, enalapril, prednisone, sertraline, mycophenolate mofetil, abatacept, belimumab	Raynaud's syndrome, lupus nephropathy, mixed dyslipidemia	2
12	10	29	Azathioprine, hydroxychloroquine, prednisone, omeprazole, calcifediol, ferrous sulfate, belimumab	Sjogren's syndrome, leukopenia/lymphopenia	7
13	2	45	Hydroxychloroquine, prednisone, calcifediol, levothyroxine, azathioprine		0
14	15	33	Hydroxychloroquine, azathioprine, chondroitin sulfate		4
15	3	21	Hydroxychloroquine		4
16	23	61	Symbicort, enalapril, tramadol, pregabalin, azathioprine		0
17	10	31	No treatment		4
18	11	35	Methotrexate, omeprazole, folic acid, prednisone, mycophenolate mofetil		2
19	22	41	Nifedipine, hydroxychloroquine	Mixed connective tissue disease, Raynaud's syndrome	2
20	24	56	Abatacept, furosemide, fluoxetine, lorazepam, amisulpride, omeprazole, prednisone, spironolactone	Rheumatoid arthritis, Sjogren's syndrome, autoimmune hepatitis	4
21	6	67	Hydroxychloroquine, calcifediol		0

Table 1. *Cont.*

Patient	Disease Duration (Years)	Age (Years)	Medication at the Time of the Study	Concomitant Diseases	SLEDAI-2K
22	8	62	Hydroxychloroquine, omeprazole, levothyroxine, diazepam, paroxetine		2
23	23	58	Hydroxychloroquine, prednisone, atenolol, calcifediol		4
24	7	25	Hydroxychloroquine, calcifediol, Robaxisal		10
25	4	65	Hydroxychloroquine, prednisone, atorvastatin	Arterial hypertension	8
26	9	40	Mycophenolate mofetil, prednisone, hydroxychloroquine, enalapril, denosumab, ranitidine, paroxetine, calcifediol		0
27	8	22	Mycophenolate mofetil, ursodeoxycholic acid, hydroxychloroquine, calcifediol, ranitidine	Alpha-thalassemia minor, Raynaud's syndrome, secondary hyperhidrosis	4
28	22	48	Hydroxychloroquine, prednisone, calcifediol, omeprazole, cholecalciferol		2
29	12	40	Calcifediol		2
30	18	33	Prednisone, hydroxychloroquine, calcifediol	Atrial septal aneurysm, Kikuchi-Fujimoto disease, osteonecrosis	2
31	37	52	Omeprazole, hydroxychloroquine, amitriptyline, calcifediol	Depression	4
32	15	38	Hydroxychloroquine		0

Lymphocytes, erythrocytes, granulocytes, leukocytes, and platelet counts were reduced in the patients with SLE (Table 2). The CRP, C3 and C4 levels, ESR, creatinine, proteinuria (24-h), anti-DNA, IgA, IgM, and IgG levels were determined in most of the patients (Table 2).

3.1.2. Global Hemostasis in Patients with Systemic Lupus Erythematosus

To evaluate the global hemostasis and kinetics of clot formation, a ROTEM® test was performed using whole blood. Patients with SLE showed a procoagulant profile compared with the control samples (Figure 1). In the SLE patient group, we observed a shortening of the CT and a higher alpha angle, amplitude at 15 min, and MCF. No differences were found in the clot lysis at 60 min.

In order to determine whether MPs might participate in the procoagulant profile of patients with SLE, CAT was performed with different triggers that, according to the manufacturer, discriminate between thrombin generation dependent on the PS or TF content of MPs. As shown in Table 3, the ETP and peak of thrombin associated with the TF content of MPs was increased in patients with SLE. Moreover, the peak correlated to disease duration (Spearman r = 0.4634, $p = 0.0084$).

Table 2. Biochemical parameters in the healthy controls and patients with SLE.

	Controls	SLE	p-Value	Normal Range
Lymphocytes/μL	1.9 (1.6–2.4)	1.6 (1–1.8)	0.0093 *	1.2–3.4
Erythrocytes ×10^6/μL	4.3 (4.1–4.6)	4.1 (3.8–4.4)	0.0421 *	4–6
Monocytes ×10^3/μL	0.4 (0.3–0.5)	0.4 (0.2–0.4)	0.1046	0.1–0.6
Granulocytes ×10^3/μL	4 (2.9–5.3)	2.9 (2.3–3.6)	0.0065 *	1.4–6.5
Leukocytes ×10^3/μL	6.4 (5.3–7.6)	4.8 (4.2–5.7)	0.0012 *	4.5–10.5
Hemoglobin (g/dL)	13.2 (12.3–14.2)	12.9 (11.6–13.5)	0.1226	11–18
Platelets ×10^3/μL	247 (208–284)	194 (171.5–231)	<0.0001 *	150–450
Hematocrit (%)	40.1 (38.4–43.7)	35.9 (34.4–39.8)	0.0004 *	35–60
MCV (fL)	94.6 (91.5–96.9)	92.4 (88.1–97)	0.2407	80–99.9
MCH (pg)	30.3 ± 1.6	28.6 ± 3.3	0.3037	27–31
MCHC (g/dL)	31.1 (31.3–32.9)	31.6 (30.7–32.3)	0.0976	33–37
RDW (%)	13.5 (12.8 –14.3)	14.1 (13.2–15.5)	0.1561	11.6–13.7
MPV (fL)	6.9 ± 0.8	7 ± 0.8	0.8931	7.8–11
Pct (%)	0.17 (0.15–0.19)	0.14 (0.12–0.19)	0.1210	0.190–0.36
PDW (%)	17.1 ± 0.8	17.3 ± 0.9	0.4936	0.190–0.36
CRP (mg/dL)	n.d	0.2650 (0.12–0.6)	-	0–0.5
C3 (mg/dL)	n.d	88.4 (71.5–106)	-	75–135
C4 (mg/dL)	n.d	16.3 (11.8–20.7)	-	14–60
Anti-DNA (mg/dL)	n.d.	14 (2.9–23)	-	<15.00
ESR (mm)	n.d	10.77 ± 0.6	-	2–20
Creatinine (mg/dL)	n.d	0.72 ± 0.12	-	0.5–0.9
IgG (mg/dL)	n.d.	1130 (910.5–1252)	-	725–1900
IgA (mg/dL)	n.d.	224.6 ± 92.32	-	50–350
IgM (mg/dL)	n.d.	84 (61.6–107.5)	-	45–280

Mann–Whitney or Student's t-tests were performed, and data are expressed as median (percentile 25%–percentile 75%) or mean ± SD depending on the sample distribution. A p-value ≤ 0.05 was set as significant, and * denotes significance. MCV, mean corpuscular volume; MCH, mean corpuscular hemoglobin; MCHC, mean corpuscular hemoglobin concentration; RDW, red blood cell distribution width; MPV, mean platelet volume; Pct, plateletcrit; PDW, platelet distribution width; CRP, C-reactive protein; ESR, erythrocyte sedimentation rate; n.d., not determined.

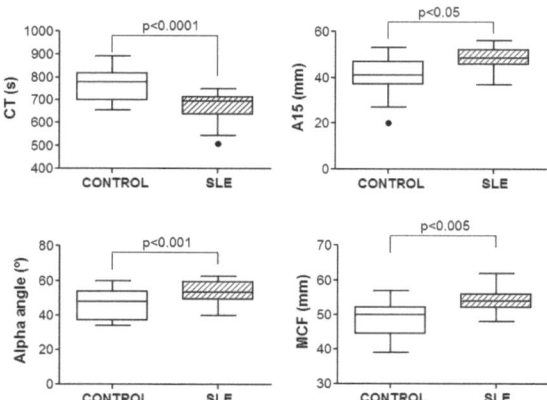

Figure 1. Procoagulant profile in patients with SLE. ROTEM® thromboelastography was performed in whole blood. Detailed procedures and measured parameters are shown in "Materials and Methods". Student's t-test or Mann–Whitney test was performed, and $p ≤ 0.05$ was set as significant. SLE, systemic lupus erythematosus; CT, clotting time; A15, amplitude at 15 min; MCF, maximum clot firmness.

Table 3. Microparticle-associated procoagulant capacity in patients with SLE.

	Controls	Patients with SLE	p
LT PRP-Reagent (min)	7.5 ± 3.8	7.8 ± 2.3	0.1280
Peak PRP-Reagent (nM)	90.5 ± 40.8	86.2 ± 52.5	0.1347
ttPeak PRP-Reagent (min)	12.1 ± 4.0	13.5 ± 3.2	0.1489
ETP PRP-Reagent (nM/min)	1021.0 ± 457.3	1107.0 ± 323.0	0.6076
LT MP-Reagent (min)	13.3 ± 3.2	13.2 ± 2.9	0.1186
Peak MP-Reagent (nM)	151.4 ± 36.5	253.8 ± 66.5	0.0021 *
ttPeak MP-Reagent (min)	16.1 ± 3.6	16.0 ± 3.3	0.1370
ETP MP-Reagent (nM/min)	1065.0 ± 241.8	1188.0 ± 313.6	0.0482 *

Data are expressed as mean ± SD. A p-value ≤ 0.05 was set as significant, and * denotes significance. Abbreviations: LT, lag time; ttPeak, time to peak; ETP, endogenous thrombin potential.

3.1.3. Platelet Activation in Patients with Systemic Lupus Erythematosus

Platelets have an essential role in clot formation; thus, we tested whether they were involved in the prothrombotic profile observed in the thromboelastogram of patients with SLE.

The platelets from patients with SLE presented basal activation, considering their increased PAC1 binding and major exposure of P-selectin and CD63 in quiescent conditions (Figure 2A). The basal activation of the platelets from patients with SLE was not the consequence of an increased expression of fibrinogen and vWF receptors on their surface (Figure S1). Moreover, we observed an increase in the platelet/leukocyte aggregate formation under basal conditions in the patients with SLE (Figure 2B). The percentage of platelet/leukocyte aggregate correlated with the ROTEM® parameters MCF (Spearman r = 0.579, p = 0.030) and alpha angle (Spearman r = 0.532, p = 0.031) and with the basal P-selectin exposure on the platelet surface (Spearman r = 0.429, p = 0.035), but did not correlate with the platelet and leukocyte counts. The platelet activation in patients with SLE did not depend on the platelet count. Moreover, the ROTEM parameters did not correlate with platelet activation markers.

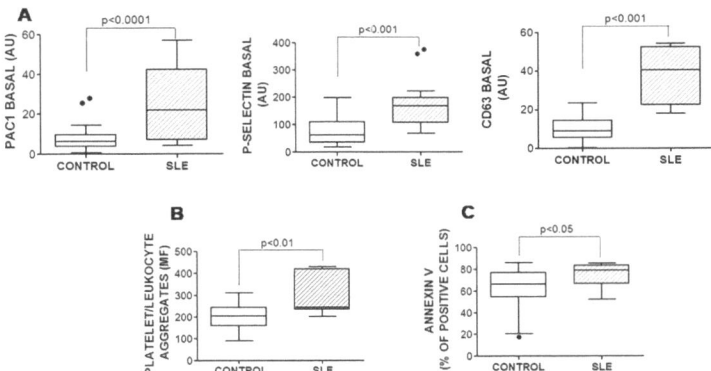

Figure 2. Basal activity of fibrinogen receptor, surface exposition of P-selectin, platelet/leukocyte aggregate formation and PS exposure. (**A**) PRP from healthy controls and patients with SLE was incubated with either FITC-PAC1, FITC anti-P-selectin mAb, or FITC anti-CD63 mAb. (**B**) To test the platelet/leukocyte aggregates, whole blood was incubated with PE anti-CD41 mAb and FITC-anti-CD45 mAb. (**C**) Annexin V binding was tested in washed platelets resuspended in the adequate buffer (see Methods). Samples were analyzed by flow cytometry. The Mann–Whitney test was performed, and p ≤ 0.05 was considered significant. Data are expressed as arbitrary units (mean fluorescence ×% of positive cells (**A**), mean fluorescence of leukocytes positive for CD41 (**B**), or percentage of positive cells (**C**)).

The response to activation with either 100 μM of TRAP or 20 μM of ADP was similar in the platelets from healthy controls and from patients with SLE (Figure S2).

3.1.4. Phosphatidylserine Exposure and Apoptosis in SLE Platelets

Platelets from patients with SLE bound more annexin on their surface than the controls, indicating an enhanced PS exposure (Figure 2C). This fact did not appear to be related to enhanced apoptosis, because the caspase activities were similar among groups (Figure S3).

3.1.5. Association between Coagulation Profile and Inflammatory State

An association between coagulation and inflammatory states has been reported [10]. Therefore, we tested the plasma levels of PAI-1, which is considered a marker of vascular inflammation [11]. The PAI-1 levels were increased in patients with SLE (Figure 3A).

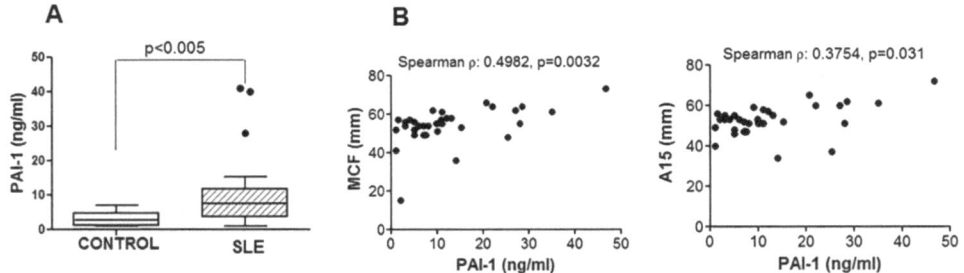

Figure 3. Plasminogen activator inhibitor-1 (PAI-1) levels in plasma and its correlation with ROTEM® parameters. Plasma levels of PAI-1 (**A**) measured with enzyme-linked immunosorbent assay correlated with A15 and MCF parameters (**B**). A Mann–Whitney test and Spearman's correlation were performed, and $p < 0.05$ was considered significant.

Furthermore, the PAI-1 levels correlated with the ROTEM® parameters A15 and MCF (Figure 3B), suggesting an association between the PAI-1 plasma levels and the procoagulant state observed in patients with SLE. On the contrary, the PAI-1 levels did not correlate with the disease activity index.

3.1.6. Thrombin Generation Associated with Neutrophil Extracellular Trap Formation

The plasma content of nucleic acids might contribute to the creation of prothrombotic profiles. We observed that the plasma from patients with SLE had increased cfDNA in fluorescence units, controls: 94.90 ± 21.29, SLE patients: 112.4 ± 26.59; $p = 0.0211$). In accordance with this observation, the neutrophils from SLE patients, but not the controls, showed NETs in basal conditions (Figure 4). Moreover, the neutrophils from these patients generated more NETs in the presence of 100 nM of PMA, as confirmed by fluorescence microscopy (Figure 4).

To evaluate whether the increment in NETs observed in patients with SLE had consequences on the hemostasis of these patients, we tested the thrombin generation of neutrophils from either patients with SLE or controls in the presence of platelets from healthy controls. The neutrophils from patients with SLE produced more thrombin than those from healthy controls under basal conditions and after stimulation with 100 nM of PMA. These increments were avoided when PRP was collected from blood samples drawn with CTI (Figure 5).

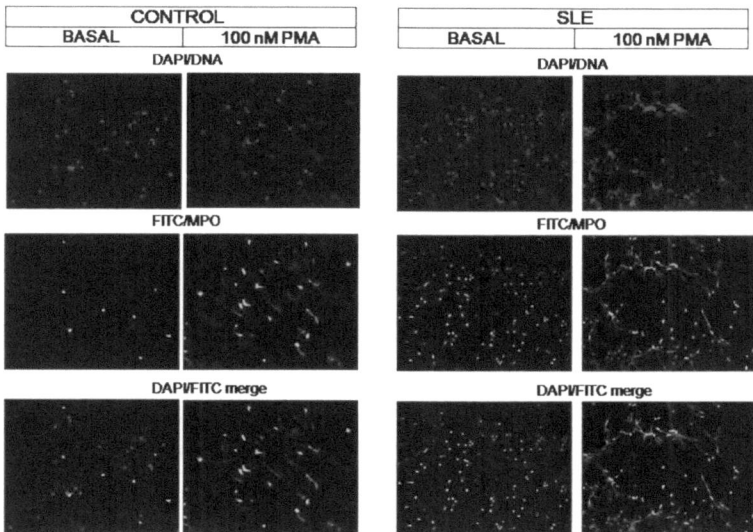

Figure 4. Formation of NETs. NETs were evaluated in basal conditions and after stimulation with 100 nM of PMA. DNA (DAPI, blue), neutrophil myeloperoxidase (MPO, FITC, green), and DAPI/FITC merge images are shown. Original magnification ×10.

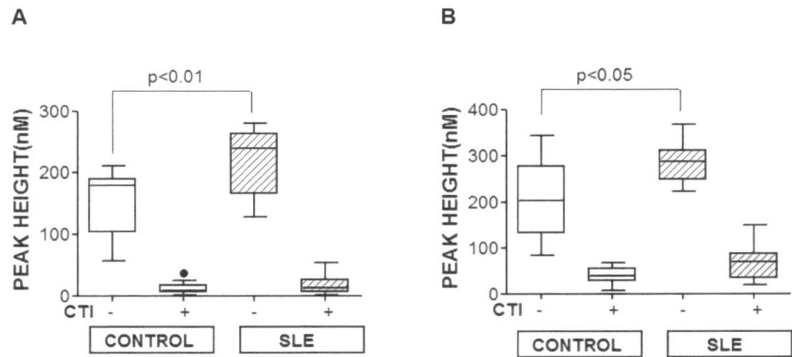

Figure 5. Thrombin generation associated with NETs. The effect of NETs on the thrombin generation was tested in either non-stimulated (**A**) or 100 nM of PMA-stimulated neutrophils (**B**) in the presence of PRP from healthy controls adjusted to 1×10^5 platelets/μL, with (+) or without (−) CTI. Detailed procedures are explained in "Materials and Methods". A Mann–Whitney test was performed, and $p < 0.05$ was considered significant.

4. Discussion

Analyses of the ROTEM® parameters in our cohort of patients showed a shortened CT and an increased alpha angle and MCF, highlighting the hypercoagulable features of these patients despite the fact that they had no antiphospholipid antibodies and no history of suffering thrombotic events. However, K.S. Collins et al. [12], who tested the kinetics of clot formation employing another global method, thromboelastography (TEG), found no differences in the TEG parameters between patients with SLE and healthy controls. This discrepancy could be due to the trigger used to induce coagulation in each case. These authors employed kaolin to activate the clotting cascade. Kaolin is a more powerful trigger, but offers a minor sensitivity in detecting mild differences in coagulation kinetics. Differently, we used the non-activated rotational thromboelastometry, NATEM®, which is sensitive to any change in the balance of the coagulation system, but has a low specificity [13]. Interestingly, other authors have evaluated coagulation by TEG in a cohort of children with SLE, and they also found a procoagulant profile; in this study, however, patients with antiphospholipid antibodies were not excluded [14].

In some of the patients from our cohort, SLE was accompanied by other syndromes such as Raynaud and Sjögren, known to induce a procoagulant state [15,16] that might overlap with that produced by SLE. Nevertheless, this does not seem to occur, because no differences were found among groups of SLE patients without and with these accompanying syndromes.

We did not find a correlation between the activity index of the disease and the patients' procoagulant profile. A similar conclusion was drawn from a systematic review and meta-analysis performed by Balloca et al. [17]. Despite the lack of correlation between the disease activity and procoagulant profile, we compared the clinical features of SLE patients with an MCF higher than the mean value + SD of MCF from healthy controls with those with an MCF within the normal range. We observed that, while both groups had similar nephrological damage, those with a high MCF had approximately 1.5 times more muscular and cardiac compromise and three times more pulmonary and nervous system clinical manifestations. Even when these data should be verified increasing the number of patients in the cohort, our observation warns about the importance of maintaining patients with hemostatic and coagulation parameters within normal ranges. Accordingly, some authors have proposed to treat patients with SLE with prophylactic oral anticoagulant therapy [18].

Platelet number and function are important determinants in the kinetics of clot formation [12,19]. The platelet counts in our SLE cohort, despite being significantly lower than in the healthy control group, were within a normal range. Thus, this difference was not expected to alter the ROTEM® parameters and, if any effect was predictable, it was a hypocoagulable one.

Treatment in SLE aims at remission or low disease activity and the prevention of flares. Our cohort of patients with SLE was treated according to the EULAR recommendations [20]. In patients without treatment, disease was in remission. Nevertheless, due to the complex and diverse nature of SLE pathogenesis, most of the patients need a combinatory therapy that may include standard immunosuppressive drugs (corticosteroids, azathioprine, methotrexate, cyclophosphamide, and mycophenolate) and monoclonal antibodies blocking CD20 (rituximab) or B-cell-activating factors (belimumab). In particular, one of our patients received at the same time rituximab and belimumab. This combination has been recently tested and demonstrated to reduce immune-complex-mediated inflammation and NETs formation [21].

Most of the patients with SLE from our cohort were treated with hydroxychloroquine, a substance known to have inhibitory effects on platelets [22]. Nevertheless, we and other authors [23] have observed that platelets from patients with SLE are basally activated. This activation could be due, at least in part, to the effect of the anti-dsDNA antibodies present in patients with SLE that may induce platelet activation, demonstrated by the enhanced P-selectin expression and morphological platelet changes [24]. However, the platelets from patients with SLE showed a reduced exposure of P-selectin after TRAP and ADP stimulation. Similarly, Frelinger et al. had reported that platelets from children with immune thrombocytopenia showed an increased P-selectin exposure in quiescent conditions but not after stimulation with agonists [25]. This observation might be because the basal activation of platelets causes either a reduction in the number or the exhaustion of secretory α-granules.

Another consequence of the basal activation of platelets from patients with SLE is the enhancement of their interaction with leukocytes (present results and other authors [26,27]) through the binding of P-selectin with the PSGL-1 present on the leukocytes' surface. Once bound, the interaction between the integrin αMβ2 on leukocytes and the GPIb on platelets produces a firm adhesion that contributes to thrombosis [28]. Moreover, platelet–leukocyte interactions induce signals that amplify proinflammatory cellular responses [29,30].

In accordance with their basal activation [31], platelets from patients with SLE exposed more PS than platelets from healthy controls (Figure 2C). Given that the PS exposition on the surface of platelets provides a negatively charged scaffold for the binding of the tenase and/or prothrombinase complexes that promote thrombin generation [32], it is tempting to speculate that this is an additional mechanism through which platelets could participate in the procoagulant profile of patients with SLE. The PS exposure on platelets from patients with SLE was due to activation and not to apoptosis [33], because the caspase activities in their quiescent platelets were similar to those observed in platelets from the healthy controls.

The procoagulant profile in patients with SLE might also be due to the presence of MPs released by cells in response to activation or apoptosis. Given that SLE is characterized by chronic inflammation and tissue damage, it is not surprising that blood from patients with SLE contains more MPs [34–36], due to both activated and damaged cells. MPs support coagulation by the exposure of negatively charged phospholipids and TF. We observed that our cohort of patients with SLE generated more thrombin associated with the TF content of MPs, whereas no differences were observed in thrombin generation linked to the PS content of MPs. These results might be explained because MPs from patients with SLE are predominantly PS-negative [37]. Nevertheless, Pereira et al. has reported an increased thrombin generation dependent on PS-associated MPs [36]. Moreover, other authors have described the augmentation of MPs in patients with SLE, measuring their PS exposure [38]. These differences might rely on the inclusion criteria for patients with SLE or/and the use of distinct technical approaches for measuring MPs. Given that the MPs in SLE exhibit unique molecular and phenotypic features, including the infrequent expression of PS, their role in the pathogenesis of SLE and their utility as biomarkers have been suggested by many authors [35,39].

On the basis of the existence of a correlation between the procoagulant profile (the peak of thrombin generation associated with MPs' TFcontent) and disease duration (but not with the disease activity index), it is tempting to speculate that chronic damage is more important than the current disease activity for the hypercoagulable state of these patients. Nevertheless, it cannot be ruled out that lack of correlation between coagulation parameters and disease activity might be due to our small sample size.

The increase in TF-bearing MPs could come from damaged endothelial cells [40]. In support of this observation, we and other authors [35,39] have observed increased plasma levels of PAI-1, a marker of endothelial dysfunction, in patients with SLE. In addition, augmented PAI-1 accompanied higher MCF values.

The damage to endothelial cells in SLE could be due, in part, to the presence of elevated levels of a pathogenic neutrophil subset known as low-density granulocytes, which have been reported to contribute to lupus pathogenesis through heightened proinflammatory responses, altered phagocytic capacity, and vascular damage [41]. Moreover, this neutrophil subset tends to release more web-like NETs [42,43], which are composed of cfDNA, histones, antimicrobial proteins, fibrinogen, FXII, and TF [43,44]. This release explains the increased levels of cfDNA found in plasma from patients with SLE. Moreover, most of the patients with SLE have a reduced ability to degrade NETs [42], and the prolonged presence of NETs in plasma could promote a rupture of immune tolerance as well as increase tissue damage [45]. These events lead to the formation of an amplification loop, in which NET components induce autoantibodies, leading to the formation of more immune complexes which, in turn, perpetuate NET formation. The experiments of Etulain et al. performed on mice showed an increase in NETs in the presence of P-selectin and PSGL1 [46]. This could explain why the neutrophils from patients with SLE were more susceptible to generating NETs due to basal platelet activation.

Moreover, enhanced NET formation has been associated with the promotion of coronary plaque formation and lipoprotein dysregulation [47].

The increased thrombin generated by non-stimulated neutrophils from patients with SLE (present results) could be explained by the fact that cfDNA triggers the intrinsic pathway of blood coagulation [48]. NETs can bind FXII and cooperate with platelets to activate the intrinsic pathway [49]. In support of this observation, NET-related thrombin generation was prevented in the presence of CTI, an inhibitor of the contact phase of coagulation activation (present results and [50]).

One of the limitations of the study is that the patients were receiving different treatments that might modify hemostasis, as mentioned above for hydroxychloroquine, and that we did not recruit enough patients for stratifying them according to the medication they were receiving.

Traditional cardiovascular risk factors do not fully explain the high rates of ischemic events in patients with SLE, and standard risk calculations underestimate the risk of developing cardiovascular disease. Previous reports have already shown similar results to those presented in this work—platelets from SLE patients are activated [27] and increments were observed in circulating MPs [36], platelets/leukocyte aggregates [26], and PAI-1 [39] and cfDNA [51] plasma levels. Importance of our work relies on the fact that all these variables were evaluated in the same cohort of patients, allowing us to detect the relationship between the different mechanisms involved. In addition, the effects observed were independent of antiphospholipid antibodies because their presence was an exclusion criterion. Another key point is that our results suggest the utility of global tests for studying hemostasis in these patients, because a procoagulant profile was detected despite the fact that they had neither antiphospholipid antibodies nor any previous thrombotic event. A global appraisal of hemostasis takes into account the relationships among all the mechanisms involved (platelets, the thrombin generation associated with MPs, cfDNA) and should, if possible, be incorporated into clinical practice to detect the risk of a thrombotic event in patients with SLE and to consequently act to prevent its occurrence, as recommended in the updated guide of EULAR [20].

Supplementary Materials: The following are available online at http://www.mdpi.com/2077-0383/9/10/3297/s1, Figure S1: Fibrinogen and von Willebrand factor (vW Factor) receptors expression on quiescent platelets. Platelets were incubated with PE-anti CD41 and FITC-anti CD61 mAbs to detect fibrinogen receptor and with FITC-anti CD42a and FITC-anti CD42b mAbs to test vW Factor receptors. Data are expressed as mean fluorescence (MF). Samples were analyzed by flow cytometry. Figure S2: Platelet's activation markers. Platelets were stimulated with either 100 μM of TRAP or 20 μM of ADP, and FITC-PAC1, FITC-anti P-selectin mAb, and FITC-anti CD63 mAb were added. Data are expressed as % of positive cells. Samples were analyzed by flow cytometry. Figure S3: Caspase activities in quiescent platelets. Data are expressed as % of positive cells. Samples were analyzed by flow cytometry.

Author Contributions: I.F.-B., E.M.M., R.J.S., and P.A.; F.J.L.-L. and Á.R.M. recruited patients and collected clinical data; I.F.-B., M.T.Á.R., V.J.Y., Á.R.M., and N.V.B. analyzed data of work, N.V.B. designed the study and wrote the manuscript. All the authors revised critically the paper and approved it. All authors have read and agreed to the published version of the manuscript.

Funding: This work was supported by grant from the FIS-FONDOS FEDER (PI19/00772, NVB). E.M.M. holds a predoctoral fellowship from Fundación Española de Trombosis y Hemostasia (FETH-SETH).

Conflicts of Interest: The authors declare no conflict of interest.

References

1. Grover-Paez, F.; Zavalza-Gomez, A.B. Endothelial dysfunction and cardiovascular risk factors. *Diabetes Res. Clin. Pract.* **2009**, *84*, 1–10. [CrossRef] [PubMed]
2. Protogerou, A.D.; Sfikakis, P.P.; Stamatelopoulos, K.S.; Papamichael, C.; Aznaouridis, K.; Karatzis, E.; Papaioannou, T.G.; Ikonomidis, I.; Kaklamanis, P.; Mavrikakis, M.; et al. Interrelated modulation of endothelial function in Behcet's disease by clinical activity and corticosteroid treatment. *Arthritis Res. Ther.* **2007**, *9*, R90. [CrossRef] [PubMed]
3. Widlansky, M.E.; Gokce, N.; Keaney, J.F., Jr.; Vita, J.A. The clinical implications of endothelial dysfunction. *J. Am. Coll. Cardiol.* **2003**, *42*, 1149–1160. [CrossRef]
4. Roman, M.J.; Crow, M.K.; Lockshin, M.D.; Devereux, R.B.; Paget, S.A.; Sammaritano, L.; Levine, D.M.; Davis, A.; Salmon, J.E. Rate and determinants of progression of atherosclerosis in systemic lupus erythematosus. *Arthritis Rheum.* **2007**, *56*, 3412–3419. [CrossRef]
5. Afeltra, A.; Vadacca, M.; Conti, L.; Galluzzo, S.; Mitterhofer, A.P.; Ferri, G.M.; Del Porto, F.; Caccavo, D.; Gandolfo, G.M.; Amoroso, A. Thrombosis in systemic lupus erythematosus: Congenital and acquired risk factors. *Arthritis Rheum.* **2005**, *53*, 452–459. [CrossRef] [PubMed]
6. Lockshin, M.D. Update on antiphospholipid syndrome. *Bull. NYU Hosp. Jt. Dis.* **2006**, *64*, 57–59.

7. Fernandez-Bello, I.; Lopez-Longo, F.J.; Arias-Salgado, E.G.; Jimenez-Yuste, V.; Butta, N.V. Behcet's disease: New insight into the relationship between procoagulant state, endothelial activation/damage and disease activity. *Orphanet J. Rare Dis.* **2013**, *8*, 81. [CrossRef]
8. Justo Sanz, R.; Monzon Manzano, E.; Fernandez Bello, I.; Teresa Alvarez Roman, M.; Martin Salces, M.; Rivas Pollmar, M.I.; Jimenez Yuste, V.; Butta, N.V. Platelet Apoptosis and PAI-1 are Involved in the Pro-Coagulant State of Immune Thrombocytopaenia Patients Treated with Thrombopoietin Receptor Agonists. *Thromb. Haemost.* **2019**, *119*, 645–659. [CrossRef]
9. Hochberg, M.C. Updating the American College of Rheumatology revised criteria for the classification of systemic lupus erythematosus. *Arthritis Rheum.* **1997**, *40*, 1725. [CrossRef]
10. Esmon, C.T. The interactions between inflammation and coagulation. *Br. J. Haematol.* **2005**, *131*, 417–430. [CrossRef]
11. Manzi, S.; Meilahn, E.N.; Rairie, J.E.; Conte, C.G.; Medsger, T.A., Jr.; Jansen-McWilliams, L.; D'Agostino, R.B.; Kuller, L.H. Age-specific incidence rates of myocardial infarction and angina in women with systemic lupus erythematosus: Comparison with the Framingham Study. *Am. J. Epidemiol.* **1997**, *145*, 408–415. [CrossRef] [PubMed]
12. Collins, K.S.; Balasubramaniam, K.; Viswanathan, G.; Natasari, A.; Tarn, J.; Lendrem, D.; Mitchell, S.; Zaman, A.; Ng, W.F. Assessment of blood clot formation and platelet receptor function ex vivo in patients with primary Sjogren's syndrome. *BMJ Open* **2013**, *3*, e002739. [CrossRef] [PubMed]
13. Trelinski, J.; Misiewicz, M.; Robak, M.; Smolewski, P.; Chojnowski, K. Assessment of rotation thromboelastometry (ROTEM) parameters in patients with multiple myeloma at diagnosis *Thromb. Res.* **2014**, *133*, 667–670. [CrossRef] [PubMed]
14. Li, Z.; Xiao, J.; Song, H.; Chen, Q.; Han, H.; Li, J.; Zhang, L.; He, Y.; Wei, M. Evaluation of coagulation disorders by thromboelastography in children with systemic lupus erythematosus. *Lupus* **2019**, *28*, 181–188. [CrossRef]
15. Avina-Zubieta, J.A.; Jansz, M.; Sayre, E.C.; Choi, H.K. The Risk of Deep Venous Thrombosis and Pulmonary Embolism in Primary Sjogren Syndrome: A General Population-based Study. *J. Rheumatol.* **2017**, *44*, 1184–1189. [CrossRef]
16. Zuk, J.; Snarska-Drygalska, A.; Malinowski, K.P.; Papuga-Szela, E.; Natorska, J.; Undas, A. Unfavourably altered plasma clot properties in patients with primary Raynaud's phenomenon: Association with venous thromboembolism. *J. Thromb. Thrombolysis* **2019**, *47*, 248–254. [CrossRef]
17. Ballocca, F.; D'Ascenzo, F.; Moretti, C.; Omede, P.; Cerrato, E.; Barbero, U.; Abbate, A.; Bertero, M.T.; Zoccai, G.B.; Gaita, F. Predictors of cardiovascular events in patients with systemic lupus erythematosus (SLE): A systematic review and meta-analysis. *Eur. J. Prev. Cardiol.* **2015**, *22*, 1435–1441. [CrossRef]
18. Wahl, D.G.; Bounameaux, H.; de Moerloose, P.; Sarasin, F.P. Prophylactic antithrombotic therapy for patients with systemic lupus erythematosus with or without antiphospholipid antibodies: Do the benefits outweigh the risks? A decision analysis. *Arch. Intern. Med.* **2000**, *160*, 2042–2048. [CrossRef]
19. Cid, J.; Escolar, G.; Galan, A.; Lopez-Vilchez, I.; Molina, P.; Diaz-Ricart, M.; Lozano, M.; Dumont, L.J. In vitro evaluation of the hemostatic effectiveness of cryopreserved platelets. *Transfusion* **2016**, *56*, 580–586. [CrossRef]
20. Fanouriakis, A.; Kostopoulou, M.; Alunno, A.; Aringer, M.; Bajema, I.; Boletis, J.N.; Cervera, R.; Doria, A.; Gordon, C.; Govoni, M.; et al. 2019 update of the EULAR recommendations for the management of systemic lupus erythematosus. *Ann. Rheum. Dis.* **2019**, *78*, 736–745. [CrossRef]
21. van Dam, L.S.; Osmani, Z.; Kamerling, S.W.A.; Kraaij, T.; Bakker, J.A.; Scherer, H.U.; Rabelink, T.J.; Voll, R.E.; Alexander, T.; Isenberg, D.A.; et al. A reverse translational study on the effect of rituximab, rituximab plus belimumab, or bortezomib on the humoral autoimmune response in SLE. *Rheumatology* **2020**, *59*, 2734–2745. [CrossRef] [PubMed]
22. Dyer, M.R.; Alexander, W.; Hassoune, A.; Chen, Q.; Brzoska, T.; Alvikas, J.; Liu, Y.; Haldeman, S.; Plautz, W.; Loughran, P.; et al. Platelet-derived extracellular vesicles released after trauma promote hemostasis and contribute to DVT in mice. *J. Thromb. Haemost.* **2019**, *17*, 1733–1745. [CrossRef] [PubMed]
23. Linge, P.; Fortin, P.R.; Lood, C.; Bengtsson, A.A.; Boilard, E. The non-haemostatic role of platelets in systemic lupus erythematosus. *Nat. Rev. Rheumatol.* **2018**, *14*, 195–213. [CrossRef] [PubMed]
24. Andrianova, I.A.; Ponomareva, A.A.; Mordakhanova, E.R.; Le Minh, G.; Daminova, A.G.; Nevzorova, T.A.; Rauova, L.; Litvinov, R.I.; Weisel, J.W. In systemic lupus erythematosus anti-dsDNA antibodies can promote thrombosis through direct platelet activation. *J. Autoimmun.* **2019**, 102355. [CrossRef]

25. Frelinger, A.L., 3rd; Grace, R.F.; Gerrits, A.J.; Carmichael, S.L.; Forde, E.E.; Michelson, A.D. Platelet Function in ITP, Independent of Platelet Count, Is Consistent Over Time and Is Associated with Both Current and Subsequent Bleeding Severity. *Thromb. Haemost.* **2018**, *118*, 143–151. [CrossRef]
26. Joseph, J.E.; Harrison, P.; Mackie, I.J.; Isenberg, D.A.; Machin, S.J. Increased circulating platelet-leucocyte complexes and platelet activation in patients with antiphospholipid syndrome, systemic lupus erythematosus and rheumatoid arthritis. *Br. J. Haematol.* **2001**, *115*, 451–459. [CrossRef]
27. Nhek, S.; Clancy, R.; Lee, K.A.; Allen, N.M.; Barrett, T.J.; Marcantoni, E.; Nwaukoni, J.; Rasmussen, S.; Rubin, M.; Newman, J.D.; et al. Activated Platelets Induce Endothelial Cell Activation via an Interleukin-1beta Pathway in Systemic Lupus Erythematosus. *Arter. Thromb. Vasc. Biol.* **2017**, *37*, 707–716. [CrossRef]
28. Wang, Y.; Gao, H.; Shi, C.; Erhardt, P.W.; Pavlovsky, A.; Soloviev, D.A.; Bledzka, K.; Ustinov, V.; Zhu, L.; Qin, J.; et al. Leukocyte integrin Mac-1 regulates thrombosis via interaction with platelet GPIbalpha. *Nat. Commun.* **2017**, *8*, 15559. [CrossRef]
29. Libby, P.; Simon, D.I. Inflammation and thrombosis: The clot thickens. *Circulation* **2001**, *103*, 1718–1720. [CrossRef]
30. Sreeramkumar, V.; Adrover, J.M.; Ballesteros, I.; Cuartero, M.I.; Rossaint, J.; Bilbao, I.; Nacher, M.; Pitaval, C.; Radovanovic, I.; Fukui, Y.; et al. Neutrophils scan for activated platelets to initiate inflammation. *Science* **2014**, *346*, 1234–1238. [CrossRef]
31. Schoenwaelder, S.M.; Yuan, Y.; Josefsson, E.C.; White, M.J.; Yao, Y.; Mason, K.D.; O'Reilly, L.A.; Henley, K.J.; Ono, A.; Hsiao, S.; et al. Two distinct pathways regulate platelet phosphatidylserine exposure and procoagulant function. *Blood* **2009**, *114*, 663–666. [CrossRef] [PubMed]
32. Fager, A.M.; Wood, J.P.; Bouchard, B.A.; Feng, P.; Tracy, P.B. Properties of procoagulant platelets: Defining and characterizing the subpopulation binding a functional prothrombinase. *Arterioscler. Thromb. Vasc. Biol.* **2010**, *30*, 2400–2407. [CrossRef] [PubMed]
33. Mason, K.D.; Carpinelli, M.R.; Fletcher, J.I.; Collinge, J.E.; Hilton, A.A.; Ellis, S.; Kelly, P.N.; Ekert, P.G.; Metcalf, D.; Roberts, A.W.; et al. Programmed anuclear cell death delimits platelet life span. *Cell* **2007**, *128*, 1173–1186. [CrossRef] [PubMed]
34. Lopez, P.; Rodriguez-Carrio, J.; Martinez-Zapico, A.; Caminal-Montero, L.; Suarez, A. Circulating microparticle subpopulations in systemic lupus erythematosus are affected by disease activity. *Int. J. Cardiol.* **2017**, *236*, 138–144. [CrossRef]
35. Mobarrez, F.; Svenungsson, E.; Pisetsky, D.S. Microparticles as autoantigens in systemic lupus erythematosus. *Eur. J. Clin. Investig.* **2018**, *48*, e13010. [CrossRef]
36. Pereira, J.; Alfaro, G.; Goycoolea, M.; Quiroga, T.; Ocqueteau, M.; Massardo, L.; Perez, C.; Saez, C.; Panes, O.; Matus, V.; et al. Circulating platelet-derived microparticles in systemic lupus erythematosus. Association with increased thrombin generation and procoagulant state. *Thromb. Haemost.* **2006**, *95*, 94–99.
37. Mobarrez, F.; Vikerfors, A.; Gustafsson, J.T.; Gunnarsson, I.; Zickert, A.; Larsson, A.; Pisetsky, D.S.; Wallen, H.; Svenungsson, E. Microparticles in the blood of patients with systemic lupus erythematosus (SLE): Phenotypic characterization and clinical associations. *Sci. Rep.* **2016**, *6*, 36025. [CrossRef]
38. Sellam, J.; Proulle, V.; Jungel, A.; Ittah, M.; Miceli Richard, C.; Gottenberg, J.E.; Toti, F.; Benessiano, J.; Gay, S.; Freyssinet, J.M.; et al. Increased levels of circulating microparticles in primary Sjogren's syndrome, systemic lupus erythematosus and rheumatoid arthritis and relation with disease activity. *Arthritis Res. Ther.* **2009**, *11*, R156. [CrossRef]
39. Somers, E.C.; Marder, W.; Kaplan, M.J.; Brook, R.D.; McCune, W.J. Plasminogen activator inhibitor-1 is associated with impaired endothelial function in women with systemic lupus erythematosus. *Ann. N. Y. Acad. Sci.* **2005**, *1051*, 271–280. [CrossRef]
40. Shustova, O.N.; Antonova, O.A.; Golubeva, N.V.; Khaspekova, S.G.; Yakushkin, V.V.; Aksuk, S.A.; Alchinova, I.B.; Karganov, M.Y.; Mazurov, A.V. Differential procoagulant activity of microparticles derived from monocytes, granulocytes, platelets and endothelial cells: Impact of active tissue factor. *Blood Coagul. Fibrinolysis* **2017**, *28*, 373–382. [CrossRef]
41. Carmona-Rivera, C.; Kaplan, M.J. Low-density granulocytes: A distinct class of neutrophils in systemic autoimmunity. *Semin. Immunopathol.* **2013**, *35*, 455–463. [CrossRef] [PubMed]
42. Leffler, J.; Ciacma, K.; Gullstrand, B.; Bengtsson, A.A.; Martin, M.; Blom, A.M. A subset of patients with systemic lupus erythematosus fails to degrade DNA from multiple clinically relevant sources. *Arthritis Res. Ther.* **2015**, *17*, 205. [CrossRef]

43. Villanueva, E.; Yalavarthi, S.; Berthier, C.C.; Hodgin, J.B.; Khandpur, R.; Lin, A.M.; Rubin, C.J.; Zhao, W.; Olsen, S.H.; Klinker, M.; et al. Netting neutrophils induce endothelial damage, infiltrate tissues, and expose immunostimulatory molecules in systemic lupus erythematosus. *J. Immunol.* **2011**, *187*, 538–552. [CrossRef] [PubMed]
44. Perdomo, J.; Leung, H.H.L.; Ahmadi, Z.; Yan, F.; Chong, J.J.H.; Passam, F.H.; Chong, B.H. Neutrophil activation and NETosis are the major drivers of thrombosis in heparin-induced thrombocytopenia. *Nat. Commun.* **2019**, *10*, 1322. [CrossRef] [PubMed]
45. Pruchniak, M.P.; Ostafin, M.; Wachowska, M.; Jakubaszek, M.; Kwiatkowska, B.; Olesinska, M.; Zycinska, K.; Demkow, U. Neutrophil extracellular traps generation and degradation in patients with granulomatosis with polyangiitis and systemic lupus erythematosus. *Autoimmunity* **2019**, *52*, 126–135. [CrossRef] [PubMed]
46. Etulain, J.; Martinod, K.; Wong, S.L.; Cifuni, S.M.; Schattner, M.; Wagner, D.D. P-selectin promotes neutrophil extracellular trap formation in mice. *Blood* **2015**, *126*, 242–246. [CrossRef] [PubMed]
47. O'Neil, L.J.; Kaplan, M.J.; Carmona-Rivera, C. The Role of Neutrophils and Neutrophil Extracellular Traps in Vascular Damage in Systemic Lupus Erythematosus. *J. Clin. Med.* **2019**, *8*, 1325. [CrossRef]
48. Swystun, L.L.; Mukherjee, S.; Liaw, P.C. Breast cancer chemotherapy induces the release of cell-free DNA, a novel procoagulant stimulus. *J. Thromb. Haemost.* **2011**, *9*, 2313–2321. [CrossRef]
49. von Bruhl, M.L.; Stark, K.; Steinhart, A.; Chandraratne, S.; Konrad, I.; Lorenz, M.; Khandoga, A.; Tirniceriu, A.; Coletti, R.; Kollnberger, M.; et al. Monocytes, neutrophils, and platelets cooperate to initiate and propagate venous thrombosis in mice in vivo. *J. Exp. Med.* **2012**, *209*, 819–835. [CrossRef]
50. Gould, T.J.; Vu, T.T.; Swystun, L.L.; Dwivedi, D.J.; Mai, S.H.; Weitz, J.I.; Liaw, P.C. Neutrophil extracellular traps promote thrombin generation through platelet-dependent and platelet-independent mechanisms. *Arterioscler. Thromb. Vasc. Biol.* **2014**, *34*, 1977–1984. [CrossRef]
51. Zhang, S.; Lu, X.; Shu, X.; Tian, X.; Yang, H.; Yang, W.; Zhang, Y.; Wang, G. Elevated plasma cfDNA may be associated with active lupus nephritis and partially attributed to abnormal regulation of neutrophil extracellular traps (NETs) in patients with systemic lupus erythematosus. *Intern. Med.* **2014**, *53*, 2763–2771. [CrossRef] [PubMed]

Publisher's Note: MDPI stays neutral with regard to jurisdictional claims in published maps and institutional affiliations.

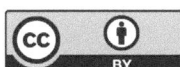

© 2020 by the authors. Licensee MDPI, Basel, Switzerland. This article is an open access article distributed under the terms and conditions of the Creative Commons Attribution (CC BY) license (http://creativecommons.org/licenses/by/4.0/).

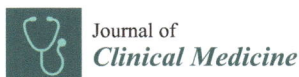

Article

Serum Levels of T Cell Immunoglobulin and Mucin-Domain Containing Molecule 3 in Patients with Systemic Lupus Erythematosus

Tomoyuki Asano, Naoki Matsuoka, Yuya Fujita, Haruki Matsumoto, Jumpei Temmoku, Makiko Yashiro-Furuya, Shuzo Sato, Eiji Suzuki, Hiroko Kobayashi, Hiroshi Watanabe and Kiyoshi Migita *

Department of Rheumatology, Fukushima Medical University School of Medicine, 1 Hikarigaoka, Fukushima, Fukushima 960-1295, Japan; asanovic@fmu.ac.jp (T.A.); naoki-11@fmu.ac.jp (N.M.); fujita31@fmu.ac.jp (Y.F.); haruki91@fmu.ac.jp (H.M.); temmoku@fmu.ac.jp (J.T.); myashiro@fmu.ac.jp (M.Y.-F.); shuzo@fmu.ac.jp (S.S.); azsuzuki@ohta-hp.or.jp (E.S.); hkoba@fmu.ac.jp (H.K.); chiehiro@fmu.ac.jp (H.W.)
* Correspondence: migita@fmu.ac.jp; Tel.: +81-24-547-1171; Fax: +81-24-547-1172

Received: 8 October 2020; Accepted: 2 November 2020; Published: 5 November 2020

Abstract: Objective: T cell immunoglobulin and mucin-domain-containing molecule 3 (TIM-3) is implicated in the development of various autoimmune diseases. We aimed to investigate the levels of soluble TIM-3 (sTIM-3) and their associations between clinical parameters in patients with systemic lupus erythematosus (SLE). Methods: Serum samples were collected from 65 patients with SLE and 35 age-matched healthy controls (HCs). The SLE Disease Activity Index 2000 (SLEDAI-2K) and the Systemic Lupus International Collaborating Clinics (SLICC) damage index (SDI) were used to assess SLE disease activity and SLE-related organ damage. British Isles Lupus Assessment Group (BILAG)-2004 index was also used to assess SLE disease activity. Soluble TIM-3 (sTIM-3) in sera from patients with SLE and HCs were evaluated by enzyme-linked immunosorbent assay (ELISA). The results were compared with the clinical parameters of SLE including SLE disease activity. Results: Serum sTIM-3 levels in patients with SLE (median 2123 pg/mL (interquartile range (IQR), 229–7235)) were significantly higher than those in HCs (1363 pg/mL; IQR, 1097–1673; $p = 0.0015$). Serum levels of sTIM-3 were correlated with disease activity of SLE using the SLEDAI-2K score ($p < 0.001$, $r = 0.53$). The serum sTIM-3 levels in SLE patients with active renal disease (BILAG renal index A-B) were significantly higher than those without the active renal disease (BILAG renal index C–E). However, no significant difference was observed in serum sTIM-3 levels between SLE patients with and without active involvement in other organs (BILAG index). Serum sTIM-3 levels were significantly elevated in SLE patients with organ damage (2710 pg/mL; IQR, 256–7235) compared to those without organ damage (1532 pg/mL; IQR, 228–5274), as assessed by the SDI ($p = 0.0102$). Conclusions: Circulating sTIM-3 levels are elevated in SLE patients, and serum sTIM-3 levels are associated with SLE disease activity and SLE-related organ damage. The data indicate a possible link between the TIM-3/Gal-9 pathway and SLE clinical phenotypes, and further investigation of the TIM-3 pathway in SLE pathophysiology is warranted.

Keywords: galectin 9; systemic lupus erythematosus; T cell immunoglobulin domain and mucin-domain-containing molecule 3

1. Introduction

Immune checkpoint receptors of co-inhibitory or co-stimulatory molecules are major components of the immune system [1]. As a negative checkpoint receptor, T cell immunoglobulin and mucin-domain-containing molecule 3 (TIM-3) and its ligand galectin 9 (Gal-9) are thought to be involved with the pathogenesis of autoimmune diseases [2]. TIM-3 is a transmembrane glycoprotein mainly expressed in Th1 and Th17 cells [3]. TIM-3 plays a central role in immune tolerance because the TIM-3/Gal-9 pathway regulates Th1 immunity through apoptosis induction [4], and blocking this interaction results in exacerbated autoimmunity [5]. Systemic lupus erythematosus (SLE) is a systemic autoimmune disease characterized by autoantibody production, immune complex deposition, and cytokine activation [6]. Although the etiology of SLE is complex, it is thought that disrupted self-tolerance leads to activate autoreactive T cells, which subsequently promote auto-antibody production by autoreactive B cells [7]. The role of immune co-inhibitory or co-inhibitory systems in anti-tumor immune responses has been demonstrated to be important by the recent success of immune checkpoint blockade in cancer therapy [8]. However, blocking inhibitory immune checkpoint receptors often causes immune-mediated adverse events (irAEs), which are similar to autoimmune diseases [9]. Conversely, blocking immune responses by enhancing co-inhibitory signals or blocking co-stimulatory signals is a promising therapeutic approach for treating autoimmune diseases [10]. In SLE patients, the TIM-3 ligand, Gal-9, is upregulated and correlates with interferon-signature gene expression [11]. These findings indicate that the TIM-3/Gal-9 pathway plays an important role in Th1 and Th17 immune response and blockage of the TIM-3/Gal-9 interaction results in exacerbated autoimmune diseases [12]. Expression of TIM-3 on peripheral blood mononuclear cells (PBMCs) isolated from SLE patients is associated with SLE disease activity [13]. TIM-3 can be shed from the cell surface by a-disintegrin-like and metalloproteinase with thrombospondin type 1 motifs (ADAM) 10 or ADAM17-mediated cleavage within the TIM-3 stalk region, resulting in a soluble form of TIM-3 (sTIM-3) [14], which is elevated in the sera of patients with autoimmune diseases [15]. In the present study, we quantified circulating sTIM-3 in both patients with SLE and healthy control subjects. We also investigated the associations between circulating sTIM-3 and clinical parameters of SLE, including disease activity.

2. Materials and Methods

2.1. Patients and Clinical Evaluations

All patients enrolled in this cohort study were diagnosed with SLE at the Department of Rheumatology, Fukushima Medical University Hospital, from June 2009 to September 2019. The enrolled SLE patients had to be older than 17 years to be diagnosed as SLE according to the American College of Rheumatology (ACR) 1997 criteria [16]. A total of 65 Japanese patients with SLE were recruited within 32 months (mean 18 months, range 0–32) from diagnosis with SLE. In patients with SLE, their medical histories and clinical findings were collected by reviewing electronic medical records. Disease activity of SLE was assessed according to the Systemic Lupus Erythematosus Disease Activity Index (SLEDAI) [17]. Chronic organ damage was assessed by the Systemic Lupus International Collaborating Clinics (SLICC) damage index (SDI) [18]. Disease activity of SLE was also assessed using the British Isles Lupus Assessment Group (BILAG)-2004 index, which was proposed to assess the disease activity of SLE using eight systems [19]. The total BILAG-2004 index was calculated by assigning the following numerical values to each BILAG index (BILAG Grade $A = 12$, $B = 5$, $C = 1$, $D = 0$, $E = 0$). Thirty-five healthy controls (HCs) (14 men, 21 women (median age 42 years); interquartile range (IQR), 35–52) were included in this cohort. Ethical approval was obtained for this study from the Committee of Fukushima Medical University International Review Board (No. 30285). Written informed consent was obtained from each individual. All research was performed under the principles of the Declaration of Helsinki.

2.2. Enzyme-Linked Immunosorbent Assay for Soluble TIM-3

Serum sTIM-3 levels from patients with SLE and HCs were measured by the human enzyme-linked immunosorbent assay (ELISA) kit (R&D Systems, Inc. Minneapolis, MN, USA), according to the manufacturer's instructions.

2.3. Statistical Analysis

Results were non-normally distributed, and they are presented as median and 25th and 75th percentiles (median (IQR)). A nonparametric test by Mann–Whitney's U test was used to determine the statistical significance of the data. Spearman's rank correlation test was used to test the correlations between serial variables.

3. Results

3.1. Demographic and Clinical Characteristics of SLE Patients

Sixty-five patients with SLE and 35 healthy control subjects (HCs) were included in this study. The overall baseline demographic and clinical characteristics of the SLE patients are summarized in Table 1. Of these, 55 (84%) of SLE patients were women and 10 (16%) were men, median age was 33 years (range 16–79), and median disease duration was 55 months (range 1–420). Sixty (92%) patients had baseline SLEDAI-2K > 4 and 37 (57%) patients had organ damage (SDI ≥ 1). There were no statistically significant differences in sex or age distribution between patients with SLE and HCs.

Table 1. General characteristics of 65 Japanese systemic lupus erythematosus patients.

Characteristics	n = 65
Sex	
Female, n (%)	56 (84)
Male, n (%)	11 (16)
Median age (range), years	33 (16–79)
Median disease duration of SLE (range), months	55 (1–420)
Untreated patients, n (%)	55 (83)
Items of SLE classification criteria, n (%)	
Rash	32 (48)
Alopecia	3 (4)
Oral ulcer	5 (7)
Arthritis	22 (33)
Serositis	17 (25)
Renal disorder	38 (57)
Laboratory findings, n (%)	
Leukocytopenia	25 (37)
Thrombocytopenia	18 (27)
Anti-double stranded-DNA antibody positive	52 (78)
Anti-smith antibody positive	31 (46)
Anti-phospholipid antibody positive	28 (42)
Median SLEDAI, index (range)	14 (0–50)
Median SDI, index (range)	1 (0–4)

SLE: systemic lupus erythematosus, SLEDAI: SLE disease activity index, SDI: Systemic Lupus International Collaborating Clinics (SLICC) damage index.

3.2. Correlation between Serum sTIM-3 Levels and Disease Activity of SLE

sTIM-3 levels in sera were determined by ELISA in patients with SLE and HCs. Soluble TIM-3 levels were significantly higher in patients with SLE (2123 pg/mL (IQR, 229–7235)) than those in HCs (1363 pg/mL; IQR, 1097–1673; $p = 0.0015$; Figure 1). We also analyzed the correlations between sTIM-3 levels and SLE disease activity. Serum sTIM-3 levels showed a significant correlation with disease activity when using the SLEDAI-2K (Figure 2A, $p < 0.001$, $r = 0.53$). Serum sTIM-3 levels showed a negative correlation with serum levels of complement (C) 3 (Figure 2B, $p = 0.038$, $r = -0.26$) and complement (C) 4 (Figure 2C, $p = 0.047$, $r = -0.25$), but not with anti-double stranded-DNA antibody titer (Figure 2D, $p = 0.085$, $r = 0.21$).

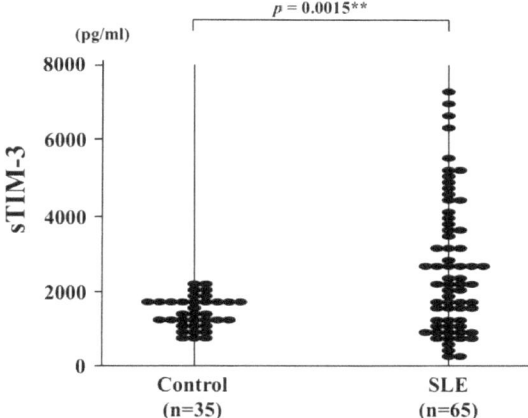

Figure 1. Serum sTIM-3 levels in SLE patients ($n = 65$) and healthy controls ($n = 35$). Soluble TIM-3 levels of SLE patients were significantly higher than those in healthy controls. Median sTIM-3 levels (bar) are displayed and statistical analysis was conducted using the Mann–Whitney's U test. sTIM-3: soluble T cell immunoglobulin and mucin-domain-containing molecule 3, SLE: systemic lupus erythematosus. ** $p < 0.01$ is considered as statistically significant.

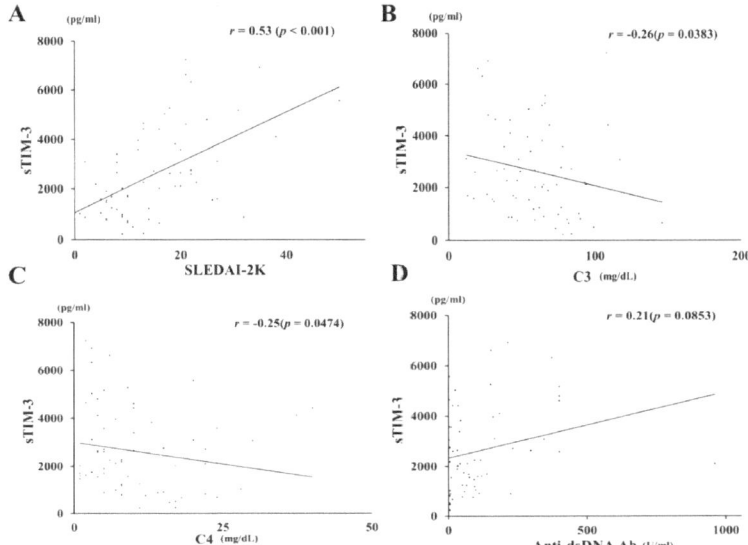

Figure 2. Correlations between serum sTIM-3 levels and clinical parameters in SLE patients. Serum sTIM-3 levels were significantly positively correlated with SLEDAI-2K (**A**) and negatively correlated with serum levels of C3 (**B**) and C4 (**C**). No significant correlation was observed between serum sTIM-3 levels and anti-double-stranded (ds) DNA antibodies (**D**). Statistics and regression lines are shown by solid lines. sTIM-3: soluble T-cell immunoglobulin and mucin-domain-containing molecule 3, SLEDAI-2K: Systemic Lupus Erythematosus Disease Activity Index 2000, C3: complement 3, C4: complement 4.

3.3. Serum Levels of sTIM-3 and Organ Involvement Measured by the BILAG-2004 Index

The BILAG-2004 index categorizes disease activity into five different levels from A to E, in which A represents the most active form of the disease and E implies the system has never been active [20].

Among the eight BILAG grading domains, active organ involvement was identified mainly in the renal, neurological, and hematological domains (Table 2). The serum sTIM-3 levels in SLE patients with active renal involvement (BILAG index A–B) were significantly elevated compared to those without active renal involvement (BILAG index C–E) (Figure 3). However, no significant difference was observed in serum sTIM-3 levels between SLE patients with or without active neurological or hematological involvement.

Table 2. Disease activity of SLE patients using the British Isles Lupus Assessment Group (BILAG)-2004 index.

BILAG Manifestations	Grade ($n = 65$)				
	A	B	C	D	E
General	3	14	16	4	29
Mucocutaneous	1	5	19	6	35
Neurological	2	10	1	1	52
Musculoskeletal	2	4	14	4	42
Cardiovascular/respiratory	0	6	9	3	48
Abdominal	1	7	0	1	57
Renal	15	6	6	5	34
Hematological	2	15	36	3	10
Ophthalmic	1	4	6	2	53

BILAG grades A: severe, B: intermediate, C: mild, D: inactive, E: no activity.

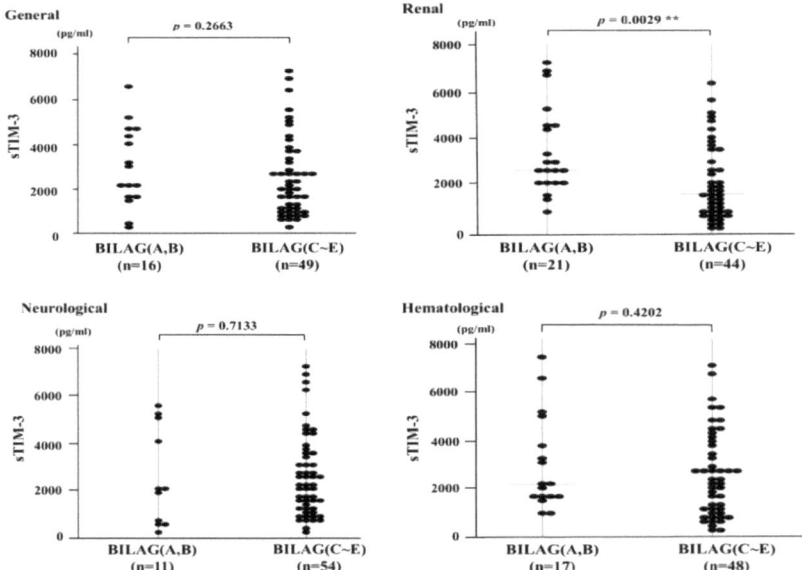

Figure 3. Serum sTIM-3 levels in patients SLE (systemic lupus erythematosus) patients with or without active organ involvement. Comparison of serum sTIM-3 levels between SLE patients with active organ involvement (BILAG general, renal, neurological, and hematological indexes A–B) and without active organ involvements (BILAG index C–E). BILAG: British Isles lupus assessment Group, sTIM-3: soluble T cell immunoglobulin and mucin-domain-containing molecule 3. **, $p < 0.01$ is considered as statistically significant.

We compared the serum levels of sTIM-3 between SLE patients with and without proteinuria. Serum levels of sTIM-3 were significantly higher in SLE patients with proteinuria compared to those without proteinuria (proteinuria negative; $n = 20$; 1361 pg/mL; IQR, 889–2114, versus proteinuria positive; $n = 35$; 2711 pg/mL; IQR, 2108–4536; $p < 0.001$). Similarly, serum levels of sTIM-3 were significantly elevated in SLE patients with microhematuria compared to those without microhematuria (microhematuria negative; $n = 39$, 1693 pg/mL, IQR, 896–2644, versus microhematuria positive; $n = 26$; 2911 pg/mL; IQR, 2156–5139; $p < 0.001$).

3.4. Circulating Levels of sTIM-3 and Organ Damage Measured by the SDI

Finally, we compared serum sTIM-3 levels between SLE patients with or without organ damage (Figure 4). SLE patients were subdivided into two groups based on the presence of at least one organ damage (SDI ≥ 1) ($n = 37$). In SLE patients with SDI ≥ 1, involvement of the ocular ($n = 11$, 29%), renal ($n = 8$, 21%), neuropsychiatric ($n = 6$, 16%), musculoskeletal ($n = 5$, 13%), and respiratory ($n = 5$, 13%) domains were most prevalent. Serum sTIM-3 levels were significantly elevated in SLE patients having at least one organ damaged (SDI ≥ 1) (2710 pg/mL; IQR, 256–7235) than those without organ damage (SDI = 0) (1532 pg/mL; IQR, 228–5274; $p = 0.0102$).

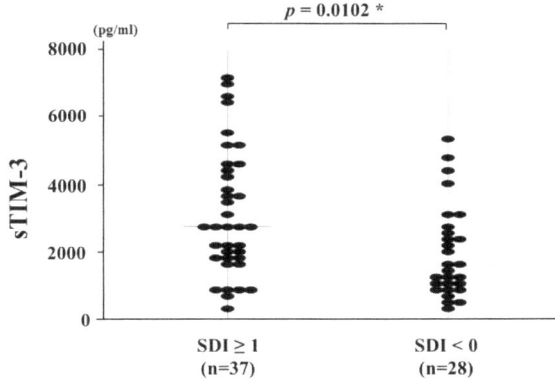

Figure 4. Serum sTIM-3 levels in SLE patients with or without organ damage. Comparison of serum sTIM-3 levels between SLE patients with at least one organ damaged (SDI ≥ 1) and those without organ damage (SDI = 0). Raised serum sTIM-3 levels were shown in SLE patients with at least one organ damage compared with those without organ damage. sTIM-3: soluble T-cell immunoglobulin and mucin-domain-containing molecule 3, SDI: Systemic Lupus International Collaborating Clinics/American College of Rheumatology Damage Index. *, $p < 0.05$ is considered as statistically significant.

4. Discussion

TIM-3 is expressed on the surface of terminally differentiated T cells and has been implicated in the pathogenesis of Th1-driven autoimmune diseases by negatively regulating the T cell response [21]. The identification of Gal-9 as a ligand for TIM-3 revealed that the TIM-3/Gal-9 pathway is an important regulator of Th1 immunity and immune tolerance [22]. SLE is a Th1-dependent human autoimmune disease that is characterized by autoantibody production and immune complex deposition [23]. Although relationships between SLE and immune co-signaling pathways have been identified, TIM-3/Gal-9 interactions in the pathogenesis of SLE have yet to be clarified.

In the present study, we demonstrated that serum sTIM-3 levels were significantly higher in SLE patients than in HCs. We found a positive correlation between serum sTIM-3 levels and SLE disease activity. Additionally, serum sTIM-3 levels were significantly higher in SLE patients with active renal involvement compared with patients without renal lesions. Thus, the relationship between serum sTIM-3 and SLE disease activity or SLE-related organ involvement indicates that serum sTIM-3 can reflect the SLE disease activity. Higher disease activity in SLE patients can increase the risk of subsequent organ damage [24]. Furthermore, circulating sTIM-3 levels can be used to discriminate between SLE patients with and those without organ damage, as measured by the SDI. Accumulated organ damage, which was measured with the SDI, seems to be related to cumulative disease activity over time or the frequency of severe disease flares. However, this damage index can be influenced by causes that are disease- or treatment-related or the result of concomitant disease. The results indicated that serum levels of sTIM-3 are notable as a clinically useful biomarker and can be a predictor for SLE disease activity.

The TIM-3/Gal-9 coinhibitory pathway is thought to be an important modulator of autoimmunity [5]. In SLE patients, the $CD3^+CD4^+TIM3^+$ T cell subset was shown to be increased compared with those in HCs, and TIM-3 expression on T cells correlates with SLE disease activity [25]. Elevated serum levels of Gal-9 were also demonstrated in SLE patients [11,26]. It can be concluded that the TIM-3/Gal-9 pathway activation works in SLE patients as an anti-immune mediator. The administration of intraperitoneal Gal-9 to lupus-prone mice ameliorated their proteinuria and arthritis by decreasing anti-double stranded-DNA antibody levels [27]. However, this pathway can be modulated by the sTIM-3 that is shed from TIM-3 expressed on the surface of the immune cells [28]. TIM-3/Gal-9 interaction may result in T cell exhaustion; in contrast, sTIM-3 seems to have alternative effects against this feedback mechanism. Of note, a soluble form of a receptor may not always result in receptor blockage; further studies are needed to determine the source of serum sTIM-3 and the role of sTIM-3 in SLE pathophysiology.

Jin et al. found an increased level of serum sTIM-3 in SLE patients that was correlated with increased serum IL-17 levels [29]. They also reported that serum sTIM-3 levels were significantly lower in SLE patients with lupus nephritis and that there was no significant correlation between sTIM-3 levels and SLEDAI scores [29]. In contrast, our data showed a positive correlation between serum levels of sTIM-3 and SLEDAI scores or active renal involvement determined by BILAG-2004 scores. These discrepancies could be caused by the variations in the demographic data of the SLE patients studied; in our study, we enrolled untreated patients and patients with active SLE. A further longitudinal study with a large number of SLE patients with different disease phenotypes is required to determine the role of sTIM-3 in SLE pathophysiology.

However, three major limitations should be noted in the present study. First, the sample size was relatively small, which limited the statistical power of this study. Second, our study did not address the organ damage of SLE specifically, which would require a repeated assessment of SLE disease activity over a longer period. Third, the mechanism through which TIM-3/Gal-9 pathway contributes to the pathogenesis of SLE was not clarified. Further research involving a large sample size is required to evaluate the usefulness of sTIM-3 determination in patients with SLE.

5. Conclusions

Our data indicate that patients with SLE have higher circulating levels of sTIM-3 compared with healthy subjects and that sTIM-3 levels correlate with SLE disease activity. These findings indicate a close association between circulating sTIM-3 and active SLE or particular SLE-related organ involvement. This highlights the need for future research to clarify how this association contributes to the development of SLE.

Author Contributions: Conceptualization, T.A., Y.F., N.M., J.T., S.S., H.M., M.Y.-F., E.S., H.K., and H.W.; methodology, T.A. and K.M.; validation, T.A. and K.M.; formal analysis, T.A., Y.F., and N.M.; investigation, T.A., Y.F., and N.M.; resources, T.A., Y.F., and N.M.; data curation, T.A.; writing—original draft preparation, T.A. and K.M.; writing—review and editing, T.A. and K.M.; visualization, K.M.; supervision, K.M.; project administration, K.M.; funding acquisition, K.M. All authors have read and agreed to the published version of the manuscript.

Funding: The study was supported by the Japan Grant-in-Aid for Scientific Research (20K08777).

Acknowledgments: We would like to thank Sachiyo Kanno who provided us technical assistance in this study.

Conflicts of Interest: K.M. has received research grants from Chugai, Pfizer, Eli Lilly, and AbbVie. The rest of the authors declare that they have no competing interests.

Abbreviations

ADAMTS	a disintegrin and metalloproteinase with a thrombospondin type 1 motif
BILAG-2004	British Isles Lupus Assessment Group 2004
IQR	Interquartile range
Gal-9	Galectin-9
SLE	Systemic lupus erythematosus
SLEDAI	Systemic Lupus Erythematosus Disease Activity Index
SLICC	Systemic Lupus International Collaborating Clinics
TIM-3	T cell immunoglobulin and mucin-domain containing 3

References

1. Zhang, Q.; Vignali, D.A. Co-stimulatory and Co-inhibitory pathways in autoimmunity. *Immunity* **2016**, *44*, 1034–1051. [CrossRef] [PubMed]
2. Anderson, A.C.; Anderson, D.E. TIM-3 in autoimmunity. *Curr. Opin. Immunol.* **2006**, *18*, 665–669. [CrossRef] [PubMed]
3. Sánchez-Fueyo, A.; Tian, J.; Picarella, D.; Domenig, C.; Zheng, X.X.; Sabatos, C.A.; Manlongat, N.; Bender, O.; Kamradt, T.; Kuchroo, V.K.; et al. Tim-3 inhibits T helper type 1-mediated auto—and alloimmune responses and promotes immunological tolerance. *Nat. Immunol.* **2003**, *4*, 1093–1101. [CrossRef] [PubMed]
4. Zhu, C.; Anderson, A.C.; Schubart, A.; Xiong, H.; Imitola, J.; Khoury, S.J.; Zheng, X.X.; Strom, T.B.; Kuchroo, V.K. The Tim-3 ligand galectin-9 negatively regulates T helper type 1 immunity. *Nat. Immunol.* **2005**, *6*, 1245–1252. [CrossRef] [PubMed]
5. Pan, H.F.; Zhang, N.; Li, W.X.; Tao, J.H.; Ye, D.Q. TIM-3 as a new therapeutic target in systemic lupus erythematosus. *Mol. Biol. Rep.* **2010**, *37*, 395–398. [CrossRef] [PubMed]
6. Katsuyama, T.; Tsokos, G.C.; Moulton, V.R. Aberrant T cell signaling and subsets in systemic lupus erythematosus. *Front. Immunol.* **2018**, *9*, 1088. [CrossRef] [PubMed]
7. Tsokos, G.C.; Lo, M.S.; Costa Reis, P.; Sullivan, K.E. New insights into the immunopathogenesis of systemic lupus erythematosus. *Nat. Rev. Rheumatol* **2016**, *12*, 716–730. [CrossRef]
8. Ni, L.; Dong, C. New checkpoints in cancer immunotherapy. *Immunol. Rev.* **2017**, *276*, 52–65. [CrossRef]
9. Sebastiani, G.D.; Scirocco, C.; Galeazzi, M. Rheumatic immune related adverse events in patients treated with checkpoint inhibitors for immunotherapy of cancer. *Autoimmun. Rev.* **2019**, *18*, 805–813. [CrossRef]
10. Boenisch, O.; D'Addio, F.; Watanabe, T.; Elyaman, W.; Magee, C.N.; Yeung, M.Y.; Padera, R.F.; Rodig, S.J.; Murayama, T.; Tanaka, K.; et al. TIM-3: A novel regulatory molecule of alloimmune activation. *J. Immunol.* **2010**, *185*, 5806–5819. [CrossRef]
11. Van den Hoogen, L.L.; van Roon, J.A.G.; Mertens, J.S.; Wienke, J.; Lopes, A.P.; de Jager, W.; Rossato, M.; Pandit, A.; Wichers, C.G.K.; van Wijk, F.; et al. Galectin-9 is an easy to measure biomarker for the interferon signature in systemic lupus erythematosus and antiphospholipid syndrome. *Ann. Rheum. Dis.* **2018**, *77*, 1810–1814. [CrossRef] [PubMed]
12. Sakuishi, K.; Jayaraman, P.; Behar, S.M.; Anderson, A.C.; Kuchroo, V.K. Emerging Tim-3 functions in antimicrobial and tumor immunity. *Trends Immunol.* **2011**, *32*, 345–349. [CrossRef]
13. Song, L.J.; Wang, X.; Wang, X.P.; Li, D.; Ding, F.; Liu, H.X.; Yu, X.; Li, X.F.; Shu, Q. Increased Tim-3 expression on peripheral T lymphocyte subsets and association with higher disease activity in systemic lupus erythematosus. *Diagn. Pathol.* **2015**, *10*, 71. [CrossRef] [PubMed]
14. Möller-Hackbarth, K.; Dewitz, C.; Schweigert, O.; Trad, A.; Garbers, C.; Rose-John, S.; Scheller, J. A disintegrin and metalloprotease (ADAM) 10 and ADAM17 are major sheddases of T cell immunoglobulin and mucin domain 3 (Tim-3). *J. Biol. Chem.* **2013**, *288*, 34529–34544. [CrossRef]
15. Chiba, M.; Yanaba, K.; Hayashi, M.; Yoshihara, Y.; Nakagawa, H. Clinical significance of serum soluble T-cell immunoglobulin and mucin domain 3 levels in systemic sclerosis: Association with disease severity. *J. Derm.* **2017**, *44*, 194–197. [CrossRef]
16. Hochberg, M.C. Updating the American College of Rheumatology revised criteria for the classification of systemic lupus erythematosus. *Arthritis Rheum.* **1997**, *40*, 1725. [CrossRef] [PubMed]

17. Bombardier, C.; Gladman, D.D.; Urowitz, M.B.; Caron, D.; Chang, C.H. Derivation of the SLEDAI. A disease activity index for lupus patients. The Committee on Prognosis Studies in SLE. *Arthritis Rheum.* **1992**, *35*, 630–640. [CrossRef]
18. Gladman, D.; Ginzler, E.; Goldsmith, C.; Fortin, P.; Liang, M.; Urowitz, M.; Bacon, P.; Bombardieri, S.; Hanly, J.; Hay, E.; et al. The development and initial validation of the systemic lupus international collaborating clinics/American College of Rheumatology damage index for systemic lupus erythematosus. *Arthritis Rheum.* **1996**, *39*, 363–369. [CrossRef] [PubMed]
19. Isenberg, D.A.; Rahman, A.; Allen, E.; Farewell, V.; Akil, M.; Bruce, I.N.; D'Cruz, D.; Griffiths, B.; Khamashta, M.; Maddison, P.; et al. BILAG 2004. Development and initial validation of an updated version of the british isles lupus assessment group's disease activity index for patients with systemic lupus erythematosus. *Rheumatology* **2005**, *44*, 902–906. [CrossRef] [PubMed]
20. Stoll, T.; Stucki, G.; Malik, J.; Pyke, S.; Isenberg, D.A. Further validation of the BILAG disease activity index in patients with systemic lupus erythematosus. *Ann. Rheum. Dis.* **1996**, *55*, 756–760. [CrossRef]
21. Monney, L.; Sabatos, C.A.; Gaglia, J.L.; Ryu, A.; Waldner, H.; Chernova, T.; Manning, S.; Greenfield, E.A.; Coyle, A.J.; Sobel, R.A.; et al. Th1-specific cell surface protein Tim-3 regulates macrophage activation and severity of an autoimmune disease. *Nature* **2002**, *415*, 536–541. [CrossRef]
22. Kuchroo, V.K.; Umetsu, D.T.; DeKruyff, R.H.; Freeman, G.J. The TIM gene family: Emerging roles in immunity and disease. *Nat. Rev. Immunol.* **2003**, *3*, 454–462. [CrossRef]
23. Moulton, V.R.; Suarez-Fueyo, A.; Meidan, E.; Li, H.; Mizui, M.; Tsokos, G.C. Pathogenesis of human systemic lupus erythematosus: A cellular perspective. *Trends Mol. Med.* **2017**, *23*, 615–635. [CrossRef]
24. Rao, V.; Gordon, C. Advances in the assessment of lupus disease activity and damage. *Curr. Opin. Rheumatol.* **2014**, *26*, 510–519. [CrossRef]
25. Jiao, Q.; Qian, Q.; Zhao, Z.; Fang, F.; Hu, X.; An, J.; Wu, J.; Liu, C. Expression of human T cell immunoglobulin domain and mucin-3 (TIM-3) and TIM-3 ligands in peripheral blood from patients with systemic lupus erythematosus. *Arch. Derm. Res.* **2016**, *308*, 553–561. [CrossRef] [PubMed]
26. Matsuoka, N.; Fujita, Y.; Temmoku, J.; Furuya, M.Y.; Asano, T.; Sato, S.; Matsumoto, H.; Kobayashi, H.; Watanabe, H.; Suzuki, E.; et al. Galectin-9 as a biomarker for disease activity in systemic lupus erythematosus. *PLoS ONE* **2020**, *15*, e0227069. [CrossRef] [PubMed]
27. Moritoki, M.; Kadowaki, T.; Niki, T.; Nakano, D.; Soma, G.; Mori, H.; Kobara, H.; Masaki, T.; Kohno, M.; Hirashima, M. Galectin-9 ameliorates clinical severity of MRL/lpr lupus-prone mice by inducing plasma cell apoptosis independently of Tim-3. *PLoS ONE* **2013**, *8*, e60807. [CrossRef]
28. Geng, H.; Zhang, G.M.; Li, D.; Zhang, H.; Yuan, Y.; Zhu, H.G.; Xiao, H.; Han, L.F.; Feng, Z.H. Soluble form of T cell Ig mucin 3 is an inhibitory molecule in T cell-mediated immune response. *J. Immunol.* **2006**, *176*, 1411–1420. [CrossRef]
29. Jin, L.; Bai, R.; Zhou, J.; Shi, W.; Xu, L.; Sheng, J.; Peng, H.; Jin, Y.; Yuan, H. Association of serum T cell immunoglobulin domain and Mucin-3 and Interleukin-17 with systemic lupus erythematosus. *Med. Sci. Monit. Basic Res.* **2018**, *24*, 168–176. [CrossRef] [PubMed]

Publisher's Note: MDPI stays neutral with regard to jurisdictional claims in published maps and institutional affiliations.

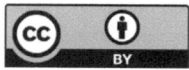

© 2020 by the authors. Licensee MDPI, Basel, Switzerland. This article is an open access article distributed under the terms and conditions of the Creative Commons Attribution (CC BY) license (http://creativecommons.org/licenses/by/4.0/).

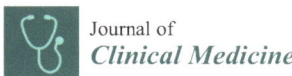 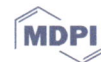

Review

The Main Challenges in Systemic Lupus Erythematosus: Where Do We Stand?

Matteo Piga [1] and Laurent Arnaud [2,3,*]

1. Rheumatology Unit, AOU University Clinic and University of Cagliari, 09042 Cagliari, Italy; matteopiga@unica.it
2. Service de Rhumatologie, Hôpitaux Universitaires de Strasbourg, Université de Strasbourg, 67000 Strasbourg, France
3. Centre National de Références des Maladies Systémiques et Auto-immunes Rares Est Sud-Ouest (RESO), 67000 Strasbourg, France
* Correspondence: Laurent.arnaud@chru-strasbourg.fr

Abstract: Systemic lupus erythematosus (SLE) is an immune-mediated multi-systemic disease characterized by a wide variability of clinical manifestations and a course frequently subject to unpredictable flares. Despite significant advances in the understanding of the pathophysiology and optimization of medical care, patients with SLE still have significant mortality and carry a risk of progressive organ damage accrual and reduced health-related quality of life. New tools allow earlier classification of SLE, whereas tailored early intervention and treatment strategies targeted to clinical remission or low disease activity could offer the opportunity to reduce damage, thus improving long-term outcomes. Nevertheless, the early diagnosis of SLE is still an unmet need for many patients. Further disentangling the SLE susceptibility and complex pathogenesis will allow to identify more accurate biomarkers and implement new ways to measure disease activity. This could represent a major step forward to find new trials modalities for developing new drugs, optimizing the use of currently available therapeutics and minimizing glucocorticoids. Preventing and treating comorbidities in SLE, improving the management of hard-to-treat manifestations including management of SLE during pregnancy are among the remaining major unmet needs. This review provides insights and a research agenda for the main challenges in SLE.

Keywords: systemic lupus erythematosus; review; disease activity; damage; glucocorticoids

Citation: Piga, M.; Arnaud, L. The Main Challenges in Systemic Lupus Erythematosus: Where Do We Stand? *J. Clin. Med.* **2021**, *10*, 243. https://doi.org/10.3390/jcm10020243

Received: 16 December 2020
Accepted: 8 January 2021
Published: 11 January 2021

Publisher's Note: MDPI stays neutral with regard to jurisdictional claims in published maps and institutional affiliations.

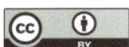

Copyright: © 2021 by the authors. Licensee MDPI, Basel, Switzerland. This article is an open access article distributed under the terms and conditions of the Creative Commons Attribution (CC BY) license (https://creativecommons.org/licenses/by/4.0/).

1. Introduction

Despite great improvements in treatment strategies leading to an improved prognosis [1–3], numerous challenges and unmet needs remain for the diagnosis and therapeutic management of Systemic Lupus Erythematosus (SLE) [4,5]. In this review we will provide an overview of the main unmet needs in the field of SLE (Figure 1), as a way to inform physicians, policy makers, funding institutions, and more generally the broad scientific community about the challenges and opportunities which remain in SLE research and clinical care.

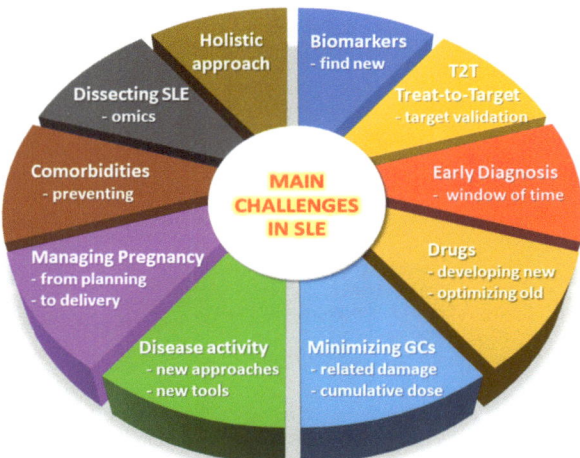

Figure 1. Overview of the main unmet needs in the field of Systemic Lupus Erythematosus (SLE).

2. Promoting Early Diagnosis

SLE is a complex disease with variable phenotypes and clinical manifestations. SLE onset is often insidious, with clinically evident disease developing over years. In addition, a variety of conditions may mimic SLE [6], including infectious and hematologic diseases, and for all these reasons the diagnosis may be delayed. It should not be surprising the median reported delay in SLE diagnosis is approximately 2 years.

It is common feeling that the early diagnosis of SLE can be beneficial by allowing early intervention and potentially improving short and long-term outcomes [5]. There is few evidence supporting this assumption and mainly derives from administrative database analysis showing that the patients with early diagnosis (<6 months between probable SLE onset and diagnosis) had lower rates of flares and hospitalizations compared with the late diagnosis patients ($\geq$6 months) [7]. However, a clear identification of an early time frame between onset and diagnosis by which there are superior clinical responses and higher rate of remission in SLE patients has not been identified. Therefore, it is not proven that a window of opportunity really exists in SLE and a generally accepted definition of early disease is still lacking.

The identification of clinical and serological features useful in the differential diagnosis of patients with recent SLE onset [8] has facilitated the definition of classification criteria with greater sensitivity and specificity for early SLE compared to the previous validated criteria set [9]. Nonetheless, a recent single-center retrospective study suggested that 7–17% of patients diagnosed as having early SLE are not correctly classified using the EULAR/ACR 2019 [9], SLICC 2012 [10] and ACR 1982/1997 [11] criteria individually, while the combined use of all three sets of criteria ensured the classification of 94–98% of patients [12]. New tools for SLE classification are a major step forward for scientific purpose and may help in the earlier recognition of the disease, but they are not developed and should not be used for diagnostic purpose.

One major challenge is to implement effective strategies for earlier SLE diagnosis. These would take on greater value if a window of opportunity for SLE patients will be found and proven to improve outcomes including damage, death, recurrent flares, and Health-Related Quality of Life (HRQoL) measures.

3. Targeting Disease Remission (or Low Disease Activity)

Preventing flares and reducing damage accrual trough control of disease activity and reduction or withdrawn of glucocorticoids (GCs) are major challenges in SLE management and represents some of the objectives of the treat-to-target strategy for SLE (T2T/SLE) [13]. The T2T/SLE identified remission or low disease activity as the most important targets in SLE treatment, while it was recognized that there was no clear definitions for them. Recent advances in T2T/SLE include relevant definitions of clinical remission (CR) on treatment [14,15] and Lupus Low Disease Activity State (LLDAS) [16]. These definitions recognize the importance of durable absence or residual of disease activity measured using validated tools (SLEDAI, PGA), together with a stable treatment with antimalarials and/or immunosuppressants and a low GCs dose (prednisone ≤ 5 mg/day in CR and ≤ 7.5 mg/day in LLDAS). Although there is an ongoing debate around the potential overlap between CR and LLDAS definitions [17], they have been widely studied and resulted predictive of lower damage accrual in both newly diagnosed and long-standing SLE cohorts [18–21]. Interestingly, CR and LLDAS resulted independently associated with lower early damage accrual in an inception SLE cohort [22], confirming that CR is recommended as the primary treatment target in SLE and LLDAS represents a valid alternative also in the early stage of SLE management. Recently, the LLDAS has been prospectively validated as a SLE treatment endpoint in a multicenter international cohort demonstrating significant protection against flare and damage accrual [23].

Although LLDAS may represent a sufficiently validated outcome to be applied in clinical practice and trials, we still believe that treatment in SLE should aim at remission unless otherwise possible. Therefore, a major challenge is represented by the need to adequately validate existing definitions of CR in order to identify an attainable remission treatment endpoint, which should be indeed predictive of outcomes including damage, recurrent flares and death. Moreover, further data are needed on the role of CR and LLDAS in predicting better HRQoL outcome.

4. Considering New Ways to Assess Disease Activity

The quantification of disease activity in SLE represents a complex multi-dimensional concept, encompassing the physician evaluation of specific clinical manifestations attributed to SLE, the efficacy and response to prescribed medications and the patient personal feelings.

There are several physician-centered indices for disease activity assessment in SLE. Well-established measures exist to assess disease activity in specific organ (e.g., the Cutaneous Lupus Erythematosus Disease Area and Severity Index) but lack in others (e.g., musculoskeletal or renal manifestations). On the other hand, several tools have been developed to assess the overall disease activity. The most used include the SLE disease activity index (SLEDAI) and its evolutions, the British Isles Lupus Assessment Group (BILAG) and its revision, the European Consensus Lupus Assessment Measure (ECLAM), and the physician's global assessment (PGA) by visual analogue scale. None of them have shown sufficient accuracy and sensitivity to change to be used alone as primary endpoints in RCTs. The PGA also suffers from reduced reliability suggesting the major need for standardization of its scoring [24,25]. We have therefore initiated an international collaboration to standardize the rating of the PGA in SLE (the PISCOS Study). Accordingly, novel composite outcomes such as the SLE responder index (SRI), which is based on the improvement of the SLEDAI with no worsening of the BILAG and the PGA, have appeared. Despite being considered more accurate in evaluate responsiveness to treatment, the SRI carries disadvantages of the individual indices from which it is composed, not least the need for clinician to judge if each manifestation is due to SLE or not. Recently, the SLE disease activity score (SLE-DAS), a continuous global score showing higher sensitivity to change and specificity than SLEDAI-2K [26], has been developed and is waiting for extensive validation. The patient component of disease assessment in SLE is not straightforward as patients tend to assess fatigue and pain, which are hardly related to disease activity.

Lupus patients and physicians are facing the need for more objective, reliable and reproducible ways to assess disease activity. Identifying new biomarkers of overall and organ specific disease activity and implementing their use in composite index may represent a major step forward. The application of deep machine-learning approaches would be helpful in the early identification of unfavorable individual patient trajectories among large SLE cohorts.

5. Minimizing the Use of Glucocorticoids

GCs still play a pivotal role in the treatment of SLE, especially in case of severe manifestations. However, several studies have emphasized the detrimental effects of chronic GCs therapy, particularly the increased risk for irreversible organ damage accrual. It has remained unclear which, if any, daily prednisone (equivalent) dose best prevent damage. Although <7.5 mg/day seem to minimize risk, even lower daily doses (4.4–6 mg/day) have been associated with a significant increase of damage [27]. In a recent multicenter Italian inception study, GC-related damage was independently associated with cumulative dose and steadily increased over time despite the reduced median daily prednisone dose below 5 mg since 12-month of follow-up [28]. However, it is not yet understood if and when GSs can be withdrawn [29]. In a survey by the SLICC group, almost 33% of patients never discontinued GCs after a mean follow-up of 7.26 years [30]. An observational study suggested that GC withdrawal is an achievable goal in SLE and may be attempted after a long-term remission or LLDAS to protect the patient from disease flares [31]. Contrarily, a randomized control trial (RCT) showed that patients with quiescent SLE who discontinued low-dose prednisone (5 mg/day) experienced significantly more flares than those who maintained this treatment [32].

Several challenges about the use of GCs in SLE emerged from these findings. Future RCTs should specifically address strategies to design effective GC tapering scheme enabling the use of the minimal possible dose of GCs for the shortest duration while minimizing the risk of flare. Moreover, when testing the efficacy of newly developed medication for the management of SLE, steroid sparing should be included in the assessment by means of cumulative GC doses or GC-related adverse events.

6. Developing More Effective Drugs and Optimizing the Use of Those Currently Available

The therapeutic management and global prognosis [33] of SLE have profoundly evolved over the years [2]. Following the discovery of GCs by Hench in the 40′, post-WW2 chemistry has brought many conventional immunosuppressive agents such as cyclosporine, azathioprine, cyclophosphamide, and more recently mycophenolate mofetil. Some adverse events have also taught us that some treatments can paradoxically induce lupus [34]. Antimalarials, the mainstay of SLE treatments have very favourable properties in lupus, but their efficacy to control disease activity and prevent flares is limited when used alone [35]. This has led to the need for the development of new treatments in SLE [36–38]. Unfortunately, effective therapeutics beyond GCs and classical immunosuppressive agents are limited [3]. Randomized controlled trials of rituximab and of at least 18 other molecules have failed in SLE, mostly due to issues associated with disease heterogeneity and trial design [39]. Therefore, there is only weak evidence upon which to base recommendations in many situations [40]. Optimizing the use of currently available therapeutics may represent a breakthrough. Belimumab has recently been tested in a 2-year RCT (BLISS-LN) in lupus nephritis and proved safe and effective when associated with the standard of care, while so far it was tested only in patients without active nephritis [41]. In an observational prospective study (BeRLiSS) treatment with belimumab early in the disease lead to better outcomes [42], which may suggest addressing the use of this agent as part of the first-line therapy for selected patients in innovative RCTs. Moreover, it appears urgent to develop more effective treatments in SLE, either through innovative trials of new agents [43] or of immunosuppressive drugs previously not tested in SLE (e.g., repository trials). Voclosporin, a next-generation calcineurin inhibitor, added to standard of care for induction therapy of active lupus nephritis resulted in a superior renal response but higher rates of adverse events including death were observed [44] Among the most recent advances is the better understanding of the role of interferons in the pathogenesis of SLE, which allowed for the development of drugs directly or indirectly targeting these pathways, such as interferon receptor blockers [36] or JAK inhibitors. Cellular therapy has shown interesting preliminary data and should also be improved [45] while new approaches, such as the use of low-dose IL-2 to expand regulatory T cells have emerged and appear promising [46]. Altogether, it is crucial to optimize the use of currently available therapeutics and develop new molecules assessing their efficacy through adequately designed trials using validated and robust outcomes.

7. Dissecting the Heterogeneity of the Disease

Environmental factors play a significant role in SLE development [47] but the interplay between genetic and environmental factors remains poorly understood at the patient level [3]. Also, epidemiology studies across different ethnic backgrounds are needed to understand better the polygenic basis and environmental influences upon disease risk, phenotypes and prognosis [3,8]. A large amount of evidence highlight that SLE has 3–4 times higher incidence, higher rate of lupus nephritis, worse severity in terms of damage accrual, HRQoL outcomes and three times greater mortality among African-Americans and other ethnic groups then in Caucasians. Although the LUMINA and Hopkins Lupus cohorts in the USA proved that socio-economic status play a major role in such ethnic disparities it is also conceivable that biologic differences might be responsible for distinct phenotypes. The SLE burden, mortality, outcomes, and quality of care and insights into health disparities and possible remedies across different ethnic backgrounds have been reviewed elsewhere [48–50].

Understanding the genetic component of SLE is complex because most patients have polygenic disease [51–53]. Genome-Wide Association Studies (GWAS) have allowed the description of more than 100 susceptibility Single Nucleotide Polymorphisms (SNPs) for SLE [52,53]. Most of those SNPs individually confer only a slight increase in the risk of SLE, making them of limited clinical utility for the diagnosis of the disease. Also, variants identified by GWAS explain only a fraction of overall heritability of SLE. Therefore, there is a missing heritability which could be explained notably by epigenetics, which remains poorly known in SLE. Finally, although very rare, the monogenic forms must be considered in the study of SLE genetics [6]. One major challenge is to develop efficient tools for characterizing patient and ethnic background heterogeneity using multi-omics. This will allow the development of personalized medicine for SLE patients. Currently, most teams are still using inaccurate biomarkers and the most recent advances are far from being implemented in most center.

8. Identifying Relevant Biomarkers for Individualized Treatment

Biomarkers to predict disease prognosis, disease remission and long-term adverse events are truly lacking in SLE [3]. The reliable identification of the right treatment for the right patient currently remains one of the most important challenges in SLE. In daily practice, the list of biomarkers which can be used in SLE has remained very limited, and includes mostly anti-dsDNA antibodies, complement factor proteins or leukopenia. Those are now insufficient to progress in the management of the disease and it is therefore crucial to identify reliable and advanced biomarkers. The era of multi-omics, biological analysis approach in which data from multiple "-omes" (such as the genome, transcriptome, proteome, epigenome, metabolome and microbiome), theoretically opens the door for highly integrated and individualized approaches [54]. At a proteomic level, cytokine profiles could be used as potential biomarkers. The most emblematic example is type I interferon gene signature found in the sera of 70–80% of active SLE patients. Blood interferon-alpha levels have been associated with the risk of subsequent flares in SLE [36]. Another approach is to assess urinary biomarkers in case of lupus nephritis [55], as this could be a better reflect of the local inflammation than when using blood-based markers. Pioneering studies tried to incorporate clinical characteristics into personalized immune-transcriptional data enabling patient stratification based on the immune networks best correlating with disease activity and providing a rationale for tailored therapeutic interventions [56]. One of the main current challenges is to integrate the vast amount of data available at the patient-level to make accurate predictions. This will require an in-depth interaction between clinical specialists, researchers in biomedicine and data scientists, with the help of artificial intelligence (Figure 2).

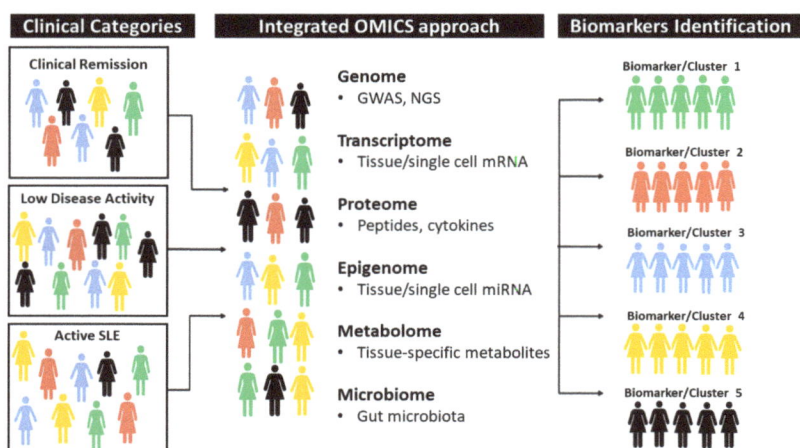

Figure 2. A hypothetical example illustrating how an integrated clinical and OMICS approach, driven by artificial intelligence, might help distinguishing homogeneous clusters from current heterogeneous phenotypes observed in Systemic Lupus Erythematosus (SLE). The example suggests that the way to identify new clusters with specific disease biomarkers should be tailored to the specific molecular events or pathways associated with disease activity and clinical phenotypes, providing a rationale for personalized therapeutic interventions.

9. Managing Pregnancy in SLE

Pregnancy is a major challenge in SLE, and is generally managed by a tandem of a rheumatologist and obstetrician with significant experience with high-risk pregnancies, especially in case of antiphospholipid syndrome [57]. Pregnancy should be carefully anticipated in SLE, and pre-pregnancy multidisciplinary counseling is important to estimate the risk of maternal and fetal complications [58]. SLE is usually not associated with infertility unless the patient has been treated with cyclophosphamide, and ovarian protection strategies using GnRH agonists or ovarian preservation can be used, if needed. It is commonly recommended that the disease has been quiescent for at least 6 months (some experts suggest one year in case of lupus nephritis) before pregnancy is allowed because active SLE at the time of conception is a strong predictor of maternal and fetal complications. Also, positivity for antiphospholipid antibodies or SSA/SSB antibodies is associated with worst obstetrical outcomes, including prematurity, growth retardation, fetal death, neonatal lupus and congenital heat block [57,59]. One of the critical issues in managing women with SLE during pregnancy is choosing the right medication to treat the mother without harming the baby. Unfortunately, most medications used in SLE are potentially harmful or contraindicated during pregnancy and must be reviewed when planning pregnancy. However, there are safe options such as hydroxychloroquine (HCQ) and low dose aspirin (LDA) which demonstrated effective in reducing disease flares, obstetric and new-born complications [60,61]. Nevertheless, recent surveys found that the use of these drugs in pregnant women with SLE is still limited (HCQ 58% and LDA 25% of pregnancies) and should be increased [61,62]. Among the main challenges, ensuring fertility and proper course of pregnancy is of outstanding importance, especially in case of antiphospholipid syndrome, and remains one of the most important clinical challenges in SLE.

10. Preventing Comorbidities

Comorbidities, such as cardiovascular disease (CVD) and infections, are major responsible of increased mortality in patients with SLE. CVD is the leading cause of mortality in SLE regardless of time to occurrence after diagnosis [63]. The higher burden of CVD in SLE patients is mosly related to accelerated atherosclerosis, which leads to CV events at an earlier age compared to the general population. Accelerated atherosclerosis is driven by the interplay between inflammation, autoimmunity, medications and traditional risk factors. No surprisingly, the traditional CV risk factors are not sufficient to fully explain the increased number of CV events observed in SLE [64], which leads to an underestimation of the actual risk using existing tools validated in the general population. Recommendations for the management of CV risk factors in SLE patients exists [65], including the widespread use of hydroxychloroquine [66]. A major challenge we have to face is the need of validated tools for estimation of the CV risk in SLE, which represents the first step for conducting therapeutic trials to provide more evidence-based data on how to manage CV risk in SLE patients.

Infections are risk factor higher than disease activity for mortality in SLE patients [63,67]. GCs use, immunosuppressive therapy and lupus nephritis are the most important risk factor for infections in SLE patients. GCs related risk of infection increases by 12% for each mg/day of prednisone, thus is already high at 7.5 mg/day which is considered relatively safe for damage accrual [68]. In a recent meta-analysis, GCs were associated with an increased risk of COVID-19 in patients with autoimmune diseases including SLE [69]. A number of prophylactic measures against infections should be recommended in SLE. A recent audit of the British Society for Rheumatology estimated 34.3% of SLE patients need to adopt extreme social distancing measures ("shielding") to minimize the risk of SARS-Cov2 infection [70]. Vaccination campaign should be implemented as vaccine administration rates remain low in SLE, in particular for vaccine against pneumococcus and influenza [71]. These are inactivated vaccines and therefore can be used at any time in SLE even though their immunogenicity may be substantially reduced if patient is taking immunosuppressant or high dose GCs. On the other hand, live attenuated vaccines are contraindicated in patients taking more than 10 mg/day of prednisone or immunosuppressant. The risk of SLE flare after vaccination is not confirmed, but vaccination should be avoided in patients with active disease. In order to reduce serious infections, besides the requirement to reduce chronic use of GCs there is an urgent need to strengthen the immunization coverage in patients with SLE. New vaccine strategies need to be evaluated and validated specifically in SLE also given the forthcoming availability of vaccination against Sars-Cov2.

11. Favoring a Global and Comprehensive Disease Management

An important challenge in SLE is to favor holistic medicine, which is the use of therapeutic strategies that attempt to treat the patient as a whole person. Feedback from SLE patients is essential. Patient-reported outcomes (PROs) capture patients' perceptions of their health condition, HRQoL [72], well-being, and other aspects. Those encompass many crucial domains such as fatigue, anxiety, and depression among many others [73]. The use of PROs in daily clinical practice currently remains limited while those tools are essential for better characterizing the impact of SLE at the individual patient level [74]. Of note, the management of common, hard-to-treat manifestations, such as fatigue and depression should be clarified in SLE, according to EULAR [3]. For instance, we found that fatigue was reported by more than two-thirds patients and severe fatigue by more than one third in the large international FATILUP study [73]. We have also shown that the association between fatigue, anxiety and depression is very strong in SLE patients with inactive disease [75]. Therefore, we should conduct more and better designed trials to evaluate psycho-behavioral interventions as well as pharmacological interventions for the management of fatigue in SLE, targeting depression and anxiety. In SLE, just as in any other chronic disease, the proportion of patients not adhering fully to the prescribed treatments is very high [76] and can lead to apparently refractory disease [77]. The main predictors of non-adherence are a younger age, non-white ethnic background, low social-economic level, lower education level, unemployment, never-use of GCs, polymedication, mood disorders such as depression and rural residency [76,78]. Non-adherence contributes to worse patient outcomes, including an increased number of flares, visits to emergency departments and, importantly, mortality [76]. Also, disease prevalence, activity and severity is strongly increased in SLE smokers compared to non-smokers [79], while therapeutic responses are decreased [80]. It is therefore crucial to encourage SLE patients to stop tobacco. Also, physical inactivity is common in SLE with up to 72% of patients who do not meet the WHO recommendations [81]. Systematic reviews suggested that exercise reduces fatigue and depression, improves cardiorespiratory capacity without affecting disease activity [82,83]. Altogether, SLE should be managed globally as a chronic disease, understanding the patient's perspective in her own holistic context.

12. Conclusions

Altogether, these challenges may be considered as an SLE roadmap for clinicians, researchers and health policy makers who wish to contribute to an improved and integrated management of this rare and complex disease.

Author Contributions: M.P. and L.A. contributed equally to conceptualization, methodology, investigation, data analysis and writing. All authors have read and agreed to the published version of the manuscript.

Funding: This research received no external funding.

Acknowledgments: The authors wish to thank Sylvie Thuong for her invaluable assistance in the handling of the manuscript.

Conflicts of Interest: Matteo PIGA has received honoraria and/or funding from BMS, GSK, Novartis, Pfizer. Laurent ARNAUD has received honoraria and/or funding from Amgen, Astra-Zeneca, GSK, Janssen-Cilag, LFB, Lilly, Menarini France, Novartis, Pfizer, Roche-Chugai, UCB.

References

1. Arnaud, L.; Fagot, J.P.; Mathian, A.; Paita, M.; Fagot-Campagna, A.; Amoura, Z. Prevalence and incidence of systemic lupus erythematosus in France: A 2010 nation-wide population-based study. *Autoimmun. Rev.* **2014**, *13*, 1082–1089. [CrossRef] [PubMed]
2. Felten, R.; Lipsker, D.; Sibilia, J.; Chasset, F.; Arnaud, L. The history of lupus throughout the ages. *J. Am. Acad. Dermatol.* **2020**, *20*, 30772–30776. [CrossRef] [PubMed]
3. RheumaMap. A Research Roadmap to Transform the Lives of People with Rheumatic and Musculoskeletal Diseases. Available online: https://www.eular.org/myUploadData/files/eular_rheumamap_2019.pdf (accessed on 16 December 2020).
4. Tamirou, F.; Arnaud, L.; Talarico, R.; Scirè, C.A.; Alexander, T.; Amoura, Z.; Avcin, T.; Bortoluzzi, A.; Cervera, R.; Conti, F.; et al. Systemic lupus erythematosus: State of the art on clinical practice guidelines. *RMD Open* **2018**, *4*, e000793. [CrossRef] [PubMed]
5. Arnaud, L.; Tektonidou, M.G. Long-term outcomes in systemic lupus erythematosus: Trends over time and major contributors. *Rheumatology* **2020**, *59 S5*, v29–v38. [CrossRef]
6. Chasset, F.; Richez, C.; Martin, T.; Belot, A.; Korganow, A.-S.; Arnaud, L. Rare diseases that mimic Systemic Lupus Erythematosus (Lupus mimickers). *Jt. Bone Spine* **2019**, *86*, 165–171. [CrossRef] [PubMed]
7. Oglesby, A.; Korves, C.; Laliberté, F.; Dennis, G.; Rao, S.; Suthoff, E.D.; Wei, R.; Sheng Duh, M. Impact of early versus late systemic lupus erythematosus diagnosis on clinical and economic outcomes. *Appl. Health Econ. Health Policy* **2014**, *12*, 179–190. [CrossRef]
8. Mosca, M.; Costenbader, K.H.; Johnson, S.R.; Lorenzoni, V.; Sebastiani, G.D.; Hoyer, B.F.; Navarra, S.; Bonfa, E.; Ramsey-Goldman, R.; Medina-Rosas, J.; et al. Brief Report: How Do Patients with Newly Diagnosed Systemic Lupus Erythematosus Present? A Multicenter Cohort of Early Systemic Lupus Erythematosus to Inform the Development of New Classification Criteria. *Arthritis Rheumatol.* **2019**, *71*, 91–98. [CrossRef]
9. Aringer, M.; Costenbader, K.; Daikh, D.; Brinks, R.; Mosca, M.; Ramsey-Goldman, R.; Smolen, J.S.; Wofsy, D.; Boumpas, D.T.; Kamen, D.L.; et al. 2019 European League Against Rheumatism/American College of Rheumatology classification criteria for systemic lupus erythematosus. *Ann. Rheum. Dis.* **2019**, *78*, 1151–1159. [CrossRef]
10. Petri, M.; Orbai, A.-M.; Alarcón, G.S.; Gordon, C.; Merrill, J.T.; Fortin, P.R.; Bruce, I.N.; Isenberg, D.; Wallace, D.J.; Nived, O.; et al. Derivation and validation of the systemic lupus in-ternational collaborating clinics classification criteria for systemic lupus erythematosus. *Arthritis Rheum.* **2012**, *64*, 2677–2686. [CrossRef]
11. Hochberg, M.C. Updating the American College of rheumatology revised criteria for the classification of systemic lupus erythematosus. *Arthritis Rheum.* **1997**, *40*, 1725. [CrossRef]

12. Adamichou, C.; Nikolopoulos, D.; Genitsaridi, I.; Bortoluzzi, A.; Fanouriakis, A.; Papastefanakis, E.; Kalogiannaki, E.; Gergianaki, I.; Sidiropoulos, P.; Boumpas, D.T.; et al. In an early SLE cohort the ACR-1997, SLICC-2012 and EULAR/ACR-2019 criteria classify non-overlapping groups of patients: Use of all three criteria ensures optimal capture for clinical studies while their modification earlier classification and treatment. *Ann. Rheum. Dis.* **2019**, *79*, 232–241. [CrossRef] [PubMed]
13. Van Vollenhoven, R.F.; Mosca, M.; Bertsias, G.; Isenberg, D.; Kuhn, A.; Lerstrøm, K.; Aringer, M.; Bootsma, H.; Boumpas, D.; Bruce, I.N.; et al. Treat-to-target in systemic lupus erythe-matosus: Recommendations from an international task force. *Ann. Rheum. Dis.* **2014**, *73*, 958–967. [CrossRef] [PubMed]
14. Zen, M.; Iaccarino, L.; Gatto, M.; Bettio, S.; Nalotto, L.; Ghirardello, A.; Punzi, L.; Doria, A. Prolonged remission in Caucasian patients with SLE: Prevalence and outcomes. *Ann. Rheum. Dis.* **2015**, *74*, 2117–2122. [CrossRef] [PubMed]
15. Van Vollenhoven, R.; Voskuyl, A.; Bertsias, G.; Aranow, C.; Aringer, M.; Arnaud, L.; Askanase, A.; Bálažová, P.; Bonfa, E.; Bootsma, H.; et al. A framework for remission in SLE: Consensus findings from a large interna-tional task force on definitions of remission in SLE (DORIS). *Ann. Rheum. Dis.* **2017**, *76*, 554–561. [CrossRef] [PubMed]
16. Franklyn, K.; Lau, C.S.; Navarra, S.V.; Louthrenoo, W.; Lateef, A.; Hamijoyo, L.; Wahono, C.S.; Le Chen, S.; Jin, O.; Morton, S.; et al. Definition and initial validation of a Lupus Low Disease Activity State (LLDAS). *Ann. Rheum. Dis.* **2016**, *75*, 1615–1621. [CrossRef]
17. Zen, M.; Iaccarino, L.; Gatto, M.; Saccon, F.; LaRosa, M.; Ghirardello, A.; Punzi, L.; Doria, A. Lupus low disease activity state is associated with a decrease in damage progression in Caucasian patients with SLE, but overlaps with remission. *Ann. Rheum. Dis.* **2018**, *77*, 104–110. [CrossRef]
18. Piga, M.; Floris, A.; Cappellazzo, G.; Chessa, E.; Congia, M.; Mathieu, A.; Cauli, A. Failure to achieve lupus low disease activity state (LLDAS) six months after diagnosis is associated with early damage accrual in Caucasian patients with systemic lupus ery-thematosus. *Arthritis Res. Ther.* **2017**, *19*, 247. [CrossRef]
19. Zen, M.; Iaccarino, L.; Gatto, M.; Bettio, S.; Saccon, F.; Ghirardello, A.; Punzi, L.; Doria, A. The effect of different durations of remission on damage accrual: Results from a prospective monocentric cohort of Caucasian patients. *Ann. Rheum. Dis.* **2017**, *76*, 562–565. [CrossRef]
20. Petri, M.; Magder, L.S. Comparison of Remission and Lupus Low Disease Activity State in Damage Prevention in a United States Systemic Lupus Erythematosus Cohort. *Arthritis Rheumatol.* **2018**, *70*, 1790–1795. [CrossRef]
21. Ugarte-Gil, M.F.; Wojdyla, D.; Pons-Estel, G.J.; Catoggio, L.J.; Drenkard, C.; Sarano, J.; Berbotto, G.A.; Borba, E.F.; Sato, E.I.; Brenol, J.C.T.; et al. Remission and Low Disease Activity Status (LDAS) protect lupus patients from damage occurrence: Data from a multiethnic, multinational Latin American Lupus Cohort (GLADEL). *Ann. Rheum. Dis.* **2017**, *76*, 2071–2074. [CrossRef]
22. Floris, A.; Piga, M.; Perra, D.; Chessa, E.; Congia, M.; Mathieu, A.; Cauli, A. Treatment Target in Newly Diagnosed Systemic Lupus Ery-thematosus: The Association of Lupus Low Disease Activity State and Remission with Lower Accrual of Early Damage. *Arthritis Care Res.* **2020**, *72*, 1794–1799. [CrossRef] [PubMed]
23. Golder, V.; Kandane-Rathnayake, R.; Huq, M.; Nim, H.T.; Louthrenoo, W.; Luo, S.F.; Wu, Y.-J.J.; Lateef, A.; Sockalingam, S.; Navarra, S.V.; et al. Lupus low disease activity state as a treatment endpoint for systemic lupus erythematosus: A prospective validation study. *Lancet Rheumatol.* **2019**, *1*, e95–e102. [CrossRef]
24. Chessa, E.; Piga, M.; Floris, A.; Devilliers, H.; Cauli, A.; Arnaud, L. Use of Physician Global Assessment in systemic lupus erythema-tosus: A systematic review of its psychometric properties. *Rheumatology* **2020**, *59*, 3622–3632. [CrossRef] [PubMed]
25. Chessa, E.; Piga, M.; Arnaud, L. Physician global assessment in systemic lupus erythematosus: Can we rely on its reliability? *Ann. Rheum. Dis.* **2020**. [CrossRef] [PubMed]
26. Jesus, D.; Matos, A.; Henriques, C.; Zen, M.; LaRosa, M.; Iaccarino, L.; Ap Da Silva, J.; Doria, A.; Inês, L.S. Derivation and validation of the SLE Disease Activity Score (SLE-DAS): A new SLE continuous measure with high sensitivity for changes in disease activity. *Ann. Rheum. Dis.* **2019**, *78*, 365–371. [CrossRef]
27. Apostolopoulos, D.; Kandane-Rathnayake, R.; Raghunath, S.; Hoi, A.; Nikpour, M.; Morand, E.F. Independent association of gluco-corticoids with damage accrual in SLE. *Lupus Sci. Med.* **2016**, *3*, e000157. [CrossRef]
28. Piga, M.; Floris, A.; Sebastiani, G.D.; Prevete, I.; Iannone, F.; Coladonato, L.; Govoni, M.; Bortoluzzi, A.; Mosca, M.; Tani, C.; et al. Risk factors of damage in early diagnosed systemic lupus erythematosus: Results of the Italian multicentre Early Lupus Project inception cohort. *Rheumatology* **2019**, *59*, 2272–2281. [CrossRef]
29. Felten, R.; Arnaud, L. Is it possible to stop glucocorticoids in systemic lupus? *Jt. Bone Spine* **2020**, *87*, 528–530. [CrossRef]
30. Little, J.; Parker, B.; Lunt, M.; Hanly, J.G.; Urowitz, M.B.; Clarke, A.E.; Romero-Díaz, J.; Gordon, C.; Bae, S.-C.; Bernatsky, S.; et al. Glucocorticoid use and factors associated with variability in this use in the Systemic Lupus International Collaborating Clinics Inception Cohort. *Rheumatology* **2018**, *57*, 677–687. [CrossRef]
31. Tani, C.; Elefante, E.; Signorini, V.; Zucchi, D.; Lorenzoni, V.; Carli, L.; Stagnaro, C.; Ferro, F.; Mosca, M. Glucocorticoid withdrawal in systemic lupus erythematosus: Are remission and low disease activity reliable starting points for stopping treatment? A real-life experience. *RMD Open* **2019**, *5*, e000916. [CrossRef]
32. Mathian, A.; Pha, M.; Haroche, J.; Cohen-Aubart, F.; Hié, M.; De Chambrun, M.P.; Du Boutin, T.H.; Miyara, M.; Gorochov, G.; Yssel, H.; et al. Withdrawal of low-dose prednisone in SLE patients with a clinically quiescent disease for more than 1 year: A randomised clinical trial. *Ann. Rheum. Dis.* **2019**, *79*, 339–346. [CrossRef] [PubMed]
33. Scherlinger, M.; Mertz, P.; Sagez, F.; Meyer, A.; Felten, R.; Chatelus, E.; Javier, R.-M.; Sordet, C.; Martin, T.; Korganow, A.-S.; et al. Worldwide trends in all-cause mortality of auto-immune systemic diseases between 2001 and 2014. *Autoimmun. Rev.* **2020**, *19*, 102531. [CrossRef] [PubMed]

34. Arnaud, L.; Mertz, P.; Gavand, P.E.; Martin, T.; Chasset, F.; Tebacher-Alt, M.; Lambert, A.; Muller, C.; Sibilia, J.; Vignes-Lebrun, B.; et al. Drug-induced systemic lupus: Revisiting the ev-er-changing spectrum of the disease using the WHO pharmacovigilance database. *Ann. Rheum. Dis.* **2019**, *78*, 504–508. [CrossRef] [PubMed]
35. Chasset, F.; Bouaziz, J.-D.; Costedoat-Chalumeau, N.; Francès, C.; Arnaud, L. Efficacy and comparison of antimalarials in cutaneous lupus erythematosus subtypes: A systematic review and meta-analysis. *Br. J. Dermatol.* **2017**, *177*, 188–196. [CrossRef]
36. Chasset, F.; Arnaud, L. Targeting interferons and their pathways in systemic lupus erythematosus. *Autoimmun. Rev.* **2018**, *17*, 44–52. [CrossRef]
37. Felten, R.; Dervovic, E.; Chasset, F.; Gottenberg, J.-E.; Sibilia, J.; Scher, F.; Arnaud, L. The 2018 pipeline of targeted therapies under clinical development for Systemic Lupus Erythematosus: A systematic review of trials. *Autoimmun. Rev.* **2018**, *17*, 781–790. [CrossRef]
38. Felten, R.; Scher, F.; Sagez, F.; Chasset, F.; Arnaud, L. Spotlight on anifrolumab and its potential for the treatment of moder-ate-to-severe systemic lupus erythematosus: Evidence to date. *Drug Des. Dev. Ther.* **2019**, *13*, 1535–1543. [CrossRef]
39. Touma, Z.; Gladman, D.D. Current and future therapies for SLE: Obstacles and recommendations for the development of novel treatments. *Lupus Sci. Med.* **2017**, *4*, e000239. [CrossRef]
40. Fernandes Moca Trevisani, V.; Castro, A.A.; Ferreira Neves Neto, J.; Atallah, A.N. Cyclophosphamide versus methylprednisolone for treating neuropsychiatric involvement in systemic lupus erythematosus. *Cochrane Database Syst. Rev.* **2013**, *28*, CD002265. [CrossRef]
41. Furie, R.; Rovin, B.H.; Houssiau, F.; Malvar, A.; Teng, Y.O.; Contreras, G.; Amoura, Z.; Yu, X.; Mok, C.-C.; Santiago, M.B.; et al. Two-Year, Randomized, Controlled Trial of Belimumab in Lupus Nephritis. *N. Engl. J. Med.* **2020**, *383*, 1117–1128. [CrossRef]
42. Gatto, M.; Saccon, F.; Zen, M.; Regola, F.; Fredi, M.; Andreoli, L.; Tincani, A.; Urban, M.L.; Emmi, G.; Ceccarelli, F.; et al. Early Disease and Low Baseline Damage as Predictors of Re-sponse to Belimumab in Patients with Systemic Lupus Erythematosus in a Real-Life Setting. *Arthritis Rheumatol.* **2020**, *72*, 1314–1324. [CrossRef] [PubMed]
43. Felten, R.; Sagez, F.; Gavand, P.-E.; Martin, T.; Korganow, A.-S.; Sordet, C.; Javier, R.-M.; Soulas-Sprauel, P.; Rivière, M.; Scher, F.; et al. 10 most important contemporary challenges in the management of SLE. *Lupus Sci. Med.* **2019**, *6*, e000303. [CrossRef] [PubMed]
44. Rovin, B.H.; Solomons, N.; Pendergraft, W.F., III; Dooley, M.A.; Tumlin, J.; Romero-Diaz, J.; Lysenko, L.; Navarra, S.V.; Huizinga, R.B.; AURA-LV Study Group. A randomized, controlled double-blind study comparing the efficacy and safety of dose-ranging voclosporin with placebo in achieving remission in patients with active lupus nephritis. *Kidney Int.* **2019**, *95*, 219–231. [CrossRef] [PubMed]
45. Deng, D.; Zhang, P.; Guo, Y.; Lim, T.O. A randomised double-blind, placebo-controlled trial of allogeneic umbilical cord-derived mesenchymal stem cell for lupus nephritis. *Ann. Rheum. Dis.* **2017**, *76*, 1436–1439. [CrossRef] [PubMed]
46. He, J.; Zhang, R.; Shao, M.; Zhao, X.; Miao, M.; Chen, J.; Liu, J.; Zhang, X.; Zhang, X.; Jin, Y.; et al. Efficacy and safety of low-dose IL-2 in the treatment of systemic lupus erythematosus: A randomised, double-blind, placebo-controlled trial. *Ann. Rheum. Dis.* **2020**, *79*, 141–149. [CrossRef] [PubMed]
47. Drenkard, C.; Lim, S.S. Update on lupus epidemiology: Advancing health disparities research through the study of minority populations. *Curr. Opin. Rheumatol.* **2019**, *31*, 689–696. [CrossRef] [PubMed]
48. Williams, E.M.; Bruner, L.; Adkins, A.; Vrana, C.; Logan, A.; Kamen, D.; Oates, J.C. I too, am America: A review of research on systemic lupus erythematosus in African-Americans. *Lupus Sci. Med.* **2016**, *3*, e000144. [CrossRef] [PubMed]
49. Demas, K.L.; Costenbader, K.H. Disparities in lupus care and outcomes. *Curr. Opin. Rheumatol.* **2009**, *21*, 102–109. [CrossRef] [PubMed]
50. Al-Maini, M.; Jeyalingam, T.; Brown, P.; Lee, J.J.Y.; Li, L.; Su, J.; Gladman, D.D.; Fortin, P.R. A Hot Spot for Systemic Lupus Erythematosus, but Not for Psoriatic Arthritis, Identified by Spatial Analysis Suggests an Interaction Between Ethnicity and Place of Residence. *Arthritis Rheum.* **2013**, *65*, 1579–1585. [CrossRef] [PubMed]
51. Moser, K.L.; Kelly, J.A.; Lessard, C.J.; Harley, J.B. Recent insights into the genetic basis of systemic lupus erythematosus. *Genes Immun.* **2009**, *10*, 373–379. [CrossRef] [PubMed]
52. Teruel, M.; Alarcón-Riquelme, M.E. The genetic basis of systemic lupus erythematosus: What are the risk factors and what have we learned. *J. Autoimmun.* **2016**, *74*, 161–175. [CrossRef] [PubMed]
53. Deng, Y.; Tsao, B.P. Updates in Lupus Genetics. *Curr. Rheumatol. Rep.* **2017**, *19*, 68. [CrossRef] [PubMed]
54. Moulton, V.R.; Suarez-Fueyo, A.; Meidan, E.; Li, H.; Mizui, M.; Tsokos, G.C. Pathogenesis of Human Systemic Lupus Erythematosus: A Cellular Perspective. *Trends Mol. Med.* **2017**, *23*, 615–635. [CrossRef] [PubMed]
55. Mejía-Vilet, J.M.; Zhang, X.L.; Cruz, C.; Cano-Verduzco, M.L.; Shapiro, J.P.; Nagaraja, H.N.; Morales-Buenrostro, L.E.; Rovin, B.H. Urinary Soluble CD163: A Novel Noninvasive Biomarker of Activity for Lupus Nephritis. *J. Am. Soc. Nephrol.* **2020**, *31*, 1335–1347. [CrossRef] [PubMed]
56. Banchereau, R.; Hong, S.; Cantarel, B.; Baldwin, N.; Baisch, J.; Edens, M.; Cepika, A.-M.; Acs, P.; Turner, J.; Anguiano, E.; et al. Personalized Immunomonitoring Uncovers Molecular Networks that Stratify Lupus Patients. *Cell* **2016**, *165*, 551–565, Erratum in **2016**, *165*, 1548–1550. [CrossRef] [PubMed]
57. Alijotas-Reig, J.; Esteve-Valverde, E.; Ferrer-Oliveras, R.; Sáez-Comet, L.; Lefkou, E.; Mekinian, A.; Belizna, C.; Ruffatti, A.; Tincani, A.; Marozio, L.; et al. The European Registry on Obstetric Antiphospholipid Syndrome (EUROAPS): A survey of 1000 consecutive cases. *Autoimmun. Rev.* **2019**, *18*, 406–414. [CrossRef] [PubMed]

58. Buyon, J.P.; Kim, M.Y.; Guerra, M.M.; Laskin, C.A.; Petri, M.; Lockshin, M.D.; Sammaritano, L.; Ware Branch, D.; Flint Porter, T.; Sawitzke, A.; et al. Predictors of Pregnancy Outcomes in Patients with Lupus: A Cohort Study. *Ann. Intern. Med.* **2015**, *163*, 153–163. [CrossRef]
59. Fredi, M.; Andreoli, L.; Bacco, B.; Bertero, T.; Bortoluzzi, A.; Breda, S.; Cappa, V.; Ceccarelli, F.; Cimaz, R.; De Vita, S.; et al. First Report of the Italian Registry on Immune-Mediated Congenital Heart Block (Lu.Ne Registry). *Front. Cardiovasc. Med.* **2019**, *6*, 11. [CrossRef]
60. Barsalou, J.; Costedoat-Chalumeau, N.; Berhanu, A.; Fors-Nieves, C.; Shah, U.; Brown, P.; Laskin, C.A.; Morel, N.; Levesque, K.; Buyon, J.P.; et al. Effect of in utero hydroxychloroquine exposure on the development of cutaneous neonatal lupus erythematosus. *Ann. Rheum. Dis.* **2018**, *77*, 1742–1749. [CrossRef]
61. Eudy, A.M.; Siega-Riz, A.M.; Engel, S.M.; Franceschini, N.; Howard, A.G.; Clowse, M.E.B.; Petri, M. Effect of pregnancy on disease flares in patients with systemic lupus erythematosus. *Ann. Rheum. Dis.* **2018**, *77*, 855–860. [CrossRef]
62. Mendel, A.; Bernatsky, S.B.; Hanly, J.G.; Urowitz, M.B.; Clarke, A.E.; Romero-Diaz, J.; Gordon, C.; Bae, S.-C.; Wallace, D.J.; Merrill, J.T.; et al. Low aspirin use and high prevalence of pre-eclampsia risk factors among pregnant women in a multinational SLE inception cohort. *Ann. Rheum. Dis.* **2019**, *78*, 1010–1012. [CrossRef] [PubMed]
63. Thomas, G.; Mancini, J.; Jourde-Chiche, N.; Sarlon, G.; Amoura, Z.; Harlé, J.R.; Jougla, E.; Chiche, L. Mortality associated with systemic lupus ery-thematosus in France assessed by multiple-cause-of-death analysis. *Arthritis Rheumatol.* **2014**, *66*, 2503–2511. [CrossRef] [PubMed]
64. Esdaile, J.M.; Abrahamowicz, M.; Grodzicky, T.; Li, Y.; Panaritis, C.; du Berger, R.; Côté, R.; Grover, S.A.; Fortin, P.R.; Clarke, A.E.; et al. Traditional Framingham risk factors fail to fully account for accelerated atherosclerosis in systemic lupus erythematosus. *Arthritis Rheum.* **2001**, *44*, 2331–2337. [CrossRef]
65. Arnaud, L.; Mathian, A.; Adoue, D.; Bader-Meunier, B.; Baudouin, V.; Belizna, C.; Bonnotte, B.; Boumdeine, F.; Chaib, A.; Groupe France Lupus Érythémateux sys-Témique Réseau (FLEUR) et les Centres de Référence et de Compétence des Lupus et Syndromes des Antiphospholipides; et al. Dépistage et prise en charge du risque cardiovasculaire au cours du lupus systémique: Élaboration de recommandations pour la pratique clinique, à partir d'une analyse de la littérature et de l'avis d'experts [Screening and management of cardiovascular risk factors in systemic lupus erythematosus: Recommendations for clinical practice based on the literature and expert opinion]. *Rev. Med. Interne* **2015**, *36*, 372–380. [PubMed]
66. Floris, A.; Piga, M.; Mangoni, A.A.; Bortoluzzi, A.; Erre, G.L.; Cauli, A. Protective Effects of Hydroxychloroquine against Accelerated Atherosclerosis in Systemic Lupus Erythematosus. *Mediat. Inflamm.* **2018**, *2018*, 1–11. [CrossRef]
67. Feldman, C.H.; Hiraki, L.T.; Winkelmayer, W.C.; Marty, F.M.; Franklin, J.M.; Kim, S.C.; Costenbader, K.H. Serious Infections Among Adult Medicaid Beneficiaries with Systemic Lupus Erythematosus and Lupus Nephritis. *Arthritis Rheumatol.* **2015**, *67*, 1577–1585. [CrossRef]
68. Porta, S.; Danza, A.; Arias Saavedra, M.; Carlomagno, A.; Goizueta, M.C.; Vivero, F.; Ruiz-Irastorza, G. Glucocorticoids in Systemic Lupus Erythematosus. Ten Questions and Some Issues. *J. Clin. Med.* **2020**, *9*, 2709. [CrossRef]
69. Akiyama, S.; Hamdeh, S.; Micic, D.; Sakuraba, A. Prevalence and clinical outcomes of COVID-19 in patients with autoimmune diseases: A systematic review and meta-analysis. *Ann. Rheum. Dis.* **2020**. [CrossRef]
70. Mackie, S.L.; Dejaco, C.; Appenzeller, S.; Camellino, D.; Duftner, C.; Gonzalez-Chiappe, S.; Mahr, A.; Mukhtyar, C.; Reynolds, G.; De Souza, A.W.S.; et al. British Society for Rheumatology guideline on diagnosis and treatment of giant cell arteritis: Executive summary. *Rheumatology* **2020**, *59*, 487–494. [CrossRef]
71. Lawson, E.F.; Trupin, L.; Yelin, E.H.; Yazdany, J. Reasons for failure to receive pneumococcal and influenza vaccinations among immunosuppressed patients with systemic lupus erythematosus. *Semin. Arthritis Rheum.* **2015**, *44*, 666–671. [CrossRef]
72. Jolly, M.; Annapureddy, N.; Arnaud, L.; Devilliers, H. Changes in quality of life in relation to disease activity in systemic lupus erythematosus: Post-hoc analysis of the BLISS-52 Trial. *Lupus* **2019**, *28*, 1628–1639. [CrossRef] [PubMed]
73. Arnaud, L.; Gavand, P.E.; Voll, R.; Schwarting, A.; Maurier, F.; Blaison, G.; Magy-Bertrand, N.; Pennaforte, J.-L.; Peter, H.-H.; Kieffer, P.; et al. Predictors of fatigue and severe fatigue in a large international cohort of patients with systemic lupus erythematosus and a systematic review of the literature. *Rheumatology* **2019**, *58*, 987–996. [CrossRef] [PubMed]
74. Mertz, P.; Schlencker, A.; Schneider, M.; Gavand, P.-E.; Martin, T.; Arnaud, L. Towards a practical management of fatigue in systemic lupus erythematosus. *Lupus Sci. Med.* **2020**, *7*, e000441. [CrossRef] [PubMed]
75. Arnaud, L.; Mertz, P.; Amoura, Z.; Voll, R.E.; Schwarting, A.; Maurier, F.; Blaison, G.; Bonnotte, B.; Poindron, V.; Fiehn, C.; et al. Patterns of fatigue and association with disease activity and clinical manifestations in systemic lupus erythematosus. *Rheumatology* **2020**. [CrossRef]
76. Costedoat-Chalumeau, N.; Houssiau, F.; Izmirly, P.; Le Guern, V.; Navarra, S.; Jolly, M.; Ruiz-Irastorza, G.; Baron, G.; Hachulla, E.; Agmon-Levin, N.; et al. Note of Republication: A Prospective International Study on Adherence to Treatment in 305 Patients With Flaring SLE: Assessment by Drug Levels and Self-Administered Questionnaires. *Clin. Pharmacol. Ther.* **2017**, *103*, 1074–1082. [CrossRef] [PubMed]
77. Arnaud, L.; Zahr, N.; Ea, H.; Amoura, Z. The importance of assessing medication exposure to the definition of refractory disease in systemic lupus erythematosus. *Autoimmun. Rev.* **2011**, *10*, 674–678. [CrossRef]
78. Feldman, C.H.; Collins, J.; Zhang, Z.; Subramanian, S.V.; Solomon, D.H.; Kawachi, I.; Costenbader, K.H. Dynamic patterns and predictors of hy-droxychloroquine nonadherence among Medicaid beneficiaries with systemic lupus erythematosus. *Semin. Arthritis Rheum.* **2018**, *48*, 205–213. [CrossRef]

79. Parisis, D.; Bernier, C.; Chasset, F.; Arnaud, L. Impact of tobacco smoking upon disease risk, activity and therapeutic response in systemic lupus erythematosus: A systematic review and meta-analysis. *Autoimmun. Rev.* **2019**, *18*, 102393. [CrossRef]
80. Chasset, F.; Francès, C.; Barete, S.; Amoura, Z.; Arnaud, L. Influence of smoking on the efficacy of antimalarials in cutaneous lupus: A meta-analysis of the literature. *J. Am. Acad. Dermatol.* **2015**, *72*, 634–639. [CrossRef]
81. Mancuso, C.A.; Perna, M.; Sargent, A.B.; Salmon, J.E. Perceptions and measurements of physical activity in patients with systemic lupus erythematosus. *Lupus* **2011**, *20*, 231–242. [CrossRef]
82. Margiotta, D.P.E.; Basta, F.; Dolcini, G.; Batani, V.; Vullo, M.L.; Vernuccio, A.; Navarini, L.; Afeltra, A. Physical activity and sedentary behavior in patients with Systemic Lupus Erythematosus. *PLoS ONE* **2018**, *13*, e0193728. [CrossRef] [PubMed]
83. O'Dwyer, T.; Durcan, L.; Wilson, F. Exercise and physical activity in systemic lupus erythematosus: A systematic review with meta-analyses. *Semin. Arthritis Rheum.* **2017**, *47*, 204–215. [CrossRef] [PubMed]

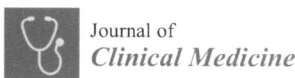

Review

Management of Lupus Nephritis

Farah Tamirou * and Frédéric A. Houssiau

Department of Rheumatology, Cliniques Universitaires Saint-Luc and Institut de Recherche Expérimentale et Clinique, UCLouvain, 1200 Bruxelles, Belgium; frederic.houssiau@uclouvain.be
* Correspondence: farah.tamirou@uclouvain.be

Abstract: Lupus nephritis (LN) is a frequent and severe manifestation of systemic lupus erythematosus. The main goal of the management of LN is to avoid chronic kidney disease (CKD). Current treatment strategies remain unsatisfactory in terms of complete renal response, prevention of relapses, CKD, and progression to end-stage kidney disease. To improve the prognosis of LN, recent data suggest that we should *(i)* modify our treat-to-target approach by including, in addition to a clinical target, a pathological target and *(ii)* switch from conventional sequential therapy to combination therapy. Here, we also review the results of recent controlled randomized trials.

Keywords: lupus nephritis; treat-to-target approach; repeat kidney biopsy; combination therapy

1. Introduction

Lupus nephritis (LN) occurs in 12 to 69% of patients suffering from systemic lupus erythematosus (SLE), depending on case series [1]. Based on clinical and laboratory findings, it affects around 50% of SLE patients, while the rates of biopsy-proven LN are somewhat lower [2]. LN is more prevalent in Asian than in African or Hispanic and European patients [3].

2. Pathophysiology of Lupus Nephritis

Immune complexes (IC), produced in lymph nodes, spleen, or other lymphoid tissues are deposited in the glomeruli of LN patients [4]. Their detection, by direct immunofluorescence techniques on kidney biopsies, is part of the diagnosis of LN [5]. Antibodies also cross-react with glomerular antigens (DNA, histones, and nucleosomes) [6,7], in particular from the basement membrane [8]. The location of IC deposits explains the clinical phenotype. Subendothelial IC induce endothelial dysfunction and recruitment of macrophages and T cells into crescents, which also contain proliferating cells from the parietal layer of Bowman's capsule, thereby causing the so-called "proliferative" variants. Monocytes are recruited from the blood and differentiate into $CD16^+$ inflammatory macrophages. Subepithelial IC cause damage to podocytes, but pro-inflammatory cell recruitment is more limited because the glomerular basement membrane prevents contact with the intravascular space. There is less glomerular inflammation, thereby less kidney failure. By contrast, the enlargement of basement membrane pores explains the (usually massive) proteinuria. Those proliferative variants with subendothelial immune deposits correspond to class III/IV LN, based on the International Society of Nephrology/Renal Pathology Society (ISN/RPS) classification [9], while subepithelial immune deposits correspond to class V LN. Beyond this first wave of immune effectors which mainly target the glomeruli, LN is also characterized by tubulointerstitial lesions which do not result from passive deposition of IC but are part of an adaptive immune response. Myeloid and plasmacytoid dendritic cells and lymphocytes are recruited in the tubulointerstitium. Antigens can be presented to T cells. T–B cell interactions promote differentiation of B cells into plasma cells that secrete antibodies against renal antigens, such as vimentin [10]. Tubulo-interstitial inflammation and hypoxia induce metabolic dysfunction and atrophy of tubular cells [11].

The lupus-affected kidney not only is the passive victim of an innate immunological attack against the glomeruli, but also participates as an actor to promote a pan-nephritis.

3. Clinical and Pathological Diagnosis of Lupus Nephritis

LN, which is clinically silent for a long time, is usually revealed by proteinuria and, in proliferative variants, by abnormal urinalysis and/or renal impairment. High blood pressure, edema secondary to hypoalbuminemia, and salt and water retention may complete the clinical picture.

In case of suspicion of LN, the proteinuria threshold at which a kidney biopsy is indicated is not defined. In practice, this procedure is proposed when the proteinuria level is ≥500 mg/day. Observational data show that proteinuria between 500 and 1000 mg/day is already associated with significant kidney damage [12] and also that "low-grade" proteinuria does not exclude significant kidney injury in LN [13]. Furthermore, it is well established that early management of LN improves the prognosis of the disease [14], an additional argument in favor of an early biopsy. The most common lesion observed in LN is glomerulonephritis with immune deposits. A kidney biopsy has several goals: *(i)* to characterize the type of glomerular involvement and thereby guide immunosuppression; *(ii)* to consider other mechanisms of renal injury such as thrombotic microangiopathy or podocytopathy, which require a different therapeutic approach; and *(iii)* to assess the chronicity and therefore the irreversibility of the lesions. The discovery of tubulointerstitial nephritis is not exceptional [15] and is also associated with a worse prognosis, independent of glomerular lesions [16].

The histological description of LN is based on classification criteria defined by the ISN/RPS [9], whose main goal is to guide treatment decisions. However, the ISN/RPS classification is a simplified view of the process and does not allow, at the onset of the disease, to capture with sufficient accuracy the very patients who will progress to chronic kidney disease (CKD). Thus, it has been indeed demonstrated that the long-term prognosis of classes III, IV-S, and IV-G LN is similar [17]. The pitfall probably stems from the glomerulocentric nature of this classification, which does not take into account tubulointerstitial lesions, known to be a major driver of renal impairment [18]. A recent revision of the ISN/RPS classification recommends their inclusion [19].

4. Treatment of Lupus Nephritis

4.1. Global Therapeutic Strategy

The ultimate goal of LN treatment is to prevent nephron loss and, thereby, CKD, especially end-stage kidney disease (ESKD). Since the risk of kidney impairment is greater in patients with proliferative LN, immunosuppressants (IS) play a pivotal role in the treatment of ISN/RPS Classes III and IV LN. To prevent CKD, the therapeutic goal in the short term is to achieve complete, at least partial, resolution of the clinical and laboratory signs of LN. At diagnosis, the kidneys are already severely damaged by glomerular deposits of immune complexes and tubulointerstitial inflammation. Patients must therefore be treated with powerful and promptly efficacious anti-inflammatory agents, such as glucocorticoids (GCs), combined with another IS agent to interrupt autoimmune processes. Immunosuppression should be maintained for several years. The standard immunosuppressive strategy consists of a formerly called "induction phase" followed by a "maintenance phase". These terms are now replaced by "initial treatment" and "subsequent treatment", which are more appropriate.

4.2. Current Therapeutic Recommendations

Th therapy of LN is based on the joint recommendations of the European League Against Rheumatism (EULAR) and the European Renal Association-European Dialysis and Transplant Association (ERA-EDTA) [20]. Proposals are based on the results of controlled randomized trials summarized in Table 1. The decision to treat LN and the choice of the treatment regimen is based on the ISN/RPS classification criteria [16].

In addition to optimal nephroprotection (angiotensin-converting enzyme inhibitor (ACEI) or angiotensin receptor blocker (ARBs)) and hydroxychloroquine (HCQ; 5 mg/kg/day, except in cases of severe kidney impairment for which the dose is reduced), the initial treatment of classes III/IV ($\pm$V) LN includes GCs administered intravenously (IV) (total dose of 500 to 2500 mg of IV methylprednisolone) and then orally (prednisolone 0.3–0.5mg/kg/d until week 4, reduced to $\leq$5–10 mg/d at month 3), in combination with either mycophenolate mofetil (MMF; target dose 2 g/d) or IV cyclophosphamide (CY), according to the Euro-Lupus regimen (EL; 6 fortnightly doses of 500 mg IV CY) [21]. An alternative is a combination of MMF (dose of 1 g) with a calcineurin inhibitor (CNI; tacrolimus 4 mg/day). In case of acute kidney injury, cellular crescents, and/or fibrinoid necrosis, the aforementioned regimens are also recommended, but higher doses of IV CY can also be proposed according to the National Institutes of Health (NIH) regimen [22].

Subsequent treatment, for at least 3 years, of Classes III/IV ($\pm$V) LN is based on MMF (2 g/day) or azathioprine (AZA) (2 mg/kg/day), in addition to HCQ and the lowest possible dose of oral prednisolone (2.5–5 mg/day, ideally not administered to patients with complete response) [20].

Of note, the management of GCs in LN is based more on convention than on evidence, although recent studies support the use of lower doses with the same efficacy but less secondary effects [23,24].

Beyond immunosuppression and nephroprotection, the treatment of LN also includes optimal pharmacological control of blood pressure and preventive measures to avoid the side effects of GCs, such as prescription of calcium salts, vitamin D3 supplements, immunization against pneumococcus and influenza, and exercise.

While it is true that this approach has ensured an overall survival of 80% at 5 years, the rate of complete renal response (CRR) at 6–12 months is only 20–40%, and up to 5–20% of patients will progress, often late, to ESKD, while an additional percentage will develop CKD. Even in patients achieving CRR after treatment, an increase in chronic lesions is observed on repeat renal biopsies [25]. Relapses, occurring in approximately 20–25% of patients within 3 to 5 years [26,27], constitute a significant risk factor for the development or progression of CKD [28]. Overall, the current treatment strategies remain unsatisfactory.

Table 1. Pivotal trials for immunosuppressant treatment of patients with lupus nephritis.

Reference	Trial	N Patients	ISN/RPS Class of LN	Treatment	Follow Up	Primary Endpoint	Results
Austin HA, NEJM 1986 [22]	NIH	107	All	High dose GC vs. NIH IV CY	Median 7 years	Time to end-stage kidney disease (ESKD)	NIH IV CY > high dose GC
Houssiau FA, A&R 2002 [21]	ELNT	90	III, IV, Vc, Vd	EL IV CY vs. NIH IV CY as induction treatment	Median 41 months	Treatment failure regarding kidney function, proteinuria, relapses	No difference observed between EL IV CY and NIH IV CY
					Mean 115 months (Houssiau, ARD 2010 [29])	Time to major event: death, ESKD, doubling of serum creatinine	No difference observed between EL IV CY and NIH IV CY
Appel GB, JASN 2009 [30]		370	III, IV et/ou V	MMF vs. IV CY as induction treatment	24 weeks	Proteinuria decrease (UPC ratio)	No difference observed between MMF and IV CY
Dooley MA, NEJM 2011 [26]	ALMS	227	III, IV ou V	AZA vs. MMF as maintenance treatment after induction by MMF or IV CY	36 months	Time to first event: death, end-stage-kidney disease, renal relapse, need of a rescue therapy	MMF > AZA Relapses: 16.4% in MMF group vs. 32.4% in AZA group
Houssiau FA, ARD 2010 [31]	MAINTAIN	105	III, IV, Vc, Vd	AZA vs. MMF as maintenance treatment after induction by EL IV CY	Mean 48 months	Time to first renal relapse	No difference observed between MMF and AZA Relapses: 19% in MMF group vs. 25% in AZA group
		87			Median 110 months (Tamirou F, ARD 2016 [32])	Time to renal flare	No difference observed between MMF and AZA Relapses: 45% in MMF group vs. 49% in AZA group
Liu Z, AIM 2015 [33]		310	III-IV ± V, V	Tacrolimus + MMF vs. NIH IV CY	24 weeks	Complete remission	Tacrolimus + MMF (45.9%) > NIH IV CY (25.6%)

NIH: National Institutes of Health, GC: glucocorticoids, ELNT: Euro-Lupus Nephritis Trial, EL: Euro-Lupus, AZA: azathioprine, MMF: mycophenolate mofetil, IV CY: intravenous cyclophosphamide, ALMS: Aspreva Lupus Assessment Study, UPC: urine protein/creatinine ratio.

5. How to Improve the Prognosis of Lupus Nephritis?

We suggest that the outcome of LN could be improved by the adoption of a treat-to-target approach and by switching from sequential to combination therapy.

5.1. Treat-to-Target Approach

The treat-to-target approach is a very fashionable concept in inflammatory and autoimmune diseases. As far as LN is concerned, we can define several types of targets: clinical, pathological, or even immunological targets at the level of the tissue, i.e., the kidneys.

5.1.1. Clinical Target

The best early predictor of a good long-term kidney outcome in LN is a prompt fall in proteinuria. Thus, we demonstrated that achieving a proteinuric target of <0.7 g/day after one year of treatment has a remarkable positive predictive value for a good long-term kidney outcome (94%) [32,34]. These data are robust because they were confirmed in two additional cohorts [35,36]. Alas, the negative predictive value (NPV) of achieving this target is only 31%, which means that 69% of patients not meeting the target will still (and fortunately!) achieve a good long-term kidney outcome. The challenge is therefore to identify those very patients (one-third) who do not reach the target and will suffer from kidney impairment in the long term in order to optimize their treatment, by switching to another IS or by adding a biotherapy, always after evaluating patients' adherence to the treatment [37]. For some cases, the kinetics of the proteinuria fall provides an argument for a "wait-and-see" attitude. Thus, in nephrotic patients at diagnosis, the failure to reach the proteinuric target should be put into perspective, and the right attitude might consists in allowing a few additional months of observation before making a therapeutic decision, certainly if the kinetics of the proteinuria decrease suggests that the target is in sight.

Attempts to add other clinical parameters (kidney function, disappearance of microhaematuria) to the proteinuric target to improve the NPV have failed. Conversely, inclusion of urinalysis (red blood cells) to the target reduced sensitivity from 71 to 41%, implying that 59% of the patients who will experience a good long-term kidney outcome would not be identified at month 12 if persistent hematuria is included in the target, while only 29% would be missed if proteinuria alone is used as criteria [34,35].

Considering that urinary proteins might be more specific for nephritis than serum proteins [38], urinary biomarkers have stimulated much research, the more so as proteomic mass spectrometry has facilitated their detection [39]. Several urinary proteins have been reported as potential predictors of LN activity, in particular NGAL (neutrophil gelatinase-associated lipocalin), MCP-1 (monocyte chemoattractant protein-1), TWEAK (tumor necrosis factor-like weak inducer of apoptosis), and PTGDS (prostaglandin D synthase) [40–46]. Unfortunately, their presence usually correlates with proteinuria, thereby compromising their interest. Moreover, very few studies have evaluated their long-term prognostic value.

Overall, clinical parameters, readily measurable in blood or urine, will probably not help to capture patients who need treatment optimization amongst those who have not reached the proteinuric target.

5.1.2. Pathological and Immunological Target

Together with other groups, we suggest that per protocol repeat kidney biopsies performed after 12 months of IS treatment might contribute to the identification of patients who require treatment intensification. Several studies have indeed shown that signs of histological activity of LN may persist in patients with CRR after IS treatment [25,47–50]. Furthermore, we recently demonstrated in a retrospective analysis performed on incident cases of LN that residual histological activity, i.e., a NIH activity index score >3, in per protocol repeat biopsies predicted subsequent renal relapse and that chronic damage, i.e., a NIH chronicity index score >3, predicted long-term kidney impairment [51]. It is worth noting that active lesions in the glomeruli mostly accounted for the association with relapses, whereas chronic damage in the tubulointerstitial compartment was found to be a more important contributor to the association with long-term renal function.

To evaluate the value of per protocol repeat biopsy after one year of treatment, we designed a prospective international study, *REBIOLUP* (www.rebiolup.com) (accessed on 31 January 2021), illustrated in Figure 1. Patients with incident LN will be treated for one year according to current standard of care (SOC), based on shared patient's and physician's decision. At baseline, they will be randomized in two groups, undergoing—or not—a per protocol control kidney biopsy at one year. The control group, without re-biopsy, will be treated according to clinical parameters, whereas histologic findings will drive treatment decisions in the re-biopsy group. Thus, if the NIH activity index at re-biopsy remains superior to 3/24 [51], immunosuppressive therapy will be intensified, again according to shared patient's and physician's decision. The goal of the study is to demonstrate that: *(i)* the percentage of patients in CRR at 2 years (primary endpoint) will be higher in the re-biopsy group; and *(ii)* conversely, that the percentage of patients with decreased kidney function at 5 years will be lower. Should these hypotheses be confirmed, a systematic one-year repeat kidney biopsy would become an integral part of LN management, hopefully leading to a significant decrease in the number of patients suffering from CKD.

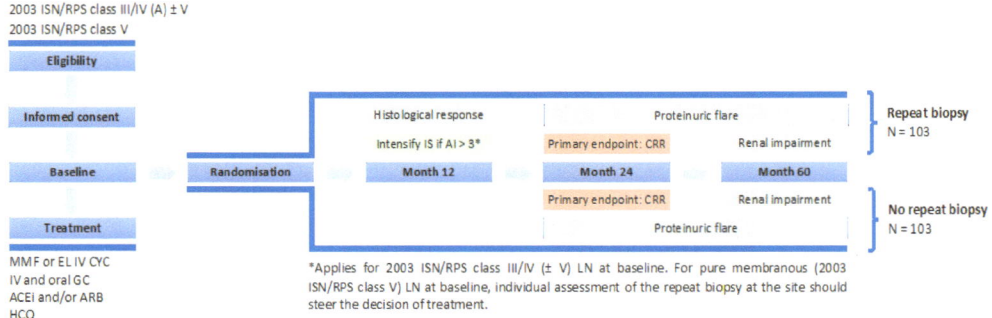

Figure 1. REBIOLUP flowchart.

REBIOLUP will also address the question of in situ immunological response or even remission after one year of treatment, by assessing the reduction or disappearance of immune deposits, as detected by electron microscopy.

5.2. Combination Therapy

Based on the conclusion that many patients suffering from LN do not achieve short-term remission and experience CKD with the current regimens, we propose a new treatment paradigm, which consists in switching from sequential to combination therapy. So far, three successful combinations have been reported with CNIs (tacrolimus (TAC) and voclosporine (VOC)), anti-BlyS/BAFF belimumab, and anti-CD20 obinutuzumab.

The first reported successful combination therapy for LN was an association of MMF and TAC. Thus, a large Chinese study demonstrated that the rate of CRR at 6 months almost doubled for patients treated with a combination of MMF and TAC compared to patients given NIH IV CY, namely, a starting dose of 0.75 (adjusted to 0.5 to 1.0) g/m^2 of body surface area every 4 weeks for 6 months (45.9% versus 25.6%, respectively), without additional adverse effects [33]. This regimen has been reported mainly for Asian patients, and the findings may not be generalizable to other populations. After 6 months of treatment, patients randomized in the MMF/TAC arm stayed on the same regimen (although the daily TAC dose was reduced from 4 to 2 mg), while patients who received NIH IV CY were treated with AZA. Interestingly, the two groups reached a similar rate of CRR after 18 months [52], thereby suggesting that the anti-proteinuric effect of TAC may be responsible for most of the early benefit noticed at month 6.

Interesting results were observed with the combination of MMF and VOC. VOC is a more potent CNI than cyclosporine A, has more predictable pharmacodynamics (thereby avoiding repeated drug monitoring), and presents a faster elimination of metabolites (thereby is likely less responsible for adverse events). In a phase 2 (*AURA*) and a phase 3 trial (*AURORA*), where steroids were very promptly tapered, it was shown that, compared to MMF alone, the combination of MMF and VOC induced a higher CRR at 6 and 12 months (in the AURA trial, 27.3% versus 32.6% and in the AURORA trial, 22.5% versus 40.8%, in the two groups, respectively) [53–55]. Despite these results being clinically significant and obtained without additional serious adverse events, most likely leading to labeling of VOC for LN by the medical agencies in the next months, some caveats must be addressed. The beneficial effect of VOC might be explained by its anti-proteinuric action through stabilization of the podocyte cytoskeleton rather than a true synergistic IS effect. This raises concerns about a rebound effect when stopping the medication. Second, only short-term results (maximum 12 months) have been reported so far. Long-term toxicity data are eagerly awaited. Recently, the U.S. Food and Drug Administration (FDA) had approved voclosporin in combination with a background immunosuppressive therapy to treat patients with active LN. It is the first FDA-approved oral therapy for LN [56].

Anti-BlyS/BAFF belimumab (BEL) is the first biologic approved for SLE, based on several pivotal trials, such as BLISS 52 [57] and BLISS 76 [58]. In these trials, patients with major kidney involvement were excluded. Yet, analysis of the subset of patients with some degree of proteinuria revealed a benefit from BEL with respect to SOC in terms of proteinuria decrease [59], which led to the design of a controlled specific LN trial (BLISS-LN), whose results were recently released [60]. In this trial, the largest and the longest ever performed for LN, 448 patients with active LN were randomized to receive either BEL (one injection every month for two years) or placebo (PBO), as an add-on therapy superimposed on SOC. The SOC was left to the decision of the physician and the patient and consisted in MMF or EL IV CY followed by AZA. The primary endpoint, which was the primary efficacy renal response at week 104 (defined as a urinary protein-to-creatinine ratio ≤ 0.7 g/g, an estimated glomerular filtration rate (eGFR) no worse than 20% below the pre-flare value or ≥ 60 mL/min/1.73 m^2, and no use of rescue therapy), was reached by significantly more patients in the BEL group than in the PBO group (43% versus 32%, respectively). Intriguingly, the beneficial effect of BEL was only observed in conjunction with MMF and not with EL IV CY followed by AZA. The reasons for this difference are unclear, but the CY-treated patients were more severely affected at baseline (higher level of urinary protein, lower eGFR, lower complement concentrations, longer disease duration, and greater exposure to previous treatment for LN, suggesting a greater kidney damage accrual in patients who received CY as SOC), which might explain why these patients did not benefit from the addition of BEL. The time to renal events (ESKD, doubling of serum creatinine, death, and renal flares) was different, again favouring BEL against PBO. The side effects did not differ between between the two groups. The results of a 6-month open-label extension study performed in *BLISS LN* completers should be released very soon and will tell us whether further improvement is observed with time with BEL treatment. Interestingly, some real-life observations indicated a possible appearance of active LN during treatment with BEL in patients who did not have a renal phenotype of SLE prior to BEL initiation [61–65].

Obinutuzumab (OBI) is an anti-CD20 monoclonal antibody that has been glycoengineered to increase antibody-dependent cytotoxicity. It has a type II binding conformation which leads to a greater direct cell death effect and more limited internalization of the monoclonal antibody. These characteristics result in a much more pronounced and sustained B cell depletion compared to rituximab (RTX) [66]. Since better B cell depletion, especially in the kidneys themselves, may increase the rate of CRR, OBI was tested in a small phase II trial, called *NOBILITY* [67]. The study drug (1000 mg administered on days 1, 15, 168, and 182) was compared to PBO on a MMF background and a moderate dose of promptly tapered GCs. At week 52, 76, and 104, the percentage of patients achieving CRR was higher for patients given OBI compared to those receiving PBO, reaching 35% (versus 23%) at week 76 and 41% (versus 23%) at week 104. Almost all patients still had very low peripheral B cell counts (CD19$^+$ count ≤5 cells/μL) at week 52, a finding much different from that of the *LUN*AR trial where only half of RTX-treated patients had undetectable peripheral B cells after one year of treatment [68]. The side effects were comparable in both groups, without additional toxicity due to the combination therapy. Of note, *NOBILITY* is a small trial mainly performed in Hispanic patients. Confirmation might come from a global phase III trial, called *REGENCY* (ClinicalTrials.gov NCT04221477), in which six doses of OBI/PBO will be given to LN patients, with CRR as primary outcome measured at week 76.

These recent trials, *AURA, AURORA, BLISS-LN, NOBILITY*, testing three different drugs and using very similar definitions of CRR, led to the same conclusion: a combination therapy is superior to SOC (GC/MMF or GC/EL IV CY/AZA). The PBO response in these three trials was consistently low, between 20% and 25% CRR after 6 months to 2 years of follow-up. The effect of VOC was prompter, which is consistent with its mode of action. We eagerly await the results (expected in 2021) of the LN anifrolumab trial, called *TULIP-LN* (ClinicalTrials.gov NCT02547922) aimed at testing the efficacy of a human monoclonal antibody against type I interferon receptor subunit 1.

Of note, we decided to focus only on trials demonstrating positive results, but many other biologics were previously tested for LN. They were not developed due to side effects or ineffectiveness. Some failures are probably explained by design flaws [69].

6. Conclusions

We suggest to adopt a treat-to-target approach for LN to limit nephron loss and thereby prevent CKD. Per protocol kidney biopsies performed after one year of treatment might be part of this strategy, which will be tested in *REBIOLUP* (www.rebiolup.com) (accessed on 31 January 2021). The current SOC does not meet patient's and physician's expectations. A combination therapy, instead of a sequential therapy, might become the new paradigm, based on recent trials. Which combination should be prescribed to which patients is currently not clear, but better knowledge of patients' molecular profiling, including at the level of the kidney itself, might possibly be helpful at the bedside.

Author Contributions: Both authors: Writing—Original Draft Preparation, Writing—Review & Editing. All authors have read and agreed to the published version of the manuscript.

Funding: This research received no external funding.

Conflicts of Interest: The authors declare no conflict of interest.

References

1. Rovin, B.H.; Stillman, I. Kidney. In *Systemic Lupus Erythematosus*, 5th ed.; Lahita, R., Ed.; Academic Press: San Diego, CA, USA, 2011; pp. 769–814.
2. Wang, H.; Ren, Y.L.; Chang, J.; Gu, L.; Sun, L.Y. A systematic review and meta-analysis of prevalence of biopsy-proven lupus nephritis. *Arch. Rheumatol.* **2017**, *33*, 17–25. [CrossRef]
3. Seligman, V.A.; Suarez, C.; Lum, R.; Inda, S.E.; Lin, D.; Li, H.; Olson, J.L.; Seldin, M.F.; Criswell, L.A. The Fcgamma receptor IIIA-158F allele is a major risk factor for the development of lupus nephritis among Caucasians but not non-Caucasians. *Arthritis Rheum.* **2001**, *44*, 618–625. [CrossRef]
4. Lech, M.; Anders, H.J. The pathogenesis of lupus nephritis. *J. Am. Soc. Nephrol.* **2013**, *24*, 1357–1366. [CrossRef] [PubMed]
5. Tojo, T.; Friou, G.J. Lupus nephritis: Varying complement-fixing properties of immunoglobulin G antibodies to antigens of cell nuclei. *Science* **1968**, *161*, 904–906. [CrossRef]
6. Kramers, C.; Hylkema, M.N.; van Bruggen, M.C.; van de Lagemaat, R.; Dijkman, H.B.; Assmann, K.J.; Smeenk, R.J.; Berden, J.H. Anti-nucleosome antibodies complexed to nucleosomal antigens show anti-DNA reactivity and bind to rat glomerular basement membrane in vivo. *J. Clin. Investig.* **1994**, *94*, 568–577. [CrossRef]
7. Mjelle, J.E.; Rekvig, O.P.; Van Der Vlag, J.; Fenton, K.A. Nephritogenic antibodies bind in glomeruli through interaction with exposed chromatin fragments and not with renal cross-reactive antigens. *Autoimmunity* **2011**, *44*, 373–383. [CrossRef] [PubMed]
8. Hahn, B.H. Antibodies to DNA. *N. Engl. J. Med.* **1998**, *338*, 1359–1368. [CrossRef] [PubMed]

9. Weening, J.J.; D'Agati, V.D.; Schwartz, M.M.; Seshan, S.V.; Alpers, C.E.; Appel, G.B.; Balow, J.E.; Bruijn, J.A.; Cook, T.; Ferrario, F.; et al. The classification of glomerulonephritis in systemic lupus erythematosus revisited. *Kidney Int.* **2004**, *65*, 521–530. [CrossRef]
10. Chang, A.; Henderson, S.G.; Brandt, D.; Liu, N.; Guttikonda, R.; Hsieh, C.; Kaverina, N.; Utset, T.O.; Meehan, S.M.; Quigg, R.J.; et al. In situ B cell-mediated immune responses and tubulointerstitial inflammation in human lupus nephritis. *J. Immunol.* **2011**, *186*, 1849–1860. [CrossRef]
11. Maria, N.I.; Davidson, A. Protecting the kidney in systemic lupus erythematosus: From diagnosis to therapy. *Nat. Rev. Rheumatol.* **2020**, *16*, 255–267. [CrossRef]
12. Christopher-Stine, L.; Siedner, M.; Lin, J.; Haas, M.; Parekh, H.; Petri, M.; Fine, D.M. Renal biopsy in lupus patients with low levels of proteinuria. *J. Rheumatol.* **2007**, *34*, 332–335.
13. De Rosa, M.; Rocha, A.S.; De Rosa, G.; Dubinsky, D.; Almaani, S.J.; Rovin, B.H. Low-grade proteinuria does not exclude significant kidney injury in lupus nephritis. *Kidney Int. Rep.* **2020**, *5*, 1066–1068. [CrossRef] [PubMed]
14. Fiehn, C.; Hajjar, Y.; Mueller, K.; Waldherr, R.; Ho, A.D.; Andrassy, K. Improved clinical outcome of lupus nephritis during the past decade: Importance of early diagnosis and treatment. *Ann. Rheum. Dis.* **2003**, *62*, 435–439. [CrossRef]
15. Singh, A.K.; Ucci, A.; Madias, N.E. Predominant tubulointerstitial lupus nephritis. *Am. J. Kidney Dis.* **1996**, *27*, 273–278. [CrossRef]
16. Leatherwood, C.; Speyer, C.B.; Feldman, C.H.; D'Silva, K.; Gómez-Puerta, J.A.; Hoover, P.J.; Waikar, S.S.; McMahon, G.M.; Rennke, H.G.; Costenbader, K.H. Clinical characteristics and renal prognosis associated with interstitial fibrosis and tubular atrophy (IFTA) and vascular injury in lupus nephritis biopsies. *Semin. Arthritis Rheum.* **2019**, *49*, 396–404. [CrossRef]
17. Vandepapelière, J.; Aydin, S.; Cosyns, J.P.; Depresseux, G.; Jadoul, M.; Houssiau, F.A. Prognosis of proliferative lupus nephritis subsets in the Louvain Lupus Nephritis inception Cohort. *Lupus* **2014**, *23*, 159–165. [CrossRef]
18. Hsieh, C.; Chang, A.; Brandt, D.; Guttikonda, R.; Utset, T.O.; Clark, M.R. Predicting outcomes of lupus nephritis with tubulointerstitial inflammation and scarring. *Arthritis Care Res.* **2011**, *63*, 865–874. [CrossRef] [PubMed]
19. Bajema, I.M.; Wilhelmus, S.; Alpers, C.E.; Bruijn, J.A.; Colvin, R.B.; Cook, H.T.; D'Agati, V.D.; Ferrario, F.; Haas, M.; Jennette, J.C.; et al. Revision of the International Society of Nephrology/Renal Pathology Society classification for lupus nephritis: Clarification of definitions, and modified National Institutes of Health activity and chronicity indices. *Kidney Int.* **2018**, *93*, 789–796. [CrossRef] [PubMed]
20. Fanouriakis, A.; Kostopoulou, M.; Cheema, K.; Anders, H.J.; Aringer, M.; Bajema, I.; Boletis, J.; Frangou, E.; Houssiau, F.A.; Hollis, J.; et al. 2019 Update of the Joint European League Against Rheumatism and European Renal Association-European Dialysis and Transplant Association (EULAR/ERA-EDTA) recommendations for the management of lupus nephritis. *Ann. Rheum. Dis.* **2020**, *79*, 713–723. [CrossRef]
21. Houssiau, F.A.; Vasconcelos, C.; D'Cruz, D.; Sebastiani, G.D.; Garrido Ed, E.; Danieli, M.G.; Abramovicz, D.; Blockmans, D.; Mathieu, A.; Direskeneli, H.; et al. Immunosuppressive therapy in lupus nephritis: The Euro-Lupus Nephritis Trial, a randomized trial of low-dose versus high-dose intravenous cyclophosphamide. *Arthritis Rheum.* **2002**, *46*, 2121–2131. [CrossRef]
22. Austin, H.A., III; Klippel, J.H.; Balow, J.E.; le Riche, N.G.; Steinberg, A.D.; Plotz, P.H.; Decker, J.L. Therapy of lupus nephritis. Controlled trial of prednisone and cytotoxic drugs. *N. Engl. J. Med.* **1986**, *314*, 614–619. [CrossRef]
23. Zeher, M.; Doria, A.; Lan, J.; Aroca, G.; Jayne, D.; Boletis, I.; Hiepe, F.; Prestele, H.; Bernhardt, P.; Amoura, Z. Efficacy and safety of enteric-coated mycophenolate sodium in combination with two glucocorticoid regimens for the treatment of active lupus nephritis. *Lupus* **2011**, *20*, 1484–1493. [CrossRef] [PubMed]
24. Lightstone, L.; Doria, A.; Wilson, H.; Ward, F.L.; Larosa, M.; Bargman, J.M. Can we manage lupus nephritis without chronic corticosteroids administration? *Autoimmun. Rev.* **2018**, *17*, 4–10. [CrossRef]
25. Malvar, A.; Pirruccio, P.; Alberton, V.; Lococo, B.; Recalde, C.; Fazini, B.; Nagaraja, H.; Indrakanti, D.; Rovin, B.H. Histologic versus clinical remission in proliferative lupus nephritis. *Nephrol. Dial. Transplant.* **2017**, *32*, 1338–1344. [CrossRef] [PubMed]
26. Dooley, M.A.; Jayne, D.; Ginzler, E.M.; Isenberg, D.; Olsen, N.J.; Wofsy, D.; Eitner, F.; Appel, G.B.; Contreras, G.; Lisk, L.; et al. Mycophenolate versus azathioprine as maintenance therapy for lupus nephritis. *N. Engl. J. Med.* **2011**, *365*, 1886–1895. [CrossRef] [PubMed]
27. El Hachmi, M.; Jadoul, M.; Lefèbvre, C.; Depresseux, G.; Houssiau, F.A. Relapses of lupus nephritis: Incidence, risk factors, serology and impact on outcome. *Lupus* **2003**, *12*, 692–696. [CrossRef]
28. Parikh, S.V.; Nagaraja, H.N.; Hebert, L.; Rovin, B.H. Renal flare as a predictor of incident and progressive CKD in patients with lupus nephritis. *Clin. J. Am. Soc. Nephrol.* **2014**, *9*, 279–284. [CrossRef]
29. Houssiau, F.A.; Vasconcelos, C.; D'Cruz, D.; Sebastiani, G.D.; de Ramon Garrido, E.; Danieli, M.G.; Abramovicz, D.; Blockmans, D.; Cauli, A.; Direskeneli, H.; et al. The 10-year follow-up data of the Euro-Lupus Nephritis Trial comparing low-dose and high-dose intravenous cyclophosphamide. *Ann. Rheum. Dis.* **2010**, *69*, 61–64. [CrossRef]
30. Appel, G.B.; Contreras, G.; Dooley, M.A.; Ginzler, E.M.; Isenberg, D.; Jayne, D.; Li, L.S.; Mysler, E.; Sánchez-Guerrero, J.; Solomons, N.; et al. Mycophenolate mofetil versus cyclophosphamide for induction treatment of lupus nephritis. *J. Am. Soc. Nephrol.* **2009**, *20*, 1103–1112. [CrossRef]
31. Houssiau, F.A.; D'Cruz, D.; Sangle, S.; Remy, P.; Vasconcelos, C.; Petrovic, R.; Fiehn, C.; de Ramon Garrido, E.; Gilboe, I.M.; Tektonidou, M.; et al. Azathioprine versus mycophenolate mofetil for long-term immunosuppression in lupus nephritis: Results from the MAINTAIN Nephritis Trial. *Ann. Rheum. Dis.* **2010**, *69*, 2083–2089. [CrossRef] [PubMed]

32. Tamirou, F.; D'Cruz, D.; Sangle, S.; Remy, P.; Vasconcelos, C.; Fiehn, C.; Ayala Guttierez, M.; Gilboe, I.M.; Tektonidou, M.; Blockmans, D.; et al. Long-term follow-up of the MAINTAIN Nephritis Trial, comparing azathioprine and mycophenolate mofetil as maintenance therapy of lupus nephritis. *Ann. Rheum. Dis.* **2016**, *75*, 526–531. [CrossRef] [PubMed]
33. Liu, Z.; Zhang, H.; Liu, Z.; Xing, C.; Fu, P.; Ni, Z.; Chen, J.; Lin, H.; Liu, F.; He, Y.; et al. Multitarget therapy for induction treatment of lupus nephritis: A randomized trial. *Ann. Intern. Med.* **2015**, *162*, 18–26. [CrossRef] [PubMed]
34. Tamirou, F.; Lauwerys, B.R.; Dall'Era, M.; Mackay, M.; Rovin, B.; Cervera, R.; Houssiau, F.A.; MAINTAIN Nephritis Trial Investigators. A proteinuria cut-off level of 0.7 g/day after 12 months of treatment best predicts long-term renal outcome in lupus nephritis: Data from the MAINTAIN Nephritis Trial. *Lupus Sci. Med.* **2015**, *2*, e000123. [CrossRef]
35. Dall'Era, M.; Cisternas, M.G.; Smilek, D.E.; Straub, L.; Houssiau, F.A.; Cervera, R.; Rovin, B.H.; Mackay, M. Predictors of long-term renal outcome in lupus nephritis trials: Lessons learned from the Euro-Lupus Nephritis cohort. *Arthritis Rheumatol.* **2015**, *67*, 1305–1313. [CrossRef]
36. Ugolini-Lopes, M.R.; Seguro, L.; Castro, M.; Daffre, D.; Lopes, A.C.; Borba, E.F.; Bonfá, E. Early proteinuria response: A valid real-life situation predictor of long-term renal outcome in an ethnically diverse group with severe biopsy-proven nephritis? *Lupus Sci. Med.* **2017**, *4*, e000213. [CrossRef]
37. Costedoat-Chalumeau, N.; Amoura, Z.; Hulot, J.S.; Aymard, G.; Leroux, G.; Marra, D.; Lechat, P.; Piette, J.C. Very low blood hydroxychloroquine concentration as an objective marker of poor adherence to treatment of systemic lupus erythematosus. *Ann. Rheum. Dis.* **2007**, *66*, 821–824. [CrossRef]
38. Reyes-Thomas, J.; Blanco, I.; Putterman, C. Urinary biomarkers in lupus nephritis. *Clin. Rev. Allergy Immunol.* **2011**, *40*, 138–150. [CrossRef] [PubMed]
39. Korte, E.A.; Gaffney, P.M.; Powell, D.W. Contributions of mass spectrometry-based proteomics to defining cellular mechanisms and diagnostic markers for systemic lupus erythematosus. *Arthritis Res. Ther.* **2012**, *14*, 204. [CrossRef]
40. Rubinstein, T.; Pitashny, M.; Levine, B.; Schwartz, N.; Schwartzman, J.; Weinstein, E.; Pego-Reigosa, J.M.; Lu, T.Y.; Isenberg, D.; Rahman, A.; et al. Urinary neutrophil gelatinase-associated lipocalin as a novel biomarker for disease activity in lupus nephritis. *Rheumatology.* **2010**, *49*, 960–971. [CrossRef]
41. Torres-Salido, M.T.; Cortés-Hernández, J.; Vidal, X.; Pedrosa, A.; Vilardell-Tarrés, M.; Ordi-Ros, J. Neutrophil gelatinase-associated lipocalin as a biomarker for lupus nephritis. *Nephrol. Dial. Transplant.* **2014**, *29*, 1740–1749. [CrossRef] [PubMed]
42. Rosa, R.F.; Takei, K.; Araújo, N.C.; Loduca, S.M.; Szajubok, J.C.; Chahade, W.H. Monocyte chemoattractant-1 as a urinary biomarker for the diagnosis of activity of lupus nephritis in Brazilian patients. *J. Rheumatol.* **2012**, *39*, 1948–1954. [CrossRef]
43. Schwartz, N.; Rubinstein, T.; Burkly, L.C.; Collins, C.E.; Blanco, I.; Su, L.; Hojaili, B.; Mackay, M.; Aranow, C.; Stohl, W.; et al. Urinary TWEAK as a biomarker of lupus nephritis: A multicenter cohort study. *Arthritis Res. Ther.* **2009**, *11*, R143. [CrossRef] [PubMed]
44. Somparn, P.; Hirankarn, N.; Leelahavanichkul, A.; Khovidhunkit, W.; Thongboonkerd, V.; Avihingsanon, Y. Urinary proteomics revealed prostaglandin H(2)D-isomerase, not Zn-α2-glycoprotein, as a biomarker for active lupus nephritis. *J. Proteom.* **2012**, *75*, 3240–3247. [CrossRef]
45. Gupta, R.; Yadav, A.; Misra, R.; Aggarwal, A. Urinary prostaglandin D synthase as biomarker in lupus nephritis: A longitudinal study. *Clin. Exp. Rheumatol.* **2015**, *33*, 694–698. [PubMed]
46. Vanarsa, K.; Soomro, S.; Zhang, T.; Strachan, B.; Pedroza, C.; Nidhi, M.; Cicalese, P.; Gidley, C.; Dasari, S.; Mohan, S.; et al. Quantitative planar array screen of 1000 proteins uncovers novel urinary protein biomarkers of lupus nephritis. *Ann. Rheum. Dis.* **2020**, *79*, 1349–1361. [CrossRef]
47. Alvarado, A.S.; Malvar, A.; Lococo, B.; Alberton, V.; Toniolo, F.; Nagaraja, H.N.; Rovin, B.H. The value of repeat kidney biopsy in quiescent Argentinian lupus nephritis patients. *Lupus* **2014**, *23*, 840–847. [CrossRef]
48. Alsuwaida, A.; Husain, S.; Alghonaim, M.; AlOudah, N.; Alwakeel, J.; Ullah, A.; Kfoury, H. Strategy for second kidney biopsy in patients with lupus nephritis. *Nephrol. Dial. Transplant.* **2012**, *27*, 1472–1478. [CrossRef]
49. Alsuwaida, A.O. The clinical significance of serial kidney biopsies in lupus nephritis. *Mod. Rheumatol.* **2014**, *24*, 453–456. [CrossRef]
50. Zickert, A.; Sundelin, B.; Svenungsson, E.; Gunnarsson, I. Role of early repeated renal biopsies in lupus nephritis. *Lupus Sci. Med.* **2014**, *1*, e000018. [CrossRef]
51. Parodis, I.; Adamichou, C.; Aydin, S.; Gomez, A.; Demoulin, N.; Weinmann-Menke, J.; Houssiau, F.A.; Tamirou, F. Per-protocol repeat kidney biopsy portends relapse and long-term outcome in incident cases of proliferative lupus nephritis. *Rheumatology* **2020**, *59*, 3424–3434. [CrossRef] [PubMed]
52. Zhang, H.; Liu, Z.; Zhou, M.; Liu, Z.; Chen, J.; Xing, C.; Lin, H.; Ni, Z.; Fu, P.; Liu, F.; et al. Multitarget Therapy for Maintenance Treatment of Lupus Nephritis. *J. Am. Soc. Nephrol.* **2017**, *28*, 3671–3678. [CrossRef]
53. Rovin, B.H.; Solomons, N.; Pendergraft, W.F., III; Dooley, M.A.; Tumlin, J.; Romero-Diaz, J.; Lysenko, L.; Navarra, S.V.; Huizinga, R.B.; AURA-LV Study Group. A randomized, controlled double-blind study comparing the efficacy and safety of dose-ranging voclosporin with placebo in achieving remission in patients with active lupus nephritis. *Kidney Int.* **2019**, *95*, 219–231. [CrossRef]
54. Arriens, C.; Polyakova, S.; Adzerikho, I.; Randhawa, S.; Solomons, N. OP0277 AURORA phase 3 study demonstrates voclosporin statistical superiority over standard of care in lupus nephritis. *Ann. Rheum. Dis.* **2020**, *79*, 172–173. [CrossRef]

55. Dooley, M.A.; Pendergraft, W., III; Ginzler, E.M.; Olsen, N.J.; Tumlin, J.; Rovin, B.H.; Houssiau, F.A.; Wofsy, D.; Isenberg, D.A.; Solomons, N.; et al. Speed of remission with the use of voclosporin, MMF and low dose steroids: Results of a global lupus nephritis study (abstract). *Arthritis Rheumatol.* **2016**, *68* (Suppl. 10).
56. Aurinia. FDA Approves Aurinia Pharmaceuticals' LUPKYNIS (Voclosporin) for Adult Patients with Active Lupus Nephritis [Press Release]. Available online: https://ir.auriniapharma.com/press-releases/detail/210/fda-approves-aurinia-pharmaceuticals-lupkynis (accessed on 22 January 2021).
57. Navarra, S.V.; Guzmán, R.M.; Gallacher, A.E.; Hall, S.; Levy, R.A.; Jimenez, R.E.; Li, E.K.; Thomas, M.; Kim, H.Y.; León, M.G.; et al. Efficacy and safety of belimumab in patients with active systemic lupus erythematosus: A randomised, placebo-controlled, phase 3 trial. *Lancet* **2011**, *377*, 721–731. [CrossRef]
58. Furie, R.; Petri, M.; Zamani, O.; Cervera, R.; Wallace, D.J.; Tegzová, D.; Sanchez-Guerrero, J.; Schwarting, A.; Merrill, J.T.; Chatham, W.W.; et al. A phase III, randomized, placebo-controlled study of belimumab, a monoclonal antibody that inhibits B lymphocyte stimulator, in patients with systemic lupus erythematosus. *Arthritis Rheum.* **2011**, *63*, 3918–3930. [CrossRef] [PubMed]
59. Dooley, M.A.; Houssiau, F.; Aranow, C.; D'Cruz, D.P.; Askanase, A.; Roth, D.A.; Zhong, Z.J.; Cooper, S.; Freimuth, W.W.; Ginzler, E.M.; et al. Effect of belimumab treatment on renal outcomes: Results from the phase 3 belimumab clinical trials in patients with SLE. *Lupus* **2013**, *22*, 63–72. [CrossRef]
60. Furie, R.; Rovin, B.H.; Houssiau, F.; Malvar, A.; Teng, Y.; Contreras, G.; Amoura, Z.; Yu, X.; Mok, C.C.; Santiago, M.B.; et al. Two-Year, Randomized, Controlled Trial of Belimumab in Lupus Nephritis. *N. Engl. J. Med.* **2020**, *383*, 1117–1128. [CrossRef] [PubMed]
61. Sjöwall, C.; Cöster, L. Belimumab may not prevent lupus nephritis in serologically active patients with ongoing non-renal disease activity. *Scand. J. Rheumatol.* **2014**, *43*, 428–430. [CrossRef]
62. Hui-Yuen, J.S.; Reddy, A.; Taylor, J.; Li, X.; Eichenfield, A.H.; Bermudez, L.M.; Starr, A.J.; Imundo, L.F.; Buyon, J.; Furie, R.A.; et al. Safety and Efficacy of Belimumab to Treat Systemic Lupus Erythematosus in Academic Clinical Practices. *J. Rheumatol.* **2015**, *42*, 2288–2295. [CrossRef] [PubMed]
63. Staveri, C.; Karokis, D.; Liossis, S.C. New onset of lupus nephritis in two patients with SLE shortly after initiation of treatment with belimumab. *Semin. Arthritis Rheum.* **2017**, *46*, 788–790. [CrossRef]
64. Anjo, C.; Mascaró, J.M., Jr.; Espinosa, G.; Cervera, R. Effectiveness and safety of belimumab in patients with systemic lupus erythematosus in a real-world setting. *Scand. J. Rheumatol.* **2019**, *48*, 469–473. [CrossRef]
65. Parodis, I.; Vital, E.M.; Hassan, S.U.; Jönsen, A.; Bengtsson, A.A.; Eriksson, P.; Leonard, D.; Gunnarsson, I.; Rönnblom, L.; Sjöwall, C. De novo lupus nephritis during treatment with belimumab. *Rheumatology* **2020**, keaa796. [CrossRef]
66. Reddy, V.; Klein, C.; Isenberg, D.A.; Glennie, M.J.; Cambridge, G.; Cragg, M.S.; Leandro, M.J. Obinutuzumab induces superior B-cell cytotoxicity to rituximab in rheumatoid arthritis and systemic lupus erythematosus patient samples. *Rheumatology* **2017**, *56*, 1227–1237. [CrossRef] [PubMed]
67. Furie, R.; Aroca, G.; Alvarez, A.; Fragoso-Loyo, H.; Zuta Santillan, E.; Rovin, B.; Brunetta, P.; Schindler, T.; Hassan, I.; Cascino, M.; et al. Two-year results from a randomized, controlled study of obinutuzumab for proliferative lupus nephritis (abstract). *Arthritis Rheumatol.* **2020**, *72* (Suppl. 10).
68. Rovin, B.H.; Furie, R.; Latinis, K.; Looney, R.J.; Fervenza, F.C.; Sanchez-Guerrero, J.; Maciuca, R.; Zhang, D.; Garg, J.P.; Brunetta, P.; et al. Efficacy and safety of rituximab in patients with active proliferative lupus nephritis: The Lupus Nephritis Assessment with Rituximab study. *Arthritis Rheum.* **2012**, *64*, 1215–1226. [CrossRef] [PubMed]
69. Houssiau, F.A. Why will lupus nephritis trials not fail anymore? *Rheumatology* **2017**, *56*, 677–678. [CrossRef] [PubMed]

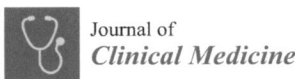

Review

Implications of Endogenous Retroelements in the Etiopathogenesis of Systemic Lupus Erythematosus

Kennedy C. Ukadike and Tomas Mustelin *

Division of Rheumatology, Department of Medicine, University of Washington School of Medicine, 750 Republican Street, Seattle, WA 98109, USA; kukadike@uw.edu
* Correspondence: tomas2@uw.edu; Tel.: +1-(206)-313-6130

Abstract: Systemic lupus erythematosus (SLE) is a heterogeneous autoimmune disease. While its etiology remains elusive, current understanding suggests a multifactorial process with contributions by genetic, immunologic, hormonal, and environmental factors. A hypothesis that combines several of these factors proposes that genomic elements, the L1 retrotransposons, are instrumental in SLE pathogenesis. L1 retroelements are transcriptionally activated in SLE and produce two proteins, ORF1p and ORF2p, which are immunogenic and can drive type I interferon (IFN) production by producing DNA species that activate cytosolic DNA sensors. In addition, these two proteins reside in RNA-rich macromolecular assemblies that also contain well-known SLE autoantigens like Ro60. We surmise that cells expressing L1 will exhibit all the hallmarks of cells infected by a virus, resulting in a cellular and humoral immune response similar to those in chronic viral infections. However, unlike exogenous viruses, L1 retroelements cannot be eliminated from the host genome. Hence, dysregulated L1 will cause a chronic, but perhaps episodic, challenge for the immune system. The clinical and immunological features of SLE can be at least partly explained by this model. Here we review the support for, and the gaps in, this hypothesis of SLE and its potential for new diagnostic, prognostic, and therapeutic options in SLE.

Keywords: systemic lupus erythematosus; retroelements; L1; LINE-1; reverse transcriptase; type I interferons; autoimmunity

Citation: Ukadike, K.C.; Mustelin, T. Implications of Endogenous Retroelements in the Etiopathogenesis of Systemic Lupus Erythematosus. *J. Clin. Med.* **2021**, *10*, 856. https://doi.org/10.3390/jcm10040856

Academic Editor: Philippe Guilpain
Received: 31 December 2020
Accepted: 13 February 2021
Published: 19 February 2021

Publisher's Note: MDPI stays neutral with regard to jurisdictional claims in published maps and institutional affiliations.

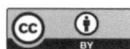

Copyright: © 2021 by the authors. Licensee MDPI, Basel, Switzerland. This article is an open access article distributed under the terms and conditions of the Creative Commons Attribution (CC BY) license (https://creativecommons.org/licenses/by/4.0/).

1. Introduction

Systemic lupus erythematosus (SLE) is a varied and often debilitating autoimmune disease that affects at least 5 million people worldwide, and women more than men with a striking gender bias of 9:1. The precise etiology of SLE remains elusive despite many decades of research to better understand it. Current knowledge suggests a multifactorial etiology with contributions from genetic, immunologic, hormonal, and environmental factors [1,2]. Even at that, the exact extent to which each of these factors contribute to SLE pathogenesis is not known. While we focus here on a specific emerging mechanism that combines genomic/genetic and immunologic factors, with hormonal and environmental contributions, we wish to first place it in the context of the broader genetic associations of SLE.

Genome-wide association studies have identified many genes with polymorphisms and copy number variants that are associated with SLE [3–7]. The most significant associations are found in the major histocompatibility complex II (MHC II), which include alleles of *HLA-DR2*, *HLA-DR3*, and *HLA-DQ2* [8–10]. Deficiencies of the complement components C1q [11], C2, C4A, and C4B, which confer an even higher risk for SLE, are relatively rare [12]. Similarly, rare polymorphisms or mutations in DNases *TREX1* [13] and *DNASE1* [14] also confer significant risk of SLE. Deletion of *trex1* in mice results in accumulation of single-stranded DNA derived from reverse transcription of retroelement RNA, elevated type I interferon production, and severe autoimmunity [15]. In humans, loss-of-function mutations in *DNASE1L3* also result in a SLE-like disease [16]. This gene encodes for an active DNase that is secreted by innate immune cells to degrade chromatin released passively (apoptosis and necrosis) or actively (NETosis) from dying cells. Together, these genes imply a pathogenic role of cytosolic DNA originating from retroelements, and the importance of effective clearance of DNA in immune complexes and cellular debris.

In agreement with this notion, several genes with a role in IFN signaling, such as *IRF5*, *IRAK1*, *STAT4*, *SPP1*, *TNFAIP3*, and *PTPN22*, also have SLE-predisposing variants, which are associated with high levels of type I IFNs and increased expression of IFN-inducible genes [17–21]. Polymorphisms in genes involved upstream of IFNs, such as *IFIH1* [22] and *TLR7* [23], have also been documented. Other genes implicated in the adaptive immune system, including *PTPN22*, *PDCD1* (encodes PD-1) [24], *BANK-1* [25], *BLK*, *LYN*, and *TNFRSF4* (OX40L), indicate that the threshold for activation of B and T cells is important in SLE [26–29]. The MHC association also supports this notion. Unlike the rare complement deficiencies and DNase mutations, these gene polymorphisms individually confer a very modest risk (odds ratio <2) for SLE, suggesting that they are not directly causative, but in aggregate increase the susceptibility to SLE, presumably in combination with the absence of protective gene variants [30,31], genomic hypomethylation, altered epigenetic control, changes in microRNAs (miRNAs) [32–36], and the presence of environmental or endogenous triggers [34–36].

In accordance with the genetics of SLE summarized above, we focus in this review on an emerging concept that is well compatible with the genetic associations, namely the notion that endogenous virus-like sequences may play a part in the pathogenesis of SLE and other related diseases [37–40]. These genomic sequences are either remnants of exogenous retroviruses that infected our ancestors millions of years ago [40–42], or ancient descendants of retroviruses that retained the ability to embed and replicate within the germline genome to become extremely abundant throughout the human genome [40,43]. Although the vast majority of all these sequences are now inactive due to mutations and truncations, a number of them are still more or less intact and able to create extrachromosomal DNA, trigger type I IFNs, and provoke an antiviral type of immune response. The biology of these retroelements and the evidence for their involvement in SLE are discussed here.

2. Transposable Elements in the Human Genome

Colloquially known as "jumping genes" or "parasitic DNA" [44], transposable elements (or transposons) are genomic DNA sequences that have the ability to move within the genome, thereby altering its organization, incrementally increasing its size, and creating duplications and redundancy [45]. There are two broad classes of transposons: Class I transposons, also known as retrotransposons, and class II or DNA transposons [46]. The former propagate using a "copy-and-paste" mechanism that consists of a reverse transcriptase (RT) that uses its own RNA transcript as a template to generate a cDNA copy, which is inserted into the genome. The latter move by a "cut-and-paste" mechanism by their encoded transposase enzyme. To the best of our knowledge, only class I transposons have been implicated in the autoimmune disease and will be discussed further here.

To illustrate the sheer volume of retrotransposons in our genome, compared to all the exons of our 20,000 genes, which occupy approximately 1% of our 3-billion base-pair genome, the retroelements occupy close to 50% of it [44,47]. There are over 3 million retroelements in our genome [48]. They fall into three categories: the over 440,000 long terminal repeat (LTR) retrotransposons, also known as human endogenous retroviruses (HERVs), the 800,000 autonomous non-LTR retrotransposons termed long interspersed nuclear elements (LINEs), and the 1,500,000 copies of the short interspersed nuclear elements (SINEs), which are non-autonomous and include over 1 million Alu elements [49] (Figure 1).

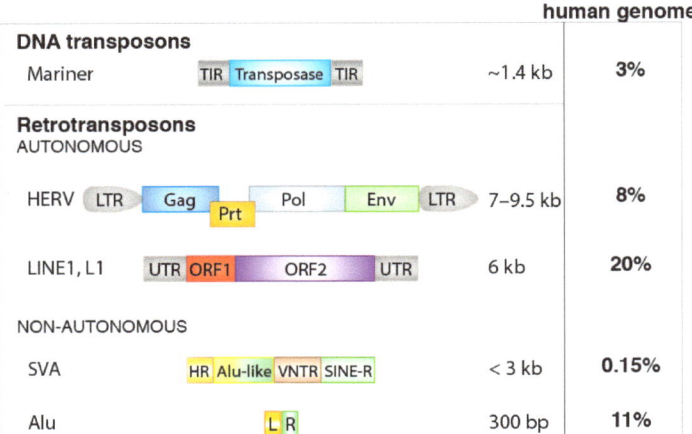

Figure 1. Classes and examples of transposable elements. Abbreviations: TIR, terminal inverted repeats; LTR, long terminal repeats (transcriptional control sequence); Gag, group antigen; Prt, protease; Pol, polymerase; Env, envelope; UTR, untranslated region; ORF, open reading frame; HR, hexamer repeat; VNTR, variable number tandem repeats; SINE-R, Alu right monomer; SVA, SINE-R/VNTR/Alu composite; L, left monomer; R, right monomer.

Before delving into the immunological impacts of retroelements, it should be stated that the retrotransposition mechanism itself can cause genomic damage and result in human disease [50]. New retrotransposon insertions in or near exonic genes can result in altered transcription [51], disrupted mRNA splicing, premature termination of translation, and loss of protein expression or function. Besides sporadic genetic diseases [52] caused by new retrotranspositions, this biology is accelerated in malignant cells [53] and is a major contributor to the activation of oncogenes [54], the inactivation of tumor suppressors [55,56], and larger chromosomal abnormalities [50,57–59]. Retroelements are also abundant around chromosome fragile sites, such as FRA3B on chromosome 3p14 and FRA16D on chromosome 16q23 [60,61].

2.1. HERVs

The HERVs are the very definition of autonomous retrotransposons in that they resulted from germline infections by exogenous retroviruses that upon cell entry reverse-transcribed their RNA genome and inserted it into the host cell genome. The resulting HERVs were subsequently passed on to offspring in a Mendelian fashion and most of them exist in all now living humans [62]. Transcription of such newly formed HERVs result in a polycistronic transcript that, after splicing, encodes for all the proteins necessary for the formation of new infectious virions [63]. However, because HERVs are not under positive selection pressures (but rather the opposite), they accumulate random mutations, deletions, insertions, recombinations, and other genetic alterations over evolutionary time [62]. The modern human genome does not appear to contain any fully intact and functional HERVs anymore [62,64,65], but there still are about a dozen HERVs that encode for proteins that have some, or all, of their original functions [63–67]. Some of the youngest (=most recently incorporated) HERVs can still form virions [68], even though they lack measurable infectivity.

The HERVs in our genome belong to three classes: gammaretroviruses (class I), betaretroviruses (class II), and spumaretroviruses (class III) [69]. The published literature proposes various roles for class I (HERV-E, and to a lesser extent -W, and -H) and class II (HERV-K) HERVs in autoimmune diseases [70–73]. A common denominator among these papers is the idea that their transcriptional upregulation will trigger various aspects of an antiviral immune response, including autoantibodies against retroviral proteins [74–77].

A popular suggestion is that HERV proteins may trigger autoimmunity by molecular mimicry [70,78] through accidental similarities between these proteins and other self-proteins. However, we believe that an immune response against HERV proteins already constitutes "autoimmunity" whether any cross-reactivity exists with proteins encoded by exonic genes, or not.

It should also be kept in mind that even HERVs that have lost their ability to encode for proteins often still possess their strong transactivating long-terminal repeats (LTRs) [79], which can influence the transcription of nearby protein-coding genes [51]. This appears to be a driver of altered gene expression in cancer [80,81], where demethylated LTRs can respond to transcription factors, including those activated by sex hormones. Demethylation of LTR sequences reportedly upregulates HERV expression also in autoimmune diseases like SLE [82,83]. An example of this is the influence on RAB4 gene expression exerted by the demethylated LTR of a truncated class I HERV element, termed HRES-1 [78]. RAB4, in turn, downregulates surface CD4 expression, which together with the immunogenic 28-kDa Gag protein of HRES-1 can contribute to the self-reactivity of T and B cells in SLE [78]. Interestingly, polymorphisms in the HRES-I LTR are associated with SLE [84].

2.2. L1 Retrotransposons

Intact and functional LINE retrotransposons are also autonomous in that they encode all the components needed for their own retrotransposition [44,85,86]. This machinery is also responsible for the retrotranspositions of the non-autonomous retrotransposons [87], and for creating all our pseudogenes [44]. Research has focused primarily on LINE-1 (or L1), which not only are abundant, but also include members that have retained all or some of their biological functions. In contrast, the LINE-2 and LINE-3 groups, although still prevalent, are all inactive, but can serve as templates for regulatory RNA species [88].

As depicted in Figure 2, the L1 transcript is bicistronic and encodes for two proteins, the 40-kDa RNA-binding protein ORF1p and the 149-kDa endonuclease [89] and reverse transcriptase ORF2p [90], which assemble in approximately a 20:1 stoichiometry into complexes with high affinity for RNA, particularly L1 mRNA, but also Alu RNA and other small RNAs [85]. To execute retrotransposition, these ORF1p/ORF2p/RNA translocate to the nucleus, where the endonuclease activity of ORF2p cuts the genome at a poly-dT tract, allowing the poly-A tail of the L1 transcript to align, enabling the reverse transcriptase activity of ORF2p to synthesize a cDNA copy of the associated RNA, followed by DNA repair [85] (Figure 2). As a result, the genome now has a new 6-kb L1 element identical to the one that created it. New Alu elements and pseudogenes are generated by the exact same mechanism [44].

While there is presently no conclusive evidence that retrotransposition of L1 plays any role in autoimmunity (and no evidence that it does not), there are several other aspects of L1 biology that make these elements prime suspects in the pathogenesis of SLE and related autoimmune diseases characterized by elevated type I IFNs.

2.3. Non-Autonomous Retroelements

The enormous abundance of Alu elements with over one million copies throughout our genome, all generated by the L1 retrotransposition machinery, bears witness to the period of very active genome remodeling during hominid evolution. Alu elements are found abundantly within introns and in regulatory regions of genes and in intergenic space. The generation of new Alu and SVA elements is still ongoing and can result in positive or negative changes in the transcriptional control of genes. As such, this mechanism can contribute to human disease, conceivably including autoimmune diseases like lupus. An example of this was the discovery of an Alu insertion into an intron of the FAS/CD95 gene, which resulted in mis-splicing of its transcript, loss of functional FAS protein, and lymphoproliferative disease [91]. Alu transcripts also have the potential to form double-stranded structures, which can be recognized by RNA sensors to induce type I IFNs [92]. This danger is normally reduced by adenosine-to-inosine editing by the ADAR1 enzyme [93], the loss of which causes the interferonopathy Aicardi–Goutières syndrome, discussed in Section 3.2. This RNA editing also appears to be defective in patients with multiple sclerosis [94].

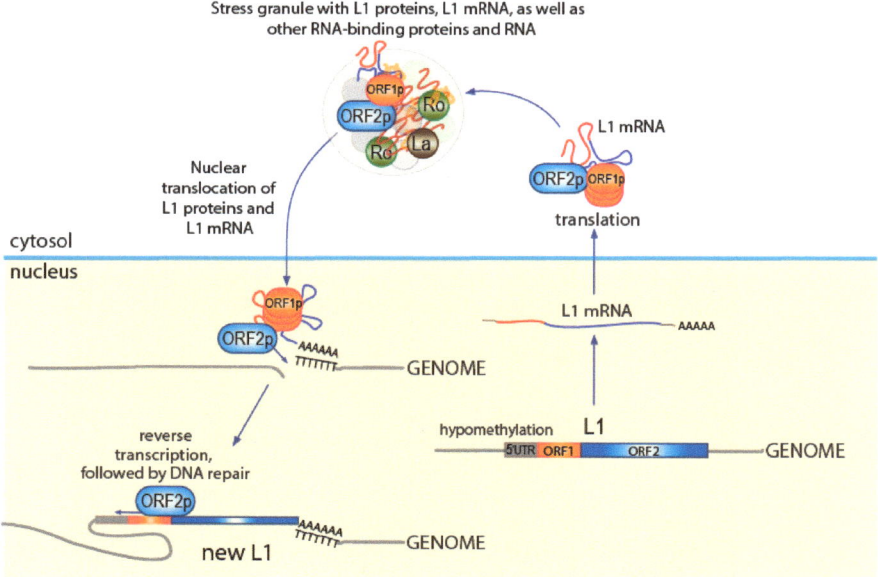

Figure 2. The L1 retrotransposition process. A similar figure is in [40].

Alu elements have also gained interest in lupus research due to the association of Alu-derived RNA with Ro60 [95–97], a well-recognized SLE autoantigen. In a 2015 paper [97], immune complexes formed by anti-Ro60 autoantibodies where isolated from SLE patients and the bound RNA sequenced, revealing that much of it was Alu- and L1-derived. We will discuss the protein and RNA complexes that contain Ro60, known as stress granules, more below.

3. How L1 Retrotransposons May Trigger IFN-Positive SLE

There are several reasons to ask whether L1 retrotransposons play an important role in the pathogenesis and flares of SLE. Increased L1 transcripts and ORF1p protein have been detected in kidney biopsies from patients with lupus nephritis and in salivary gland biopsies from Sjögren's syndrome patients [98]. In healthy individuals, L1 transcripts are low or undetectable, but can be induced by demethylating drugs like 5-aza-deoxycytosine [99], including those known to cause drug-induced lupus [100,101], e.g., hydralazine and procainamide. Reduced methylation of the 5′ regulatory ("promoter") region of L1 has been reported in both adult and pediatric lupus patients [102]. UV light, a well-known trigger of lupus flares [103,104], also causes DNA demethylation, in addition to causing direct DNA damage and cell death at higher exposures. L1 expression also responds to other environmental and microbial factors [105,106].

Essentially all patients with SLE have IgG autoantibodies against ORF1p [107,108], which correlate with disease activity measured by the SLE disease activity index (SLEDAI), the presence of lupus nephritis, complement consumption, increased anti-dsDNA, and higher type I IFN activity [107]. Importantly, there anti-ORF1p autoantibodies do not represent anti-DNA reactivity, as free dsDNA did not compete (while free ORF1p did), DNase treatment did not affect them (while it eliminated anti-dsDNA reactivity), and ORF1p was recognized even when mixed with whole cell lysates. Presumably related to this finding, ORF1p and ORF2p reside in cells in macromolecular assemblies referred to as "stress-granules" [109], which are rich in RNA and RNA-binding proteins, including Ro60 and other SLE autoantigens [110].

Importantly, L1 expression has been shown to induce type I IFNs [111–113], which are a hallmark of SLE [114–118]. This can reportedly occur by two different mechanism [111–113,119], which are not mutually exclusive: (i) cytosolic DNA generated by reverse transcription by ORF2p activates DNA sensors [111], such as cyclic guanosine adenosine monophosphate synthase (cGAS), which through the stimulator of interferon genes (STING) adapter protein [120] activates the TBK1 protein kinase [121], which phosphorylates the IRF3 transcription factor leading to type 1 IFN production. Indeed, cGAS activation was documented in some 17% of SLE in a recent study [122]; (ii) double-stranded RNA species [113], perhaps related to bidirectional L1 promoter activity, activates RNA sensors that initiate the same kinase-transcription factor pathway to type I IFNs. While this second pathway is not restricted to L1 transcripts, either, or both, of these mechanisms can explain the elevated expression of IFN-inducible genes, referred to as the "IFN signature" [116,123] in SLE and related autoimmune diseases, such as idiopathic inflammatory myopathies and primary Sjögren's syndrome [124].

Taking all these observations together, it appears that L1 elements with intact ORF1 and ORF2 are derepressed by reduced DNA methylation (and other epigenetic mechanisms that depend on it) and, therefore, transcribed at elevated levels compared to healthy individuals. Indeed, decreased DNA methylation has been documented in SLE, including specifically in the 5′ regulatory regions of L1 [102]. However, there are also reports that L1 methylation is not altered, but one has to keep in mind that such measures are a composite of numerous L1 elements and does not necessarily represent the relatively small number of L1 loci that are transcriptionally activated in SLE. The epigenetic regulation of L1 elements also varies between cell types. Even different immune cell lineages have distinct patterns of active L1 elements (our unpublished observation).

Translation of these elevated L1 transcripts leads to accumulation of ORF1p and ORF2p in stress granules [109], which, because they contain immunogenic ORF1p protein and lots of RNA, seem to be of special interest to the immune system in SLE patients. We surmise that cells expressing L1, containing triggered DNA and/or RNA sensors, and producing type I IFNs, will appear virally infected to the host immune system and drive a chronic and/or episodic systemic inflammation, which will escalate every time L1 transcription increases. Since the culprit L1 elements cannot be eradicated from the genome, the frustrated immune response will increase in magnitude with time and eventually be diagnosed as SLE.

This model (Figure 3) illustrates how L1 may contribute to many of the well-recognized aspects of SLE: its long prediagnosis development [125] and gradual presentation, its unpredictable and relapsing/remitting nature, the high type I interferons, its sensitivity to demethylating drugs and UV, and the focus of the autoimmune response towards nucleic acids and proteins associated with them. These features also explain the typical symptoms of SLE, such as fever, fatigue, arthralgias, and the multitude of organ manifestations related to the accumulation of immune complexes.

3.1. HERVs and Other Non-L1 Retrotransposons in SLE

Elevated expression [67,126] of many HERVs and autoantibodies against HERV-K and HERV-E Gag and Env proteins [40,72,74–76] have been reported in SLE [127] and other autoimmune diseases [71]. The broader genomic hypomethylation observed in SLE may well explain the upregulation of HERV transcription, but since most HERVs have lost their ability to encode full-length retroviral proteins, only a few of these transcripts are capable of supporting autoantibody production. The resulting autoantibodies may synergize with anti-L1 immunity, for example, in the formation of immune complexes that drive tissue inflammation and organ damage. HERVs with an intact pol gene, encoding for their reverse transcriptase, can, in principle, produce DNA species that trigger DNA sensors like cGAS or ZBP-1 to induce type I IFN production. However, the retroviral life-cycle involves a protected reverse transcription of the RNA genome only upon cell entry and in the confines of the nucleocapsid [128,129]. Hence, HERVs are not likely to generate pathogenic DNA in SLE, but they may well generate double-stranded RNA transcripts that can trigger RNA sensors.

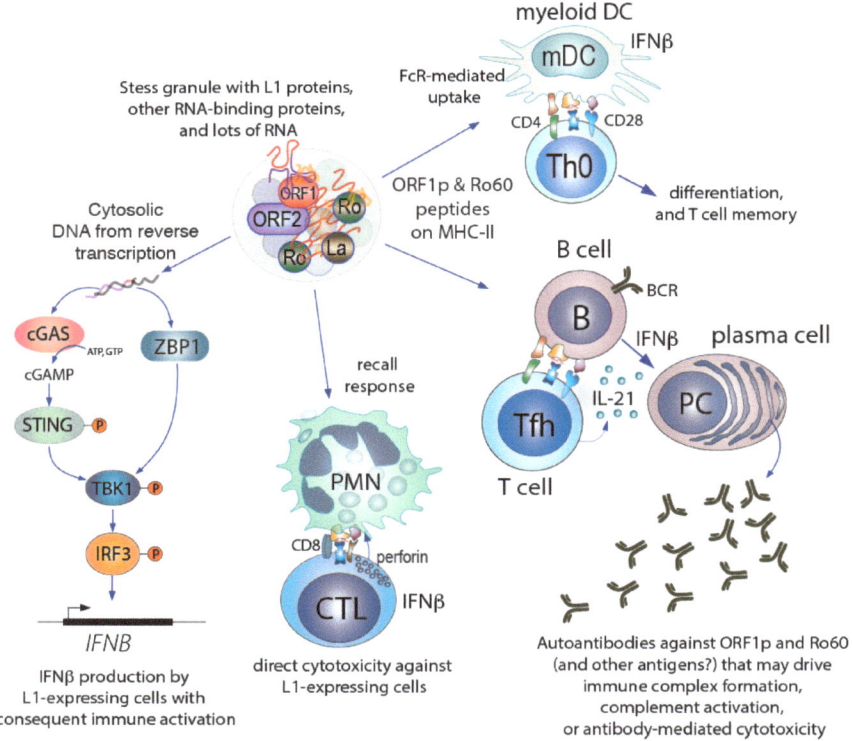

Figure 3. How the L1-containing stress granule may participate in driving SLE-related autoimmunity. The initial priming of T cells likely occurs by dendritic cells, which can take up stress granules, process their contents, and present peptides on class II MHC. The production of autoantibodies against ORF1p and Ro60 likely involves T cells primed by DC, followed by differentiation into follicular or peripheral helper T cells. CD8 T cells derived by cross-priming likely can recognized L1-expressing cells by virtue of ORF1p (and Ro60) derived peptides on class I MHC. Intracellularly, the reverse transcription of L1 transcripts into DNA will trigger IFNβ production and secretion. The secreted IFNβ will further stimulate monocyte differentiation to myeloid DC, plasma cell differentiation, and the differentiation and activation of CD8 T cells to become cytotoxic. Some cells do not express cGAS, but instead have other DNA sensors, such as Z-DNA binding protein 1, ZBP1, which also induce IFNβ production. Lastly (and not specifically illustrated), immune complexes that contain ORF1p, Ro60, and RNA (i.e., stress granules) will be taken up by plasmacytoid dendritic cells and B cells to trigger TLR-mediated IFNα production.

3.2. Are Defenses Against L1 and HERVs Defective in SLE?

Although many components of the model presented above are well documented, it still contains significant gaps. Why does L1 become hypomethylated in individuals who develop SLE? Why is ORF1p so immunogenic? What prevents this from occurring in healthy individuals?

Since majority of people never develop SLE, there must be effective mechanisms to counteract the biology of L1 and HERVs to prevent their deleterious effects on our health. Indeed, numerous defenses exist against all retrotransposons [130,131], many discovered during research into the infectivity of human immunodeficiency virus (HIV). These defenses operate at every step of the life-cycle of retrotransposons and HERVs, and exogenous retroviruses. Some of these defense mechanisms also operate to combat other exogenous RNA and DNA viruses.

Epigenetic regulation is a fundamental mechanism employed by cells to silence genes whose actions are either not needed or are potentially deleterious [132]. This mechanism of transcriptional repression operates on L1 [132] and HERVs and is initiated by DNA methyltransferase 1 (DNMT1) [133], which methylates the 5-position of cytosine in genomic CpG islands, attracting several silencing factors such as the human silencing hub (HUSH) complex [134] and histone modifiers [135] to effectively suppress transcription. Next, RNA interference and silencing activities of small interfering RNAs (siRNAs), miRNAs, and Piwi-interacting RNAs (piRNAs) act to prevent retrotransposon mRNA translation [136]. Of these, the piRNA system is particularly important for protecting the integrity of the germline genome against retrotransposons [137,138].

Hypomethylation of the genome [139] and specific hypomethylation of L1 elements and HERVs have been documented in SLE [140,141] and Sjögren's syndrome [139,141]. The epigenetic mechanisms of L1 repression may also be influenced by environmental factors [142,143]. It is intriguing that drugs known to cause drug-induced lupus, such as hydralazine and procainamide [144,145], and UV light exposure (a well-known trigger of lupus flares [104]), are demethylating agents [146] and increase L1 and HERV expression.

In concert with the above mechanisms, the cytosolic DNase TREX1 [147] and the heterotrimeric RNaseH2 enzyme [148] act to remove cytosolic DNA [15] and RNA species, respectively. Both enzymes are particularly active against DNA:RNA hybrids [149], the intermediate stage of reverse transcription. Indeed, loss of TREX1 results in accumulation of L1-catalyzed DNA in cytosolic granules [149,150]. The importance of these nucleic acid degrading enzymes is perhaps best illustrated by their loss-of-function mutations [151] in Aicardi–Goutières syndrome (AGS) a devastating disease characterized by constitutively high production of type I IFNs, neurologic deficits due to IFN toxicity, and autoimmunity with all the hallmarks and autoantibodies of SLE [152]. L1 expression is high in AGS [153] and type I IFN production can be reduced by administering reverse transcriptase inhibitors that are active against ORF2p [154]. The form of SLE caused by TREX1 mutations [13] likely involves the same overproduction of ORF2p-generated DNA.

The function of retrotransposon proteins is also targeted by defense mechanisms, such as translational inhibition by the ATP-dependent RNA helicase Moloney leukemia virus 10 (MOV10) protein [155–157], which coexists with ORF1p in stress granules [110]. Exactly how MOV10 works is not well understood. Another L1-associated protein identified by proteomics [110,158] is zinc finger CCHC domain-containing 3 (ZCCHC3), a cofactor for both DNA and RNA sensors [159,160]. The *SAMHD1* gene, loss-of-function mutations of which also lead to AGS [161], encodes a phosphohydrolase that dephosphorylates the deoxy-nucleotide triphosphates required for reverse transcription. In addition, the retrotransposition process is directly disrupted by mutation-inducing members of the apolipoprotein B mRNA editing catalytic polypeptide-like 3 (APOBEC3) family of enzymes [162,163], which deaminate cytosines to uracil, and adenosine deaminase of RNA 1 (ADAR1) [93], which deaminates adenosines to inosine. As a result of these mechanisms, the majority of all retrotranspositions result in mutated and severely 5′ truncated new copies (reverse transcription starts in the 3′ end). Most importantly, these mechanisms counteract the production of IFN-inducing DNA and other aspects of L1 biology that can lead to immune activation. Future work will determine if any of these mechanisms are defective in SLE.

3.3. Subsets of SLE with Distinct Mechanisms

The therapeutic options for the management of SLE are limited and often fail to control the disease without unacceptable adverse events. Numerous candidate drugs have failed in clinical trials, for reasons that likely include its molecular heterogeneity and the inaccuracy of tools to assess disease activity. It is quite possible that no single drug will be effective and safe in all SLE patients, but that the precision medicine concept of "the right medicine for the right patient" is particularly relevant in SLE.

Based on biochemical and available clinical trial data, we proposed recently that SLE consists of at least four distinct molecular "endotypes" [164]. The first of these is the IFN-independent form of SLE, "SLE1", defined as the patients who meet the diagnostic criteria for SLE, but consistently lack an IFN signature, i.e., IFN-induced genes are expressed at normal low levels. The remaining three endotypes are characterized by a positive IFN signature, but differ in which nucleic acid sensors have been activated and, consequently, which isotypes of type I IFNs are overproduced.

We define SLE2 as the form in which extracellular immune complexes that contain nucleic acids (e.g., L1-containing stress granules) activate endosomal toll-like receptors (TLRs) 3, 7, 8, or 9 to induce type I IFN production [165]. Due to the predominant expression of TLRs in immune cells, particularly plasmacytoid [166], but also myeloid dendritic cells, macrophages, monocytes, and B cells, the spectrum of induced IFNs include numerous isotypes of IFNα with lesser contributions by IFNβ and type III IFNs [123]. This form of SLE was previously thought to be the main form [167], but the failures in phase 2 clinical trials of multiple TLR7/9 antagonists and antibodies like rontalizumab and sifalimumab that effectively neutralize IFNα, indicate that only 10% or less of SLE patients have SLE2. Most telling, the elevated IFN-inducible genes in the blood of treated patients only declined marginally in patients treated with sifalimumab.

SLE3 is an IFNβ-predominant endotype with activated cytosolic DNA and/or RNA sensors, representing the two alternative mechanisms by which L1 can drive type I IFNs. This biology can occur in any cell type that expresses L1 and/or produces pathogenic double-stranded RNA and this is also how exogenous DNA or RNA viruses initiate an antiviral immune response.

We consider it plausible that SLE typically starts as a pure SLE3 endotype, but that the immune response eventually escalates to a stage where circulating immune complexes with L1-containing, or other, RNA-rich particles accumulate and begin to trigger TLRs on immune cells, i.e., inducing the SLE2 endotype mechanism for type I IFN production. We designated this overlap as SLE4, in which all type I IFNs are at play and both cytosolic and endosomal nucleic acid sensors are active. We estimated that SLE1 represents 10–30%, SLE2 less than 10%, and SLE3 and SLE4 together 60–80% of all SLE patients.

Support for this molecular classification comes from clinical trials with drugs that target IFNs, such as rontalizumab (anti-IFNα), sifalimumab (anti-IFNα), and anifrolumab (antitype I IFN receptor) [168–170], bearing in mind that average outcomes are not as illuminating as a more detailed responder vs. non-responder assessment. Indeed, it is likely that many clinical trial failures in SLE, e.g., with TLR7 antagonists, are the results of too few patients of the responding endotype. In this scenario, the patients with non-responding endotypes diluted out the therapeutic effects beyond the statistical analysis of the entire intent-to-treat cohort.

3.4. L1- and HERV-Related Biomarkers

Whether the above classification is relevant or not, SLE is clearly a heterogeneous disease in its clinical manifestations and response to therapy [1,2]. Many tools have been developed and revised over the years to help guide the diagnosis and management of patients with SLE, and to measure therapeutic effects of drugs during clinical trials. They include various high-sensitivity and high-specificity clinical- and laboratory-based classification criteria (e.g., SLICC criteria) and disease activity indices (e.g., SLEDAI). Despite all these tools, however, the management of SLE, especially in severe disease states, remains one of the biggest challenges in rheumatology. There is often discordance between laboratory evidence of immunologic activity and clinical evidence of disease activity. New diagnostic tools or biomarkers might help narrow the gap.

As we recently demonstrated, the titers of IgG autoantibodies against L1 ORF1p correlate significantly with disease phenotypes, SLEDAI, markers of disease activity, and IFN score [107]. These autoantibodies could conceivably aid in the diagnosis and prognosis of the disease, perhaps guiding which endotype of SLE an individual patient has and, hence, which treatment regimen might be most effective. High titers of anti-ORF1p autoantibodies may also help identify patients who progress to end organ damage, such as lupus nephritis, and may benefit from earlier optimization of their treatment. This would need to be rigorously tested in prospective clinical studies.

Another set of biomarkers would be tests for the activation of the DNA and RNA sensors. Quantitation of the unique second messenger that cGAS produces, cyclic-guanosine adenosine-2,3-monophosphate (cGAMP) by mass spectrometry is probably too cumbersome for use in clinical practice, but newer high-sensitivity ELISAs are under development. For example, it would make sense to consider cGAS inhibitors specifically in those patients that are positive for cGAMP. Another biomarker to reveal the activation of the RNA sensors could be useful. When triggered, these sensors cause the oligomerization of the mitochondrial antiviral signaling (MAVS) adaptor protein, a response that is readily detectable on non-denaturing gels as an ultrahigh-molecular weight species [171]. Representative individual isotypes of the 17 type I IFNs can be quantitated by the ultra-sensitive single-molecule array (SIMOA) platform [172].

3.5. Novel Therapeutic Opportunities Related to L1

New effective and safe drugs are urgently needed for SLE. It stands to reason that drugs that selectively interfere with the molecular pathways that drive SLE, rather than broadly suppress the immune system, would be both more effective and better tolerated than current treatments. The L1 mechanisms we discussed above offer a new option, at least for the SLE3 and SLE4 endotypes, namely the inhibition of ORF2p-catalyzed reverse transcription, which is upstream of type I IFN production, and all the other biological responses induced by activated DNA sensors, such as the upregulation of MHC and costimulatory molecules. Of the FDA-approved reverse transcriptase inhibitors used for the treatment of HIV, some nucleoside RTIs (NRTIs) are equally or near-equally potent on ORF2p as on HIV RT, while others, including the non-nucleoside reverse transcriptase inhibitors, are not. Studies in Trex1-deficient mice, which suffer from severe autoimmune myocarditis and high type I IFNs similar to AGS, have shown that these mice can be rescued by treatment with a three-drug NRTI combination (emtricitabine, tenofovir, and nevirapine). Even more striking, patients with AGS treated with an FDA-approved three-drug NRTI regimen (abacavir, lamivudine, and zidovudine) showed marked reduction in the levels of IFNα proteins and IFN-inducible genes, and an improvement in cerebral blood flow. Several other novel treatments are being explored for AGS, as well as SLE, including inhibitors of cGAS [173], and tyrosine kinase 2 (TYK2), which mediates IFN receptor signaling. Notably, the suppression of inflammation mediated by type I IFNs (potentially triggered by L1 DNA) is a common theme among these potential SLE therapies.

Based on the biology of L1 and HERVs, agents that promote genomic CpG island methylation or other suppressive epigenetic events, or that prevent the translation of their transcripts, e.g., siRNAs, could also be developed for a more uniquely targeted treatment of SLE. The testing of such agents would also go a long way to validate, or refute, the pathogenic relevance of retrotransposons. Lastly, to the best of our knowledge, there is nothing in the drug development pipeline specifically for type I IFN-independent SLE, which mechanistically remains an enigma.

4. Concluding Remarks

The very modest successes in SLE drug development in modern times, and the shortcomings of mainstream models for its etiopathogenesis, make it apparent that new ideas are needed. A more reliable early diagnosis, more accurate prognostication, and the development of more effective treatments with better safety profiles, are all highly needed.

To this end, the emerging evidence of endogenous retroelement involvement in SLE offers a tantalizing promise of progress.

While a broader set of retrotransposons may have varying degrees of involvement in initiating and perpetuating SLE and its flares, current evidence suggests that the L1 retrotransposon is likely the most consequential. However, a true causative role will need to be demonstrated by clinical trials using drugs that interfere with relevant aspects of L1 biology, e.g., reverse transcriptase inhibitors.

Author Contributions: K.C.U. and T.M. contributed equally to the writing of this review and share accountability for its content. All authors have read and agreed to the published version of the manuscript.

Funding: This research was funded by NIH, research grants T32 AR007108 to K.C.U., and R21 AR075134, R21 AR077266 and R01 AR074939 to T.M.

Institutional Review Board Statement: Our work with patient samples has been approved by the University of Washington Institutional Review Board, approval number STUDY00006196, and informed written consent was obtained from all participants according to the Declaration of Helsinki.

Informed Consent Statement: Not applicable.

Data Availability Statement: Not applicable.

Acknowledgments: We thank John LaCava, Marty Taylor, and Christian Lood for valuable suggestions and discussions.

Conflicts of Interest: K.C.U. declares no financial conflicts of interest. T.M. has received consulting fees from Cugene, Kiniksa, Miro Bio, and QiLu Pharmaceuticals, research funding from Gilead Sciences, and has an ownership share in Amdax. These organizations had no role in the design of our studies; in the collection, analyses, or interpretation of data; in the writing of this manuscript, or in the decision to publish study results.

References

1. Wang, L.; Wang, F.S.; Gershwin, M.E. Human autoimmune diseases: A comprehensive update. *J. Intern. Med.* **2015**, *278*, 369–395. [CrossRef] [PubMed]
2. Lockshin, M.D.; Barbhaiya, M.; Izmirly, P.; Buyon, J.P.; Crow, M.K. SLE: Reconciling heterogeneity. *Lupus Sci. Med.* **2019**, *6*, e000280. [CrossRef]
3. Rullo, O.J.; Tsao, B.P. Recent insights into the genetic basis of systemic lupus erythematosus. *Ann. Rheum. Dis.* **2013**, *72* (Suppl. S2), ii56–ii61. [CrossRef]
4. Hom, G.; Graham, R.R.; Modrek, B.; Taylor, K.E.; Ortmann, W.; Garnier, S.; Lee, A.T.; Chung, S.A.; Ferreira, R.C.; Pant, P.V.; et al. Association of systemic lupus erythematosus with C8orf13-BLK and ITGAM-ITGAX. *N. Engl. J. Med.* **2008**, *358*, 900–909. [CrossRef]
5. Graham, R.R.; Hom, G.; Ortmann, W.; Behrens, T.W. Review of recent genome-wide association scans in lupus. *J. Intern. Med.* **2009**, *265*, 680–688. [CrossRef]
6. Nath, S.K.; Han, S.; Kim-Howard, X.; Kelly, J.A.; Viswanathan, P.; Gilkeson, G.S.; Chen, W.; Zhu, C.; McEver, R.P.; Kimberly, R.P.; et al. A nonsynonymous functional variant in integrin-alpha(M) (encoded by ITGAM) is associated with systemic lupus erythematosus. *Nat. Genet.* **2008**, *40*, 152–154. [CrossRef] [PubMed]
7. Boackle, S.A. Advances in lupus genetics. *Curr. Opin. Rheumatol.* **2013**, *25*, 561–568. [CrossRef] [PubMed]
8. Barcellos, L.F.; May, S.L.; Ramsay, P.P.; Quach, H.L.; Lane, J.A.; Nititham, J.; Noble, J.A.; Taylor, K.E.; Quach, D.L.; Chung, S.A.; et al. High-density SNP screening of the major histocompatibility complex in systemic lupus erythematosus demonstrates strong evidence for independent susceptibility regions. *PLoS Genet.* **2009**, *5*, e1000696. [CrossRef]
9. International MHC, and Autoimmunity Genetics Network; Rioux, J.D.; Goyette, P.; Vyse, T.J.; Hammarstrom, L.; Fernando, M.M.; Green, T.; De Jager, P.L.; Foisy, S.; Wang, J.; et al. Mapping of multiple susceptibility variants within the MHC region for 7 immune-mediated diseases. *Proc. Natl. Acad. Sci. USA* **2009**, *106*, 18680–18685. [CrossRef] [PubMed]
10. Graham, R.R.; Ortmann, W.; Rodine, P.; Espe, K.; Langefeld, C.; Lange, E.; Williams, A.; Beck, S.; Kyogoku, C.; Moser, K.; et al. Specific combinations of HLA-DR2 and DR3 class II haplotypes contribute graded risk for disease susceptibility and autoantibodies in human SLE. *Eur. J. Hum. Genet.* **2007**, *15*, 823–830. [CrossRef]
11. Bowness, P.; Davies, K.A.; Norsworthy, P.J.; Athanassiou, P.; Taylor-Weideman, J.; Borysiewicz, L.K.; Meyer, P.A.R.; Walport, M.J. Hereditary C1q deficiency and systemic lupus erythematosus. *Quart. J. Med.* **1994**, *87*, 455–464.
12. Truedsson, L.; Bengtsson, A.A.; Sturfelt, G. Complement deficiencies and systemic lupus erythematosus. *Autoimmunity* **2007**, *40*, 560–566. [CrossRef] [PubMed]

13. Namjou, B.; Kothari, P.H.; Kelly, J.A.; Glenn, S.B.; Ojwang, J.O.; Adler, A.; Alarcon-Riquelme, M.E.; Gallant, C.J.; Boackle, S.A.; Criswell, L.A.; et al. Evaluation of the TREX1 gene in a large multi-ancestral lupus cohort. *Genes Immun.* **2011**, *12*, 270–279. [CrossRef]
14. Gaipl, U.S.; Beyer, T.D.; Heyder, P.; Kuenkele, S.; Bottcher, A.; Voll, R.E.; Kalden, J.R.; Herrmann, M. Cooperation between C1q and DNase I in the clearance of necrotic cell-derived chromatin. *Arthritis Rheum.* **2004**, *50*, 640–649. [CrossRef] [PubMed]
15. Stetson, D.B.; Ko, J.S.; Heidmann, T.; Medzhitov, R. Trex1 prevents cell-intrinsic initiation of autoimmunity. *Cell* **2008**, *134*, 587–598. [CrossRef] [PubMed]
16. Al-Mayouf, S.M.; Sunker, A.; Abdwani, R.; Abrawi, S.A.; Almurshedi, F.; Alhashmi, N.; Al Sonbul, A.; Sewairi, W.; Qari, A.; Abdallah, E.; et al. Loss-of-function variant in DNASE1L3 causes a familial form of systemic lupus erythematosus. *Nat. Genet.* **2011**, *43*, 1186–1188. [CrossRef] [PubMed]
17. Bronson, P.G.; Chaivorapol, C.; Ortmann, W.; Behrens, T.W.; Graham, R.R. The genetics of type I interferon in systemic lupus erythematosus. *Curr. Opin. Immunol.* **2012**, *24*, 530–537. [CrossRef]
18. Kariuki, S.N.; Kirou, K.A.; MacDermott, E.J.; Barillas-Arias, L.; Crow, M.K.; Niewold, T.B. Cutting edge: Autoimmune disease risk variant of STAT4 confers increased sensitivity to IFN-alpha in lupus patients in vivo. *J. Immunol.* **2009**, *182*, 34–38. [CrossRef]
19. Banchereau, R.; Hong, S.; Cantarel, B.; Baldwin, N.; Baisch, J.; Edens, M.; Cepika, A.M.; Acs, P.; Turner, J.; Anguiano, E.; et al. Personalized Immunomonitoring Uncovers Molecular Networks that Stratify Lupus Patients. *Cell* **2016**, *165*, 551–565. [CrossRef]
20. Niewold, T.B.; Kelly, J.A.; Flesch, M.H.; Espinoza, L.R.; Harley, J.B.; Crow, M.K. Association of the IRF5 risk haplotype with high serum interferon-alpha activity in systemic lupus erythematosus patients. *Arthritis Rheum.* **2008**, *58*, 2481–2487. [CrossRef]
21. Kariuki, S.N.; Crow, M.K.; Niewold, T.B. The PTPN22 C1858T polymorphism is associated with skewing of cytokine profiles toward high interferon-alpha activity and low tumor necrosis factor alpha levels in patients with lupus. *Arthritis Rheum.* **2008**, *58*, 2818–2823. [CrossRef] [PubMed]
22. Gorman, J.A.; Hundhausen, C.; Errett, J.S.; Stone, A.E.; Allenspach, E.J.; Ge, Y.; Arkatkar, T.; Clough, C.; Dai, X.; Khim, S.; et al. The A946T variant of the RNA sensor IFIH1 mediates an interferon program that limits viral infection but increases the risk for autoimmunity. *Nat. Immunol.* **2017**, *18*, 744–752. [CrossRef] [PubMed]
23. Tian, J.; Ma, Y.; Li, J.; Cen, H.; Wang, D.G.; Feng, C.C.; Li, R.J.; Leng, R.X.; Pan, H.F.; Ye, D.Q. The TLR7 7926A>G polymorphism is associated with susceptibility to systemic lupus erythematosus. *Mol. Med. Rep.* **2012**, *6*, 105–110. [CrossRef]
24. Prokunina, L.; Castillejo-Lopez, C.; Oberg, F.; Gunnarsson, I.; Berg, L.; Magnusson, V.; Brookes, A.J.; Tentler, D.; Kristjansdottir, H.; Grondal, G.; et al. A regulatory polymorphism in PDCD1 is associated with susceptibility to systemic lupus erythematosus in humans. *Nat. Genet.* **2002**, *32*, 666–669. [CrossRef] [PubMed]
25. Kozyrev, S.V.; Abelson, A.K.; Wojcik, J.; Zaghlool, A.; Linga Reddy, M.V.; Sanchez, E.; Gunnarsson, I.; Svenungsson, E.; Sturfelt, G.; Jonsen, A.; et al. Functional variants in the B-cell gene BANK1 are associated with systemic lupus erythematosus. *Nat. Genet.* **2008**, *40*, 211–216. [CrossRef] [PubMed]
26. Namjou, B.; Kim-Howard, X.; Sun, C.; Adler, A.; Chung, S.A.; Kaufman, K.M.; Kelly, J.A.; Glenn, S.B.; Guthridge, J.M.; Scofield, R.H.; et al. PTPN22 association in systemic lupus erythematosus (SLE) with respect to individual ancestry and clinical sub-phenotypes. *PLoS ONE* **2013**, *8*, e69404. [CrossRef]
27. Curran, C.S.; Gupta, S.; Sanz, I.; Sharon, E. PD-1 immunobiology in systemic lupus erythematosus. *J. Autoimmun.* **2019**, *97*, 1–9. [CrossRef]
28. Jiang, S.H.; Athanasopoulos, V.; Ellyard, J.I.; Chuah, A.; Cappello, J.; Cook, A.; Prabhu, S.B.; Cardenas, J.; Gu, J.; Stanley, M.; et al. Functional rare and low frequency variants in BLK and BANK1 contribute to human lupus. *Nat. Commun.* **2019**, *10*, 2201. [CrossRef]
29. Jacquemin, C.; Schmitt, N.; Contin-Bordes, C.; Liu, Y.; Narayanan, P.; Seneschal, J.; Maurouard, T.; Dougall, D.; Davizon, E.S.; Dumortier, H.; et al. OX40 Ligand Contributes to Human Lupus Pathogenesis by Promoting T Follicular Helper Response. *Immunity* **2015**, *42*, 1159–1170. [CrossRef]
30. Orru, V.; Tsai, S.J.; Rueda, B.; Fiorillo, E.; Stanford, S.M.; Dasgupta, J.; Hartiala, J.; Zhao, L.; Ortego-Centeno, N.; D'Alfonso, S.; et al. A loss-of-function variant of PTPN22 is associated with reduced risk of systemic lupus erythematosus. *Hum. Mol. Genet.* **2009**, *18*, 569–579. [CrossRef]
31. Hawn, T.R.; Wu, H.; Grossman, J.M.; Hahn, B.H.; Tsao, B.P.; Aderem, A. A stop codon polymorphism of Toll-like receptor 5 is associated with resistance to systemic lupus erythematosus. *Proc. Natl. Acad. Sci. USA* **2005**, *102*, 10593–10597. [CrossRef]
32. Altorok, N.; Sawalha, A.H. Epigenetics in the pathogenesis of systemic lupus erythematosus. *Curr. Opin. Rheumatol.* **2013**, *25*, 569–576. [CrossRef] [PubMed]
33. Costenbader, K.H.; Gay, S.; Alarcon-Riquelme, M.E.; Iaccarino, L.; Doria, A. Genes, epigenetic regulation and environmental factors: Which is the most relevant in developing autoimmune diseases? *Autoimmun. Rev.* **2012**, *11*, 604–609. [CrossRef] [PubMed]
34. Yeung, K.S.; Chung, B.H.; Choufani, S.; Mok, M.Y.; Wong, W.L.; Mak, C.C.; Yang, W.; Lee, P.P.; Wong, W.H.; Chen, Y.A.; et al. Genome-Wide DNA Methylation Analysis of Chinese Patients with Systemic Lupus Erythematosus Identified Hypomethylation in Genes Related to the Type I Interferon Pathway. *PLoS ONE* **2017**, *12*, e0169553. [CrossRef] [PubMed]
35. Patel, D.R.; Richardson, B.C. Dissecting complex epigenetic alterations in human lupus. *Arthritis Res. Ther.* **2013**, *15*, 201. [CrossRef]
36. Shen, N.; Liang, D.; Tang, Y.; de Vries, N.; Tak, P.P. MicroRNAs–novel regulators of systemic lupus erythematosus pathogenesis. *Nat. Rev. Rheumatol.* **2012**, *8*, 701–709. [CrossRef] [PubMed]

37. Stetson, D.B. Endogenous retroelements and autoimmune disease. *Curr. Opin. Immunol.* **2012**, *24*, 692–697. [CrossRef]
38. Crow, M.K. Long interspersed nuclear elements (LINE-1): Potential triggers of systemic autoimmune disease. *Autoimmunity* **2010**, *43*, 7–16. [CrossRef]
39. Tugnet, N.; Rylance, P.; Roden, D.; Trela, M.; Nelson, P. Human Endogenous Retroviruses (HERVs) and Autoimmune Rheumatic Disease: Is There a Link? *Open Rheumatol. J.* **2013**, *7*, 13–21. [CrossRef]
40. Mustelin, T.; Ukadike, K.C. How Retroviruses and Retrotransposons in Our Genome May Contribute to Autoimmunity in Rheumatological Conditions. *Front. Immunol.* **2020**, *11*, 593891. [CrossRef]
41. Belshaw, R.; Pereira, V.; Katzourakis, A.; Talbot, G.; Paces, J.; Burt, A.; Tristem, M. Long-term reinfection of the human genome by endogenous retroviruses. *Proc. Natl. Acad. Sci. USA* **2004**, *101*, 4894–4899. [CrossRef]
42. Nelson, P.N.; Hooley, P.; Roden, D.; Davari Ejtehadi, H.; Rylance, P.; Warren, P.; Martin, J.; Murray, P.G.; Molecular Immunology Research, G. Human endogenous retroviruses: Transposable elements with potential? *Clin. Exp. Immunol.* **2004**, *138*, 1–9. [CrossRef] [PubMed]
43. Kano, H.; Godoy, I.; Courtney, C.; Vetter, M.R.; Gerton, G.L.; Ostertag, E.M.; Kazazian, H.H., Jr. L1 retrotransposition occurs mainly in embryogenesis and creates somatic mosaicism. *Genes Dev.* **2009**, *23*, 1303–1312. [CrossRef]
44. Goodier, J.L.; Kazazian, H.H., Jr. Retrotransposons revisited: The restraint and rehabilitation of parasites. *Cell* **2008**, *135*, 23–35. [CrossRef]
45. Bourque, G.; Burns, K.H.; Gehring, M.; Gorbunova, V.; Seluanov, A.; Hammell, M.; Imbeault, M.; Izsvak, Z.; Levin, H.L.; Macfarlan, T.S.; et al. Ten things you should know about transposable elements. *Genome Biol.* **2018**, *19*, 199. [CrossRef] [PubMed]
46. Wicker, T.; Sabot, F.; Hua-Van, A.; Bennetzen, J.L.; Capy, P.; Chalhoub, B.; Flavell, A.; Leroy, P.; Morgante, M.; Panaud, O.; et al. A unified classification system for eukaryotic transposable elements. *Nat. Rev. Genet.* **2007**, *8*, 973–982. [CrossRef] [PubMed]
47. Lander, E.S.; Linton, L.M.; Birren, B.; Nusbaum, C.; Zody, M.C.; Baldwin, J.; Devon, K.; Dewar, K.; Doyle, M.; FitzHugh, W.; et al. Initial sequencing and analysis of the human genome. *Nature* **2001**, *409*, 860–921. [CrossRef] [PubMed]
48. Mandal, P.K.; Kazazian, H.H., Jr. SnapShot: Vertebrate transposons. *Cell* **2008**, *135*, 192–192.e1. [CrossRef] [PubMed]
49. Deininger, P. Alu elements: Know the SINEs. *Genome Biol.* **2011**, *12*, 236. [CrossRef]
50. Hancks, D.C.; Kazazian, H.H., Jr. Roles for retrotransposon insertions in human disease. *Mob. DNA* **2016**, *7*, 9. [CrossRef]
51. Karamitros, T.; Hurst, T.; Marchi, E.; Karamichali, E.; Georgopoulou, U.; Mentis, A.; Riepsaame, J.; Lin, A.; Paraskevis, D.; Hatzakis, A.; et al. Human Endogenous Retrovirus-K HML-2 integration within RASGRF2 is associated with intravenous drug abuse and modulates transcription in a cell-line model. *Proc. Natl. Acad. Sci. USA* **2018**, *115*, 10434–10439. [CrossRef]
52. Batista, R.L.; Yamaguchi, K.; Rodrigues, A.D.S.; Nishi, M.Y.; Goodier, J.L.; Carvalho, L.R.; Domenice, S.; Costa, E.M.F.; Kazazian, H.H.; Mendonca, B.B. Mobile DNA in Endocrinology: LINE-1 Retrotransposon Causing Partial Androgen Insensitivity Syndrome. *J. Clin. Endocrinol. Metab.* **2019**, *104*, 6385–6390. [CrossRef]
53. Ardeljan, D.; Taylor, M.S.; Ting, D.T.; Burns, K.H. The Human Long Interspersed Element-1 Retrotransposon: An Emerging Biomarker of Neoplasia. *Clin. Chem.* **2017**, *63*, 816–822. [CrossRef]
54. Xia, Z.; Cochrane, D.R.; Anglesio, M.S.; Wang, Y.K.; Nazeran, T.; Tessier-Cloutier, B.; McConechy, M.K.; Senz, J.; Lum, A.; Bashashati, A.; et al. LINE-1 retrotransposon-mediated DNA transductions in endometriosis associated ovarian cancers. *Gynecol. Oncol.* **2017**, *147*, 642–647. [CrossRef]
55. Qian, Y.; Mancini-DiNardo, D.; Judkins, T.; Cox, H.C.; Brown, K.; Elias, M.; Singh, N.; Daniels, C.; Holladay, J.; Coffee, B.; et al. Identification of pathogenic retrotransposon insertions in cancer predisposition genes. *Cancer Genet.* **2017**, *216–217*, 159–169. [CrossRef] [PubMed]
56. Scott, E.C.; Gardner, E.J.; Masood, A.; Chuang, N.T.; Vertino, P.M.; Devine, S.E. A hot L1 retrotransposon evades somatic repression and initiates human colorectal cancer. *Genome Res.* **2016**, *26*, 745–755. [CrossRef]
57. Xue, B.; Sechi, L.A.; Kelvin, D.J. Human Endogenous Retrovirus K (HML-2) in Health and Disease. *Front. Microbiol.* **2020**, *11*, 1690. [CrossRef] [PubMed]
58. Kemp, J.R.; Longworth, M.S. Crossing the LINE Toward Genomic Instability: LINE-1 Retrotransposition in Cancer. *Front. Chem.* **2015**, *3*, 68. [CrossRef]
59. Rodić, N.; Sharma, R.; Sharma, R.; Zampella, J.; Dai, L.; Taylor, M.S.; Hruban, R.H.; Iacobuzio-Donahue, C.A.; Maitra, A.; Torbenson, M.S.; et al. Long Interspersed Element-1 Protein Expression Is a Hallmark of Many Human Cancers. *Am. J. Pathol.* **2014**, *184*, 1280–1286. [CrossRef] [PubMed]
60. Ma, K.; Qiu, L.; Mrasek, K.; Zhang, J.; Liehr, T.; Quintana, L.G.; Li, Z. Common fragile sites: Genomic hotspots of DNA damage and carcinogenesis. *Int. J. Mol. Sci.* **2012**, *13*, 11974–11999. [CrossRef]
61. Fungtammasan, A.; Walsh, E.; Chiaromonte, F.; Eckert, K.A.; Makova, K.D. A genome-wide analysis of common fragile sites: What features determine chromosomal instability in the human genome? *Genome Res.* **2012**, *22*, 993–1005. [CrossRef] [PubMed]
62. Subramanian, R.P.; Wildschutte, J.H.; Russo, C.; Coffin, J.M. Identification, characterization, and comparative genomic distribution of the HERV-K (HML-2) group of human endogenous retroviruses. *Retrovirology* **2011**, *8*, 90. [CrossRef]
63. Dewannieux, M.; Harper, F.; Richaud, A.; Letzelter, C.; Ribet, D.; Pierron, G.; Heidmann, T. Identification of an infectious progenitor for the multiple-copy HERV-K human endogenous retroelements. *Genome Res.* **2006**, *16*, 1548–1556. [CrossRef]
64. Hohn, O.; Hanke, K.; Bannert, N. HERV-K(HML-2), the Best Preserved Family of HERVs: Endogenization, Expression, and Implications in Health and Disease. *Front. Oncol.* **2013**, *3*, 246. [CrossRef]

65. Garcia-Montojo, M.; Doucet-O'Hare, T.; Henderson, L.; Nath, A. Human endogenous retrovirus-K (HML-2): A comprehensive review. *Crit. Rev. Microbiol.* **2018**, *44*, 715–738. [CrossRef]
66. Jha, A.R.; Nixon, D.F.; Rosenberg, M.G.; Martin, J.N.; Deeks, S.G.; Hudson, R.R.; Garrison, K.E.; Pillai, S.K. Human endogenous retrovirus K106 (HERV-K106) was infectious after the emergence of anatomically modern humans. *PLoS ONE* **2011**, *6*, e20234. [CrossRef]
67. Ehlhardt, S.; Seifert, M.; Schneider, J.; Ojak, A.; Zang, K.D.; Mehraein, Y. Human endogenous retrovirus HERV-K(HML-2) Rec expression and transcriptional activities in normal and rheumatoid arthritis synovia. *J. Rheumatol.* **2006**, *33*, 16–23.
68. Boller, K.; Schonfeld, K.; Lischer, S.; Fischer, N.; Hoffmann, A.; Kurth, R.; Tonjes, R.R. Human endogenous retrovirus HERV-K113 is capable of producing intact viral particles. *J. Gen. Virol.* **2008**, *89*, 567–572. [CrossRef] [PubMed]
69. Nelson, P.N.; Carnegie, P.R.; Martin, J.; Davari Ejtehadi, H.; Hooley, P.; Roden, D.; Rowland-Jones, S.; Warren, P.; Astley, J.; Murray, P.G. Demystified. Human endogenous retroviruses. *Mol. Pathol.* **2003**, *56*, 11–18. [CrossRef] [PubMed]
70. Perl, A.; Fernandez, D.; Telarico, T.; Phillips, P.E. Endogenous retroviral pathogenesis in lupus. *Curr. Opin. Rheumatol.* **2010**, *22*, 483–492. [CrossRef] [PubMed]
71. Mameli, G.; Erre, G.L.; Caggiu, E.; Mura, S.; Cossu, D.; Bo, M.; Cadoni, M.L.; Piras, A.; Mundula, N.; Colombo, E.; et al. Identification of a HERV-K env surface peptide highly recognized in Rheumatoid Arthritis (RA) patients: A cross-sectional case-control study. *Clin. Exp. Immunol.* **2017**, *189*, 127–131. [CrossRef]
72. Talotta, R.; Atzeni, F.; Laska, M.J. The contribution of HERV-E clone 4-1 and other HERV-E members to the pathogenesis of rheumatic autoimmune diseases. *APMIS* **2020**, *128*, 367–377. [CrossRef] [PubMed]
73. Karimi, A.; Esmaili, N.; Ranjkesh, M.; Zolfaghari, M.A. Expression of human endogenous retroviruses in pemphigus vulgaris patients. *Mol. Biol. Rep.* **2019**, *46*, 6181–6186. [CrossRef]
74. Bengtsson, A.; Blomberg, J.; Nived, O.; Pipkorn, R.; Toth, L.; Sturfelt, G. Selective antibody reactivity with peptides from human endogenous retroviruses and nonviral poly(amino acids) in patients with systemic lupus erythematosus. *Arthritis Rheum.* **1996**, *39*, 1654–1663. [CrossRef] [PubMed]
75. Blomberg, J.; Nived, O.; Pipkorn, R.; Bengtsson, A.; Erlinge, D.; Sturfelt, G. Increased antiretroviral antibody reactivity in sera from a defined population of patients with systemic lupus erythematosus. Correlation with autoantibodies and clinical manifestations. *Arthritis Rheum.* **1994**, *37*, 57–66. [CrossRef] [PubMed]
76. Talal, N.; Garry, R.F.; Schur, P.H.; Alexander, S.; Dauphinee, M.J.; Livas, I.H.; Ballester, A.; Takei, M.; Dang, H. A conserved idiotype and antibodies to retroviral proteins in systemic lupus erythematosus. *J. Clin. Investig.* **1990**, *85*, 1866–1871. [CrossRef] [PubMed]
77. Pelton, B.K.; North, M.; Palmer, R.G.; Hylton, W.; Smith-Burchnell, C.; Sinclair, A.L.; Malkovsky, M.; Dalgleish, A.G.; Denman, A.M. A search for retrovirus infection in systemic lupus erythematosus and rheumatoid arthritis. *Ann. Rheum. Dis.* **1988**, *47*, 206–209. [CrossRef]
78. Perl, A.; Nagy, G.; Koncz, A.; Gergely, P.; Fernandez, D.; Doherty, E.; Telarico, T.; Bonilla, E.; Phillips, P.E. Molecular mimicry and immunomodulation by the HRES-1 endogenous retrovirus in SLE. *Autoimmunity* **2009**, *41*, 287–297. [CrossRef]
79. Montesion, M.; Williams, Z.H.; Subramanian, R.P.; Kuperwasser, C.; Coffin, J.M. Promoter expression of HERV-K (HML-2) provirus-derived sequences is related to LTR sequence variation and polymorphic transcription factor binding sites. *Retrovirology* **2018**, *15*, 57. [CrossRef]
80. Zhou, F.; Li, M.; Wei, Y.; Lin, K.; Lu, Y.; Shen, J.; Johanning, G.L.; Wang-Johanning, F. Activation of HERV-K Env protein is essential for tumorigenesis and metastasis of breast cancer cells. *Oncotarget* **2016**, *7*, 84093–84117. [CrossRef]
81. Goering, W.; Schmitt, K.; Dostert, M.; Schaal, H.; Deenen, R.; Mayer, J.; Schulz, W.A. Human endogenous retrovirus HERV-K(HML-2) activity in prostate cancer is dominated by a few loci. *Prostate* **2015**, *75*, 1958–1971. [CrossRef] [PubMed]
82. Kelly, M.; Lihua, S.; Zhe, Z.; Li, S.; Yoselin, P.; Michelle, P.; Sullivan Kathleen, E. Transposable element dysregulation in systemic lupus erythematosus and regulation by histone conformation and Hsp90. *Clin. Immunol.* **2018**, *197*, 6–18. [CrossRef] [PubMed]
83. Elbarbary, R.A.; Lucas, B.A.; Maquat, L.E. Retrotransposons as regulators of gene expression. *Science* **2016**, *351*, aac7247. [CrossRef] [PubMed]
84. Pullmann, R., Jr.; Bonilla, E.; Phillips, P.E.; Middleton, F.A.; Perl, A. Haplotypes of the HRES-1 endogenous retrovirus are associated with development and disease manifestations of systemic lupus erythematosus. *Arthritis Rheum.* **2008**, *58*, 532–540. [CrossRef]
85. Ostertag, E.M.; Kazazian, H.H., Jr. Biology of mammalian L1 retrotransposons. *Annu. Rev. Genet.* **2001**, *35*, 501–538. [CrossRef]
86. Brouha, B.; Schustak, J.; Badge, R.M.; Lutz-Prigge, S.; Farley, A.H.; Moran, J.V.; Kazazian, H.H., Jr. Hot L1s account for the bulk of retrotransposition in the human population. *Proc. Natl. Acad. Sci. USA* **2003**, *100*, 5280–5285. [CrossRef]
87. Richardson, S.R.; Doucet, A.J.; Kopera, H.C.; Moldovan, J.B.; Garcia-Perez, J.L.; Moran, J.V. The Influence of LINE-1 and SINE Retrotransposons on Mammalian Genomes. *Microbiol. Spectr.* **2015**, *3*, MDNA3-0061-2014. [CrossRef]
88. Petri, R.; Brattas, P.L.; Sharma, Y.; Jonsson, M.E.; Pircs, K.; Bengzon, J.; Jakobsson, J. LINE-2 transposable elements are a source of functional human microRNAs and target sites. *PLoS Genet.* **2019**, *15*, e1008036. [CrossRef] [PubMed]
89. Feng, Q.; Moran, J.V.; Kazazian, H.H., Jr.; Boeke, J.D. Human L1 retrotransposon encodes a conserved endonuclease required for retrotransposition. *Cell* **1996**, *87*, 905–916. [CrossRef]
90. Mathias, S.L.; Scott, A.F.; Kazazian, H.H., Jr.; Boeke, J.D.; Gabriel, A. Reverse transcriptase encoded by a human transposable element. *Science* **1991**, *254*, 1808–1810. [CrossRef]

91. Tighe, P.J.; Stevens, S.E.; Dempsey, S.; Le Deist, F.; Rieux-Laucat, F.; Edgar, J.D. Inactivation of the Fas gene by Alu insertion: Retrotransposition in an intron causing splicing variation and autoimmune lymphoproliferative syndrome. *Genes Immun.* **2002**, *3* (Suppl. 1), S66–S70. [CrossRef]
92. Heinrich, M.J.; Purcell, C.A.; Pruijssers, A.J.; Zhao, Y.; Spurlock, C.F., 3rd; Sriram, S.; Ogden, K.M.; Dermody, T.S.; Scholz, M.B.; Crooke, P.S., 3rd; et al. Endogenous double-stranded Alu RNA elements stimulate IFN-responses in relapsing remitting multiple sclerosis. *J. Autoimmun.* **2019**, *100*, 40–51. [CrossRef] [PubMed]
93. Rice, G.I.; Kasher, P.R.; Forte, G.M.; Mannion, N.M.; Greenwood, S.M.; Szynkiewicz, M.; Dickerson, J.E.; Bhaskar, S.S.; Zampini, M.; Briggs, T.A.; et al. Mutations in ADAR1 cause Aicardi-Goutieres syndrome associated with a type I interferon signature. *Nat. Genet.* **2012**, *44*, 1243–1248. [CrossRef]
94. Tossberg, J.T.; Heinrich, R.M.; Farley, V.M.; Crooke, P.S., 3rd; Aune, T.M. Adenosine-to-Inosine RNA Editing of Alu Double-Stranded (ds)RNAs Is Markedly Decreased in Multiple Sclerosis and Unedited Alu dsRNAs Are Potent Activators of Proinflammatory Transcriptional Responses. *J. Immunol.* **2020**, *205*, 2606–2617. [CrossRef] [PubMed]
95. Shen, C.K.; Maniatis, T. The organization, structure, and in vitro transcription of Alu family RNA polymerase III transcription units in the human alpha-like globin gene cluster: Precipitation of in vitro transcripts by lupus anti-La antibodies. *J. Mol. Appl. Genet.* **1982**, *1*, 343–360.
96. Kole, R.; Fresco, L.D.; Keene, J.D.; Cohen, P.L.; Eisenberg, R.A.; Andrews, P.G. Alu RNA-protein complexes formed in vitro react with a novel lupus autoantibody. *J. Biol. Chem.* **1985**, *260*, 11781–11786. [CrossRef]
97. Hung, T.; Pratt, G.A.; Sundararaman, B.; Townsend, M.J.; Chaivorapol, C.; Bhangale, T.; Graham, R.R.; Ortmann, W.; Criswell, L.A.; Yeo, G.W.; et al. The Ro60 autoantigen binds endogenous retroelements and regulates inflammatory gene expression. *Science* **2015**, *350*, 455–459. [CrossRef] [PubMed]
98. Mavragani, C.P.; Sagalovskiy, I.; Guo, Q.; Nezos, A.; Kapsogeorgou, E.K.; Lu, P.; Liang Zhou, J.; Kirou, K.A.; Seshan, S.V.; Moutsopoulos, H.M.; et al. Expression of Long Interspersed Nuclear Element 1 Retroelements and Induction of Type I Interferon in Patients With Systemic Autoimmune Disease. *Arthritis Rheumatol.* **2016**, *68*, 2686–2696. [CrossRef]
99. Richardson, B.C.; Strahler, J.R.; Pivirotto, T.S.; Quddus, J.; Bayliss, G.E.; Gross, L.A.; O'Rourke, K.S.; Powers, D.; Hanash, S.M.; Johnson, M.A. Phenotypic and functional similarities between 5-azacytidine-treated T cells and a T cell subset in patients with active systemic lupus erythematosus. *Arthritis Rheum.* **1992**, *35*, 647–662. [CrossRef]
100. Goldstein, N.; Leider, M.; Baer, R.L. Drug eruptions from anticonvulsant drugs. Observations on drug-induced lesions that were fixed and lupus-erythematosus-like, and on cross-reactivity between several drugs involved. *Arch. Dermatol.* **1963**, *87*, 612–617. [CrossRef]
101. Zingale, S.B.; Minzer, L.; Rosenberg, B.; Lee, S.L. Drug induced lupus-like syndrome. Clinical and laboratory syndrome similar to systemic lupus erythematosus following antituberculous therapy: Report of a case. *Arch. Intern. Med.* **1963**, *112*, 63–66. [CrossRef] [PubMed]
102. Huang, X.; Su, G.; Wang, Z.; Shangguan, S.; Cui, X.; Zhu, J.; Kang, M.; Li, S.; Zhang, T.; Wu, F.; et al. Hypomethylation of long interspersed nucleotide element-1 in peripheral mononuclear cells of juvenile systemic lupus erythematosus patients in China. *Int. J. Rheum. Dis.* **2014**, *17*, 280–290. [CrossRef] [PubMed]
103. Everett, M.A.; Olson, R.L. Response of Cutaneous Lupus Erythematosus to Ultraviolet Light. *J. Invest. Dermatol.* **1965**, *44*, 133–138. [CrossRef]
104. Bijl, M.; Kallenberg, C.G. Ultraviolet light and cutaneous lupus. *Lupus* **2006**, *15*, 724–727. [CrossRef] [PubMed]
105. Del Re, B.; Giorgi, G. Long INterspersed element-1 mobility as a sensor of environmental stresses. *Environ. Mol. Mutagen.* **2020**, *61*, 465–493. [CrossRef] [PubMed]
106. Leffers, H.C.B.; Lange, T.; Collins, C.; Ulff-Moller, C.J.; Jacobsen, S. The study of interactions between genome and exposome in the development of systemic lupus erythematosus. *Autoimmun. Rev.* **2019**, *18*, 382–392. [CrossRef]
107. Carter, V.; LaCava, J.; Taylor, M.S.; Liang, S.Y.; Mustelin, C.; Ukadike, K.C.; Bengtsson, A.; Lood, C.; Mustelin, T. High Prevalence and Disease Correlation of Autoantibodies Against p40 Encoded by Long Interspersed Nuclear Elements in Systemic Lupus Erythematosus. *Arthritis Rheumatol.* **2020**, *72*, 89–99. [CrossRef]
108. Crow, M.K. Reactivity of IgG with the p40 Protein Encoded by the Long Interspersed Nuclear Element 1 Retroelement: Comment on the Article by Carter et al. *Arthritis Rheumatol.* **2020**, *72*, 374–376. [CrossRef]
109. Goodier, J.L.; Zhang, L.; Vetter, M.R.; Kazazian, H.H., Jr. LINE-1 ORF1 protein localizes in stress granules with other RNA-binding proteins, including components of RNA interference RNA-induced silencing complex. *Mol. Cell. Biol.* **2007**, *27*, 6469–6483. [CrossRef]
110. Taylor, M.S.; LaCava, J.; Mita, P.; Molloy, K.R.; Huang, C.R.; Li, D.; Adney, E.M.; Jiang, H.; Burns, K.H.; Chait, B.T.; et al. Affinity proteomics reveals human host factors implicated in discrete stages of LINE-1 retrotransposition. *Cell* **2013**, *155*, 1034–1048. [CrossRef]
111. De Cecco, M.; Ito, T.; Petrashen, A.P.; Elias, A.E.; Skvir, N.J.; Criscione, S.W.; Caligiana, A.; Brocculi, G.; Adney, E.M.; Boeke, J.D.; et al. L1 drives IFN in senescent cells and promotes age-associated inflammation. *Nature* **2019**, *566*, 73–78. [CrossRef]
112. Jiao, H.; Wachsmuth, L.; Kumari, S.; Schwarzer, R.; Lin, J.; Eren, R.O.; Fisher, A.; Lane, R.; Young, G.R.; Kassiotis, G.; et al. Z-nucleic-acid sensing triggers ZBP1-dependent necroptosis and inflammation. *Nature* **2020**, *580*, 391–395. [CrossRef]
113. Wang, R.; Li, H.; Wu, J.; Cai, Z.Y.; Li, B.; Ni, H.; Qiu, X.; Chen, H.; Liu, W.; Yang, Z.H.; et al. Gut stem cell necroptosis by genome instability triggers bowel inflammation. *Nature* **2020**, *580*, 386–390. [CrossRef]

114. Bengtsson, A.A.; Sturfelt, G.; Truedsson, L.; Blomberg, J.; Alm, G.; Vallin, H.; Ronnblom, L. Activation of type I interferon system in systemic lupus erythematosus correlates with disease activity but not with antiretroviral antibodies. *Lupus* **2000**, *9*, 664–671. [CrossRef] [PubMed]
115. Baechler, E.C.; Batliwalla, F.M.; Karypis, G.; Gaffney, P.M.; Ortmann, W.A.; Espe, K.J.; Shark, K.B.; Grande, W.J.; Hughes, K.M.; Kapur, V.; et al. Interferon-inducible gene expression signature in peripheral blood cells of patients with severe lupus. *Proc. Natl. Acad. Sci. USA* **2003**, *100*, 2610–2615. [CrossRef] [PubMed]
116. Bennett, L.; Palucka, A.K.; Arce, E.; Cantrell, V.; Borvak, J.; Banchereau, J.; Pascual, V. Interferon and granulopoiesis signatures in systemic lupus erythematosus blood. *J. Exp. Med.* **2003**, *197*, 711–723. [CrossRef] [PubMed]
117. Crow, M.K.; Kirou, K.A.; Wohlgemuth, J. Microarray analysis of interferon-regulated genes in SLE. *Autoimmunity* **2003**, *36*, 481–490. [CrossRef] [PubMed]
118. Ronnblom, L.; Alm, G.V.; Eloranta, M.L. Type I interferon and lupus. *Curr. Opin. Rheumatol.* **2009**, *21*, 471–477. [CrossRef]
119. Zhao, K.; Du, J.; Peng, Y.; Li, P.; Wang, S.; Wang, Y.; Hou, J.; Kang, J.; Zheng, W.; Hua, S.; et al. LINE1 contributes to autoimmunity through both RIG-I- and MDA5-mediated RNA sensing pathways. *J. Autoimmun.* **2018**, *90*, 105–115. [CrossRef]
120. Melki, I.; Rose, Y.; Uggenti, C.; Van Eyck, L.; Fremond, M.L.; Kitabayashi, N.; Rice, G.I.; Jenkinson, E.M.; Boulai, A.; Jeremiah, N.; et al. Disease-associated mutations identify a novel region in human STING necessary for the control of type I interferon signaling. *J. Allergy Clin. Immunol.* **2017**, *140*, 543–552.e5. [CrossRef]
121. Bodewes, I.L.A.; Huijser, E.; van Helden-Meeuwsen, C.G.; Tas, L.; Huizinga, R.; Dalm, V.; van Hagen, P.M.; Groot, N.; Kamphuis, S.; van Daele, P.L.A.; et al. TBK1: A key regulator and potential treatment target for interferon positive Sjogren's syndrome, systemic lupus erythematosus and systemic sclerosis. *J. Autoimmun.* **2018**, *91*, 97–102. [CrossRef]
122. An, J.; Durcan, L.; Karr, R.M.; Briggs, T.A.; Rice, G.I.; Teal, T.H.; Woodward, J.J.; Elkon, K.B. Expression of Cyclic GMP-AMP Synthase in Patients with Systemic Lupus Erythematosus. *Arthritis Rheumatol.* **2017**, *69*, 800–807. [CrossRef] [PubMed]
123. Ronnblom, L.; Eloranta, M.L.; Alm, G.V. The type I interferon system in systemic lupus erythematosus. *Arthritis Rheum.* **2006**, *54*, 408–420. [CrossRef] [PubMed]
124. Ronnblom, L. The importance of the type I interferon system in autoimmunity. *Clin. Exp. Rheumatol.* **2016**, *34*, 21–24. [PubMed]
125. Arbuckle, M.R.; McClain, M.T.; Rubertone, M.V.; Scofield, R.H.; Dennis, G.J.; James, J.A.; Harley, J.B. Development of autoantibodies before the clinical onset of systemic lupus erythematosus. *N. Engl. J. Med.* **2003**, *349*, 1526–1533. [CrossRef]
126. Reynier, F.; Verjat, T.; Turrel, F.; Imbert, P.E.; Marotte, H.; Mougin, B.; Miossec, P. Increase in human endogenous retrovirus HERV-K (HML-2) viral load in active rheumatoid arthritis. *Scand. J. Immunol.* **2009**, *70*, 295–299. [CrossRef]
127. Talal, N.; Flescher, E.; Dang, H. Are endogenous retroviruses involved in human autoimmune disease? *J. Autoimmun.* **1992**, *5* (Suppl. SA), 61–66. [CrossRef]
128. Barat, C.; Schatz, O.; Le Grice, S.; Darlix, J.L. Analysis of the interactions of HIV1 replication primer tRNA(Lys,3) with nucleocapsid protein and reverse transcriptase. *J. Mol. Biol.* **1993**, *231*, 185–190. [CrossRef]
129. Ji, X.; Klarmann, G.J.; Preston, B.D. Effect of human immunodeficiency virus type 1 (HIV-1) nucleocapsid protein on HIV-1 reverse transcriptase activity in vitro. *Biochemistry* **1996**, *35*, 132–143. [CrossRef]
130. Ariumi, Y. Guardian of the Human Genome: Host Defense Mechanisms against LINE-1 Retrotransposition. *Front. Chem.* **2016**, *4*, 28. [CrossRef]
131. Yang, F.; Wang, P.J. Multiple LINEs of retrotransposon silencing mechanisms in the mammalian germline. *Semin. Cell Dev. Biol.* **2016**, *59*, 118–125. [CrossRef] [PubMed]
132. Tsutsumi, Y. Hypomethylation of the retrotransposon LINE-1 in malignancy. *Jpn. J. Clin. Oncol.* **2000**, *30*, 289–290. [CrossRef] [PubMed]
133. Nawrocki, M.J.; Majewski, D.; Puszczewicz, M.; Jagodzinski, P.P. Decreased mRNA expression levels of DNA methyltransferases type 1 and 3A in systemic lupus erythematosus. *Rheumatol. Int.* **2017**, *37*, 775–783. [CrossRef] [PubMed]
134. Tunbak, H.; Enriquez-Gasca, R.; Tie, C.H.C.; Gould, P.A.; Mlcochova, P.; Gupta, R.K.; Fernandes, L.; Holt, J.; van der Veen, A.G.; Giampazolias, E.; et al. The HUSH complex is a gatekeeper of type I interferon through epigenetic regulation of LINE-1s. *Nat. Commun.* **2020**, *11*, 5387. [CrossRef]
135. Hunter, R.G.; Murakami, G.; Dewell, S.; Seligsohn, M.; Baker, M.E.; Datson, N.A.; McEwen, B.S.; Pfaff, D.W. Acute stress and hippocampal histone H3 lysine 9 trimethylation, a retrotransposon silencing response. *Proc. Natl. Acad. Sci. USA* **2012**, *109*, 17657–17662. [CrossRef]
136. Wang, X.; Jiang, C.; Fu, B.; Zhu, R.; Diao, F.; Xu, N.; Chen, Z.; Tao, W.; Li, C.J. MILI, a PIWI family protein, inhibits melanoma cell migration through methylation of LINE1. *Biochem. Biophys. Res. Commun.* **2015**, *457*, 514–519. [CrossRef]
137. Kuramochi-Miyagawa, S.; Watanabe, T.; Gotoh, K.; Totoki, Y.; Toyoda, A.; Ikawa, M.; Asada, N.; Kojima, K.; Yamaguchi, Y.; Ijiri, T.W.; et al. DNA methylation of retrotransposon genes is regulated by Piwi family members MILI and MIWI2 in murine fetal testes. *Genes Dev.* **2008**, *22*, 908–917. [CrossRef]
138. Russell, S.J.; Stalker, L.; LaMarre, J. PIWIs, piRNAs and Retrotransposons: Complex battles during reprogramming in gametes and early embryos. *Reprod. Domest. Anim.* **2017**, *52* (Suppl. 4), 28–38. [CrossRef]
139. Imgenberg-Kreuz, J.; Sandling, J.K.; Almlof, J.C.; Nordlund, J.; Signer, L.; Norheim, K.B.; Omdal, R.; Ronnblom, L.; Eloranta, M.L.; Syvanen, A.C.; et al. Genome-wide DNA methylation analysis in multiple tissues in primary Sjogren's syndrome reveals regulatory effects at interferon-induced genes. *Ann. Rheum. Dis.* **2016**, *75*, 2029–2036. [CrossRef]

140. Sukapan, P.; Promnarate, P.; Avihingsanon, Y.; Mutirangura, A.; Hirankarn, N. Types of DNA methylation status of the interspersed repetitive sequences for LINE-1, Alu, HERV-E and HERV-K in the neutrophils from systemic lupus erythematosus patients and healthy controls. *J. Hum. Genet.* **2014**, *59*, 178–188. [CrossRef]
141. Mavragani, C.P.; Nezos, A.; Sagalovskiy, I.; Seshan, S.; Kirou, K.A.; Crow, M.K. Defective regulation of L1 endogenous retroelements in primary Sjogren's syndrome and systemic lupus erythematosus: Role of methylating enzymes. *J. Autoimmun.* **2018**, *88*, 75–82. [CrossRef]
142. Lee, J.; Kalia, V.; Perera, F.; Herbstman, J.; Li, T.; Nie, J.; Qu, L.R.; Yu, J.; Tang, D. Prenatal airborne polycyclic aromatic hydrocarbon exposure, LINE1 methylation and child development in a Chinese cohort. *Environ. Int.* **2017**, *99*, 315–320. [CrossRef]
143. Breton, C.V.; Yao, J.; Millstein, J.; Gao, L.; Siegmund, K.D.; Mack, W.; Whitfield-Maxwell, L.; Lurmann, F.; Hodis, H.; Avol, E.; et al. Prenatal Air Pollution Exposures, DNA Methyl Transferase Genotypes, and Associations with Newborn LINE1 and Alu Methylation and Childhood Blood Pressure and Carotid Intima-Media Thickness in the Children's Health Study. *Environ. Health Perspect.* **2016**, *124*, 1905–1912. [CrossRef]
144. Cornacchia, E.; Golbus, J.; Maybaum, J.; Strahler, J.; Hanash, S.; Richardson, B. Hydralazine and procainamide inhibit T cell DNA methylation and induce autoreactivity. *J. Immunol.* **1988**, *140*, 2197–2200.
145. Yung, R.L.; Quddus, J.; Chrisp, C.E.; Johnson, K.J.; Richardson, B.C. Mechanism of drug-induced lupus. I. Cloned Th2 cells modified with DNA methylation inhibitors in vitro cause autoimmunity in vivo. *J. Immunol.* **1995**, *154*, 3025–3035. [PubMed]
146. Lieberman, M.W.; Beach, L.R.; Palmiter, R.D. Ultraviolet radiation-induced metallothionein-I gene activation is associated with extensive DNA demethylation. *Cell* **1983**, *35*, 207–214. [CrossRef]
147. Yang, Y.G.; Lindahl, T.; Barnes, D.E. Trex1 exonuclease degrades ssDNA to prevent chronic checkpoint activation and autoimmune disease. *Cell* **2007**, *131*, 873–886. [CrossRef] [PubMed]
148. Pokatayev, V.; Hasin, N.; Chon, H.; Cerritelli, S.M.; Sakhuja, K.; Ward, J.M.; Morris, H.D.; Yan, N.; Crouch, R.J. RNase H2 catalytic core Aicardi-Goutieres syndrome-related mutant invokes cGAS-STING innate immune-sensing pathway in mice. *J. Exp. Med.* **2016**, *213*, 329–336. [CrossRef] [PubMed]
149. Thomas, C.A.; Tejwani, L.; Trujillo, C.A.; Negraes, P.D.; Herai, R.H.; Mesci, P.; Macia, A.; Crow, Y.J.; Muotri, A.R. Modeling of TREX1-Dependent Autoimmune Disease using Human Stem Cells Highlights L1 Accumulation as a Source of Neuroinflammation. *Cell Stem Cell* **2017**, *21*, 319–331.e8. [CrossRef]
150. Lim, Y.W.; Sanz, L.A.; Xu, X.; Hartono, S.R.; Chedin, F. Genome-wide DNA hypomethylation and RNA:DNA hybrid accumulation in Aicardi-Goutieres syndrome. *Elife* **2015**, *4*. [CrossRef]
151. Crow, Y.J.; Chase, D.S.; Lowenstein Schmidt, J.; Szynkiewicz, M.; Forte, G.M.; Gornall, H.L.; Oojageer, A.; Anderson, B.; Pizzino, A.; Helman, G.; et al. Characterization of human disease phenotypes associated with mutations in TREX1, RNASEH2A, RNASEH2B, RNASEH2C, SAMHD1, ADAR, and IFIH1. *Am. J. Med. Genet. A* **2015**, *167A*, 296–312. [CrossRef] [PubMed]
152. Crow, Y.J.; Manel, N. Aicardi-Goutieres syndrome and the type I interferonopathies. *Nat. Rev. Immunol.* **2015**, *15*, 429–440. [CrossRef] [PubMed]
153. Li, P.; Du, J.; Goodier, J.L.; Hou, J.; Kang, J.; Kazazian, H.H., Jr.; Zhao, K.; Yu, X.F. Aicardi-Goutieres syndrome protein TREX1 suppresses L1 and maintains genome integrity through exonuclease-independent ORF1p depletion. *Nucleic Acids Res.* **2017**, *45*, 4619–4631. [CrossRef] [PubMed]
154. Rice, G.I.; Meyzer, C.; Bouazza, N.; Hully, M.; Boddaert, N.; Semeraro, M.; Zeef, L.A.H.; Rozenberg, F.; Bondet, V.; Duffy, D.; et al. Reverse-Transcriptase Inhibitors in the Aicardi-Goutieres Syndrome. *N. Engl. J. Med.* **2018**, *379*, 2275–2277. [CrossRef] [PubMed]
155. Li, X.; Zhang, J.; Jia, R.; Cheng, V.; Xu, X.; Qiao, W.; Guo, F.; Liang, C.; Cen, S. The MOV10 helicase inhibits LINE-1 mobility. *J. Biol. Chem.* **2013**, *288*, 21148–21160. [CrossRef]
156. Arjan-Odedra, S.; Swanson, C.M.; Sherer, N.M.; Wolinsky, S.M.; Malim, M.H. Endogenous MOV10 inhibits the retrotransposition of endogenous retroelements but not the replication of exogenous retroviruses. *Retrovirology* **2012**, *9*, 53. [CrossRef]
157. Choi, J.; Hwang, S.Y.; Ahn, K. Interplay between RNASEH2 and MOV10 controls LINE-1 retrotransposition. *Nucleic Acids Res.* **2018**, *46*, 1912–1926. [CrossRef]
158. Taylor, M.S.; LaCava, J.; Dai, L.; Mita, P.; Burns, K.H.; Rout, M.P.; Boeke, J.D. Characterization of L1-Ribonucleoprotein Particles. *Methods Mol. Biol.* **2016**, *1400*, 311–338. [CrossRef]
159. Lian, H.; Wei, J.; Zang, R.; Ye, W.; Yang, Q.; Zhang, X.N.; Chen, Y.D.; Fu, Y.Z.; Hu, M.M.; Lei, C.Q.; et al. ZCCHC3 is a co-sensor of cGAS for dsDNA recognition in innate immune response. *Nat. Commun.* **2018**, *9*, 3349. [CrossRef]
160. Lian, H.; Zang, R.; Wei, J.; Ye, W.; Hu, M.M.; Chen, Y.D.; Zhang, X.N.; Guo, Y.; Lei, C.Q.; Yang, Q.; et al. The Zinc-Finger Protein ZCCHC3 Binds RNA and Facilitates Viral RNA Sensing and Activation of the RIG-I-like Receptors. *Immunity* **2018**, *49*, 438–448.e5. [CrossRef]
161. Rice, G.I.; Bond, J.; Asipu, A.; Brunette, R.L.; Manfield, I.W.; Carr, I.M.; Fuller, J.C.; Jackson, R.M.; Lamb, T.; Briggs, T.A.; et al. Mutations involved in Aicardi-Goutieres syndrome implicate SAMHD1 as regulator of the innate immune response. *Nat. Genet.* **2009**, *41*, 829–832. [CrossRef]
162. Bogerd, H.P.; Wiegand, H.L.; Doehle, B.P.; Lueders, K.K.; Cullen, B.R. APOBEC3A and APOBEC3B are potent inhibitors of LTR-retrotransposon function in human cells. *Nucleic Acids Res.* **2006**, *34*, 89–95. [CrossRef] [PubMed]
163. Refsland, E.W.; Harris, R.S. The APOBEC3 family of retroelement restriction factors. *Curr. Top. Microbiol. Immunol.* **2013**, *371*, 1–27. [CrossRef] [PubMed]

164. Mustelin, T.; Lood, C.; Giltiay, N.V. Sources of Pathogenic Nucleic Acids in Systemic Lupus Erythematosus. *Front. Immunol.* **2019**, *10*, 1028. [CrossRef]
165. Barrat, F.J.; Meeker, T.; Gregorio, J.; Chan, J.H.; Uematsu, S.; Akira, S.; Chang, B.; Duramad, O.; Coffman, R.L. Nucleic acids of mammalian origin can act as endogenous ligands for Toll-like receptors and may promote systemic lupus erythematosus. *J. Exp. Med.* **2005**, *202*, 1131–1139. [CrossRef]
166. Ronnblom, L.; Alm, G.V. A pivotal role for the natural interferon alpha-producing cells (plasmacytoid dendritic cells) in the pathogenesis of lupus. *J. Exp. Med.* **2001**, *194*, F59–F63. [CrossRef] [PubMed]
167. Lloyd, W.; Schur, P.H. Immune complexes, complement, and anti-DNA in exacerbations of systemic lupus erythematosus. *Medicine* **1981**, *60*, 208–217. [CrossRef]
168. Kalunian, K.C.; Merrill, J.T.; Maciuca, R.; McBride, J.M.; Townsend, M.J.; Wei, X.; Davis, J.C., Jr.; Kennedy, W.P. A Phase II study of the efficacy and safety of rontalizumab (rhuMAb interferon-alpha) in patients with systemic lupus erythematosus (ROSE). *Ann. Rheum. Dis.* **2016**, *75*, 196–202. [CrossRef]
169. Khamashta, M.; Merrill, J.T.; Werth, V.P.; Furie, R.; Kalunian, K.; Illei, G.G.; Drappa, J.; Wang, L.; Greth, W.; on behalf of the CD1067 Study Investigators. Sifalimumab, an anti-interferon-alpha monoclonal antibody, in moderate to severe systemic lupus erythematosus: A randomised, double-blind, placebo-controlled study. *Ann. Rheum. Dis.* **2016**, *75*, 1909–1916. [CrossRef]
170. Tanaka, Y.; Tummala, R. Anifrolumab, a monoclonal antibody to the type I interferon receptor subunit 1, for the treatment of systemic lupus erythematosus: An overview from clinical trials. *Mod. Rheumatol.* **2020**, *30*, 1–12. [CrossRef]
171. Shao, W.H.; Shu, D.H.; Zhen, Y.; Hilliard, B.; Priest, S.O.; Cesaroni, M.; Ting, J.P.; Cohen, P.L. Prion-like Aggregation of Mitochondrial Antiviral Signaling Protein in Lupus Patients Is Associated with Increased Levels of Type I Interferon. *Arthritis Rheumatol.* **2016**, *68*, 2697–2707. [CrossRef] [PubMed]
172. Rodero, M.P.; Decalf, J.; Bondet, V.; Hunt, D.; Rice, G.I.; Werneke, S.; McGlasson, S.L.; Alyanakian, M.A.; Bader-Meunier, B.; Barnerias, C.; et al. Detection of interferon alpha protein reveals differential levels and cellular sources in disease. *J. Exp. Med.* **2017**, *214*, 1547–1555. [CrossRef] [PubMed]
173. An, J.; Woodward, J.J.; Minie, M.; Sasaki, T.; Elkon, K.B. Novel Anti-Malarial Drug Derivative Inhibited Type I Interferon Production and Autoimmune Inflammation through Inhibition of CGAS-Sting Pathway in Trex1-/- Mouse (abstract 2984). *Arthritis Rheumatol.* **2016**, *68*. Available online: https://acrabstracts.org/abstract/novel-anti-malarial-drug-derivative-inhibited-type-i-interferon-production-and-autoimmune-inflammation-through-inhibition-of-cgas-sting-pathway-in-trex1-mouse/ (accessed on 13 February 2021).

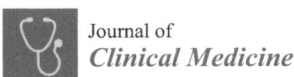

Article

High Comorbidity Burden in Patients with SLE: Data from the Community-Based Lupus Registry of Crete

Irini Gergianaki [1,2,3], Panagiotis Garantziotis [4,5], Christina Adamichou [1,2], Ioannis Saridakis [1,2], Georgios Spyrou [1,2], Prodromos Sidiropoulos [1,2,3] and George Bertsias [1,2,3,*]

1. Department of Rheumatology and Clinical Immunology, University of Crete School of Medicine, 71500 Giofirakia, Greece; iriniger@hotmail.com (I.G.); christina.adamichou@gmail.com (C.A.); sar_giannis@outlook.com.gr (I.S.); gergianakii@gmail.com (G.S.); sidiropp@uoc.gr (P.S.)
2. Department of Rheumatology and Clinical Immunology, University Hospital of Heraklion, 71500 Heraklion, Greece
3. Institute of Molecular Biology and Biotechnology, Foundation for Research and Technology-Hellas (FORTH), 70013 Heraklion, Greece
4. Laboratory of Immune Regulation and Tolerance, Autoimmunity and Inflammation, Biomedical Research Foundation of the Academy of Athens, 11527 Athens, Greece; garantziotis.p@gmail.com
5. Division of Immunology and Rheumatology, Hannover Medical University, 30625 Hannover, Germany
* Correspondence: gbertsias@uoc.gr; Tel.: +30-2810-394635

Citation: Gergianaki, I.; Garantziotis, P.; Adamichou, C.; Saridakis, I.; Spyrou, G.; Sidiropoulos, P.; Bertsias, G. High Comorbidity Burden in Patients with SLE: Data from the Community-Based Lupus Registry of Crete. *J. Clin. Med.* **2021**, *10*, 998. https://doi.org/10.3390/jcm10050998

Academic Editor: Matteo Piga

Received: 2 January 2021
Accepted: 22 February 2021
Published: 2 March 2021

Publisher's Note: MDPI stays neutral with regard to jurisdictional claims in published maps and institutional affiliations.

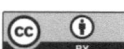

Copyright: © 2021 by the authors. Licensee MDPI, Basel, Switzerland. This article is an open access article distributed under the terms and conditions of the Creative Commons Attribution (CC BY) license (https://creativecommons.org/licenses/by/4.0/).

Abstract: Comorbidities and multimorbidity, often complicating the disease course of patients with chronic inflammatory rheumatic diseases, may be influenced by disease-intrinsic and extrinsic determinants including regional and social factors. We analyzed the frequency and co-segregation of self-reported comorbid diseases in a community-based Mediterranean registry of patients (*n* = 399) with systemic lupus erythematosus (SLE). Predictors for multimorbidity were identified by multivariable logistic regression, strongly-associated pairs of comorbidities by the Cramer's V-statistic, and comorbidities clusters by hierarchical agglomerative clustering. Among the most prevalent comorbidities were thyroid (45.6%) and metabolic disorders (hypertension: 24.6%, dyslipidemia: 33.3%, obesity: 35.3%), followed by osteoporosis (22.3%), cardiovascular (20.8%), and allergic (20.6%) disorders. Mental comorbidities were also common, particularly depression (26.7%) and generalized anxiety disorder (10.7%). Notably, 51.0% of patients had ≥3 physical and 33.1% had ≥2 mental comorbidities, with a large fraction (*n* = 86) displaying multimorbidity from both domains. Sociodemographic (education level, marital status) and clinical (disease severity, neurological involvement) were independently associated with physical or mental comorbidity. Patients were grouped into five distinct clusters of variably prevalent comorbid diseases from different organs and domains, which correlated with SLE severity patterns. Conclusively, our results suggest a high multimorbidity burden in patients with SLE at the community, advocating for integrated care to optimize outcomes.

Keywords: autoimmunity; metabolic risk factors; cardiovascular; mental disorders; disease severity; social factors

1. Introduction

It has long been appreciated that patients with Systemic Lupus Erythematosus (SLE) suffer from a chronic disease course burdened with comorbid conditions from multiple organs [1,2]. This was illustrated in a large case-control study utilizing data from the UK Clinical Practice Research Datalink, where SLE patients had significantly increased incidence for comorbidities with adjusted relative rates ranging from 1.31 to 7.83 [3]. These results are further supported by observational studies examining individual disorders such as infections [4–6], hypertension and metabolic risk factors [7,8], atherosclerotic vascular events [9–13], malignancies [14–16], and osteoporosis [17,18]. Psychiatric comorbidities, albeit less well studied, are also prevalent in SLE patients [19,20]. Notably, comorbid diseases may occur both at early and late stages of the disease, and tend to accumulate in individuals, also known as multimorbidity, which is an emerging frontier in autoimmune rheumatic diseases [21]. Compared to morbidity, multimorbidity represents a broader, patient-centered concept that extends beyond the coexistence of disorders and implies potential disease interaction and pathophysiological links [21].

Similar to other diseases, comorbidities have been shown to correlate with a number of adverse outcomes in patients with SLE including poor health-related quality of life [22,23], reduced work productivity [24], irreversible end-organ damage [25], increased hospitalizations and healthcare costs [26,27], and excess mortality [28]. Accordingly, clinical management of SLE should focus on strategies for preventing or mitigating the impact of comorbidities [1,29], also emphasized in the recommendations issued by regulatory committees such as the European League Against Rheumatism (EULAR) [30–32] and the American College of Rheumatology (ACR) [32].

Although incompletely understood, occurrence of comorbidity and multimorbidity might be due to the inflammatory (e.g., soluble mediators) and clinical (e.g., pain) burden of the underlying index disease (SLE), the effect of administered treatments (e.g., glucocorticoids), and shared pathogenic risk factors [33]. In this context, very few studies have examined the association between lupus activity and severity patterns and comorbidities in patients with SLE [34]. Importantly, development of comorbidities may be influenced by parameters such as race and ethnicity [35,36], access to medical care [37] and other social determinants [38]. Accordingly, examining the prevalence of comorbid diseases and their associated factors in different settings is important to obtain a comprehensive view of the clinical burden of SLE and unravel medical needs at regional level.

To this end, we recently established the Cretan Lupus Epidemiclogy and Surveillance Registry in order to examine SLE occurrence trends and disease characteristics in Crete, the fifth largest Mediterranean island [39,40]. This is a community-based registry of patients who reside both at rural and urban districts and receive care from the primary to tertiary level. Therefore, a wide spectrum of disease presentations is captured ranging from milder to severe forms of SLE [39,40]. Herein, we report on the frequency of comorbid diseases based on patient-reported data collected during face interviews upon enrolment to the registry, and we explore demographic and clinical variables associated with the presence of multiple comorbidities. Driven by our results showing co-segregation of comorbidities in SLE patients, we performed cluster analysis to determine phenotypes of comorbidities in our dataset. Our findings suggest a high burden of comorbid diseases and multimorbidity within SLE patients encountered at the community, related to both disease and sociodemographic characteristics.

2. Materials and Methods

2.1. Source Population and Setting

Crete is the southernmost and largest island of Greece with a relatively stable population of 623,065 inhabitants (2011 National Census). About 61% of the residents live in rural ($\leq$10,000 dwellers) and the remaining 39% in urban (>10,000 dwellers) regions. The health system is mixed public and private, and patients can visit a specialist at the hospital or privately. The Department of Rheumatology, Clinical Immunology at the University Hospital of Heraklion (Panepistimiou, Iraklio, Greece) serves as a referral centre for patients with autoimmune rheumatic diseases, connects to private rheumatologists and general physicians working in rural health centers, and provides inpatient and outpatient services from primary to tertiary level [39,40]. Access to primary and specialized care is generally not considered to be hampered in Crete [41].

2.2. The Cretan Community-Based Lupus Registry

Details on the registry and its methodology are provided elsewhere [39,40]. Briefly, the main inclusion criterion was any definite or possible case of SLE aged >15 years at the time of enrolment, and the primary aim was to estimate the frequency and burden of SLE in the community. Cases were diagnosed by experienced rheumatologists and ascertained by the American College of Rheumatology (ACR) 1997 [42] and Systemic Lupus International Collaborating Clinics (SLICC) 2012 [43] classification criteria. To achieve the highest possible patient enrolment from all four prefectures of the island, from the community to the tertiary centre, and reduce the risk of selection bias for the more severe, hospital-based cases, we pursued active multisource recruitment from all hospital departments (Rheumatology, Dermatology, Nephrology; inpatient and outpatient clinics) caring for lupus patients and also, private rheumatology practices across the island. Patients were enrolled between April 2012 and December 2015 with a stable enrolment rate of 8 to 12 patients per week and an acceptance rate > 95%. Upon inclusion, patients were assessed clinically and completed a structured questionnaire regarding residential history, lifestyle factors, and disease characteristics [39,40]. A review of the medical charts, supervised by trained researchers with data cross-checking and quality control was conducted to reduce possible misclassification and information bias. Administrative data were used regarding hospitalizations. A total of 460 patients were enrolled, following informed consent, and gave face interviews except for five patients who could not stay after their visit to the outpatient clinic and were instead phone interviewed. This sample corresponds to more than half of the previously identified, community-based prevalent SLE cases in Crete (n = 753) [40]. In total, 61 cases were excluded as they did not fulfil the classification criteria or had incomplete information, thus resulting in a final dataset of 399 patients.

2.3. Variables and Comorbidities

We assessed for the presence of comorbid disease using patient-reported data obtained during the structured face interviews, as several studies have previously demonstrated high concordance between self-reported and medical record- or hospital-based comorbidities data [44–47]. Specifically, questionnaires were used to collect information on: gender, ethnicity, education level ($\leq$ or >12 years), marital status, employment status, and descent (Cretan (for at least three past generations), other), place of current and upbringing residency and any translocations (urban-rural), smoking (current, never, ever, pack-years), body mass index (BMI; kg/m^2), use of cosmetics and pesticides (frequent, ever, no use) [39]. The following comorbidities were also assessed by means of predefined questionnaire and were further ascertained by medical charts screening and use of relevant medications: allergies (allergic rhinitis, asthma, urticaria, drug allergies), diabetes mellitus, hypertension, dyslipidemia, thyroid disease (cancer, nodules, autoimmune thyroiditis), osteoporosis or osteoporotic fracture, heart disease, neurologic condition, cancer, kidney disease, lung disease, liver or gallbladder disease, peptic ulcer disease, blood disorders or thalassemia trait, skin diseases. Latent (tuberculosis, HIV) or recurrent urinary tract infections were assessed by self-reporting or medical charts screening and no confirmatory essay was used. The following mental conditions were assessed: depression, generalized anxiety disorder, bipolar disorder, memory and cognitive disorder, eating disorders, alcohol dependence, illicit drug dependence, suicidal attempt. The age-adjusted Charlson Comorbidity Index (CCI) [48] was calculated for each patient.

2.4. Clinical Data Abstracted from the Medical Records

The following data were extracted from the medical charts: clinical diagnosis and date of diagnosis, SLE classification criteria [42,43], biopsy-proven lupus nephritis, neuropsychiatric lupus (NPSLE) (defined by multidisciplinary consensus and attribution models [49]), organ damage (assessed by the SLICC/ACR damage index (SDI) [50]). For every patient, disease was categorised as mild, moderate or severe according to the British Isles Lupus Assessment Group (BILAG) classification system [51], and as previously described [39]. Briefly, the medical charts of all patients were scrutinized to detect incident activity (at any timepoint during the disease course) from individual organs and domains. Manifestations classified as "BILAG A" were assigned as severe, "BILAG B" as moderate, and the remaining ones (e.g., polyarthritis not restricting mobility and not affecting large joints; hair loss without excessive alopecia and without scalp skin inflammation; thrombocytopenia > 50,000/µL) as mild. These data were entered into a structured sheet and were collectively evaluated by two experienced Rheumatologists (G.B., C.A.) who provided their overall assessment of disease severity.

2.5. Statistical Analysis and Hierarchical Clustering

Data are expressed as mean (±standard deviation (SD)) or percentages as appropriate. The Student's t-test or Mann–Whitney non-parametric test were applied for continuous, and the chi-squared or Fisher's exact test for categorical variables. Any missing data from the questionnaires (mainly "do not know" answers) was handled by complete case analysis method. Stepwise logistic regression analysis (adjusted for possible confounding variables including age at diagnosis, disease duration, gender, smoking, residence place (urban or rural) and number of ACR-1997 criteria) was performed to examine the association between selected demographic and clinical parameters with comorbidities outcome measures (≥ 3 physical comorbidities, ≥ 2 mental comorbidities, CCI ≥ 1) (IBM SPSS Statistics for Mac, version 22.0. Armonk, NY: IBM Corp, Armonk, NY, USA). We created a correlation matrix for comorbidities groups (according to the affected organ or domain) and used the Cramer's V statistic to determine the magnitude of pairwise associations; strong relationships were defined according to a threshold of V value > 0.10. Utilizing Gower's distance and complete linkage method, hierarchical agglomerative clustering of the patients according to their comorbidity profile was performed. Clusters statistics were analyzed using the R package (version 3.5.0, R Core Team, 2018, R Foundation for Statistical Computing, Vienna, Austria). The chi-squared statistic was used to examine whether the distribution of the comorbidities differed between the identified patient clusters. The heatmap of the frequencies of comorbidities groups across the patient clusters was created using the pheatmap package (version 1.0.12, R Core Team, 2018, R Foundation for Statistical Computing, Vienna, Austria).

3. Results

3.1. High Prevalence of Comorbid Diseases in SLE Patients at the Community

We studied 399 SLE patients (91.2% females) with an average disease duration of 10 years. At the time of assessment, approximately 11% had history of biopsy-proven nephritis and a similar proportion had neuropsychiatric disease attributed to SLE (Table 1).

Table 1. Demographic and clinical characteristics of Systemic Lupus Erythematous (SLE) patients (n = 399) at the time of enrolment.

Parameter	No. (%) or Mean ± Standard Deviation
Gender (female)	364 (91.2%)
Age at diagnosis (years)	42.8 ± 14.6
Disease duration (years)	9.9 ± 6.6
No. ACR criteria	4.7 ± 1.2
Lupus nephritis (biopsy-proven)	45 (11.3%)
Neuropsychiatric lupus	43 (10.8%)
Disease severity [1]	
Mild	190 (47.7%)
Moderate	144 (36.1%)
Severe	65 (16.2%)
Organ damage	144 (36.2%)
Residence	
Rural	172 (43.1%)
Urban and semi-urban	227 (56.9%)
Education level	
<12 years	284 (71.2%)
$\geq$12 years	115 (28.8%)

Table 1. *Cont.*

Parameter	No. (%) or Mean ± Standard Deviation
Marital status	
Single	55 (13.7%)
Married	299 (74.9%)
Divorced or separated	21 (5.3%)
Widowed	24 (6.1%)
Tobacco use	
Never	208 (55.3%) [2]
Past	55 (14.6%)
Active	113 (30.1%)

[1] See Materials and Methods for details on the definitions. [2] Data available in n = 376 patients.

Among the most prevalent physical comorbidities were thyroid (45.6%) and metabolic disorders (hypertension: 24.6%, dyslipidemia: 33.3%, obesity: 35.3%), followed by osteoporosis (22.3%) and cardiovascular diseases (20.8%) and allergic disorders (20.6%) (Table 2). Mental disorders were also common (45.1%) particularly depression (26.7%) and generalized anxiety disorder (10.7%). Female SLE patients had significantly increased frequency of thyroid diseases (51 vs. 16%, p < 0.001), allergic diseases (21 vs. 3%, p = 0.006), and osteoporosis (19 vs. 6%, p = 0.05) compared to male patients, whereas respiratory comorbidities (21 vs. 9%, p < 0.001) and alcohol abuse (3 vs. 0%, p < 0.01) were more prevalent among male patients.

Table 2. Prevalence of comorbid diseases in SLE patients at the community-based registry in Crete (n = 399).

Comorbidiy	Prevalence
Thyroid disease [1]	45.6%
Mental disorder [2]	42.1%
Depression	26.7%
Anxiety disorder	10.7%
Obesity [3]	35.3%
Dyslipidemia	33.3%
Hypertension	24.6%
Osteoporosis and osteoporotic fracture	22.3%
Cardiovascular disease [4]	20.8%
Allergic disorders [5]	20.6%
Gastrointestinal disease [6]	19.0%
Infectious disease [7]	12.8%
Neurologic disease [8]	10.3%
Cerebrovascular disease	2.5%
Kidney disease	9.5%
Respiratory disease	9.3%
Diabetes mellitus	8.8%
Malignant disease	4.8%
Skin disease	3.3%
Hematologic disease	2.3%

[1] Including autoimmune thyroiditis, hypo- or hyperthyroidism, thyroid nodules; [2] including bipolar disease, cognitive impairment, generalized anxiety disorder, major depression, alcohol dependence, eating disorder, suicidal attempt; [3] defined as body mass index $\geq$ 30 kg/m^2; [4] including coronary heart disease (angina, myocardial infarction, or coronary revascularization procedure), valvular disease, peripheral vascular disease; [5] including allergic rhinitis, asthma, urticaria; [6] including liver, gallbladder or biliary tract disease, gastroesophageal reflux disease, peptic ulcer disease, chronic diarrhea; [7] including latent hepatitis or HIV infection, recurrent urinary tract infections, chronic osteomyelitis; [8] including epilepsy, stroke, cerebrovascular disease, or other neurological diseases.

Overall, SLE patients had an average (±SD) 2.8 (±2.0) physical and 0.9 (±1.3) mental comorbidities with a mean age-adjusted CCI of 0.91 ± 1.16 (Table 3). Notably, 51.0% of patients had three or more physical comorbidities and 33.1% had two or more mental comorbidities, suggesting a high comorbidity burden in patients with SLE at the community.

Table 3. Burden of comorbidities in SLE patients at the community-based registry in Crete.

Comorbidities	Mean ± Standard Deviation or Prevalence (%)
Physical comorbidities	2.8 ± 2.0
None	9.8%
1 or 2	39.2%
≥3	51.0%
Mental comorbidities	0.94 ± 1.25
None	57.9%
1	9.0%
≥2	33.1%
Charlson Comorbidity Index (CCI)	0.91 ± 1.16
>0	50.3%

3.2. Co-Segregation of Physical and Mental Comorbidities in Patients with SLE

Driven by our findings, we carried out a correlation analysis to detect concurrent comorbidities. We noted several pairs of diseases with high prevalence in our sample, for instance, thyroid disease and dyslipidemia ($n = 71$, 18%), dyslipidemia and hypertension ($n = 59$, 15%), allergic disorders and thyroid disease ($n = 49$, 12%), gastrointestinal disorders, and thyroid disease ($n = 45$, 11%). Mental disorders (merged together into a single group) often coexisted with thyroid disease ($n = 94$, 24%), dyslipidemia ($n = 62$, 16%), and gastrointestinal disorders ($n = 45$, 11%). Next, the Cramer's V statistic was implemented to obtain a statistically robust measure of the relative strength of association between different pairs of comorbidities. We observed a substantive relationship between allergic and hematological diseases, hypertension and diabetes, dyslipidemia, and cardiovascular diseases, the latter concurring also with other comorbidities such as obesity, osteoporosis, neurologic, and respiratory disorders (Figure 1A). Other associations included thyroid disease with kidney and mental disorders, skin with gastrointestinal and neurological diseases, kidney disease with hypertension. By further examining the co-segregation of comorbidities, we found a positive correlation between an increasing number of physical and mental disorders. Specifically, within SLE patients with ≥3 physical comorbidities, a large fraction ($n = 86$) also reported multiple (≥2) mental disorders (Figure 1B). Conversely, within 39 patients with no physical comorbidity, only 5 had two or more mental disorders. Together, these results suggest a substantial multimorbidity burden in SLE patients including the co-existence of physical and mental disorders.

3.3. Predictors of Morbidity and Multimorbidity in Patients with SLE

We evaluated for factors associated with comorbidities in our SLE dataset by analyzing for the presence of multiple physical comorbidities (≥3), mental comorbidities (≥2), or CCI ≥ 1. Demographic, social and clinical features were treated as independent variables initially at univariate level, followed by multivariate logistic regression. We found that moderate vs. mild disease was associated with increased risk (adjusted odds ratio (OR) 2.30) and that higher vs. lower (≥12 years vs. <12 years) education level was associated with decreased risk (OR 0.46) for physical multimorbidity (Table 4). Disease duration correlated with the total number of physical comorbidities (Spearman's rho 0.152, $p = 0.019$) but only at univariate level. In the case of mental multimorbidity, independent predictors were the marital status (divorced or widowed patients having OR 2.76) and the ACR 1997-defined neurologic disease item (OR 6.02). Finally, morbidity defined according to CCI ≥1 was associated with the education level, marital status, and number of ACR 1997 classification criteria (OR 1.30 per 1-item). In a separate analysis, we also correlated the total number of used (ever) immunosuppressive or biological agents (azathioprine, mycophenolate, belimumab, cyclophosphamide, rituximab) with the sum of physical -but not mental-comorbidities (Spearman's rho 0.136, p = 0.036) and adjusted Charlson Comorbidity Index (Spearman's rho 0.183, p = 0.001). Altogether, both sociodemographic and clinical factors are linked to the comorbidities risk in patients with SLE at the community.

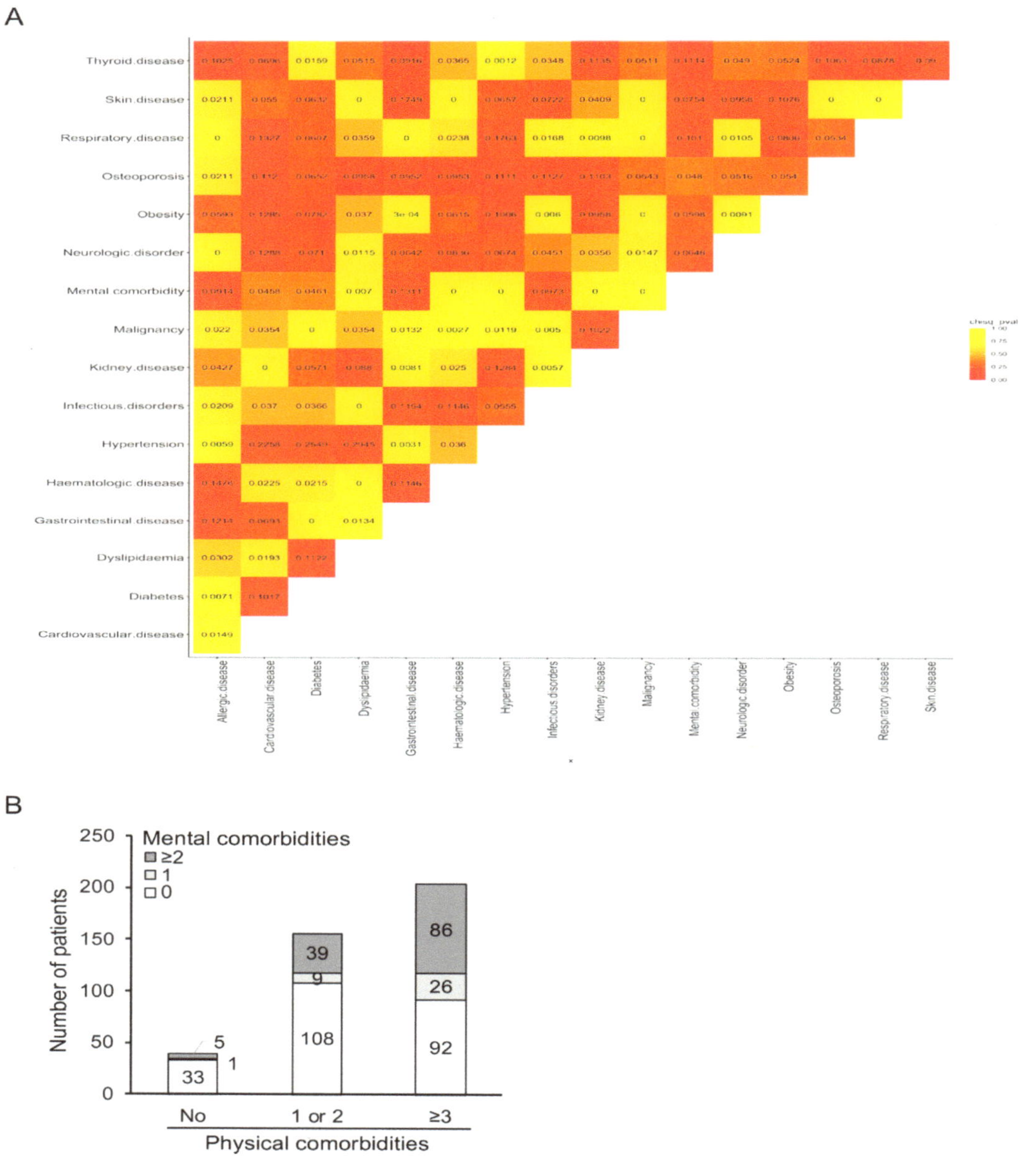

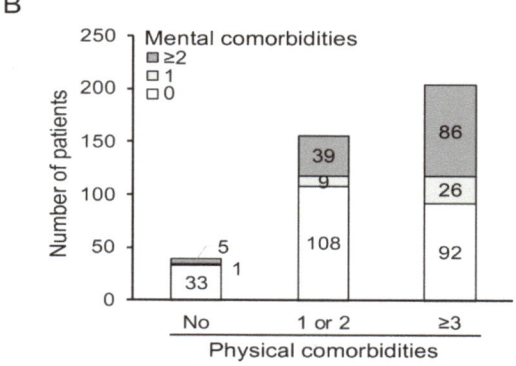

Figure 1. Co-segregation of comorbidities in patients with SLE at the community-based registry of Crete. (**A**) Correlation matrix of various comorbidities from diverse organs and domains. Numbers inside each box represents the Cramer's V statistic estimated for each pair of comorbidities with values > 0.10 signifying robust correlation. Color intensity corresponds to the chi-squared p-value for each pairwise association. (**B**) SLE patients were categorized according to the number of physical (none, 1 or 2, ≥3) and mental (none, 1, ≥2) comorbidities as described in the main text. Y axis shows the number of patients with various combinations of physical and mental comorbid disorders.

Table 4. Predictors for the presence of comorbidities in patients with SLE.

Dependent Variable [1]	Predictor (s)	OR (95% CI) [2]	p Value
≥3 physical comorbidities	Education level		
	≥12 years vs. <12 years	0.46 (0.28–0.75)	0.002
	SLE severity		
	Moderate vs. mild	2.30 (1.43–3.71)	0.001
	Severe vs. mild	1.30 (0.71–2.41)	0.398
≥2 mental comorbidities	Marital status		
	Divorced or widowed vs. single or married	2.76 (1.43–5.35)	0.003
	ACR-1997 neurologic item		
	Present vs. absent	6.02 (1.86–19.53)	0.003
Charlson comorbidity index ≥ 1	Education level		
	≥12 years vs. <12 years	0.52 (0.31–0.86)	0.011
	No. ACR-1997 criteria (per 1-item)	1.30 (1.06–1.59)	0.013
	Marital status		
	Divorced or widowed vs. single or married	2.18 (1.02–4.68)	0.045

[1] Backwards elimination model. Possible predictors included: age at diagnosis, disease duration, gender, smoking, residence place, number of ACR-1997 criteria; [2] Odds ratio (95% confidence interval).

3.4. Distinct Comorbidities Phenotypes in Patients with SLE Revealed by Cluster Analysis

We next examined whether SLE patients can be classified into distinct phenotypic groups as this may further enhance our understanding of the complexity of comorbid diseases beyond a single-disease perspective, and how these might differ according to demographic, clinical, or other determinants. Hierarchical agglomerative clustering revealed five patient clusters, each with variable prevalence of comorbid diseases from various organs and domains (Figure 2A). Cluster 1 included the majority of patients (n = 227) and was characterized by increased prevalence of thyroid disease and to lesser extent, obesity, dyslipidemia and mental comorbidities. Cluster 2 (n = 46) had high frequency of metabolic risk factors, cluster 3 (n = 43) of gastrointestinal, skin, allergic, and hematologic diseases, and cluster 4 (n = 45) of metabolic risk factors, cardiovascular, respiratory, and mental disorders. Cluster 5 included a minority (n = 6) of SLE patients with relatively increased prevalence of osteoporosis, malignant, neurologic, infectious, and kidney disorders. Identified clusters did not differ in terms of gender, residence place, education level, smoking status, age of SLE diagnosis, and disease duration. Notably, clusters 2 and 5 included patients with high frequency of biopsy-proven nephritis (28.3 and 33.3%, respectively) as compared to other clusters (p < 0.001). NPSLE had highest prevalence in clusters 4 and 5 (20.0 and 66.7%) than in clusters 1–3 (p < 0.001). Prevalence of combined lupus skin lesions (both malar and discoid rash) was higher in cluster 1 (7.6%) as compared to clusters 2 (4.5%), 3 (2.3%) and 4–5 (0.0%) (p = 0.019). No associations were detected with regards to other clinical or immunological disease features. Patterns of disease severity differed across the aforementioned groups with clusters 1 and 3 including increased fractions of patients with mild disease (47.2 and 69.0%, respectively) as compared to clusters 2 and 5 which comprised severe SLE patients (26.1 and 40.0%, respectively) (p = 0.024) (Figure 2B).

3.5. Association between Morbidities and Clinical Outcomes in Patients with SLE

Previous work has demonstrated that comorbid diseases may have an adverse impact on miscellaneous patient and disease outcomes in SLE. Analysis of our data did not reveal a statistically significant association between physical or mental multimorbidity and rates of irreversible organ damage (SDI ≥ 1), although the total number of physical comorbidities showed a trend for correlation with the SDI (Spearman's rho = 0.126, p = 0.050). Notably, patients with ≥3 physical comorbid diseases had experienced an increased number of hospitalizations due to active SLE (1.96 ± 0.40 vs. 0.91 ± 0.17 in counterparts with 0–2 morbidities, p = 0.018).

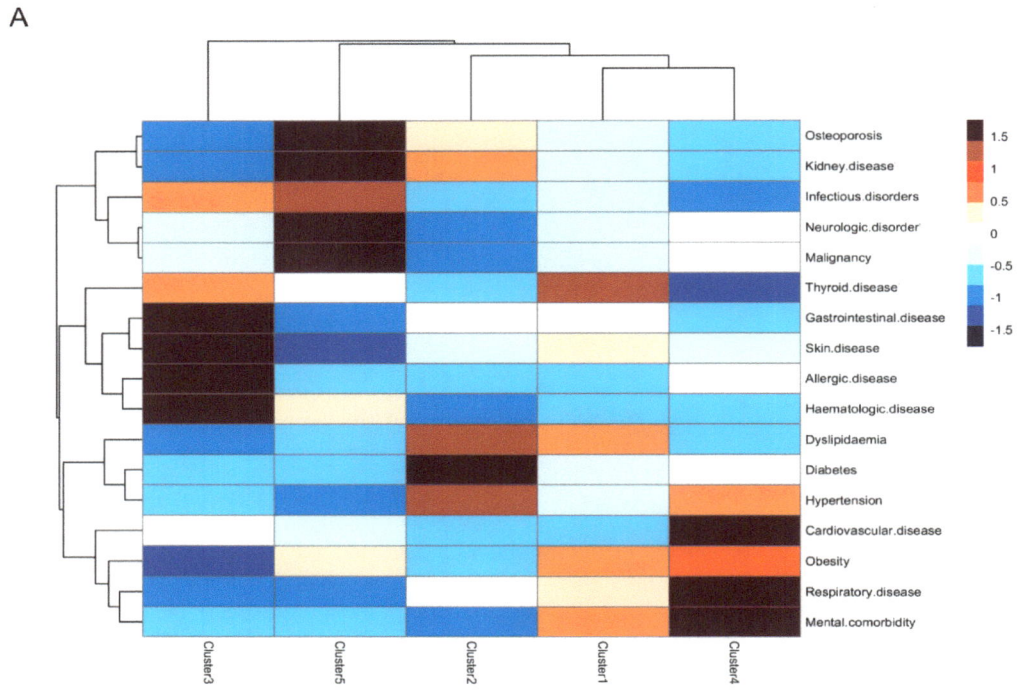

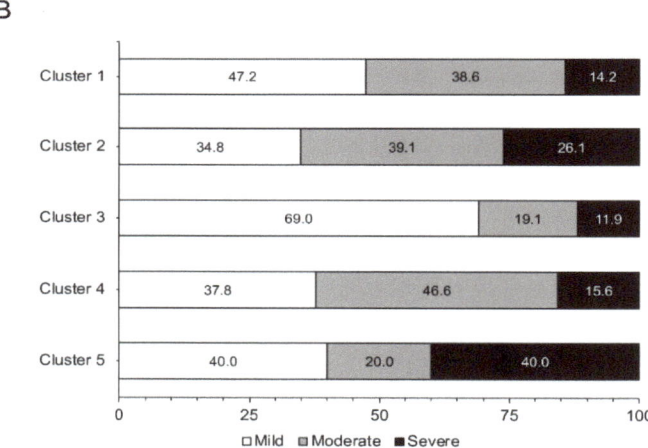

Figure 2. Distinct comorbidities phenotypes in patients with SLE revealed by cluster analysis. (**A**) Utilizing Gower's distance and complete linkage method, hierarchical agglomerative clustering of the patients according to their comorbidity profile was performed. The chi-squared statistic was used to examine whether the distribution of the comorbidities differed between the identified patient clusters. The heatmap of the frequencies of comorbidities groups across the patient clusters is shown. Legend depicts the relative frequency (ranging from −1.5 to +1.5) of each comorbidity within each cluster. (**B**) Prevalence of SLE severity patterns (mild, moderate, severe) based on the BILAG system across the identified comorbidities clusters (cluster 1 to 5). Numbers are proportions (%).

4. Discussion

Herein, we evaluated the presence of comorbid diseases and their determinants in SLE patients from a homogenous south European population. Background, race and ethnicity, and geographical characteristics are important determinants of both lupus ominosity and associated comorbid disorders [7,35,36,52,53]. Our findings, derived from a community-based, Caucasian registry that captures both severe and milder disease forms, highlights a high burden of physical and mental comorbidities among SLE patients, which tend to co-segregate and cluster into distinct phenotypic groups. Moreover, we demonstrate that comorbidities may be associated with clinical disease severity and certain sociodemographic factors, which further supports the complex nature of comorbidity in SLE and the need for holistic approach.

Our results reiterate the previously reported prevalence of numerous comorbid medical disorders in patients with SLE. Although direct comparisons are hampered due to differences in the study design, assessment and documentation methods, and the definitions used, our findings concord with published data underpinning increased occurrence of metabolic and atherosclerotic factors such as hypertension, dyslipidemia, obesity, diabetes, cardiovascular, and cerebrovascular disease as compared to the general population [7–13,54–58]. Cardiovascular burden is also increased in SLE, attributable to the interplay between demographic (e.g., gender, ethnicity), disease duration, traditional risk factors (including smoking), lupus autoimmunity such as type I interferon signaling, and the known deleterious effects of chronic glucocorticoids use [7,56,58–63]. In line with this, circumstantial non-randomized evidence suggests that attainment of low disease activity state on a minimal background dose of glucocorticoids is associated with reduced risk for cardiovascular events in SLE [64].

Disorders of the thyroid gland comprised a prevalent condition in our cohort, consistent with case-control studies indicating a statistically significant association between SLE and autoimmune and non-autoimmune thyroidopathies [65–67]. Moreover, osteoporosis, a well-established comorbidity in SLE [17,18,68] attributed to multiple factors [69], was reported by a high proportion (22.3%) of our patients. Another notable finding was the high frequency of allergic disorders (20.6%), which aligns with epidemiological evidence demonstrating that SLE patients have an estimated 1.4 to 2.3-fold increased risk for atopic dermatitis, allergic rhinitis, allergic conjunctivitis, or asthma [70,71]. Intriguingly, lupus and allergy share—to some extent—common genetic predisposition, environmental factors, and immune pathways such as increased serum immunoglobulin E levels and mast cell activation [72]. Malignant disorders are also more prevalent in SLE patients than the general population [3].

Besides physical comorbidities, a considerable number of patients in our study reported at least one mental comorbidity, in particular depression and anxiety. This concords with observational studies underlining increased prevalence of the aforementioned conditions and also, cognitive complaints, in SLE patients as compared to the general population [20,73–76]. Other psychiatric disorders including bipolar [77], suicidal ideation [78], schizophrenia [79], and sleep disturbances [80], are also encountered more frequently in SLE. To this end, fibromyalgia, which was not evaluated in our cohort, represents a common SLE comorbidity often correlating with or considered to be part of the spectrum of mental conditions [19]. Although these comorbidities are typically not attributed to direct immune insult against the central nervous system as in the case of primary neuropsychiatric SLE [49], nonetheless circumstantial evidence implicates soluble inflammatory mediators in their pathogenesis [81,82].

The multimorbidity state has been well documented in inflammatory arthritides, such as rheumatoid arthritis [21,83–85], whereas fewer reports exist in SLE [86,87]. A remarkable finding in our study was the high prevalence of multimorbidity with more than half of SLE patients reporting ≥ 3 physical and about one-third of patients reporting ≥ 2 mental comorbid diseases. In addition, we noted a positive correlation between physical and mental multimorbidity, with their synchronous presence in 21.6% of cases. Besides the apparent impact on patient well-being, the possible implication of multimorbidity on the management and outcomes of SLE remain to be determined. To this end, our analysis showed increased rates of hospitalizations due to SLE among patients with multiple physical comorbid disease, a finding that warrants further investigation in prospective studies.

Identification of morbidity predictors is valuable for recognizing high-risk patient groups and thus, adjusting medical care accordingly. Rather than focusing on isolated diseases, we analyzed for factors associated with physical and mental multimorbidity as well as CCI-defined morbid status. We found that increasing SLE severity, reflected in a BILAG-based classification of manifestations or the number of ACR 1997 classification criteria, correlated with increased odds for physical morbidity, thus corroborating evidence on the effects of high disease activity and medications (e.g., glucocorticoids) on the development of comorbid disorders [7,34,60,61,88]. This finding might be mirrored by the positive correlation between exposure to immunosuppressive and biological agents and physical comorbidities, although drug-intrinsic effects cannot be ruled out. Notably, and in agreement with studies in other patient populations [38,89,90], higher education level was linked to reduced comorbidity risk, presumably due to increased awareness, treatment adherence and better overall management of the index disease (SLE) and its complications. In the case of mental multimorbidity, neurological disorder (ACR 1997-defined) and the marital status were independent predictors. Whether the former association corresponds to increased neuropsychiatric or general inflammatory burden of SLE or is confounded by other factors is unknown. Likewise, the increased risk in widowed and separated patients could possibly be related to stressful life events or other socio-economic parameters not evaluated in the present analysis.

In view of our results demonstrating aggregation of multiple disorders from diverse organs and domains, we performed clustering analysis searching for phenotypic subgroups of clinical relevance [85,91]. Using this approach, our SLE sample was categorized into five clusters of highly coinciding comorbidities. The clusters did not differ with regards to the distribution of age, gender, other demographic and clinical factors, implying that they might be driven by other factors. Nonetheless, cluster 1, encompassing common disorders (thyroid, obesity, dyslipidemia, mental) was most prevalent in SLE patients especially those with milder disease forms. Pending confirmation in additional studies with larger patient cohorts, these findings could be helpful in the context of personalized medical care and to unravel shared underlying genetic or pathogenic links.

A number of limitations need to be acknowledged such as the fact that our study was not designed to address in detail the frequency of comorbidities and that it did not include a control group. Nonetheless, information was collected using pre-specified forms during face interviews of patients enrolled in the registry. Although self-reported and medical record- or hospital-based comorbidities data seems to correlate well [44–47], some information or misclassification errors may have occurred. As we did not monitor patient exposure to glucocorticoids, we were not able to differentiate steroid-related vs. unrelated mental disorders. Additionally, despite the fact that our sample size ($n = 399$) is generally considered sufficient, it may be underpowered to detect or evaluate infrequent disorders, differences according to gender or the autoantibodies status. To this end, our goal was not to provide an exhaustive description of isolated diseases but rather, to gain an overview of the burden of comorbidity and multimorbidity in our setting.

In conclusion, our results from a community-based, Caucasian registry highlight a considerable burden of physical and mental comorbidities in patients with SLE. Multimorbidity is a pervasive characteristic correlating both with the disease severity and sociodemographic factors such as the education and marital status, thus underscoring the need to address these factors in patient risk stratification and management. Cluster analysis of comorbidities enables the identification of distinct clinical phenotypes, which might reflect different pathophysiological processes linked to the disease. Altogether, these findings have potential implications for rheumatologists and other disciplines involved in the care of SLE patients, and emphasize the need for integrated action plans to optimize disease outcomes.

Author Contributions: I.G. was involved in the establishment of the lupus registry, performed interviews with the patients, collected data, performed initial analyses, and wrote parts of the manuscript. P.G. performed statistical analysis (correlation matrix, clustering analysis). C.A. collected data from the medical charts. G.S. developed an electronic registry for data entering, storage, and extraction. I.S. performed literature review and wrote parts of the manuscript. P.S. commented on the results and wrote parts of the manuscript. G.B. supervised the study, performed statistical analysis, and drafted the manuscript, tables, and figures. All authors have read and agreed to the published version of the manuscript.

Funding: This work was funded in part by the Pancretan Health Association and the Research Account of the University of Crete (KA 10210).

Institutional Review Board Statement: The study was conducted in accordance with the Declaration of Helsinki and the Cretan Epidemiology and Surveillance SLE Project has been approved by the Ethics Committee of the University Hospital of Heraklion.

Informed Consent Statement: Informed consent was obtained from all subjects involved in the study.

Data Availability Statement: Data are available upon reasonable request.

Acknowledgments: We would like to thank the medical and nursing staff of the Department of Rheumatology-Clinical Immunology, University Hospital of Iraklio.

Conflicts of Interest: The authors declare no conflict of interest.

References

1. Gonzalez, L.A.; Alarcon, G.S. The evolving concept of SLE comorbidities. *Expert Rev. Clin. Immunol.* **2017**, *13*, 1–16. [CrossRef]
2. Urowitz, M.B.; Bookman, A.A.; Koehler, B.E.; Gordon, D.A.; Smythe, H.A.; Ogryzlo, M.A. The bimodal mortality pattern of systemic lupus erythematosus. *Am. J. Med.* **1976**, *60*, 221–225. [CrossRef]
3. Rees, F.; Doherty, M.; Grainge, M.; Lanyon, P.; Davenport, G.; Zhang, W. Burden of comorbidity in systemic lupus erythematosus in the UK, 1999–2012. *Arthritis Care Res.* **2016**, *68*, 819–827. [CrossRef] [PubMed]
4. Kedves, M.; Kosa, F.; Kunovszki, P.; Takacs, P.; Szabo, M.Z.; Karyekar, C.; Lofland, J.H.; Nagy, G. Large-scale mortality gap between SLE and control population is associated with increased infection-related mortality in lupus. *Rheumatology* **2020**, *59*, 3443–3451. [CrossRef] [PubMed]
5. Rua-Figueroa, I.; Lopez-Longo, J.; Galindo-Izquierdo, M.; Calvo-Alen, J.; Del Campo, V.; Olive-Marques, A.; Perez-Vicente, S.; Fernandez-Nebro, A.; Andres, M.; Erausquin, C.; et al. Incidence, associated factors and clinical impact of severe infections in a large, multicentric cohort of patients with systemic lupus erythematosus. *Semin. Arthritis Rheum.* **2017**, *47*, 38–45. [CrossRef] [PubMed]
6. Tektonidou, M.G.; Wang, Z.; Dasgupta, A.; Ward, M.M. Burden of serious infections in adults with systemic lupus erythematosus: A national population-based study, 1996–2011. *Arthritis Care Res.* **2015**, *67*, 1078–1085. [CrossRef] [PubMed]
7. Parker, B.; Urowitz, M.B.; Gladman, D.D.; Lunt, M.; Bae, S.C.; Sanchez-Guerrero, J.; Romero-Diaz, J.; Gordon, C.; Wallace, D.J.; Clarke, A.E.; et al. Clinical associations of the metabolic syndrome in systemic lupus erythematosus: Data from an international inception cohort. *Ann. Rheum. Dis.* **2013**, *72*, 1308–1314. [CrossRef] [PubMed]
8. Tselios, K.; Koumaras, C.; Gladman, D.D.; Urowitz, M.B. Dyslipidemia in systemic lupus erythematosus: Just another comorbidity? *Semin. Arthritis Rheum.* **2016**, *45*, 604–610. [CrossRef] [PubMed]
9. Katz, G.; Smilowitz, N.R.; Blazer, A.; Clancy, R.; Buyon, J.P.; Berger, J.S. Systemic lupus erythematosus and increased prevalence of atherosclerotic cardiovascular disease in hospitalized patients. *Mayo Clin. Proc.* **2019**, *94*, 1436–1443. [CrossRef]
10. Urowitz, M.B.; Gladman, D.; Ibanez, D.; Bae, S.C.; Sanchez-Guerrero, J.; Gordon, C.; Clarke, A.; Bernatsky, S.; Fortin, P.R.; Hanly, J.G.; et al. Atherosclerotic vascular events in a multinational inception cohort of systemic lupus erythematosus. *Arthritis Care Res.* **2010**, *62*, 881–887. [CrossRef]
11. Chuang, Y.W.; Yu, M.C.; Lin, C.L.; Yu, T.M.; Shu, K.H.; Kao, C.H. Risk of peripheral arterial occlusive disease in patients with systemic lupus erythematosus: A nationwide population-based cohort study. *Medicine* **2015**, *94*, e2121. [CrossRef]
12. Holmqvist, M.; Simard, J.F.; Asplund, K.; Arkema, E.V. Stroke in systemic lupus erythematosus: A meta-analysis of population-based cohort studies. *RMD Open* **2015**, *1*, e000168. [CrossRef]
13. Schoenfeld, S.R.; Kasturi, S.; Costenbader, K.H. The epidemiology of atherosclerotic cardiovascular disease among patients with SLE: A systematic review. *Semin. Arthritis Rheum.* **2013**, *43*, 77–95. [CrossRef]
14. Cao, L.; Tong, H.; Xu, G.; Liu, P.; Meng, H.; Wang, J.; Zhao, X.; Tang, Y.; Jin, J. Systemic lupus erythematous and malignancy risk: A meta-analysis. *PLoS ONE* **2015**, *10*, e0122964. [CrossRef]

15. Wadstrom, H.; Arkema, E.V.; Sjowall, C.; Askling, J.; Simard, J.F. Cervical neoplasia in systemic lupus erythematosus: A nationwide study. *Rheumatology* **2017**, *56*, 613–619. [CrossRef]
16. Wu, Y.; Hou, Q. Systemic lupus erythematous increased lung cancer risk: Evidence from a meta-analysis. *J. Cancer Res. Ther.* **2016**, *12*, 721–724. [CrossRef] [PubMed]
17. Mendoza-Pinto, C.; Rojas-Villarraga, A.; Molano-Gonzalez, N.; Jimenez-Herrera, E.A.; Leon-Vazquez, M.L.; Montiel-Jarquin, A.; Garcia-Carrasco, M.; Cervera, R. Bone mineral density and vertebral fractures in patients with systemic lupus erythematosus: A systematic review and meta-regression. *PLoS ONE* **2018**, *13*, e0196113. [CrossRef] [PubMed]
18. Tedeschi, S.K.; Kim, S.C.; Guan, H.; Grossman, J.M.; Costenbader, K.H. Comparative fracture risks among United States medicaid enrollees with and those without systemic lupus erythematosus. *Arthritis Rheumatol.* **2019**, *71*, 1141–1146. [CrossRef] [PubMed]
19. Haliloglu, S.; Carlioglu, A.; Akdeniz, D.; Karaaslan, Y.; Kosar, A. Fibromyalgia in patients with other rheumatic diseases: Prevalence and relationship with disease activity. *Rheumatol. Int.* **2014**, *34*, 1275–1280. [CrossRef] [PubMed]
20. Zhang, L.; Fu, T.; Yin, R.; Zhang, Q.; Shen, B. Prevalence of depression and anxiety in systemic lupus erythematosus: A systematic review and meta-analysis. *BMC Psychiatry* **2017**, *17*, 70. [CrossRef]
21. Radner, H.; Yoshida, K.; Smolen, J.S.; Solomon, D.H. Multimorbidity and rheumatic conditions-enhancing the concept of comorbidity. *Nat. Rev. Rheumatol.* **2014**, *10*, 252–256. [CrossRef] [PubMed]
22. Balitsky, A.K.; Peeva, V.; Su, J.; Aghdassi, E.; Yeo, E.; Gladman, D.D.; Urowitz, M.B.; Fortin, P.R. Thrombovascular events affect quality of life in patients with systemic lupus erythematosus. *J. Rheumatol.* **2011**, *38*, 1017–1019. [CrossRef] [PubMed]
23. Rizk, A.; Gheita, T.A.; Nassef, S.; Abdallah, A. The impact of obesity in systemic lupus erythematosus on disease parameters, quality of life, functional capacity and the risk of atherosclerosis. *Int. J. Rheum. Dis.* **2012**, *15*, 261–267. [CrossRef] [PubMed]
24. Baker, K.; Pope, J.; Fortin, P.; Silverman, E.; Peschken, C. Work disability in systemic lupus erythematosus is prevalent and associated with socio-demographic and disease related factors. *Lupus* **2009**, *18*, 1281–1288. [CrossRef]
25. Kim, S.K.; Choe, J.Y.; Lee, S.S. Charlson comorbidity index is related to organ damage in systemic lupus erythematosus: Data from KORean lupus network (KORNET) registry. *J. Rheumatol.* **2017**, *44*, 452–458. [CrossRef]
26. Yang, Y.; Thumboo, J.; Earnest, A.; Yong, S.L.; Fong, K.Y. The effect of comorbidity on hospital mortality in patients with SLE from an Asian tertiary hospital. *Lupus* **2014**, *23*, 714–720. [CrossRef]
27. Han, G.M.; Han, X.F. Comorbid conditions are associated with emergency department visits, hospitalizations, and medical charges of patients with systemic lupus erythematosus. *J. Clin. Rheumatol.* **2017**, *23*, 19–25. [CrossRef]
28. Jonsen, A.; Clarke, A.E.; Joseph, L.; Belisle, P.; Bernatsky, S.; Nived, O.; Bengtsson, A.A.; Sturfelt, G.; Pineau, C.A. Association of the Charlson comorbidity index with mortality in systemic lupus erythematosus. *Arthritis Care Res.* **2011**, *63*, 1233–1237. [CrossRef]
29. van Vollenhoven, R.F.; Mosca, M.; Bertsias, G.; Isenberg, D.; Kuhn, A.; Lerstrom, K.; Aringer, M.; Bootsma, H.; Boumpas, D.; Bruce, I.N.; et al. Treat-to-target in systemic lupus erythematosus: Recommendations from an international task force. *Ann. Rheum. Dis.* **2014**, *73*, 958–967. [CrossRef]
30. Duru, N.; van der Goes, M.C.; Jacobs, J.W.; Andrews, T.; Boers, M.; Buttgereit, F.; Caeyers, N.; Cutolo, M.; Halliday, S.; Da Silva, J.A.; et al. EULAR evidence-based and consensus-based recommendations on the management of medium to high-dose glucocorticoid therapy in rheumatic diseases. *Ann. Rheum. Dis.* **2013**, *72*, 1905–1913. [CrossRef]
31. Fanouriakis, A.; Kostopoulou, M.; Alunno, A.; Aringer, M.; Bajema, I.; Boletis, J.N.; Cervera, R.; Doria, A.; Gordon, C.; Govoni, M.; et al. 2019 update of the EULAR recommendations for the management of systemic lupus erythematosus. *Ann. Rheum. Dis.* **2019**, *78*, 736–745. [CrossRef]
32. Mosca, M.; Tani, C.; Aringer, M.; Bombardieri, S.; Boumpas, D.; Brey, R.; Cervera, R.; Doria, A.; Jayne, D.; Khamashta, M.A.; et al. European League against Rheumatism recommendations for monitoring patients with systemic lupus erythematosus in clinical practice and in observational studies. *Ann. Rheum. Dis.* **2010**, *69*, 1269–1274. [CrossRef] [PubMed]
33. Leonard, D.; Svenungsson, E.; Dahlqvist, J.; Alexsson, A.; Arlestig, L.; Taylor, K.E.; Sandling, J.K.; Bengtsson, C.; Frodlund, M.; Jonsen, A.; et al. Novel gene variants associated with cardiovascular disease in systemic lupus erythematosus and rheumatoid arthritis. *Ann. Rheum. Dis.* **2018**, *77*, 1063–1069. [CrossRef] [PubMed]
34. Greenstein, L.; Makan, K.; Tikly, M. Burden of comorbidities in South Africans with systemic lupus erythematosus. *Clin. Rheumatol.* **2019**, *38*, 2077–2082. [CrossRef]
35. Falasinnu, T.; Chaichian, Y.; Li, J.; Chung, S.; Waitzfelder, B.E.; Fortmann, S.P.; Palaniappan, L.; Simard, J.F. Does SLE widen or narrow race/ethnic disparities in the risk of five co-morbid conditions? Evidence from a community-based outpatient care system. *Lupus* **2019**, *28*, 1619–1627. [CrossRef] [PubMed]
36. Walsh, S.J.; Algert, C.; Rothfield, N.F. Racial aspects of comorbidity in systemic lupus erythematosus. *Arthritis Care Res.* **1996**, *9*, 509–516. [CrossRef]
37. Akinyemiju, T.; Jha, M.; Moore, J.X.; Pisu, M. Disparities in the prevalence of comorbidities among US adults by state Medicaid expansion status. *Prev. Med.* **2016**, *88*, 196–202. [CrossRef]
38. Schiotz, M.L.; Stockmarr, A.; Host, D.; Glumer, C.; Frolich, A. Social disparities in the prevalence of multimorbidity—A register-based population study. *BMC Public Health* **2017**, *17*, 422. [CrossRef]
39. Gergianaki, I.; Fanouriakis, A.; Adamichou, C.; Spyrou, G.; Mihalopoulos, N.; Kazadzis, S.; Chatzi, L.; Sidiropoulos, P.; Boumpas, D.T.; Bertsias, G. Is systemic lupus erythematosus different in urban versus rural living environment? Data from the Cretan Lupus Epidemiology and Surveillance Registry. *Lupus* **2019**, *28*, 104–113. [CrossRef]

40. Gergianaki, I.; Fanouriakis, A.; Repa, A.; Tzanakakis, M.; Adamichou, C.; Pompieri, A.; Spirou, G.; Bertsias, A.; Kabouraki, E.; Tzanakis, I.; et al. Epidemiology and burden of systemic lupus erythematosus in a Southern European population: Data from the community-based lupus registry of Crete, Greece. *Ann. Rheum. Dis.* **2017**, *76*, 1992–2000. [CrossRef]
41. Chatziarsenis, M.; Lionis, C.; Faresjo, T.; Fioretos, M.; Trell, E. Community-based medical systems advancement in a hospital-primary health care centre in Crete, Greece: Concepts, methods, and the new role of the general practitioner. *J. Med. Syst.* **1998**, *22*, 173–188. [CrossRef]
42. Hochberg, M.C. Updating the American College of Rheumatology revised criteria for the classification of systemic lupus erythematosus. *Arthritis Rheum.* **1997**, *40*, 1725. [CrossRef] [PubMed]
43. Petri, M.; Orbai, A.M.; Alarcon, G.S.; Gordon, C.; Merrill, J.T.; Fortin, P.R.; Bruce, I.N.; Isenberg, D.; Wallace, D.J.; Nived, O.; et al. Derivation and validation of the Systemic Lupus International Collaborating Clinics classification criteria for systemic lupus erythematosus. *Arthritis Rheum.* **2012**, *64*, 2677–2686. [CrossRef] [PubMed]
44. Chaudhry, S.; Jin, L.; Meltzer, D. Use of a self-report-generated Charlson Comorbidity Index for predicting mortality. *Med. Care* **2005**, *43*, 607–615. [CrossRef]
45. Ho, P.J.; Tan, C.S.; Shawon, S.R.; Eriksson, M.; Lim, L.Y.; Miao, H.; Png, E.; Chia, K.S.; Hartman, M.; Ludvigsson, J.F.; et al. Comparison of self-reported and register-based hospital medical data on comorbidities in women. *Sci. Rep.* **2019**, *9*, 3527. [CrossRef] [PubMed]
46. Ng, X.; Low, A.H.; Thumboo, J. Comparison of the Charlson Comorbidity Index derived from self-report and medical record review in Asian patients with rheumatic diseases. *Rheumatol. Int.* **2015**, *35*, 2005–2011. [CrossRef] [PubMed]
47. Olomu, A.B.; Corser, W.D.; Stommel, M.; Xie, Y.; Holmes-Rovner, M. Do self-report and medical record comorbidity data predict longitudinal functional capacity and quality of life health outcomes similarly? *BMC Health Serv. Res.* **2012**, *12*, 398. [CrossRef] [PubMed]
48. Charlson, M.E.; Pompei, P.; Ales, K.L.; MacKenzie, C.R. A new method of classifying prognostic comorbidity in longitudinal studies: Development and validation. *J. Chronic Dis.* **1987**, *40*, 373–383. [CrossRef]
49. Fanouriakis, A.; Pamfil, C.; Rednic, S.; Sidiropoulos, P.; Bertsias, G.; Boumpas, D.T. Is it primary neuropsychiatric systemic lupus erythematosus? Performance of existing attribution models using physician judgment as the gold standard. *Clin. Exp. Rheumatol.* **2016**, *34*, 910–917. [PubMed]
50. Sutton, E.J.; Davidson, J.E.; Bruce, I.N. The systemic lupus international collaborating clinics (SLICC) damage index: A systematic literature review. *Semin. Arthritis Rheum.* **2013**, *43*, 352–361. [CrossRef] [PubMed]
51. Isenberg, D.A.; Rahman, A.; Allen, E.; Farewell, V.; Akil, M.; Bruce, I.N.; D'Cruz, D.; Griffiths, B.; Khamashta, M.; Maddison, P.; et al. BILAG 2004. Development and initial validation of an updated version of the British Isles Lupus Assessment Group's disease activity index for patients with systemic lupus erythematosus. *Rheumatology* **2005**, *44*, 902–906. [CrossRef]
52. Barbhaiya, M.; Feldman, C.H.; Guan, H.; Chen, S.K.; Fischer, M.A.; Solomon, D.H.; Everett, B.M.; Costenbader, K.H. Racial/ethnic variation in stroke rates and risks among patients with systemic lupus erythematosus. *Semin. Arthritis Rheum.* **2019**, *48*, 840–846. [CrossRef] [PubMed]
53. Brown, E.A.; Gebregziabher, M.; Kamen, D.L.; White, B.M.; Williams, E.M. Examining racial differences in access to primary care for people living with lupus: Use of ambulatory care sensitive conditions to measure access. *Ethn. Dis.* **2020**, *30*, 611–620. [CrossRef] [PubMed]
54. Avina-Zubieta, J.A.; To, F.; Vostretsova, K.; De Vera, M.; Sayre, E.C.; Esdaile, J.M. Risk of myocardial infarction and stroke in newly diagnosed systemic lupus erythematosus: A general population-based study. *Arthritis Care Res.* **2017**, *69*, 849–856. [CrossRef]
55. Katz, P.; Gregorich, S.; Yazdany, J.; Trupin, L.; Julian, L.; Yelin, E.; Criswell, L.A. Obesity and its measurement in a community-based sample of women with systemic lupus erythematosus. *Arthritis Care Res.* **2011**, *63*, 261–268. [CrossRef]
56. Nived, O.; Ingvarsson, R.F.; Joud, A.; Linge, P.; Tyden, H.; Jonsen, A.; Bengtsson, A.A. Disease duration, age at diagnosis and organ damage are important factors for cardiovascular disease in SLE. *Lupus Sci. Med.* **2020**, *7*, e000398. [CrossRef] [PubMed]
57. Sabio, J.M.; Vargas-Hitos, J.A.; Navarrete-Navarrete, N.; Mediavilla, J.D.; Jimenez-Jaimez, J.; Diaz-Chamorro, A.; Jimenez-Alonso, J.; Grupo Lupus Virgen de las, N. Prevalence of and factors associated with hypertension in young and old women with systemic lupus erythematosus. *J. Rheumatol.* **2011**, *38*, 1026–1032. [CrossRef] [PubMed]
58. Tselios, K.; Gladman, D.D.; Su, J.; Ace, O.; Urowitz, M.B. Evolution of risk factors for atherosclerotic cardiovascular events in systemic lupus erythematosus: A longterm prospective study. *J. Rheumatol.* **2017**, *44*, 1841–1849. [CrossRef]
59. Magder, L.S.; Petri, M. Incidence of and risk factors for adverse cardiovascular events among patients with systemic lupus erythematosus. *Am. J. Epidemiol.* **2012**, *176*, 708–719. [CrossRef]
60. Kostopoulou, M.; Nikolopoulos, D.; Parodis, I.; Bertsias, G. Cardiovascular disease in systemic lupus erythematosus: Recent data on epidemiology, risk factors and prevention. *Curr. Vasc. Pharm.* **2020**, *18*, 549–565. [CrossRef] [PubMed]
61. Li, D.; Yoshida, K.; Feldman, C.H.; Speyer, C.; Barbhaiya, M.; Guan, H.; Solomon, D.H.; Everett, B.M.; Costenbader, K.H. Initial disease severity, cardiovascular events and all-cause mortality among patients with systemic lupus erythematosus. *Rheumatology* **2020**, *59*, 495–504. [CrossRef]
62. Romero-Diaz, J.; Vargas-Vorackova, F.; Kimura-Hayama, E.; Cortazar-Benitez, L.F.; Gijon-Mitre, R.; Criales, S.; Cabiedes-Contreras, J.; Iniguez-Rodriguez Mdel, R.; Lara-Garcia, E.A.; Nunez-Alvarez, C.; et al. Systemic lupus erythematosus risk factors for coronary artery calcifications. *Rheumatology* **2012**, *51*, 110–119. [CrossRef]

63. Robles-Vera, I.; Visitacion, N.; Toral, M.; Sanchez, M.; Gomez-Guzman, M.; O'Valle, F.; Jimenez, R.; Duarte, J.; Romero, M. Toll-like receptor 7-driven lupus autoimmunity induces hypertension and vascular alterations in mice. *J. Hypertens* **2020**, *38*, 1322–1335. [CrossRef]
64. Petri, M.; Magder, L.S. Comparison of remission and lupus low disease activity state in damage prevention in a United States systemic lupus erythematosus cohort. *Arthritis Rheumatol.* **2018**, *70*, 1790–1795. [CrossRef] [PubMed]
65. Ferrari, S.M.; Elia, G.; Virili, C.; Centanni, M.; Antonelli, A.; Fallahi, P. Systemic lupus erythematosus and thyroid autoimmunity. *Front. Endocrinol. (Lausanne)* **2017**, *8*, 138. [CrossRef]
66. Luo, W.; Mao, P.; Zhang, L.; Yang, Z. Association between systemic lupus erythematosus and thyroid dysfunction: A meta-analysis. *Lupus* **2018**, *27*, 2120–2128. [CrossRef]
67. Yun, J.S.; Bae, J.M.; Kim, K.J.; Jung, Y.S.; Kim, G.M.; Kim, H.R.; Lee, J.S.; Ko, S.H.; Cha, S.A.; Ahn, Y.B. Increased risk of thyroid diseases in patients with systemic lupus erythematosus: A nationwide population-based study in Korea. *PLoS ONE* **2017**, *12*, e0179088. [CrossRef]
68. Cramarossa, G.; Urowitz, M.B.; Su, J.; Gladman, D.; Touma, Z. Prevalence and associated factors of low bone mass in adults with systemic lupus erythematosus. *Lupus* **2017**, *26*, 365–372. [CrossRef]
69. Bultink, I.E.; Lems, W.F. Systemic lupus erythematosus and fractures. *RMD Open* **2015**, *1*, e000069. [CrossRef] [PubMed]
70. Hsiao, Y.P.; Tsai, J.D.; Muo, C.H.; Tsai, C.H.; Sung, F.C.; Liao, Y.T.; Chang, Y.J.; Yang, J.H. Atopic diseases and systemic lupus erythematosus: An epidemiological study of the risks and correlations. *Int. J. Environ. Res. Public Health* **2014**, *11*, 8112–8122. [CrossRef] [PubMed]
71. Wongtrakul, W.; Charoenngam, N.; Ponvilawan, B.; Ungprasert, P. Allergic rhinitis and risk of systemic lupus erythematosus: A systematic review and meta-analysis. *Int. J. Rheum. Dis.* **2020**, *23*, 1460–1467. [CrossRef]
72. Sin, E.; Anand, P.; Frieri, M. A link: Allergic rhinitis, asthma & systemic lupus erythematosus. *Autoimmun. Rev.* **2016**, *15*, 487–491. [CrossRef] [PubMed]
73. Fernandez, H.; Cevallos, A.; Jimbo Sotomayor, R.; Naranjo-Saltos, F.; Mera Orces, D.; Basantes, E. Mental disorders in systemic lupus erythematosus: A cohort study. *Rheumatol. Int.* **2019**, *39*, 1689–1695. [CrossRef] [PubMed]
74. Hesselvig, J.H.; Egeberg, A.; Kofoed, K.; Gislason, G.; Dreyer, L. Increased risk of depression in patients with cutaneous lupus erythematosus and systemic lupus erythematosus: A Danish nationwide cohort study. *Br. J. Derm.* **2018**, *179*, 1095–1101. [CrossRef] [PubMed]
75. Moustafa, A.T.; Moazzami, M.; Engel, L.; Bangert, E.; Hassanein, M.; Marzouk, S.; Kravtsenyuk, M.; Fung, W.; Eder, L.; Su, J.; et al. Prevalence and metric of depression and anxiety in systemic lupus erythematosus: A systematic review and meta-analysis. *Semin. Arthritis Rheum.* **2020**, *50*, 84–94. [CrossRef] [PubMed]
76. Abd-Alrasool, Z.A.; Gorial, F.I.; Hashim, M.T. Prevalence and severity of depression among Iraqi patients with systemic lupus rythematosus: A descriptive study. *Mediterr. J. Rheumatol.* **2017**, *28*, 142–146. [CrossRef]
77. Tiosano, S.; Nir, Z.; Gendelman, O.; Comaneshter, D.; Amital, H.; Cohen, A.D.; Amital, D. The association between systemic lupus erythematosus and bipolar disorder—A big data analysis. *Eur. Psychiatry J. Assoc. Eur. Psychiatr.* **2017**, *43*, 116–119. [CrossRef]
78. Mok, C.C.; Chan, K.L.; Cheung, E.F.; Yip, P.S. Suicidal ideation in patients with systemic lupus erythematosus: Incidence and risk factors. *Rheumatology* **2014**, *53*, 714–721. [CrossRef]
79. Tiosano, S.; Farhi, A.; Watad, A.; Grysman, N.; Stryjer, R.; Amital, H.; Comaneshter, D.; Cohen, A.D.; Amital, D. Schizophrenia among patients with systemic lupus erythematosus: Population-based cross-sectional study. *Epidemiol. Psychiatr. Sci.* **2017**, *26*, 424–429. [CrossRef] [PubMed]
80. Lillis, T.A.; Tirone, V.; Gandhi, N.; Weinberg, S.; Nika, A.; Sequeira, W.; Hobfoll, S.E.; Block, J.A.; Jolly, M. Sleep disturbance and depression symptoms mediate relationship between pain and cognitive dysfunction in lupus. *Arthritis Care Res.* **2019**, *71*, 406–412. [CrossRef]
81. Figueiredo-Braga, M.; Cornaby, C.; Cortez, A.; Bernardes, M.; Terroso, G.; Figueiredo, M.; Mesquita, C.D.S.; Costa, L.; Poole, B.D. Depression and anxiety in systemic lupus erythematosus: The crosstalk between immunological, clinical, and psychosocial factors. *Medicine* **2018**, *97*, e11376. [CrossRef]
82. Tisseverasinghe, A.; Peschken, C.; Hitchon, C. Anxiety and mood disorders in systemic lupus erythematosus: Current insights and future directions. *Curr. Rheumatol. Rep.* **2018**, *20*, 85. [CrossRef] [PubMed]
83. McQueenie, R.; Nicholl, B.I.; Jani, B.D.; Canning, J.; Macdonald, S.; McCowan, C.; Neary, J.; Browne, S.; Mair, F.S.; Siebert, S. Patterns of multimorbidity and their effects on adverse outcomes in rheumatoid arthritis: A study of 5658 UK Biobank participants. *BMJ Open* **2020**, *10*, e038829. [CrossRef] [PubMed]
84. Radner, H.; Yoshida, K.; Mjaavatten, M.D.; Aletaha, D.; Frits, M.; Lu, B.; Iannaccone, C.; Shadick, N.; Weinblatt, M.; Hmamouchi, I.; et al. Development of a multimorbidity index: Impact on quality of life using a rheumatoid arthritis cohort. *Semin. Arthritis Rheum.* **2015**, *45*, 167–173. [CrossRef]
85. Ziade, N.; El Khoury, B.; Zoghbi, M.; Merheb, G.; Abi Karam, G.; Mroue, K.; Messaykeh, J. Prevalence and pattern of comorbidities in chronic rheumatic and musculoskeletal diseases: The COMORD study. *Sci Rep.* **2020**, *10*, 7683. [CrossRef]
86. Kariniemi, S.; Rantalaiho, V.; Virta, L.J.; Puolakka, K.; Sokka-Isler, T.; Elfving, P. Multimorbidity among incident Finnish systemic lupus erythematosus patients during 2000–2017. *Lupus* **2021**, *30*, 165–171. [CrossRef] [PubMed]

87. Medhat, B.M.; Behiry, M.E.; Sobhy, N.; Farag, Y.; Marzouk, H.; Mostafa, N.; Khalifa, I.; Elkhalifa, M.; Eissa, B.M.; Hassan, E.H.E. Late-onset systemic lupus erythematosus: Characteristics and outcome in comparison to juvenile- and adult-onset patients-a multicenter retrospective cohort. *Clin. Rheumatol.* **2020**, *39*, 435–442. [CrossRef]
88. Petri, M.A.; Barr, E.; Magder, L.S. Development of a systemic lupus erythematosus cardiovascular risk equation. *Lupus Sci. Med.* **2019**, *6*, e000346. [CrossRef]
89. Kubota, Y.; Heiss, G.; MacLehose, R.F.; Roetker, N.S.; Folsom, A.R. Association of educational attainment with lifetime risk of cardiovascular disease: The atherosclerosis risk in communities study. *JAMA Intern. Med.* **2017**, *177*, 1165–1172. [CrossRef]
90. Nagel, G.; Peter, R.; Braig, S.; Hermann, S.; Rohrmann, S.; Linseisen, J. The impact of education on risk factors and the occurrence of multimorbidity in the EPIC-Heidelberg cohort. *BMC Public Health* **2008**, *8*, 384. [CrossRef]
91. Richette, P.; Clerson, P.; Perissin, L.; Flipo, R.M.; Bardin, T. Revisiting comorbidities in gout: A cluster analysis. *Ann. Rheum. Dis.* **2015**, *74*, 142–147. [CrossRef] [PubMed]

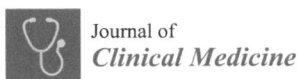

Article

Assessment of EULAR/ACR-2019, SLICC-2012 and ACR-1997 Classification Criteria in SLE with Longstanding Disease

Berta Magallares [1,2,3], David Lobo-Prat [1], Ivan Castellví [1,2,3], Patricia Moya [1,2,3], Ignasi Gich [2,4,5], Laura Martinez-Martinez [6], Hye Park [1], Ana Milena Millán [1], Ana Laiz [1,2,3], César Díaz-Torné [1,2,3], Susana Fernandez [1] and Hèctor Corominas [1,2,3],*

[1] Department of Rheumatology, Hospital de la Santa Creu i Sant Pau, 08025 Barcelona, Spain; bmagallares@santpau.cat (B.M.); Dlobo@santpau.cat (D.L.-P.); icastellvi@santpau.cat (I.C.); pmoyaa@santpau.cat (P.M.); HyeSang.Park@sanitatintegral.org (H.P.); amillana@santpau.cat (A.M.M.); alaiz@santpau.cat (A.L.); cdiazt@santpau.cat (C.D.-T.); sfernandez@santpau.cat (S.F.)
[2] Sant Pau Biomedical Research Institute (IIB Sant Pau), 08025 Barcelona, Spain; igich@santpau.cat
[3] Department of Immunology, Universitat Autònoma de Barcelona (UAB), 08193 Barcelona, Spain
[4] CIBER Epidemiología y Salud Pública (CIBERESP), 28029 Madrid, Spain
[5] Department of Clinical Epidemiology and Public Health, Hospital de la Santa Creu i Sant Pau, 08041 Barcelona, Spain
[6] Department of Immunology, Hospital de la Santa Creu i Sant Pau, 08025 Barcelona, Spain; lmartinezm@santpau.cat
* Correspondence: hcorominas@santpau.cat; Tel.: +34-932919000

Abstract: Background: Different classification criteria for systemic lupus erythematosus (SLE) have been launched over the years. Our aim was to evaluate the performance of the EULAR/ACR-2019, SLICC-2012 and ACR-1997 classification criteria in a cohort of SLE patients with longstanding disease. Methods: Descriptive observational study in 79 patients with established and longstanding SLE. The three classification criteria sets were applied to those patients. Results: Of the 79 patients, 70 were women (88.6%), with a mean age of 51.8 ± 14 years and a mean disease duration of 15.2 ± 11.5 years. The sensitivity of the different criteria were: 51.9%, 87.3% and 86.1% for ACR-1997, SLICC-2012 and EULAR/ACR-2019, respectively. In total, 68 out of 79 patients (53.7%) met all three classification criteria; 11.4% did not meet any classification criteria and were characterized by low SLEDAI (0.6 ± 0.9), low SLICC/ACR Damage Index (0.88 ± 0.56) and fulfilling only skin domains, antiphospholipid antibodies or hypocomplementemia. To fulfill EULAR/ACR-2019 criteria was associated with low complement levels ($p < 0.04$), high anti-dsDNA levels ($p < 0.001$), presence of lupus nephritis III-IV ($p < 0.05$) and arthritis ($p < 0.001$). Conclusion: The EULAR/ACR-2019 classification criteria showed high sensitivity, similar to SLICC-2012, in SLE patients with longstanding disease. Patients with serological, articular or renal involvement are more likely to fulfill SLICC-2012 or EULAR/ACR-2019 criteria.

Keywords: SLE; classification criteria; EULAR/ACR-2019; SLICC-2012; ACR-1997; longstanding lupus

Citation: Magallares, B.; Lobo-Prat, D.; Castellví, I.; Moya, P.; Gich, I.; Martinez-Martinez, L.; Park, H.; Millán, A.M.; Laiz, A.; Díaz-Torné, C.; et al. Assessment of EULAR/ACR-2019, SLICC-2012 and ACR-1997 Classification Criteria in SLE with Longstanding Disease. *J. Clin. Med.* **2021**, *10*, 2377. https://doi.org/10.3390/jcm10112377

Academic Editor: Matteo Piga

Received: 31 March 2021
Accepted: 25 May 2021
Published: 28 May 2021

Publisher's Note: MDPI stays neutral with regard to jurisdictional claims in published maps and institutional affiliations.

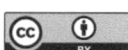

Copyright: © 2021 by the authors. Licensee MDPI, Basel, Switzerland. This article is an open access article distributed under the terms and conditions of the Creative Commons Attribution (CC BY) license (https://creativecommons.org/licenses/by/4.0/).

1. Introduction

Systemic lupus erythematosus (SLE) is a systemic autoimmune disease with a wide range of clinical manifestations occasionally leading to life-threatening organic failure [1]. The diagnosis of SLE may be challenging as several other conditions can mimic SLE and there are no specific findings to set up the diagnosis [2,3]. SLE is based on the sum of signs, symptoms, serological parameters, radiological features and histologic and pathological findings [4].

Classification criteria are essential to identify well-defined, relatively homogeneous groups of patients; they are primarily designed to be used in clinical research [5]. Classification criteria do not mean diagnostic criteria, but they are used frequently to detect patients with clinical symptoms and laboratory features of the disease [6]. Although they can provide diagnostic aids, the classification criteria are characterized by high specificity and usually lower sensitivity; therefore, patients with very recent onset of the disease or with less common manifestations may be missed [7]. Longstanding SLE cohorts should mostly meet these criteria, given the fact that they are patients with established disease and the risk of them presenting other systemic autoimmune diseases is slightly lower.

In 1971, the American College of Rheumatology (ACR) published the first preliminary criteria for SLE. These criteria were later updated in 1982 [8] and in 1997 [9]. The 1997 ACR criteria maintained the same structure, with 11 criteria, both clinical and immunological, four of which had to be present to identify patients with SLE [8,9]. Some clinical characteristics were over-represented, such as skin manifestations covering four of the 11 criteria, while immunological criteria were represented by only two criteria: positivity for Antinuclear antibodies (ANA)s on the one hand, and the presence of anti-double-stranded DNA (anti-dsDNA), anti-Sm or antiphospholipid antibodies on the other [9]. Consistently, ACR-1997 criteria have a sensitivity of 85% and specificity of 98% for classifying patients as having SLE [5,10].

Taking into account the limitations of the ACR-1997 criteria, the Systemic Lupus International Collaborating Clinics (SLICC) group published a new classification criteria proposal in 2012. The SLICC criteria were launched with 11 clinical and six immunological items. These criteria better determined each criterion and included some of the characteristic mucocutaneous manifestations and neuropsychiatric symptoms in comparison with ACR-1997 classification criteria. The most important advance in the SLICC-2012 criteria was the inclusion of specific histological findings of lupus nephritis, which along with immunological findings, are nowadays a sufficient condition to meet the classification criteria [11]. The SLICC-2012 criteria reached a sensitivity of 95% with a specificity of 95.5% [10].

Recently, a major effort to develop new criteria was led by the European League Against Rheumatism (EULAR) and ACR, and in 2019, new classification criteria came to light [12]. There are two main particularities among this new set of criteria in comparison with previous proposals: the required ANA positivity as an entry criterion and the categorization of the other criteria in different domains weighted from 2 to 10, where only the highest item of each domain is counted [11]. At least one clinical criterion is required and a total score of 10 points is necessary to be classified as having SLE [12]. Another key feature is that items are only counted towards SLE if there is no other more likely explanation [11,12]. One of the goals of these new criteria was to maintain high specificity, such as the ACR-1997 criteria, and high sensitivity, similar to the SLICC-2012 criteria. The validation data concluded that this objective was met, with a sensitivity of 96% and a specificity of 93% [13]. Since their publication, the precision of the new criteria has been evaluated in different SLE cohorts, such as early [5,14] and pediatric SLE [15,16]. Nevertheless, longstanding SLE patients represent the majority of patients in clinical practice, with various disease severities and usually exposed to several treatments. As patients with longstanding SLE are also potential candidates for clinical trials, it is crucial to evaluate how classification criteria perform in this subset of patients. Furthermore, these patients have an established disease and time is a key factor ruling out other diseases that could mimic SLE in their onset. Efforts have been made to assess the EULAR/ACR-2019 criteria in real clinical practice [17,18], but their performance and application in long-term SLE have not yet been well established.

In the present study, we aimed to assess the performance and characteristics of the EULAR/ACR-2019 in comparison with SLICC-2012 and ACR-1997 classification criteria in a cohort of SLE patients with longstanding disease.

2. Materials and Methods

The study was carried out in the Systemic Autoimmune Disease Outpatient Clinic at the Rheumatology Department of Hospital Universitari de la Santa Creu i Sant Pau. Our center is the only tertiary referral hospital in the district of AIS Dreta in Barcelona with around 308,268 inhabitants. All high complexity and severe diseases are referred to our center through the Universal Health Coverage of the Public Health System.

The inclusion criteria were patients older than 18 years with a confirmed diagnosis of SLE based on the clinical expertise of the attending rheumatologist, with a follow-up of at least 12 months. The exclusion criteria were patients who had lost follow-ups or for any reason did not provide necessary clinical or laboratory information to evaluate the classification criteria's fulfillment. Between June 2020 and August 2020, 84 patients were screened during routine clinical follow-ups. Finally, 79 consecutive patients were included.

Demographic, clinical and laboratory data were gathered. Disease activity was measured using the Systemic Lupus Erythematosus Disease Activity Index (SLEDAI) and accumulated damage was assessed using the SLICC/ACR Damage Index (SLICC/ACR DI). Each of the three sets of criteria was applied at the last follow-up after reviewing past medical records and SLE damage.

Anti-nuclear antibodies were determined by indirect immunofluorescent (IIF) assay with Hep2 cells (INOVA diagnostics). Screening dilution was over 1:80. The anti-dsDNA and anti-Sm and antibodies were tested using chemiluminescence tests (INOVA diagnostics). The cut-off of positivity was 35 Units/mL for anti-dsDNA and 20 Units/mL for anti-Sm. The quantitative determination of antiphospholipid IgG/IgM was performed using Orgentec Diagnostika GmbH (Palex) kits with the ELISA method, following the recommendations of the International Society on Thrombosis and Haemostasis. To ensure a homogeneous method of immunological examination, all tests were performed in the same laboratory and repeated before inclusion. All patients had blood tests checked at least every 6–12 months except for patients with more active disease who required more frequent examination.

The characteristics of the cohort were presented as absolute and relative frequencies [n (%)] for categorical variables, and using mean and standard deviation (mean ± SD) for quantitative variables. A study of association between criteria fulfillment and clinical and immunological data was performed using contingency tables and chi-square; to calculate concordance between the criteria, the kappa coefficient was used. Statistical significance was assumed in p values < 0.05. IBM-SPSS (V26.1) software was used for data analysis.

3. Results

A total of 79 patients were included. Seventy patients (88.6%) were women. The mean age of our cohort was 51.8 ± 14 years and they had a mean disease duration of 15.2 ± 11.5 years. All patients had a positive ANA test. The clinical and demographic characteristics of the cohort are detailed in Table 1.

Out of 79 patients, 40 (51.9%) met all three classification criteria. Figure 1 shows the proportion of patients who met the sets of different classification criteria. In our cohort, no patients met the EULAR/ACR-2019 and ACR-1997 but not the SLICC-2012, nor did we find any patients who met only the ACR-1997 criteria. Nine patients (11.4%) did not meet any SLE classification criteria. Intriguingly, those patients were characterized by meeting only skin domains (alopecia or oral ulcers), antiphospholipid antibodies or hypocomplementemia domains, and presented low SLEDAI scores (0.6 ± 0.9). In addition, they presented significantly lower SLICC/ACR Damage Index scores compared to those who met all three sets of criteria (0.88 ± 0.56 vs. 4.02 ± 0.56; $p < 0.025$).

Table 1. Demographic and clinical characteristics.

General conditions	n (79)
Age (years), mean ± SD	51.89 ± 14.04
Female, n (%)	70 (88.6%)
Disease duration (years), mean ± SD	15.22 ± 11.59
SLEDAI score, mean ± SD	2.65 ± 2.1
SLICC/ACR DI, mean ± SD	3.23 ± 1.35
Clinical features	
Fever, n (%)	2 (2.5)
Non-scarring alopecia, n (%)	18 (22.8)
Oral ulcers, n (%)	28 (35.4)
Subacute cutaneous or discoid lupus, n (%)	12 (15.2)
Acute cutaneous lupus, n (%)	16 (20.3)
Arthritis, n (%)	38 (48.1)
Seizure, n (%)	1 (1.3)
Pleural or pericardial effusion, n (%)	2 (2.5)
Acute pericarditis, n (%)	4 (5.1)
Proteinuria > 0.5 g/24 h, n (%)	11 (13.9)
Class II or V lupus nephritis, n (%)	15 (19)
Class III or IV lupus nephritis, n (%)	12 (15.2)
Leukopenia, n (%)	24 (30.4)
Thrombocytopenia, n (%)	9 (11.4)
Autoimmune hemolysis, n (%)	2 (2.5)
Immunologic features	
Anticardiolipin IgG > 40 GPL, n (%)	12 (15.2)
Anti B2 glycoprotein 1 > 40 UI, n (%)	10 (12.7)
Lupus anticoagulant, n (%)	12 (15.2)
Low C3 or low C4, n (%)	29 (36.7)
Low C3 and low C4, n (%)	28 (35.4)
Anti-dsDNA antibody, n (%)	50 (63.3)
Anti-Sm antibody, n (%)	14 (17.7)

SD: Standard deviation.

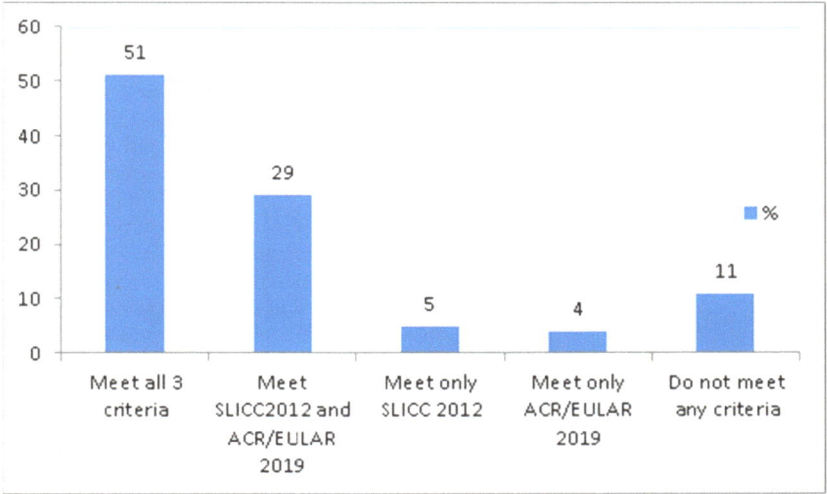

Figure 1. Proportion of patients meeting the different sets of criteria.

Seven patients only fulfilled one of the three classification criteria: three of them only met the EULAR/ACR-2019 criteria and were characterized by having hypocomplementemia or arthritis with positive anti-dsDNA and ANA. The four patients that exclusively met the SLICC-2012 criteria did not have a predilection for any domain. The cohort of patients who met the EULAR/ACR-2019 criteria had high scores, almost doubling the cut-off point for classifying in comparison with the ACR 1997 and SLICC 2012 sets of criteria. Interestingly, patients with higher scores (≥ 20) for the EULAR/ACR-2019 classification criteria were characterized by higher scores on the SLICC/ACR Damage Index (4.41 ± 1.13) compared to those with lower EULAR/ACR-2019 scores (2.54 ± 1.01 SD) ($p < 0.02$).

The percentages of patients meeting the different classification criteria are summarized in Table 2.

Table 2. Proportion of patients meeting the different classification criteria and their scores.

	Sensitivity (% Achieving Criteria)	Mean Score of Patients Classified with SLE ($\pm$SD)	Mean Score of Patients Not Classified with SLE ($\pm$SD)
ACR-1997	51.9	5 ± 0.9	2.8 ± 0.8
SLICC-2012	87.3	5.3 ± 1.4	2.8 ± 0.4
EULAR/ACR-2019	86.1	18.6 ± 5.8	6.1 ± 2.5

SD: Standard deviation.

Regarding the EULAR/ACR-2019 criteria, statistically significant associations were found between meeting the EULAR/ACR-2019 classification criteria and the presence of low C3 and C4 ($p = 0.03$), anti-dsDNA ($p < 0.01$), lupus nephritis III-IV ($p < 0.05$) and arthritis ($p < 0.01$). Only one patient with C3 and C4 hypocomplementemia did not meet any of those criteria. All patients with positive anti-dsDNA met the criteria and 73.5% of patients that met the EULAR/ACR-2019 criteria tested positive for anti-dsDNA. All patients with lupus nephritis III–IV and arthritis were classified as having SLE, and 55.9% and 17.6% of patients classified as having SLE by these criteria had arthritis or lupus nephritis III–IV, respectively. Moreover, all patients with proteinuria > 0.5 g/24 h also met the EULAR/ACR-2019 criteria.

In the SLICC-2012 evaluation, there were significant associations between meeting these criteria and the presence of arthritis ($p < 0.01$), renal involvement ($p < 0.01$), leukopenia/lymphopenia ($p < 0.01$), anti-dsDNA ($p = 0.02$) and hypocomplementemia ($p = 0.02$). Of the patients with arthritis and/or renal involvement/leukopenia/lymphopenia, 97.2% and 100% were classified as having SLE, respectively. Likewise, 94% of the patients with elevated anti-dsDNA and 93% with decreased complement also met the SLICC-2012 criteria.

Fulfillment of ACR-1997 was associated with malar rash ($p < 0.01$), discoid rash ($p = 0.05$), oral ulcers ($p = 0.03$) and presence of photosensitivity ($p < 0.01$), as well as arthritis ($p < 0.01$), serositis ($p = 0.02$) and renal ($p = 0.05$) and hematologic ($p = 0.05$) involvement. The proportions of patients in our cohort with malar rash, discoid lupus, oral ulcers or photosensitivity who met the ACR-1997 criteria were 93%, 85.7%, 67.8% and 84.6%, respectively. Of the patients with arthritis, 73.6% were classified as having SLE, as well as 100%, 68% and 72.4% of those with serositis, renal and hematologic involvement, respectively. Table 3 summarizes the different involvement associations with all sets of classification criteria.

Finally, the Kappa agreement coefficient between the three sets of classification criteria found the best concordance between the EULAR/ACR-2019 and SLICC-2012 classification criteria (K 0.61) in comparison with the agreement between the EULAR/ACR -2019 and ACR-1997 (K 0.27) and between the SLICC-2012 and ACR-1997 (K 0.30).

Table 3. Statistical associations between the clinical/immunological domains and the EULAR/ACR-2019, SLICC-2012 and ACR-1997 classification criteria.

EULAR/ACR-2019 Domains	Achieving EULAR/ACR-2019 (p)	SLICC-2012 Domains	Achieving SLICC-2012 (p)	ACR-1997 Domains	Achieving ACR-1997 (p)
Fever	0.436	Acute cutaneous lupus	0.265	Malar rash	0.000
Non-scarring alopecia	0.707	Chronic cutaneous lupus	0.130	Discoid rash	0.048
Oral ulcers	0.461	Oral or nasal ulcers	0.697	Photosensitivity	0.000
Subacute cutaneous or discoid lupus	0.770	Non-scarring alopecia	0.820	Oral ulcers	0.034
Acute cutaneous lupus	0.283	Arthritis	0.009	Arthritis	0.000
Arthritis	0.000	Serositis	0.291	Serositis	0.020
Delirium	NA	Renal involvement	0.003	Renal disorder	0.049
Psychosis	NA	Neurologic disorder	0.602	Neurologic disorder	0.957
Seizure	0.583	Hemolytic anemia	0.459	Hematologic disorder	0.005
Pleural or pericardial effusion	0.436	Leukopenia < 4000/mm^3/lymphopenia < 1000/mm^3	0.005	Immunologic disorder	0.120
Acute pericarditis	0.267	Thrombocytopenia < 100.000/mm^3	0.107	ANA	NA
Proteinuria > 0.5 g/24 h	0.059	ANA	NA		
Class II or V lupus nephritis	0.331	Anti-dsDNA	0.022		
Class III or IV lupus nephritis	0.047	Anti-Sm	0.467		
Leukopenia < 4000/mm^3	0.069	Antiphospholipid antibodies	0.796		
Thrombocytopenia < 100.000/mm^3	0.471	Low complement	0.022		
Autoimmune hemolysis	0.436	Direct Combs test	0.236		
Anticardiolipin IgG > 40 GPL	0.509				
Anti B2 glycoprotein 1 > 40 UI	0.070				
Lupus anticoagulant	0.270				
Low C3 or low C4	0.980				
Low C3 and low C4	0.031				
Anti-dsDNA antibody	0.000				
Anti-Sm antibody	0.387				

ACR: American College of Rheumatology. EULAR: European League Against Rheumatism. NA: Not applicable. SLICC: Systemic Lupus International Collaborating Clinics.

4. Discussion

We found significant differences among the three sets of SLE classification criteria and the patients' characteristics according to the achieved criteria. Only 51.9% of our patients met all three classification criteria, which is a lower proportion than that described in other cohorts [5,13,14]. This percentage is even lower than expected considering that those were patients with long-standing disease [19]. It is known that the sensitivity of each classification criteria differs among them. The EULAR/ACR-2019 classification criteria show high sensitivity in SLE patients with longstanding disease, similar to the SLICC-2012 criteria, both of which are much higher than the ACR-1997, as has been described previously in other cohorts [5,13,14]. This might be explained by the increased weight that a better understanding of SLE physiopathology provides to analytic and immunological criteria in the new sets of criteria against the relevance of dermatological manifestations in the ACR-1997 criteria.

Patients who were classified as having SLE by the EULAR/ACR-2019 classification criteria had a mean higher score and were further above the cut-off point than in the other two sets of criteria. We have not found this data described in other cohorts but we consider this finding to be positive, making it more difficult to find doubtful cases. It is worth emphasizing that high scores (≥ 20) in the EULAR/ACR-2019 criteria were associated with more accumulated damage and this might indicate a predictive role of this set of criteria for disease severity.

We also observed that patients with low SLEDAI scores were less likely to meet the classification criteria for any of the three sets. Thus, 11.4% of patients diagnosed with SLE barely classified in any of the three sets of classification criteria and were characterized by presenting low SLEDAI scores (0.6 ± 0.9). Recently, higher disease activity indices in SLE have been described in patients with increased EULAR/ACR-2019 scores and <12 months of disease course [20]. Other authors conclude that the new criteria may misclassify a small subset of SLE patients with milder disease [17].

Another interesting finding was the different weights that some features have in the different sets of classification criteria. The clinical and immunological characteristics that were statistically associated with positive EULAR/ACR-2019 criteria were renal involvement, arthritis, low C3 and C4 and a positive test for DNA, with all of those important and highly specific to SLE [21]. Those features were also associated with the SLICC-2012 classification criteria together with leukopenia/lymphopenia. None of these two sets showed a statistical association with other clinical domains such as cutaneous, serositis or constitutional syndrome. On the other hand, patients that met the ACR-1997 criteria were linked with other clinical characteristics such as in the cutaneous, serositis, arthritis or hematological domains. It is noteworthy that the magnitude of dermatological manifestations in the ACR1997 classification criteria decreased in favor of analytic and immunological parameters in the later presented classification criteria from 2012 and 2019. Partially, the explanation may lie in the different definitions used for cutaneous lupus among the three sets of criteria and the weight given to every single manifestation [11].

We also observed a low agreement among the different criteria to classify patients as having SLE, with the highest kappa coefficient between the EULAR/ACR-2019 and SLICC-2012 classification criteria (K = 0.61). This may be explained by similarities between the EULAR/ACR-2019 and SLICC-2012 classification criteria [6].

Some limitations are obvious in our study. Firstly, this is a retrospective study with the weaknesses of such types of projects. The inclusion criterion that the patients had to accomplish for us to apply every set of criteria excluded patients with previous unavailable data or there was a need to update the information on specific items. Moreover, some clinical information may have been missed or underestimated. This is associated with the second limitation of the study: the small size of the cohort did not allow us to precisely identify clinical profiles of patients diagnosed with SLE who did not meet some or any of the classification criteria. Finally, specificity has not been assessed as we did not include control subjects or patients with other diagnoses. Further research with larger, multiracial and worldwide-representative cohorts is needed, especially regarding the specificity of the EULAR/ACR-2019 criteria.

5. Conclusions

To summarize, our data support the validity of the new 2019 criteria for accurate classification of SLE in patients with longstanding disease, potentially leading to better outcomes and targeted therapies. It also expands the reliability of EULAR/ACR-2019 classification criteria in real-life conditions, in a longstanding disease cohort exposed to several treatments, sometimes with low disease activity.

Author Contributions: Conceptualization, D.L.-P., B.M. and H.C.; methodology, H.P., I.G. and B.M.; software, I.G. and C.D.-T.; validation, D.L.-P., A.L., A.M.M. and P.M.; formal analysis, D.L.-P., I.G. and B.M.; investigation, D.L.-P., P.M., S.F. and B.M.; resources, D.L.-P., L.M.-M., A.M.M. and B.M.; data curation, D.L.-P., S.F., L.M.-M. and B.M.; writing—original draft preparation, D.L.-P. and B.M.; writing—review and editing, H.C., P.M. and I.C.; visualization, I.C. H.C., B.M. and C.D.-T.; supervision, A.L., H.P., I.C. and H C.; project administration, B.M. and H.C. All authors have read and agreed to the published version of the manuscript.

Funding: This research received no external funding.

Institutional Review Board Statement: The study was conducted according to the guidelines of the Declaration of Helsinki and approved by the Ethics Committee of Hospital Universitari de la Sant Creu i Sant Pau, Barcelona (protocol code HSCSP:/20/013(R-OBS) and date of approval: 15 January 2020).

Informed Consent Statement: Oral informed consent was obtained from all subjects involved in the study.

Data Availability Statement: All data concerning the results of the study may be found in patient's clinical charts.

Acknowledgments: To all patient participants in the study and to all the staff of the Rheumatology Department from Hospital de la Santa Creu i Sant Pau, Universitat Autònoma de Barcelona (UAB).

Conflicts of Interest: The authors declare no conflict of interest.

References

1. Kaul, A.; Gordon, C.; Crow, M.K.; Touma, Z.; Urowitz, M.B.; van Vollenhoven, R.; Ruiz-Irastorza, G.; Hughes, G. Systemic lupus erythematosus. *Nat. Rev. Dis. Primers* **2016**, *2*, 16039. [CrossRef]
2. Chasset, F.; Richez, C.; Martin, T.; Belot, A.; Korganow, A.S.; Arnaud, L. Rare diseases that mimic systemic lupus erythematosus (Lupus mimickers). *Jt. Bone Spine Rev. Du Rhum.* **2019**, *86*, 165–171. [CrossRef] [PubMed]
3. Concha, J.S.S.; Tarazi, M.; Kushner, C.J.; Gaffney, R.G.; Werth, V.P. The diagnosis and classification of amyopathic dermatomyositis: A historical review and assessment of existing criteria. *Br. J. Dermatol.* **2019**, *180*, 1001–1008. [CrossRef] [PubMed]
4. Petri, M.; Orbai, A.M.; Alarcón, G.S.; Gordon, C.; Merrill, J.T.; Fortin, P.R.; Bruce, I.N.; Isenberg, D.; Wallace, D.J.; Nived, O.; et al. Derivation and validation of the systemic lupus international collaborating clinics classification criteria for systemic lupus erythematosus. *Arthritis Rheum.* **2012**, *64*, 2677–2686. [CrossRef] [PubMed]
5. Adamichou, C.; Nikolopoulos, D.; Genitsaridi, I.; Bortoluzzi, A.; Fanouriakis, A.; Papastefanakis, E.; Kalogiannaki, E.; Gergianaki, I.; Sidiropoulos, P.; Boumpas, D.T.; et al. In an early SLE cohort the ACR-1997, SLICC-2012 and EULAR/ACR-2019 criteria classify non-overlapping groups of patients: Use of all three criteria ensures optimal capture for clinical studies while their modification earlier classification and treatment. *Ann. Rheum. Dis.* **2020**, *79*, 232–241. [CrossRef] [PubMed]
6. Bertsias, G.K.; Pamfil, C.; Fanouriakis, A.; Boumpas, D.T. Diagnostic criteria for systemic lupus erythematosus: Has the time come? *Nat. Rev. Rheumatol.* **2013**, *9*, 687–694. [CrossRef]
7. Aggarwal, R.; Ringold, S.; Khanna, D.; Neogi, T.; Johnson, S.R.; Miller, A.; Brunner, H.I.; Ogawa, R.; Felson, D.; Ogdie, A.; et al. Distinctions between diagnostic and classification criteria? *Arthritis Care Res.* **2015**, *67*, 891–897. [CrossRef]
8. Tan, E.M.; Cohen, A.S.; Fries, J.F.; Masi, A.T.; McShane, D.J.; Rothfield, N.F.; Schaller, J.G.; Talal, N.; Winchester, R.J. The 1982 revised criteria for the classification of systemic lupus erythematosus. *Arthritis Rheum.* **1982**, *25*, 1271–1277. [CrossRef]
9. Hochberg, M.C. Updating the American College of Rheumatology revised criteria for the classification of systemic lupus erythematosus. *Arthritis Rheum.* **1997**, *40*, 1725. [CrossRef]

10. Hartman, E.A.R.; van Royen-Kerkhof, A.; Jacobs, J.W.G.; Welsing, P.M.J.; Fritsch-Stork, R.D.E. Performance of the 2012 systemic lupus international collaborating clinics classification criteria versus the 1997 American college of rheumatology classification criteria in adult and juvenile systemic lupus erythematosus. A systematic review and meta-analysis. *Autoimmun. Rev.* **2018**, *17*, 316–322. [CrossRef]
11. Aringer, M.; Leuchten, N.; Johnson, S.R. New Criteria for Lupus. *Curr. Rheumatol. Rep.* **2020**, *22*, 18. [CrossRef] [PubMed]
12. Aringer, M.; Costenbader, K.; Daikh, D.; Brinks, R.; Mosca, M.; Ramsey-Goldman, R.; Smolen, J.S.; Wofsy, D.; Boumpas, D.T.; Kamen, D.L.; et al. 2019 European league against rheumatism/American college of rheumatology classification criteria for systemic lupus erythematosus. *Arthritis Rheumatol.* **2019**, *71*, 1400–1412. [CrossRef] [PubMed]
13. Aringer, M. EULAR/ACR classification criteria for SLE. *Semin. Arthritis Rheum.* **2019**, *49*, S14–S17. [CrossRef] [PubMed]
14. Johnson, S.R.; Brinks, R.; Costenbader, K.H.; Daikh, D.; Mosca, M.; Ramsey-Goldman, R.; Smolen, J.S.; Wofsy, D.; Boumpas, D.T.; Kamen, D.L.; et al. Performance of the 2019 EULAR/ACR classification criteria for systemic lupus erythematosus in early disease, across sexes and ethnicities. *Ann. Rheum. Dis.* **2020**, *79*, 1333–1339. [CrossRef] [PubMed]
15. Aljaberi, N.; Nguyen, K.; Strahle, C.; Merritt, A.; Mathur, A.; Brunner, H.I. The performance of the new 2019-EULAR/ACR classification criteria for systemic lupus erythematosus in children and young adults. *Arthritis Care Res.* **2020**. [CrossRef]
16. Ma, M.; Hui-Yuen, J.S.; Cerise, J.E.; Iqbal, S.; Eberhard, B.A. Validation of the 2019 European league against rheumatism/American college of rheumatology criteria compared to the 1997 American college of rheumatology criteria and the 2012 systemic lupus international collaborating clinics criteria in pediatric systemic lupus erythematosus. *Arthritis Care Res.* **2020**, *72*, 1597–1601.
17. Rubio, J.; Krishfield, S.; Kyttaris, V.C. Application of the 2019 European league against rheumatism/American college of rheumatology systemic lupus erythematosus classification criteria in clinical practice: A single center experience. *Lupus* **2020**, *29*, 421–425. [CrossRef] [PubMed]
18. Suda, M.; Kishimoto, M.; Ohde, S.; Okada, M. Validation of the 2019 ACR/EULAR classification criteria of systemic lupus erythematosus in 100 Japanese patients: A real-world setting analysis. *Clin. Rheumatol.* **2020**, *39*, 1823–1827. [CrossRef]
19. Inês, L.; Silva, C.; Galindo, M.; López-Longo, F.J.; Terroso, G.; Romão, V.C.; Rúa-Figueroa, I.; Santos, M.J.; Pego-Reigosa, J.M.; Nero, P.; et al. Classification of systemic lupus erythematosus: Systemic lupus international collaborating clinics versus American college of rheumatology criteria. A comparative study of 2055 patients from a real-life, international systemic lupus erythematosus cohort. *Arthritis Care Res.* **2015**, *67*, 1180–1185. [CrossRef]
20. Whittall Garcia, L.P.; Gladman, D.D.; Urowitz, M.; Touma, Z.; Su, J.; Johnson, S.R. New EULAR/ACR 2019 SLE classification criteria: Defining ominosity in SLE. *Ann. Rheum. Dis.* **2021**. [CrossRef]
21. Jia, Y.; Zhao, L.; Wang, C.; Shang, J.; Miao, Y.; Dong, Y.; Zhao, Z. Anti-double-stranded DNA isotypes and anti-C1q antibody improve the diagnostic specificity of systemic lupus erythematosus. *Dis. Markers* **2018**, *2018*, 4528547. [CrossRef] [PubMed]

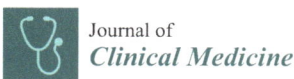

Journal of Clinical Medicine

Article

Cytomegalovirus-Associated Autoantibody against TAF9 Protein in Patients with Systemic Lupus Erythematosus

Yen-Fu Chen [1,†], Ao-Ho Hsieh [1,†], Lian-Chin Wang [1], Kuang-Hui Yu [1,*] and Chang-Fu Kuo [1,2,*]

[1] Division of Rheumatology, Allergy and Immunology, Chang Gung Memorial Hospital, Linkou Center, Taoyuan 333, Taiwan; patrichen0693@gmail.com (Y.-F.C.); mayitsu2006@gmail.com (A.-H.H.); lian.chin.wang@gmail.com (L.-C.W.)

[2] Center for Artificial Intelligence in Medicine, Chang Gung Memorial Hospital, Linkou Center, Taoyuan 333, Taiwan

* Correspondence: goutyu@gmail.com (K.-H.Y.); zandis@gmail.com (C.-F.K.)

† Equal contribution.

Abstract: Background: Evidence indicates a causal link between cytomegalovirus (CMV) infection and the triggering of systemic lupus erythematosus (SLE). Animal studies have revealed that CMV phosphoprotein 65 (pp65) induces autoantibodies against nuclear materials and causes the autoantibody attack of glomeruli. IgG eluted from the glomeruli of CMVpp65-peptide-immunized mice exhibited cross-reactivity against dsDNA and TATA-box-binding protein associated factor 9 (TAF9). Whether the elevation of anti-TAF9 IgG is associated with anti-CMV reactivity in human lupus remains unclear. **Methods**: The sera from patients with rheumatic diseases, including ankylosing spondylitis (AS), gout, rheumatoid arthritis (RA), systemic lupus erythematosus (SLE), and Sjögren syndrome (SS) were examined using ELISA for antibodies of CMV, CMVpp65, and TAF9. **Results**: In total, 83.8% of the rheumatic patients had acquired CMV infections. The SLE patients had a high prevalence of anti-CMV IgM. The highest seropositivity rates for anti-HCMVpp65 and anti-TAF9 IgG were observed in the SLE patients. Purified anti-CMVpp65 IgG from CMVpp65/TAF9 dual-positive SLE sera reacted to both TAF9 and dsDNA. An increased prevalence of proteinuria and low hemoglobin levels were found in CMV IgG- and CMVpp65 IgG-positive SLE patients. **Conclusions**: This observation suggests that immunity to CMVpp65 is associated with cross-reactivity with TAF9 and dsDNA and that it is involved in the development of clinical manifestations in SLE.

Keywords: systemic lupus erythematosus; cytomegalovirus phosphoprotein 65; TATA-box-binding protein associated factor 9; anemia; proteinuria

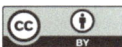

1. Introduction

Systemic lupus erythematosus (SLE) is a chronic inflammatory immune disorder characterized by widespread loss of host immune tolerance to self-nuclear antigens. Increasing evidence indicates that human cytomegalovirus (CMV) infection precedes the onset of this loss of tolerance [1]. Most people infected with CMV during childhood are asymptomatic or exhibit self-limiting manifestations. Lifelong persistence, intermittent reactivation, and the dampening of the host defenses by interference with the host's immune system are essential characteristics of CMV infection [2]. Several autoimmune disorders have been linked to CMV infection, particularly SLE [3]. Active CMV infections that are more frequently observed in SLE patients with active disease are related to the clinical manifestations and other complications [4]. CMV infection increases Ro/La protein expression on keratinocytes and laboratory cell lines [5,6]. The seroprevalence of anti-CMV and anti-U1 small nuclear ribonucleoprotein (snRNP) IgG is greater in SLE patients than healthy individuals, suggesting that CMV has a potential role in SLE development [7].

CMV phosphoprotein 65 (pp65), the major component of the extracellular viral particle, is responsible for the modulation of the host's immune system during CMV infection [8,9].

SLE patients have a higher seroprevalence of anti-CMVpp65 IgG than other rheumatic patients [10]. Glomerular cellularity, proteinuria, and anti-CMVpp65 IgG cross-reacting with dsDNA and nuclear proteins were found in mice immunized with a CMVpp65 protein fragment [11,12]. Recently, we observed that the immunoglobulin G eluted from the glomeruli of CMVpp65-peptide-immunized mice bound to dsDNA and the human TATA-box-binding protein associated factor 9 (TAF9) protein [13]. To further confirm this observation in human subjects and investigate the association between serum anti-CMV/CMVpp65 IgG and the anti-TAF9 IgG antibody and SLE disease, cross-sectional research was performed on patients with one of five common rheumatic diseases.

2. Materials and Methods

2.1. Study Subjects

We followed the method proposed in our previous study [13]. All the participants were enrolled from rheumatology clinics in the Linkou branch of Chang Gung Memorial Hospital. The definition of rheumatic diseases was based on the American College of Rheumatology classification criteria, and a rheumatologist confirmed all the diagnoses. The current study was approved by the Institutional Review Board of Chang Gung Memorial Hospital, and all the participants provided written informed consent before their inclusion as required by the Declaration of Helsinki (approval numbers #201600798B0 and 201600795B0). The follow-up sera were collected from rheumatic patients whose disease was well-controlled at 3 months after disease onset. The clinical manifestation data were monitored and analyzed at the same time.

2.2. Antibody Purification

Antibody purification from serum was conducted as previously described [11]. Briefly, cyanogen-bromide-activated Sepharose (CnBr, 0.25 g/mL; Sigma Aldrich, St. Louis, Missouri, USA; CAS Number: 68987-32-6) was activated using 15 gel volumes of 1 mM HCl at 4 °C for 1 h. After activation, the CnBr resin was washed using an ice-cold coupling buffer twice. A total of 2 mg of CMVpp65 protein (ProSpect, Rehovot, Israeli; Catalog code: CMV-215) was dissolved by gentle rotation in ice-cold coupling buffer (0.1 M $NaHCO_3$, 0.5 M NaCl, pH 8.3) with activated CnBr resin at 4 °C overnight. The free active groups on the CnBr resin were deactivated using 0.1 M Tris-HCl (pH 8.0) at room temperature for 2 h. After deactivation, the CnBr resin was washed three times with alternating buffer (0.1 M NaAc, 0.5 M NaCl, pH 4.0, and 0.1 M Tris-HCl, 0.5 M NaCl, pH 8.0) and washed with 10 mL of PBS once. For purification, 2 mL of serum from each patient with SLE and an anti-CMVpp65 IgG-positive status, in 20 mL of ice-cold PBS, was added to CMVpp65-protein-conjugated CnBr resin and incubated at 4 °C overnight. The bound antibodies were eluted using 1 mL of 0.1 M glycine (pH 2.0), and the eluted fraction was immediately neutralized with 50 µL of neutralizing buffer (1 M Tris-HCl, 2 M NaCl, pH 8.8).

2.3. ELISA Assay

The measurement of CMV IgM and CMV IgG was conducted using the Cytomegalovirus IgG/IgM ELISA Kit (Abnova, Taipei City, Taiwan; Catalog code: KA-1452 and KA-0228). The detection of serum CMV IgM and IgG was performed according to the manufacturer's instructions. For the semi-quantitative determination of the CMVpp65 IgG, TAF9, and dsDNA IgG antibody titers, ELISA was conducted as previously described with minor modifications [13]. Briefly, 100 ng/well of CMVpp65 (Prospect, Rehovot, Israeli; Catalog code: CMV-215), TAF protein (MyBiosource, San Diego, CA, USA; Catalog code: MBS1385026), or purified calf thymus dsDNA (Sigma-Aldrich, St. Louis, MO, USA; CAS Number: 73049-39-5), in phosphate buffered saline (PBS, pH 7.4), was coated on a 96-well microtiter plate (Greiner Bio-One, North Carolina, USA; Catalog Number: 655074) at 4 °C overnight. After blocking the plate with 5% skimmed milk, 100× diluted human serum or 0.5 µg of purified IgG antibody in PBS was added, and the plate was incubated at 4 °C for 2 h. Following incubation, the unbound antibody was washed away four times using

TBS with 0.05% Tween-20, and the bound antibody was incubated with 5000× diluted horseradish peroxidase (HRP)-conjugated anti-human IgG (Jackson ImmunoResearch, Pennsylvania, PA, USA; Catalog code: 109-035-088) at 4 °C for 2 h. After washing, TMB (Sigma-Aldrich, St. Louis, MO, USA) was added as the substrate, and the HRP activity was measured using a microplate ELISA reader at 450 nm (EZ read 400). Anti-CMVpp65 and anti-TAF9 positivity were defined according to the mean + 3SEM for the sera from the SLE patients.

2.4. CMV IgG Avidity Testing

The CMVIgG avidity was determined using a modified protocol [14]. The CMV IgG avidity was measured using the same CMV IgG kit with the use of TBST containing 8 M urea as a washing solution. We performed two sets of ELISA testing for CMV IgG avidity: one set was washed with TBST containing 8 M urea, and the other was washed with TBST without 8 M urea. The CMV IgG activities were used to calculate the avidity index (AI). The AI calculation was as follows: percentage of AI = (O.D.$_{450}$ absorbance value of CMV IgG activity per well with 8 M urea wash/O.D.$_{450}$ absorbance value of CMV IgG activity per well without 8 M urea wash) ×100. The cut-off value of AI >60% represented high IgG avidity, which is considered to indicate a past or recurrent infection, while the cut-off value of AI <30%, the low avidity, demonstrates primary infection.

2.5. Statistical Analysis

Statistical analyses of the titers and multiple-comparison corrections were performed using the GraphPad Prism software 8.0. Student's t and two-tailed Fisher's tests were used for these comparisons, with graphs depicting the mean ± SEM. Pearson's correlation coefficient test was used to examine these comparisons, with graphs depicting the R squared and p values. The independent t-test, Kruskal–Wallis test, and chi-squared test were used to examine the results of the serological analysis. A p value <0.05 was considered significant, and different levels of significance are reported (* $p \leq 0.05$; ** $p \leq 0.01$; *** $p \leq 0.001$).

3. Results

First, we examined the sera from patients with one of five rheumatic diseases—SLE ($n = 193$), SS ($n = 70$), RA ($n = 84$), gout ($n = 92$), and AS ($n = 68$)—for IgG and IgM antibodies against CMV (Table 1).

Table 1. Antibody responses to CMV, CMVpp65, and human TAF in rheumatic patients.

Characteristics	SLE ($n = 193$)	SS ($n = 70$)	RA ($n = 84$)	Gout ($n = 92$)	AS ($n = 68$)	p Value
Mean age, y (SD)	41.5 (12.7)	52.8 (11.1)	54.1 (12.6)	51.7 (14.1)	44.0 (12.8)	<0.0001 [a]
Gender						<0.0001 [b]
Male, n (%)	17 (8.8)	8 (11.4)	9 (10.7)	86 (93.5)	32 (47.1)	
Female, n (%)	176 (91.2)	62 (88.6)	75 (89.3)	6 (6.5)	36 (52.9)	
Anti-CMV IgG (+)	163 (84.5)	64 (91.4)	76 (90.5)	70 (76.1)	52 (76.5)	0.0063 [b]
Anti-CMVpp65 IgG [c], n (%)	61 (37.4)	12 (18.8)	10 (13.2)	13 (18.6)	17 (32.7)	0.0004 [b]
Anti-TAF9 IgG [c], n (%)	50 (30.7)	13 (20.3)	6 (7.9)	8 (11.4)	6 (11.5)	0.0001 [b]
Dual positives [c], n (%)	28 (17.2)	8 (12.5)	3 (3.9)	4 (5.7)	5 (9.6)	0.0219 [b]
Anti-CMV IgM	21 (10.9)	5 (7.1)	2 (2.4)	3 (3.3)	2 (2.9)	0.0217 [b]
Anti-CMV IgM and IgG	21 (10.9)	5 (7.1)	2 (2.4)	3 (3.3)	2 (2.9)	0.0217 [b]

SLE, systemic lupus erythematosus; SS, Sjögren syndrome; RA, rheumatoid arthritis; AS, ankylosing spondylitis; [a] Kruskal–Wallis test. [b] Chi-squared test. [c] The positive sera from patients with anti-CMV IgG antibodies. The anti-CMVpp65 and anti-TAF9 positive sera were defined according to the mean + 3SEM of the sera from SLE patients. SD, standard deviation; y, year.

Over 75% of the patients of each rheumatic cohort who had acquired immunity from past CMV infections displayed anti-CMV IgG responses (Figure 1A,B) and exhibited intermediate or high CMV IgG avidity (Supplementary Tables S1–S5). SLE patients (10.9%,

21/193) had a higher rate of CMV IgM positivity than patients with other rheumatic diseases (Table 1).

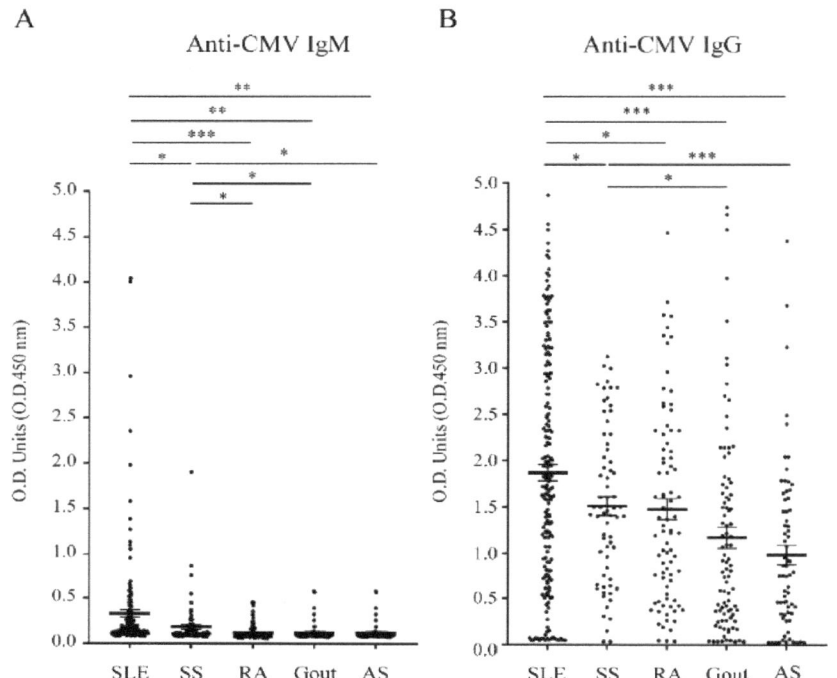

Figure 1. ELISA analysis of the antibody response to CMV using sera of patients with SLE ($n = 193$), SS ($n = 70$), RA ($n = 84$), gout ($n = 92$), and AS ($n = 68$). (**A**) Anti-CMV IgM activity. (**B**) Anti-CMV IgG activity. * $p \leq 0.05$; ** $p \leq 0.01$; *** $p \leq 0.001$.

In addition, the IgG antibody responses to CMVpp65 and the human TAF9 protein were evaluated using the sera from rheumatic patients with CMV IgG-positive statuses, including SLE ($n = 163$), SS ($n = 64$), RA ($n = 76$), gout ($n = 70$), and AS ($n = 52$). We found that the serum titers of anti-CMV IgG, anti-CMVpp65 IgG, and anti-TAF9 IgG were significantly more elevated in SLE patients than in the other rheumatic patients (Figures 1B and 2A,B).

SLE sera (37.4% and 30.7%) exhibited the highest seropositive rate for anti-CMVpp65 IgG and anti-TAF9 IgG when compared to the sera from AS (32.7% and 11.5%) and SS (18.8% and 20.3%; Table 1). Moreover, a higher prevalence of coexisting anti-CMVpp65 and anti-TAF9 IgG was found in SLE (17.2%) than in AS (9.6%) and SS (12.5%; Table 1). Therefore, we purified anti-CMVpp65 antibodies from CMVpp65/TAF9 dual-positive SLE sera and examined antibody binding to dsDNA and the TAF9 protein (Figure 3).

ELISA results showed that the purified anti-CMVpp65 IgG could recognize dsDNA and the TAF9 protein. The positive association between anti-CMVpp65, anti-TAF9, and anti-dsDNA IgG antibody activities was significant in our cross-reactivity testing.

In addition, we compared the hematological and serological changes in SLE patients in the presence or absence of the IgG antibody to CMV and/or CMVpp65. CMV IgG-seropositive SLE patients had a higher prevalence of anti-dsDNA ($p = 0.014$) and anti-SSA ($p = 0.014$) antibodies than did CMV IgG-negative SLE patients. A statistically significant decrease in hemoglobin ($p = 0.013$) and hematocrit ($p < 0.001$) levels and an increased proteinuria rate ($p = 0.026$) were found in CMV IgG-seropositive SLE patients (Table 2). A high prevalence of proteinuria (p = 0.001) and low hemoglobin level (p < 0.001) were also observed in CMVpp65 IgG-positive SLE patients.

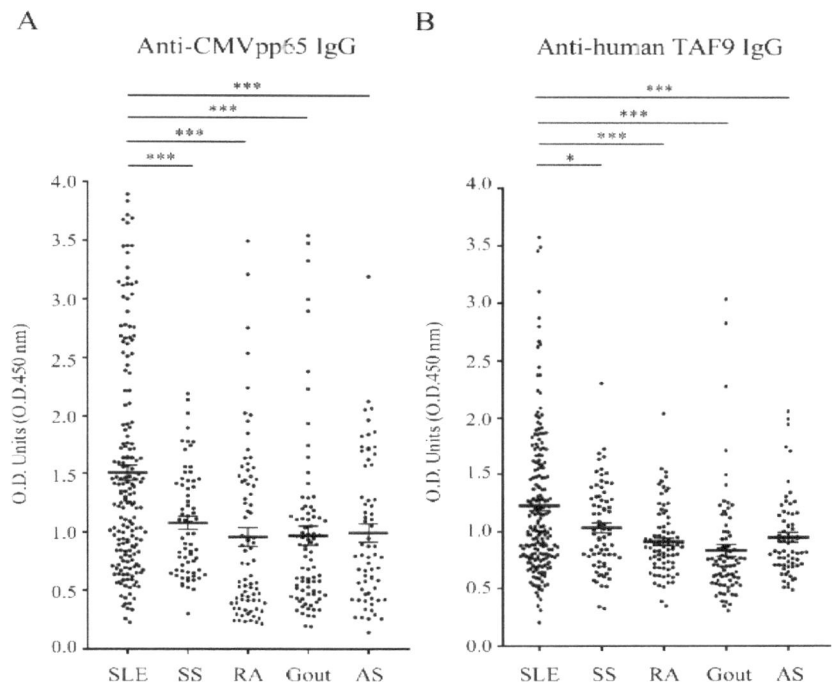

Figure 2. ELISA analysis of the antibody responses to CMVpp65 and TAF9 using sera of patients with SLE (n = 193), SS (n = 70), RA (n = 84), gout (n = 92), and AS (n = 68). (**A**) Anti-CMVpp65 IgG activity. (**B**) Anti-human TAF9 IgG activity. * $p \leq 0.05$; *** $p \leq 0.001$.

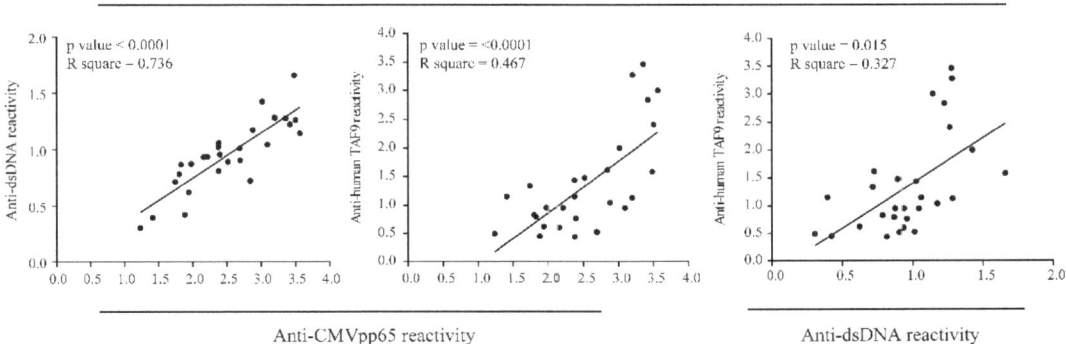

Figure 3. Analysis of the correlation between anti-CMVpp65 IgG, anti-human TAF9 IgG, and anti-dsDNA IgG by ELISA testing with anti-CMVpp65 IgG purified from CMVpp65/TAF9 dual-positive SLE sera (n = 28).

Table 2. Comparison of hematological and serological abnormalities in SLE patients in the presence or absence of IgG antibody to CMV and CMVpp65.

Characteristics	CMV IgG Negative (n = 30)	CMV IgG Positive (n = 163)	p Value	CMVpp65 IgG Negative (n = 102)	CMVpp65 IgG Positive (n = 61)	p Value
Mean age, y (SD)	43.4 (12.7)	42.9 (12.1)	0.837 [a]	42.9 (12.3)	42.8 (12.9)	0.961 [a]
Female, n (%)	26 (86.7)	150 (92.0)	0.309 [b]	94 (92.2)	56 (91.8)	1.000 [b]
Cre, n (%)	3 (10.0)	25 (15.3)	0.580 [b]	16 (15.7)	9 (14.8)	0.873 [c]
Urine protein, n (%)	3 (10.0)	48 (29.4)	0.026 [c]	21 (20.6)	27 (44.3)	0.002 [c]
WBC, n (%)	7 (23.3)	24 (14.7)	0.278 [b]	14 (13.7)	10 (16.4)	0.642 [c]
RBC, n (%)	8 (26.7)	52 (31.9)	0.569 [c]	29 (28.4)	23 (37.7)	0.219 [c]
Hb, n (%)	9 (30.0)	89 (54.6)	0.013 [c]	42 (41.2)	47 (77.1)	<0.0001 [c]
Hct, n (%)	10 (33.3)	127 (77.9)	<0.001 [c]	78 (76.5)	49 (80.3)	0.566 [c]
MCV, n (%)	4 (13.3)	29 (17.8)	0.551 [c]	18 (17.6)	11 (18.0)	0.950 [c]
MCH, n (%)	3 (10.0)	34 (20.9)	0.165 [c]	19 (18.6)	15 (24.6)	0.365 [c]
MCHC, n (%)	2 (6.7)	14 (8.6)	1.000 [b]	5 (4.9)	9 (14.8)	0.029 [c]
Platelets, n (%)	2 (6.7)	26 (16)	0.262 [b]	13 (12.7)	13 (21.3)	0.148 [c]
Low C3, n (%)	11 (36.7)	73 (44.8)	0.410 [c]	40 (39.2)	33 (54.1)	0.064 [c]
Low C4, n (%)	8 (26.7)	69 (42.3)	0.107 [c]	42 (41.2)	27 (44.3)	0.699 [c]
Autoantibodies						
Anti-dsDNA, n (%)	12 (40.0)	104 (63.8)	0.014 [b]	63 (61.8)	41 (67.2)	0.484 [c]
Anti-SSA, n (%)	4 (13.3)	59 (36.2)	0.014 [c]	36 (35.3)	23 (37.7)	0.757 [c]
Anti-SSB, n (%)	6 (20.0)	17 (10.4)	0.214 [b]	11 (10.8)	6 (9.8)	0.848 [c]
Anti-Sm, n (%)	6 (20.0)	31 (19)	0.900 [c]	19 (18.6)	12 (19.7)	0.869 [c]
Anti-RNP, n (%)	3 (10.0)	34 (20.9)	0.165 [c]	20 (19.6)	14 (23.0)	0.611 [c]
Anti-Scl70, n (%)	0 (0)	1 (0.6)	1.000 [b]	0 (0)	1 (1.6)	0.374 [b]
Anti-Jo1, n (%)	0 (0)	2 (1.2)	1.000 [b]	1 (1)	1 (1.6)	1.000 [b]
Anti-CentB, n (%)	1 (3.3)	4 (2.5)	0.575 [b]	3 (2.9)	1 (1.6)	1.000 [b]
Anti-Histone, n (%)	4 (13.3)	22 (13.5)	1.000 [b]	14 (13.7)	8 (13.1)	0.912 [c]

Normal adult reference ranges. WBC (leukocyte count, M: 3.9~10.6, F: 3.5~11, $\times 10^9$/L), RBC (erythrocyte count, M: 4.5 ~ 5.9, F: 4.0~5.2, $\times 10^{12}$/L), Hb (hemoglobin, M: 13.5~17.5, F: 12~16, g/dL), Hct (hematocrit, M: 41~53, F: 36~46%), MCV (mean corpuscular volume, 80~100, fL), MCH (mean corpuscular hemoglobin, 26~34, pg), MCHC (mean corpuscular hemoglobin concentration, 31~37%), platelet count (150~400, $\times 10^9$/L), Cre (creatinine, M: 0.64~1.27, F: 0.44~1.03, mg/dL), urine protein (>30 mg/dL), C3 (complement C3, 80~155, mg/dL), C4 (complement C4, 13~37, mg/dL). M: male; F: female. Anti-SSA, anti-Sjögren syndrome-related antigen A antibody; Anti-SSB, anti-Sjögren syndrome-related antigen B antibody; Anti-Sm, anti-Smith antibody; Anti-RNP, anti-nuclear ribonucleoprotein antibody; Anti-Scl70, anti-topoisomerase I antibody; Anti-CentB, anti-centromere B antibody. [a] Independent t test; [b] Fisher's exact test; [c] Chi-square test.

4. Discussion

In the current study, the CMV IgG seropositivity in 507 patients with rheumatic diseases was 83.8%. The CMV IgG seropositivity rate in rheumatic patients ranged from 76.1% to 91.4%, and few patients were CMV IgM positive. Our study population's seropositivity rates for CMV IgG and IgM were close to those of previous studies [15,16]. Notwithstanding the observation that those patients with SLE or SS exhibited high seropositivity for CMV IgM, the CMV IgG antibody titer had already been elevated, as the patients were diagnosed with SLE or SS. The presence of anti-CMV IgM and IgG was assumed to indicate CMV reactivation rather than primary infection.

Antibody reactivity to the CMVpp65 antigen was less frequent in healthy individuals but more frequent in patients with SLE [10,12]. We observed a similar pattern with the antibody reactivity to the TAF9 antigen. The SLE patients had greater seropositivity for the anti-TAF9 IgG antibody than the patients with AS, gout, or RA. Compared with the groups of rheumatic patients, a higher prevalence of coexisting anti-CMVpp65 IgG and anti-TAF9 IgG was found in patients with SLE. Moreover, anti-CMVpp65 IgG purified from CMVpp65/TAF9 dual-positive SLE sera recognized CMVpp65, TAF9, or dsDNA, indicating that immunity to CMVpp65 is a potential trigger inducing cross-reactive antibodies in susceptible individuals.

During CMV infection or reactivation, the replication of CMV in kidney mesangial cells is implicated in the pathogenesis of CMV-induced renal disease [17,18]. The glomerular deposition of the CMV antibody–antigen complex is a critical factor contributing to immune complex glomerulonephritis [10,19]. Our previous study observed that BALB/c mice receiving the CMVpp65 peptide developed cross-reactive antibodies, proteinuria, and immunoglobulin deposition on the glomeruli [13]. In the present study, we found that the increased incidence of proteinuria in anti-CMVpp65-positive SLE patients was higher than that in anti-CMVpp65-negative SLE patients, suggesting that the elevated anti-CMVpp65 antibodies in SLE patients may be associated with renal damage and proteinuria. However, a causal link between autoimmune hemolytic anemia and SLE risk has also been discussed. CMV infection has been reported to inhibit erythropoietin production, which induces or exacerbates anemia in patients [20,21]. Low hemoglobin and hematocrit levels were found in SLE patients with CMV IgG or CMV/CMVpp65 IgG responses. However, the pathogenesis of anemia during CMV infection remains unclear, and our results cannot explain the causative link between the presence of CMV/CMVpp65 IgG and the occurrence of anemia in SLE. A comprehensive investigation is required to verify the role of anti-CMVpp65 IgG in anemia.

ELISA is a useful tool for determining the presence of serum anti-CMV IgM and IgG antibodies for the preliminary detection of CMV; however, several limitations of qualitative detection should be mentioned. For example, for patients with positive anti-CMV IgM results, it is not possible to clearly distinguish between CMV primary infection and reactivation. Furthermore, the time for the seroconversion of CMV IgM to CMV IgG or an elevated antibody response to CMVpp65 or the TAF9 protein varied between patients, meaning that quantitative testing is not suitable for monitoring the resolution of infection, especially when considering the fact that the seroprevalence rate for CMV is around 90% in Taiwanese patients [15]. Therefore, longitudinal research may offer comprehensive insights into the resolution of viral infection and cross-reactivity occurrence in autoimmune disease. Moreover, antibody reactivity toward linear epitopes is unable to be detected by ELISA testing. This may explain the low seropositivity of IgG antibodies against CMVpp65 in the current study [12].

5. Conclusions

In the present study, we examined the seroprevalence of anti-CMV IgG/IgM, anti-CMVpp65 IgG, and anti-TAF9 IgG among patients with five common rheumatic diseases. Compared to those from individuals with other rheumatic diseases, sera from SLE patients showed the highest seropositivity for antibodies against CMVpp65 and/or TAF9. The high proportion of coexisting serum IgG antibodies to CMVpp65 and TAF9 and the occurrence of cross-reactivity in SLE sera suggested that immunity to CMVpp65 is a potential trigger inducing cross-reactive antibodies. In addition, the high prevalence of proteinuria and low hemoglobin levels present in CMV IgG- and CMVpp65 IgG-positive SLE patients implied that CMV infection or reactivation might be involved in proteinuria and anemia during the development of SLE.

Supplementary Materials: The following are available online at https://www.mdpi.com/article/10.3390/jcm10163722/s1. Table S1: The measurement of CMV IgG avidity in SLE patients with positive CMV IgG status, Table S2. The measurement of CMV IgG avidity in SS patients with positive CMV IgG status, Table S3. The measurement of CMV IgG avidity in RA patients with positive CMV IgG status, Table S4. The measurement of CMV IgG avidity in gout patients with positive CMV IgG status, Table S5. The measurement of CMV IgG avidity in AS patients with positive CMV IgG status.

Author Contributions: A.-H.H., L.-C.W., and C.-F.K. designed the project. A.-H.H., L.-C.W., and Y.-F.C. performed the experiments, acquired the data, and interpreted the results. A.-H.H., K.-H.Y., and C.-F.K. participated in the interpretation of the results and drafted and revised the manuscript. All authors have read and agreed to the published version of the manuscript.

Funding: This study was supported by the Chang Gung Memorial Hospital (CMRPG3F1703 and CMRPG3G0851) and the Taiwan Ministry of Science and Technology (108-314-B-182A-064). The funders had no role in the study design, data collection, analysis, decision to publish, or preparation of the manuscript.

Institutional Review Board Statement: The study was approved by the Institutional Review Board of Chang Gung Memorial Hospital, and all the patients provided written informed consent before inclusion as required by the Declaration of Helsinki (approval numbers #201600798B0 and 201600795B0).

Informed Consent Statement: Informed consent was obtained from all subjects recruited in the study. Written informed consent was obtained from the patients.

Data Availability Statement: The datasets analyzed during the current study are not publicly available due to our IRB policy, but they are available from the corresponding author upon reasonable request.

Acknowledgments: We greatly appreciate Wei-Ling Chang for technical support.

Conflicts of Interest: The authors declare no conflict of interest.

References

1. Berman, N.; Belmont, H.M. Disseminated cytomegalovirus infection complicating active treatment of systemic lupus erythematosus: An emerging problem. *Lupus* **2017**, *26*, 431–434. [CrossRef]
2. Dioverti, M.V.; Razonable, R.R. Cytomegalovirus. *Microbiol. Spectr.* **2016**, *4*, 1–26. [CrossRef]
3. Rozenblyum, E.V.; Levy, D.M.; Allen, U.; Harvey, E.; Hebert, D.; Silverman, E.D. Cytomegalovirus in pediatric systemic lupus erythematosus: Prevalence and clinical manifestations. *Lupus* **2015**, *24*, 730–735. [CrossRef] [PubMed]
4. Reis, A.D.; Mudinutti, C.; de Freitas Peigo, M.; Leon, L.L.; Bonon, S.H.A. Active human herpesvirus infections in adults with systemic lupus erythematosus and correlation with the SLEDAI score. *Adv. Rheumatol.* **2020**, *60*, 42. [CrossRef] [PubMed]
5. Baboonian, C.; Venables, P.J.; Booth, J.; Williams, D.G.; Roffe, L.M.; Maini, R.N. Virus infection induces redistribution and membrane localization of the nuclear antigen La (SS-B): A possible mechanism for autoimmunity. *Clin. Exp. Immunol.* **1989**, *78*, 454–459. [CrossRef] [PubMed]
6. Zhu, J. Cytomegalovirus infection induces expression of 60 KD/Ro antigen on human keratinocytes. *Lupus* **1995**, *4*, 396–406. [CrossRef] [PubMed]
7. Newkirk, M.M.; van Venrooij, W.J.; Marshall, G.S. Autoimmune response to U1 small nuclear ribonucleoprotein (U1 snRNP) associated with cytomegalovirus infection. *Arthritis Res.* **2001**, *3*, 253–258. [CrossRef]
8. Abate, D.A.; Watanabe, S.; Mocarski, E.S. Major human cytomegalovirus structural protein pp65 (ppUL83) prevents interferon response factor 3 activation in the interferon response. *J. Virol.* **2004**, *78*, 10995–11006. [CrossRef]
9. Li, T.; Chen, J.; Cristea, I.M. Human cytomegalovirus tegument protein pUL83 inhibits IFI16-mediated DNA sensing for immune evasion. *Cell Host Microbe* **2013**, *14*, 591–599. [CrossRef]
10. Chang, M.; Pan, M.R.; Chen, D.Y.; Lan, J.L. Human cytomegalovirus pp65 lower matrix protein: A humoral immunogen for systemic lupus erythematosus patients and autoantibody accelerator for NZB/W F1 mice. *Clin. Exp. Immunol.* **2006**, *143*, 167–179. [CrossRef]
11. Hsieh, A.H.; Wang, C.M.; Wu, Y.J.; Chen, A.; Chang, M.I.; Chen, J.Y. B cell epitope of human cytomegalovirus phosphoprotein 65 (HCMV pp65) induced anti-dsDNA antibody in BALB/c mice. *Arthritis Res. Ther.* **2017**, *19*, 65. [CrossRef]
12. Hsieh, A.H.; Jhou, Y.J.; Liang, C.T.; Chang, M.; Wang, S.L. Fragment of tegument protein pp65 of human cytomegalovirus induces autoantibodies in BALB/c mice. *Arthritis Res. Ther.* **2011**, *13*, R162. [CrossRef] [PubMed]
13. Hsieh, A.H.; Kuo, C.F.; Chou, I.J.; Tseng, W.Y.; Chen, Y.F.; Yu, K.H.; Luo, S.F. Human cytomegalovirus pp65 peptide-induced autoantibodies cross-reacts with TAF9 protein and induces lupus-like autoimmunity in BALB/c mice. *Sci. Rep.* **2020**, *10*, 9662. [CrossRef] [PubMed]
14. Prince, H.E.; Lape-Nixon, M. Role of cytomegalovirus (CMV) IgG avidity testing in diagnosing primary CMV infection during pregnancy. *Clin. Vaccine Immunol.* **2014**, *21*, 1377–1384. [CrossRef] [PubMed]
15. Chen, M.H.; Chen, P.C.; Jeng, S.F.; Hsieh, C.J.; Hsieh, W.S. High perinatal seroprevalence of cytomegalovirus in northern Taiwan. *J. Paediatr. Child. Health* **2008**, *44*, 166–169. [CrossRef] [PubMed]
16. Lu, S.C.; Chin, L.T.; Wu, F.M.; Hsieh, G.J. Seroprevalence of CMV antibodies in a blood donor population and premature neonates in the south-central Taiwan. *Kaohsiung J. Med. Sci.* **1999**, *15*, 603–610. [PubMed]
17. Heieren, M.H.; van der Woude, F.J.; Balfour, H.H., Jr. Cytomegalovirus replicates efficiently in human kidney mesangial cells. *Proc. Natl. Acad. Sci. USA* **1988**, *85*, 1642–1646. [CrossRef]
18. Popik, W.; Correa, H.; Khatua, A.; Aronoff, D.M.; Alcendor, D.J. Mesangial cells, specialized renal pericytes and cytomegalovirus infectivity: Implications for HCMV pathology in the glomerular vascular unit and post-transplant renal disease. *J. Transl. Sci.* **2019**, *5*, 1–27. [CrossRef] [PubMed]
19. Ozawa, T.; Stewart, J.A. Immune-complex glomerulonephritis associated with cytomegalovirus infection. *Am. J. Clin. Pathol.* **1979**, *72*, 103–107. [CrossRef] [PubMed]

20. Mo, H.Y.; Wei, J.C.C.; Chen, X.H.; Chen, H.H. Increased risk of systemic lupus erythematosus in patients with autoimmune haemolytic anaemia: A nationwide population-based cohort study. *Ann. Rheum. Dis.* **2020**, *80*, 403–404. [CrossRef]
21. Butler, L.M.; Dzabic, M.; Bakker, F.; Davoudi, B.; Jeffery, H.; Religa, P.; Bojakowski, K.; Yaiw, K.C.; Rahbar, A.; Soderberg-Naucler, C. Human cytomegalovirus inhibits erythropoietin production. *J. Am. Soc. Nephrol.* **2014**, *25*, 1669–1678. [CrossRef] [PubMed]

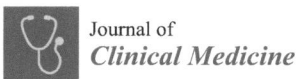

Article

Mindfulness-Based Stress Reduction for Systemic Lupus Erythematosus: A Mixed-Methods Pilot Randomized Controlled Trial of an Adapted Protocol

Renen Taub [1,*,†], Danny Horesh [1,2,†], Noa Rubin [1], Ittai Glick [3], Orit Reem [3], Gitit Shriqui [4] and Nancy Agmon-Levin [5]

1. Department of Psychology, Bar-Ilan University, Ramat Gan 5290002, Israel; danny.horesh@biu.ac.il (D.H.); badashnoa@gmail.com (N.R.)
2. Department of Psychiatry, New York University School of Medicine, 1 Park Ave., New York, NY 10016, USA
3. Shachaf Clinic for Stress Reduction, Chaim Sheba Medical Center, Tel-Hashomer, Ramat Gan 52621, Israel; ittai.glick@gmail.com (I.G.); oritreem@gmail.com (O.R.)
4. Psychodharma, 6 George Wise Street, Tel Aviv 6997705, Israel; gitit11@gmail.com
5. Clinical Immunology, Angioedema and Allergy, Center for Autoimmune Diseases, Chaim Sheba Medical Center, Tel-Hashomer, Ramat Gan 52621, Israel; nancy.Agmon-Levin@sheba.health.gov.il
* Correspondence: renentaub@gmail.com
† These authors shared first authorship.

Abstract: Background: The psychological effects of systemic lupus erythematosus (SLE) are tremendous. This pilot mixed-methods randomized controlled trial aimed to evaluate the effects of a mindfulness-based stress reduction (MBSR) adapted protocol on psychological distress among SLE patients. Methods: 26 SLE patients were randomly assigned to MBSR group therapy ($n = 15$) or a waitlist (WL) group ($n = 11$). An adapted MBSR protocol for SLE was employed. Three measurements were conducted: pre-intervention, post-intervention and 6-months follow up. A sub-sample ($n = 12$) also underwent qualitative interviews to assess their subjective experience of MBSR. Results: Compared to the WL, the MBSR group showed greater improvements in quality of life, psychological inflexibility in pain and SLE-related shame. Analysis among MBSR participants showed additional improvements in SLE symptoms and illness perception. Improvements in psychological inflexibility in pain and SLE-related shame remained stable over six months, and depression levels declined steadily from pre-treatment to follow-up. Qualitative analysis showed improvements in mindfulness components (e.g., less impulsivity, higher acceptance), as well as reduced stress following MBSR. Conclusions: These results reveal the significant therapeutic potential of MBSR for SLE patients. With its emphasis on acceptance of negative physical and emotional states, mindfulness practice is a promising treatment option for SLE, which needs to be further applied and studied.

Keywords: systemic lupus erythematosus (SLE); autoimmune diseases; mindfulness-based stress reduction (MBSR); mindfulness; psychotherapy

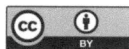

1. Introduction

Systemic Lupus Erythematosus (SLE) is an autoimmune disease, the intensity of which varies between mild and severe. Apart from classical criteria such as joint pain, arthritis, skin lesions, and photosensitivity, it involves various organ-specific manifestations, as well as chronic fatigue and reduced quality of life [1,2]. The prevalence of SLE vary by age and gender, as it predominantly affects women in their 20's and 30's [3]. Furthermore, SLE is considered a stress-related disease, and in many cases symptoms are worsened under stressful conditions [4,5].

In their model of SLE symptom types, Pisetsky et al. [6] have coined the term "Type 2" symptoms. These include symptoms such as fatigue, widespread body pain, depression, anxiety, cognitive dysfunction, and sleep disturbance. Such symptoms usually do not respond to therapy with immunosuppression or corticosteroids, even with escalation of doses. Neurological and psychiatric manifestations affect the majority of SLE patients, and several of these manifestations define a disease criterion [7]. Throughout their lives, 65% of patients with SLE are diagnosed with a mood or anxiety disorder, including major depression (47%), specific phobia (24%), panic disorder (16%), obsessive-compulsive disorder (9%), and bipolar disorder (6%). Thus, psychological effects related to SLE are significant, and exert a considerable impact on patients' quality of life [8]. SLE patients also experience cognitive impairment in various fields, and disease activity is correlated with cognitive dysfunction, along with self-reported fatigue, pain, and negative mood [9]. Type 2 symptoms of SLE are today recognized as a highly important aspect of the disease, which has yet to receive sufficient clinical attention [10]. Thus, despite these significant psychological difficulties experienced by individuals with SLE, there is a scarcity of research examining novel psychotherapeutic interventions in this field [11]. In this study, we focus on mindfulness-based therapy and its effects on different aspects of SLE.

Mindfulness involves "paying attention in a particular way: on purpose, in the present moment, and non-judgmentally" [12]. It refers to the cultivation of conscious awareness and attention on a moment-to-moment basis, with an open and non-judgmental attitude [13]. According to a growing body of evidence, mindfulness-based interventions (MBI) may improve coping with pain and psychological symptoms [14,15]. The most well-known variant of MBI is called Mindfulness–Based Stress Reduction (MBSR), a group therapy program that provides systemic training in mindfulness meditation as a self-regulation approach to stress reduction [16].

In its original version, MBSR is an eight-week program in mindfulness training. The standard program includes weekly group sessions of 2–2.5 h and one full-day session after six to seven weeks. The program's core elements consist of various mental and physical mindfulness exercises: (1) body-scan exercises (paying close attention to all body parts, from head to toe), (2) mental exercises focusing one's attention on breathing, (3) physical exercises (e.g., walking meditation) focusing on being aware of bodily sensations and one's own limits during exercises, and (4) practicing being fully aware during everyday activities. Essential to all parts of the program is developing an accepting and non-reactive attitude to what one experiences in the present moment. In each session, time is allocated for group members to reflect together on what they experience when they practice mindfulness. Between sessions, participants are instructed to listen to 30–45 min guided exercises in body-scan, sitting meditation, focusing on breathing and yoga stretching [17].

Surprisingly, despite its well-documented effects on rheumatic and autoimmune diseases [18], research on MBI among SLE has so far been very scarce, and showed notable methodological limitations. To date, there has been only one randomized controlled trial of MBSR among SLE patients, focusing on a very limited set of outcome measures, none of which included physical or psychiatric symptoms [19]. Two other previous studies applied mindfulness-based cognitive therapy (MBCT) on SLE patients [20–22]. MBCT is another variant of MBI, which was originally designed to treat depression [23], and thus is less focused on stress reduction per-se. Here too, outcome measures were quite limited in scope. Finally, a recent study applied a mindfulness protocol specifically focused on meta-cognition (i.e., one's ability to "think about one's thoughts") among individuals with SLE, showing improvements in psychological well-being, with no follow-up long-term assessment [24].

Furthermore, due to SLE patients' physical limitations, administering the generic MBSR intervention may prove as both challenging and ineffective, as individuals may feel too sick to participate or experience difficulties with prolonged sitting/meditating, which may, in turn, entail high dropout rates [25]. Thus, a newly adapted protocol is called for. Finally, in order to achieve a fuller understanding of patients' experiences in therapy, mixed-methods studies are needed, combining both quantitative and qualitative research methods.

In this study, we aim to fill these large gaps in research and clinical work, by conducting a randomized controlled trial of MBSR for SLE patients. The aims of this study were to evaluate the effects of MBSR on various psychological (i.e., "Type 2" symptoms) and physical outcomes, including reported SLE symptoms, health related quality of life, major depression and psychological inflexibility in pain, as well as SLE-related shame and illness perception. Due to the wide heterogeneity of SLE symptoms, we will also specifically assess weather changes in specific SLE symptoms following MBSR were associated with changes in psychological measures, in order to understand weather physical and mental health processes work together or separately in SLE psychotherapy. For this study, a unique MBSR protocol was constructed, to meet the specific needs of SLE patients. The study employs a mixed-methods approach, which has never been employed in SLE mindfulness research.

2. Materials and Methods

2.1. Participants and Procedure

SLE patients (Mean age = 41.62, SD = 11.78, Range: 22–64) were recruited from two major sources: 1. The Center for Autoimmune Diseases at the Sheba Medical Center in Israel. 2. Ads posted on social media (online groups and forums of SLE patients), as well as sent to organizations supporting SLE patients. A total of 85 individuals showed initial interest in the study. The first phone call presented patients with information about the intervention, and also included an initial screening-out of 26 participants, due to lack of interest after hearing about the intervention, inability to participate due to the place or time of the intervention, and lack of formal SLE diagnosis. The remaining 59 patients underwent in-depth telephone clinical interviews. Criteria for study inclusion were: (1) A recent documented clinical diagnosis of SLE given by an expert rheumatologist and/or clinical immunologist and verified via an interview with a lupus specialist from the study team. (2) Age 18 years or older (3) Hebrew speakers (4) Physical ability to attend MBSR sessions (5) Psychological ability to practice mindfulness (no serious cognitive impairments/psychosis/active suicidality/substance abuse) (6) No concurrent participation in another clinical study. *All SLE patients were diagnosed according to the American College of Rheumatology (ACR) criteria, by a lupus specialist. Upon inclusion in the study SLE diagnosis was re-confirmed* via *interviewing the patient and reviewing the medical chart for clinical and serological criteria of SLE.* 26 patients met eligibility criteria. All participants provided informed consent prior to their inclusion in the study. Patients were randomly assigned to either an MBSR group (n = 15) or a wait-list control group (WL; n = 11). Patients randomized to WL control group received no active treatment during their 10-weeks waiting period, at the end of which they received MBSR. Patients from the WL who chose to participate in the intervention after their waiting period (i.e., "delayed MBSR"; n = 5) were measured at the end of the intervention and their data were analyzed together with the original MBSR group (i.e., the "combined MBSR" group; n = 20).

The study received a Helsinki Committee approval by the ethics committee at Sheba Medical Center (No. 3296-16-SMC).

A detailed description of study procedures can be found in Figure 1 (PRISMA chart).

Table 1 presents the background characteristics of participants according to assignment group. Due to the wide heterogeneity of symptom type and severity in SLE, we also show levels of all SLE symptoms that are included in the SLAQ (Systemic Lupus Activity Questionnaire) at baseline, in Table 2.

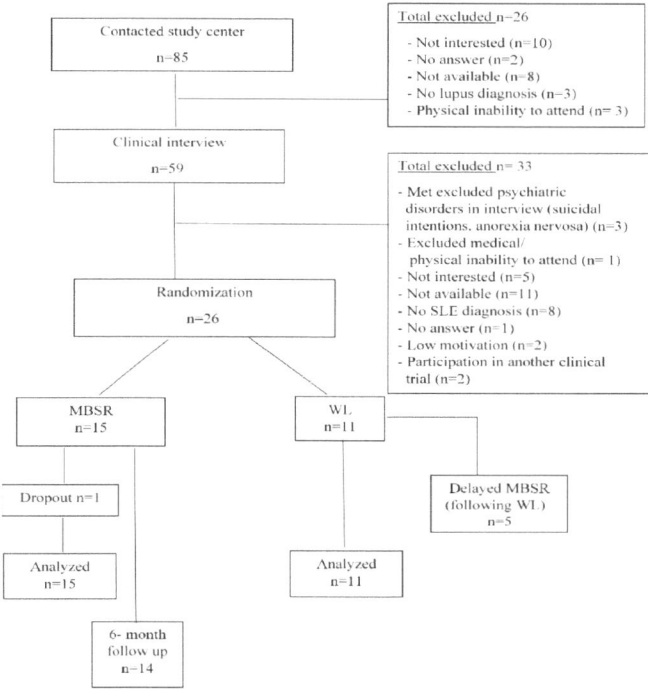

Figure 1. PRISMA flow-chart for screening and allocation process.

Table 1. Baseline characteristics according to group.

Characteristic	MBSR Group $n = 15$	Wait-List Controls $n = 11$
Gender	Male ($n = 1$, 6.67%) Female ($n = 14$, 93.33%)	Male ($n = 2$, 18.18%) Female ($n = 9$, 81.82%)
Age (in years, mean, SD)	43.93 (11.78)	38.45 (10.56)
Duration of disease (in years, mean (SD)	11.00 (10.06)	11.73 (8.73)
Disease activity during the past month	4.40 (2.47)	3.91 (2.63)
Hospitalized due to SLE complications	64% ($n = 9$)	81% ($n = 9$)
Treated by rheumatologist	100%	100%
Pharmacological treatment	100%	100%
Family status-%		
Married/ In a relationship	10 (66.67%)	7 (63.63%)
Single/Divorced	5 (33.33%)	4 (36.36%)
Education level-%		
12th grade or less	4 (26.66%)	3 (27.27%)
Currently student/Academic degree	11 (73.33%)	8 (72.72%)
Income		
Under average	3 (21.43%)	4 (36.36%)
Average and above	11 (78.57%)	7 (63.64%)

Table 2. Baseline SLE Symptoms according to the SLAQ (on a Likert scale of 0 (no problem) to 3 (Severe).

SLE Symptom	Baseline Severity Level of Symptom Mean (SD)
Flares	1.27 (0.83)
Lost weight	0.73 (1.08)
Fatigue	1.69 (1.23)
Fevers (>101 °F, 38.5 °C) taken by a thermometer	0.38 (0.64)
Sores in mouth or nose	0.73 (1.00)
Rash on cheeks (butterfly shaped)	0.73 (0.78)
Other rash	0.85 (0.97)
Dark blue or purple spots on the skin	0.96 (0.96)
Rash or feeling sick after sun exposure	1.04 (1.00)
Bald patches on scalp, or clumps of hair on pillow	0.81 (0.94)
Swollen glands (nodes) in the neck	0.58 (0.81)
Shortness of breath	0.69 (0.84)
Chest pain with a deep breath	0.92 (0.93)
Fingers or toes turning dead white or very pale in the cold (Raynaud's)	1.12 (1.11)
Stomach or belly pain	0.92 (0.98)
Persistent numbness or tingling in arms or legs	1.23 (1.03)
Seizures	0.65 (0.85)
Stroke	0.50 (0.86)
Forgetfulness	1.35 (1.02)
Feeling depressed	1.38 (1.10)
Unusual headaches	1.00 (0.89)
Muscle pain	1.35 (1.26)
Muscle weakness	1.19 (1.10)
Pain or stiffness in joints	1.23 (1.27)
Swelling in joints	0.53 (0.76)

2.2. Randomization and Measurement

Patients were randomized using the SPSS 23.0 statistical software package randomization algorithm. Patients in the WL were blind to the fact that they were allocated to the control group, as they were told that they were waiting for the next group opening. The therapists who conducted the treatment were blind to pre- and post-treatment evaluation data. Following randomization, paired-sample t-tests and Chi-square/Fisher tests were performed comparing between the WL and MBSR groups. No significant differences were found in terms of background characteristics or in any of the outcome measures. Finally, patients were asked about medical monitoring and treatment. All patients reported undergoing medical monitoring by a primary care physician or a rheumatologist and 22 patients were treated with Hydroxychloroquine; thirteen of these were from the MBSR group (86.67%) and nine were from the WL group (81.82%).

We collected data at three different stages: at baseline (before the first treatment session), at the end of the intervention (immediately after the final treatment session) and a follow-up assessment six months after treatment. The follow up assessment was conducted for the MBSR group only. Additionally, a sub sample of 12 patients took part in an in-depth qualitative interview, examining patients' subjective experience of the intervention (see more details below).

We employed an (ITT) approach for our analysis, i.e., all randomized participants were contacted post-treatment to fill out questionnaires, regardless of whether they attended the entire therapy or dropped out. This was meant to provide a complete, reliable, and externally valid picture of our patient population.

2.3. Course Attendance

Patients showed relatively high attendance rates, with only one participant requesting to discontinue therapy. On average, patients in the MBSR group (n = 15) attended eight and a half out of eleven sessions. Six participants (40%) attended ten sessions, five participants (33.3%) attended nine sessions, three participants (20.1%) attended between five to eight sessions, and one participant (6.7%) attended three sessions and dropped out of treatment.

2.4. An Adapted MBSR Protocol for SLE

In order to create an adapted treatment protocol, more suited to the unique characteristics and difficulties of SLE patients, we used the standard MBSR 8-week format (University of Massachusetts, 1979) as the basis of the intervention, and then added modifications. The standard MBSR protocol was adapted in several ways:

1. The intervention was extended into a 10-week program with 11 sessions, which included shortened 2-h weekly sessions, due to potential physical difficulties for SLE patients, such as prolonged sitting. This extension enabled a significant expansion of the psycho-education section at the beginning of the intervention, where explanations about mindfulness, stress, and SLE were presented. The full-day retreat was also shortened into a 3-h session that took place after the eighth week.

2. The protocol included shorter, more carefully paced exercises, which gradually progressed from "easy" to "hard". This was intended to facilitate SLE patients' encounter with their body and physical sensations. An emphasis was placed on the concept of "pacing", where patients were encouraged to strategize how much energy to exert according to which activities were planned for the day; "pacing" would prevent patients from being overly active when energy is available and feeling depleted by the end.

3. Therapists were instructed to pay special attention to SLE-related themes (e.g., pain and fatigue) throughout the sessions and practice, and to translate the general components of generic MBSR intervention into specific components relevant to SLE patients. For example, the issue of automatic thinking in the generic protocol would be translated into specific discourse about automatic pain-related thoughts and pain catastrophizing.

4. Therapists were instructed to specifically target maladaptive avoidance behaviors. Such behaviors are common among SLE patients, aimed to reduce physical efforts and movement and to prevent further diseases or infections.

5. Compassion, which is a vital component of MBSR, was emphasized to encourage a more flexible and accepting mindset towards the disease and the self. Further emphasis was placed in the protocol on decentering, which reflects the ability to observe one's thoughts and feelings as transient, somewhat external mental states, as opposed to reflections of the self that are necessarily "true" and stable.

The amended protocol was carefully based on the standard components of the MBSR program, which were all included in the intervention (e.g., body scan, focus on breathing, mindfulness in daily life—see above). Home practice assignments included audio recorded mindfulness exercises (e.g., body scan, sitting mindfulness exercises, breathing exercises) in the therapist's own voice. Daily home practice ranged from 5–30 min in duration, and patients were encouraged to exercise as much as possible.

The intervention was led by a licensed clinical psychologist who is an experienced MBSR teacher. Before commencing the complete RCT reported here, the study team held one pilot group which supported the feasibility of MBSR among SLE patients [11].

2.5. Measures

The systemic Lupus Activity Questionnaire (SLAQ) [26] is a 24-item questionnaire with a scoring range of 0–44. It also includes a single item (0–10) rating scale for SLE activity, and a rating scale for SLE flares (from no flare to severe flare). In the current study, SLAQ demonstrated excellent internal consistency, with a Cronbach's alpha of 0.90.

The World Health Organization Quality of Life Questionnaire-Brief Version (WHOQOL-BREF) [27] was developed based on the original 100-item WHQOL questionnaire. It is a 26-item scale, with each item rated on a scale from 1 to 5. It covers four Quality of Life domains: physical, psychological, social, and environmental, additional to a global Quality of Life item. Cronbach's alpha was very high, at 0.94.

The Patient Health Questionnaire-9 (PHQ-9) [28] is a commonly used self-reporting measure for symptoms of major depressive disorder. The scale scores each of the nine DSM-5 depression criteria from "0" (not at all) to "3" (nearly every day). It can yield either a continuous score, or a probable major depressive disorder diagnosis using a cut-off of 10. Cronbach's alpha of the PHQ-9 in this study was very good, at 0.87.

Psychological Inflexibility in Pain Scale (PIPS) [29] is a 12-item measure based on a Likert scale of 1 to 7 per item, developed to assess psychological inflexibility towards pain (i.e., one's ability or inability to manage pain in a flexible manner, not avoiding it altogether while at the same time not being "flooded" by it). The subscales measure avoidance (eight items) and cognitive fusion (four items). The total score ranges from 12 to 84. PIPS showed high reliability with Cronbach's alpha of 0.91.

In order to measure SLE-related shame and identity, two single items assessed the degree to which the patient felt: (1) shame regarding her/his SLE; and (2) the degree to which SLE affects one's personal identity. Both questions were assessed using a Visual Analog Scale (VAS), rated between 0 (minimum) to 100 (maximum), in order to allow for a wide spectrum of responses regarding these issues. The VAS has been used in numerous studies and randomized control trials in order to assess various emotional and physical symptoms among individuals suffering from chronic illnesses [30,31].

2.6. Qualitative Interviews

Out of the 26 participants, a sub-sample of 12 patients underwent a semi-structured qualitative interview regarding their subjective experience in therapy, at post treatment (60% of patients from the MBSR group; $n = 9$; 60% of patients from the delayed MBSR group; $n = 3$). The interviews were conducted on average 15 days following treatment (SD = 3.97). The average duration of the interviews was 48.25 min (SD = 4.76; range 44–55 min). The interviews were meant to explore participants' subjective experiences, in their own words, in order to acquire a deeper understanding of changes in the psychological and physical aspects. The interviews were semi-structured, leaving room for both guideline-based questions as well as a more explorative approach. They started with an open question (e.g., "What comes to mind when you think about the 10-week mindfulness program?") and then focused on the group (e.g., "How did you feel among the group?"), the experience with the instructor, intervention content ("how did you experience the exercises in the sessions?") and potential difficulties with the exercises. The next part of the interview focused on the disease and the extent towhich the intervention was relevant to its physical aspects (e.g., "Do you feel changes in your coping with SLE?"), and psychological aspects (e.g., "What changes, if any, have you noticed in your mental and psychological state since joining the intervention?").

Analysis was based on Renner and Taylor-Powell's [32] systemic approach for analyzing qualitative data, which requires categorizing the themes which emerge from the text into primary themes and sub-themes, as well as classifying the themes according to their frequency, allowing for a better understanding of not only which of the themes emerge, but also how often they do so.

In order to attain interrater reliability, two independent raters analyzed three random transcripts of interviews, categorizing the texts into main themes. Cohen's Kappa was 0.830, which indicated excellent inter-rater agreement [33].

3. Results

We will report here three types of results: (1) differences the MBSR and WL groups in changes over time (on the various outcome measures). (2) the long-term effects of MBSR, as seen in the follow-up measurement of the treatment group and (3) within-group effects in the larger MBSR group, which includes both the MBSR and delayed MBSR (e.g., post-WL) group.

3.1. Pre- to Post-Treatment Differences between the MBSR and WL Groups

In order to examine changes in outcome measures among MBSR participants compared to WL controls, we conducted a series of repeated measures multivariate analysis of covariance (MANCOVA) for Group X Time interactions, adjusting for age as a covariate (due to its important role in SLE, as well as due to the wide age range in our sample). For the sake of brevity, we report here only measures where at least some significant effects were found.

For SLE-related Shame and Illness Identity, the repeated measures MANCOVA yielded a significant effect for Time ($F(1, 22) = 5.72$, $p < 0.01$), a non-significant effect for Group ($F(1, 22) = 2.85$, n.s), and a significant Group X Time interaction ($F(1, 22) = 3.80$, $p < 0.05$). Subsequent univariate analysis for Shame yielded a significant interaction for Group X Time, while that for Illness Identity was marginally significant. The multivariate analysis for Quality of Life showed a significant effect for Time ($F(1, 24) = 2.77$, $p < 0.05$), but not for Group ($F(1, 24) = 0.83$, n.s) or for the Group X Time interaction ($F(1, 24) = 3.10$, n.s). However, due to our small sample size, as well as to the clear directionality of our hypotheses (MBSR > WL), we went on to examine the univariate interaction effects. In the subsequent univariate analysis of variance for Quality of Life, a significant interaction was found for the General subscale and for the Environmental subscale. Repeated measures univariate effect for the Physical Quality of Life subscale was marginally significant. Univariate tests for the other subscales did not reach significance. For Psychological Inflexibility in Pain, the MANCOVA was non-significant for Group X Time interaction ($F(1, 24) = 2.39$, n.s) and for Time ($F(1, 24) = 2.17$, n.s). The MANCOVA for Group was significant ($F(1, 24) = 3.68$, $p < 0.05$). As above, we went on to examine univariate interactions, where a significant effect was detected for the Fusion with Pain subscale. Univariate tests for Avoidance of Pain did not reach significance. Table 3 presents univariate effects and descriptive statistics for between-group comparisons, as well as for MBSR follow-up (discussed later).

Next, we conducted subsequent pairwise comparisons for all significant Group X Time effects, in order to establish the source of the interaction. Comparison of the MBSR versus WL groups in Physical QOL, Shame and Fusion, revealed significant improvements in the MBSR group (Physical Quality of Life: $i - j = 1.35$, SE = 0.55, $p = 0.02$; Shame: $i - j = -17.32$, SE = 5.53, $p = 0.005$; Fusion: $i - j = -3.48$, SE = 1.189, $p = 0.008$), and no significant change among WL controls group (Physical Quality of Life: $i - j = -0.33$, SE = 0.64, $p = 0.61$, Shame: $i - j = 5.9$, SE = 6.49, $p = 0.37$; Fusion: $i - j = 0.38$, SE = 1.4, $p = 0.79$). General and Environmental QOL showed non-significant improvements in the MBSR group (General QOL: $i - j = 0.79$, SE = 0.62, $p = 0.22$; Environmental QOL: $i - j = 0.65$, SE = 0.41, $p = 0.13$) and non-significant worsening in the WL group (General QOL: $i - j = -1.25$, SE = 0.72, $p = 0.1$; Environmental QOL: $i - j = -0.75$, SE = 0.48, $p = 0.13$). Thus, the interaction seemed to have stemmed from the general difference in trend in both groups (improvements/worsening). Figure 2 presents effects of all significant interactions.

Table 3. MBSR vs. WL and MBSR follow-up effects and descriptive statistics.

Outcome	Scale	MBSR (n = 15)			WL (n = 11)		Treatment Effects				6-Month Follow-Up (MBSR Alone)
		Pre	Post	6-Month Follow-Up	Pre	Post	F Time	F Group	F Univariate Time X Group	Time X Group Cohen's d	F
		Mean (SD)									
Health-Related Quality of life	General	12.93 (2.60)	13.47 (2.56)	12.71 (2.02)	11.82 (2.89)	10.9 (3.14)	5.96 *	3.91	4.49 *	0.52	0.62
	Environmental	15.20 (2.46)	15.80 (1.98)	15.39 (2.40)	15.09 (2.69)	14.41 (3.05)	0.46	0.73	4.75 *	0.49	0.27
	Physical	14.13 (3.31)	12.95 (2.82)	13.22 (3.00)	11.58 (4.22)	11.48 (3.77)	5.11 *	2.16	3.90~ (p = 0.06)	−0.28	0.40
	Social	13.51 (3.01)	13.33 (13.15)	13.71 (3.16)	12.24 (4.08)	12.97 (3.32)	0.05	0.17	0.96	−0.25	0.84
	Psychological	14.76 (3.16)	15.11 (2.74)	14.38 (2.92)	13.09 (3.54)	12.67 (3.33)	0.01	2.36	1.25	0.22	0.38
Psychological Inflexibility in Pain	Fusion with pain	29.73 (4.92)	26.47 (5.97)	27.36 (6.96)	31.82 (5.79)	31.91 (3.75)	2.73	2.53	4.32 *	−0.61	7.69 *
	Avoidance of pain	31.31 (11.98)	29.27 (6.92)	30.14 (7.40)	44.36 (14.75)	43.73 (14.4)	1.40	7.38 *	0.39	−0.10	0.91
SLE-related Shame and Illness Identity	Shame	28.00 (33.42)	11.67 (16.00)	17.86 (24.86)	45.45 (35.88)	50.00 (37.41)	2.04	5.20 *	6.78 *	−0.59	4.99 *
	Illness identity	33.33 (25.82)	18.33 (19.24)	28.57 (24.45)	56.00 (33.73)	50.00 (33.66)	11.83 **	5.05 *	3.36~ (p = 0.08)	−0.30	7.41 *

* p < 0.05; ** p < 0.01; ~marginally significant.

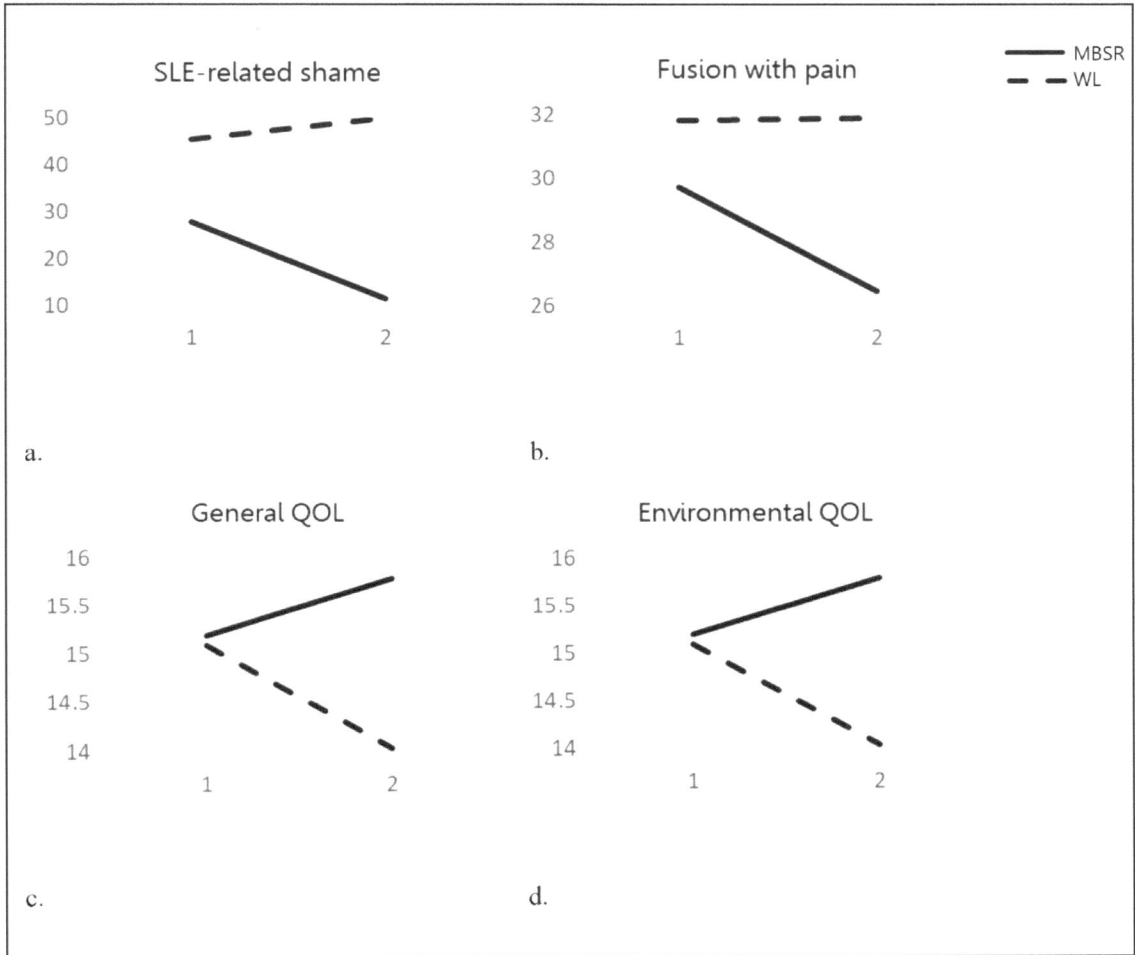

Figure 2. Pre- Intervention to Post-Intervention Differences between the MBSR and WL. Note: Pre-intervention (1); post-intervention (2). (**a**) Changes in cognitive Fusion among MBSR group and WL; (**b**) Changes in SLE-related Shame among MBSR group and WL; (**c**) Changes in General Quality of Life among MBSR group and WL; (**d**) Changes in Environmental Quality of Life among MBSR group and WL.

3.2. Long-Term Effectiveness of MBSR

To assess the long-term effect of MBSR intervention, we conducted univariate and multivariate analysis for follow up assessment six months after the last MBSR session. We base this analysis on the original MBSR group alone ($n = 15$), as this group was the only one with three assessments. We generally expected that the contrasts between pre- and post-treatment would be significant, while those between post-treatment and the 6-month follow-up will be non-significant, showing a stability of identified treatment effects over time.

A repeated measures within-group multivariate analysis of variance was conducted, with three time points-pre-MBSR, post-MBSR and six months follow-up. The within-group MANOVA for SLE-related Shame and Illness Identity was significant ($F(2, 13) = 3.99$,

$p < 0.05$), while the MANOVA for Psychological Inflexibility in Pain was marginally significant ($F(2, 13) = 3.12$, $p = 0.066$). Subsequently, univariate effects were calculated for all variables, in order to detect the source of the effect (see Table 3).

As can be seen in Table 3, univariate analysis was significant for SLE-related Shame and Illness Identity. Subsequent contrasts for Shame showed a significant effect between pre- and post- intervention assessments ($p < 0.05$, Cohen's d = 0.64) and a non-significant effect between post-intervention and follow-up ($p = 0.13$), indicating effect stability. Illness Identity showed a significant effect between pre- and post-intervention assessments ($p < 0.01$, Cohen's d = 0.83), and a significant increase again between post- intervention and follow- up ($p < 0.01$), showing that the benefit of MBSR was relatively short-lived.

Next, a univariate significant effect was found for the Fusion with Pain subscale. There was no significant effect for Avoidance of Pain. For Fusion, a significant improvement was found between pre- and post-intervention assessments ($p < 0.01$, Cohen's = 0.98), while a non-significant effect was found between post-intervention and follow-up ($p = 0.83$), indicating effect stability. Figure 3 presents the follow-up effects of Fusion with Pain and SLE-related Shame.

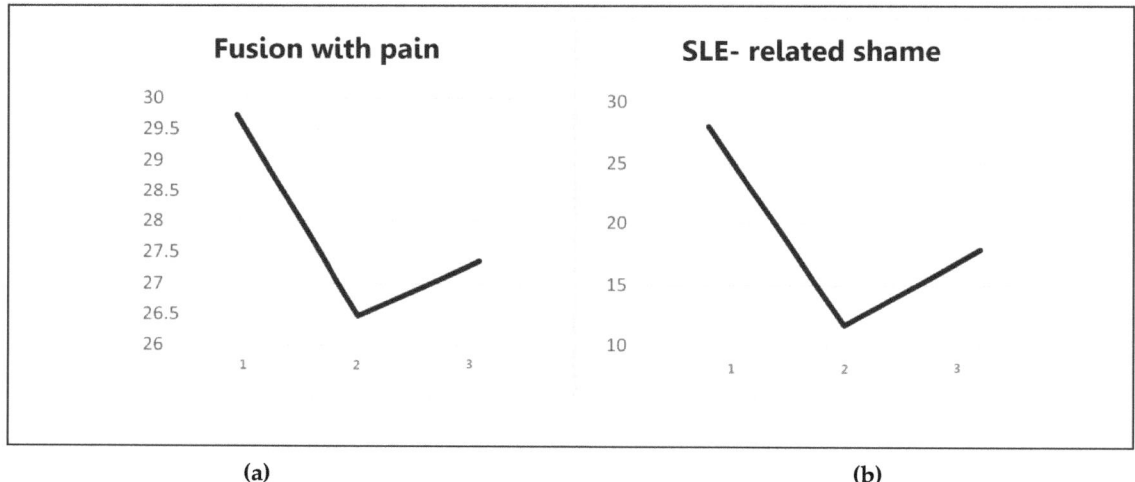

Figure 3. Long- Term effects of SLE- related Shame and Cognitive Fusion with Pain. Note: Measurements at pre- intervention (1); post-intervention (2); 6-month follow-up (3). (**a**) Follow- up effect of SLE- related shame among MBSR group; (**b**) Follow-up effect of Fusion with pain among MBSR group.

Finally, we set out to examine changes in Depression rates across time. We calculated the rates of participants who met the PHQ-9 cutoff (sum > 10) for a probable diagnosis of major depressive disorder (MDD). As can be seen in Figure 4, the analysis showed that in the original MBSR group, 40% of participants met the MDD cutoff before treatment, followed by 33% post-treatment, and 28.5% at the 6-months follow-up. Thus, rates of MDD declined consistently over time.

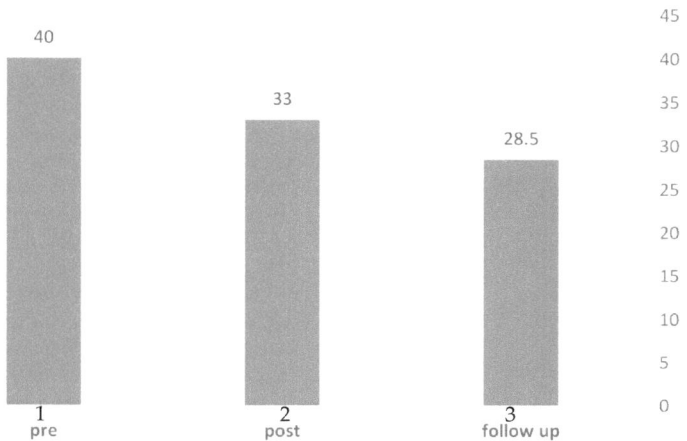

Figure 4. Rates (%) of Major Depressive Disorder in pre-, post- and follow-up assessments (MBSR group). Note: Pre-intervention (1); post-intervention (2); 6-month follow-up (3).

3.3. Pre- to Post-Intervention Changes within the Combined MBSR Group (n = 20)

In subsequent analysis, we included all participants who underwent MBSR, combining the original MBSR group with the "delayed MBSR" group (i.e., WL participants who subsequently went on to complete MBSR, and were measured pre- and post-treatment). This enabled a closer examination of all those undergoing MBSR, relaying on a larger sample ($n = 20$) to identify treatment effects.

First, repeated-measures analysis of variance for SLE symptoms (based on the SLAQ measure) showed a significant treatment effect. Next, a repeated measures multivariate analysis of variance showed a significant main effect for psychological inflexibility in pain ($F = 9.36$, $p < 0.01$), as well as for SLE-related Shame and Illness Identity ($F = 5.10$, $p < 0.05$). Subsequently, in order to examine what were the specific components that contributed to the observed changes, a univariate analysis was conducted, yielding significant treatment effects for the Fusion with Pain subscale, but not for Avoidance of Pain. Univariate analysis also showed a significant effect for SLE-related Shame and Illness Identity.

Table 4 presents main effects for the MBSR combined group (only measures with at least one significant effect are presented).

Table 4. Pre- to post-intervention changes in the combined MBSR group.

Combined MBSR (n = 20)		Pre	Post	F	Cohen's d
SLE symptoms	SLE (SLAQ)	26.05 (16.5)	20.35 (10.64)	5.32 *	**0.52**
SLE-related Shame and Illness Identity	Shame	35.91 (36.6)	27.5 (34.56)	4.79 *	0.33
	Illness Identity	43.64 (30.79)	32.05 (31.12)	10.73 **	0.57
Psychological Inflexibility in Pain	Fusion	29.9 (4.48)	26.55 (5.8)	18.18 ***	0.95
	Avoidance	33.75 (13.8)	32.4 (11.07)	0.63	0.17

Note: * $p < 0.05$; ** $p < 0.01$; *** $p < 0.001$

In order to examine more thoroughly the relationships between the change in SLE symptoms and the change in psychological outcomes following MBSR, we also calculated Pearson correlations between each SLE symptom (according to the SLAQ questionnaire) and psychological changes (e.g., Shame, Quality of Life, pain cognitions), by calculating the score at the end of the intervention minus the score at the beginning of the intervention for each measure. A correlation was then calculated between each difference score.

The change in SLE-related Shame was related to the changes in fever ($r = 0.70$, $p < 0.01$), presence of dark, blue or purple spots on the skin ($r = 0.65$, $p < 0.01$), rash or feeling sick after sun exposure ($r = 0.48$, $p < 0.05$), bald patches on scalp, or clumps of hair on pillow ($r = 0.57$, $p < 0.01$), swollen glands in the neck ($r = 0.48$, $p < 0.05$), shortness of breath ($r = 0.62$, $p < 0.01$) and forgetfulness ($r = 0.52$, $p < 0.05$). The change in General Quality of Life was related to the change in forgetfulness ($r = -0.44$, $p < 0.05$). The change in Psychological Inflexibility in Pain was related to the changes in fatigue ($r = 0.49$, $p < 0.05$), headaches ($r = 0.51$, $p < 0.05$) and muscle pain ($r = 0.49$, $p < 0.05$). The change in Pain Avoidance was related to the change in bald patches on scalp, or clumps of hair on pillow ($r = 0.54$, $p < 0.05$), muscle pain ($r = 0.50$, $p < 0.05$), and muscle weakness ($r = 0.45$, $p < 0.05$).

3.4. Qualitative Analysis of In-Depth Interviews

As noted above, 12 qualitative interviews were analyzed to identify the major recurring themes related to participants' experience during and following MBSR. Analysis of participants' transcripts generated five primary themes: (1) changes related to mindfulness; (2) stress reduction; (3) improvement in general physical functioning; (4) changes in illness identity and illness perception; and (5) the group as a mechanism of psychological change.

Changes related to mindfulness

Throughout the 12 analyzed interviews, participants commonly referred to changes related to their ability to be mindful. Mindfulness is a multi-faceted concept, and accordingly, we have identified several sub-themes in the interviews:

(a) Non-reactivity to inner experiences: Ten out of twelve participants referred to their in-creased ability, following MBSR, to be less reactive or impulsive in the face of distress. As one participant noted: " ... *I am very impulsive ... and it became worse for me ... I feel like this workshop has helped me. I don't really count 'til ten, but it did somewhat help me to delay my response and really choose it before I react one way or the other*".

(b) Observing one's negative feelings and physical sensations: 7 of 12 participants have referred to their increased ability to focus their attention on what they feel or experience in a given moment, thus being able to better understand and regulate their physical and psychological experiences. The following quote exemplifies this notion: "*(during meditation) I can sit for 20 min, even 30 min, and I don't think about when it's going to end ... I go back to feeling my breath or my sensations, and then I can remain there with a good feeling. I feel I can actually benefit from that time*".

(c) Non-judgement towards one's negative emotions or physical sensations: six of twelve participants referred to the fact that MBSR helped them feel less self-critical towards themselves as SLE patients, as well as allowing them to feel more self-compassionate about their symptoms and distress. This participant described what is happening to her during SLE flares: "*I've learned how to say 'OK, so today I wasn't able to do this or that-I am not going to give myself a hard time about it. If it doesn't work, so it doesn't work, it's all good. It gives me some kind of ... ease*".

Stress reduction

A highly prominent theme, which emerged from nine of the interviews, concerned the changes participants experienced in terms of their stress-related cognitions and reactions. Participants reported a reduction in stress following the intervention, stemming from the exercises they learned, as well as from their ability to be more mindful about their physical and emotional sensations. For example, one participant noted: "*When I feel my heart pounding, I listen to my pulse and it's simply calming it down. I can feel the pressure dropping, the lungs expanding, and I can breathe deeper"*. The improved mental skills mentioned in the interviews included participants' ability to distance themselves from distressing experiences, and leave stressful thoughts aside, while placing distressing events within a more acceptable, manageable, and less catastrophic perspective.

Improvement in general physical functioning

In line with what was found in the quantitative section of this paper, interviews also showed an improvement in physical functioning in everyday life. Five participants described having formed a new and adaptive attitude towards their body, which enabled them to function more freely and to feel less limited by their symptoms. In the words of one participant: *"When I have to brace myself and go to work, I listen to the body scan exercise and it helps me to physically pick up my body"*. In another instance, a participant noted: *"My body told me what it needed . . . There was a connection between what I was going through and what my body was going through"*.

Changes in Illness identity and perception

In line with our quantitative findings, six out of twelve interviewees reported a positive change in their identity as SLE patients following the intervention. Participants described how they developed a healthier and less stigmatic attitude towards their illness, and its accompanying symptoms. Participants also mentioned how the intervention has helped them to be less defined by their SLE, for example: *"I want to hope that my Lupus would stay calm, but if it will decide to flare, it would be a bit easier to accept the episode . . . but I don't let it define me"*.

The group as a mechanism of psychological change

Another theme strongly emerging from the interviews concerned the therapy group and its positive effect on the individual. Six participants stated that the intervention set up a unique opportunity to meet other SLE patients who were suffering from similar physical and psychological symptoms: *"It felt good to be part of this 'togetherness'. I met other strong women that have been coping with life and death for many years, and still continue to live their lives... they are mothers that gave birth with Lupus, and this gave me a lot of strength, and maybe even hope"*. The group was portrayed by participants as very important in terms of solidarity. Group members mirrored to each other their ability to cope with SLE, thus creating a strong reciprocal support system for participants.

4. Discussion

We conducted a randomized controlled trial to examine the effects of MBSR group therapy for SLE, employing both self-reporting measures and qualitative in-depth interviews. For this study, we developed an adapted MBSR protocol, specifically suited to meet the needs and symptoms of SLE patients. The results showed the positive effects of MBSR on SLE self-reported symptoms, Quality of Life, Depression, SLE-related Shame and Illness Identity, and Psychological Inflexibility in Pain. Importantly, some effects remained stable over a 6-month follow-up period.

Surprisingly, mindfulness-based interventions have been very rarely studied in the context of SLE, despite a growing body of evidence showing their effectiveness on rheumatic [34], autoimmune [35] and pain [36] conditions. In addition, to the best of our knowledge, ours is the first mixed-methods RCT of MBSR, as well as the only MBSR study of SLE to include a variety of psychological and SLE-related measures. The effectiveness of MBSR shown here may be attributed to several factors. Firstly, many studies have indicated the major role of mind-body connections in SLE. This is perhaps most apparent in the strong associations between psychological stress and SLE disease activity [4]. Thus, an intervention with proven efficacy in reducing stress could be expected to alleviate the distress of SLE patients. Secondly, and perhaps more importantly, MBSR inherently targets various aspects which have been shown to be at the heart of SLE-related distress, including impaired emotion regulation, negative mood, and difficulties in identifying and acknowledging various feelings and emotions (i.e., alexithymia; [37]). Finally, some of the core symptoms of SLE, most notably pain and chronic physical discomfort, have been shown to improve via MBSR in previous studies [38].

Furthermore, our findings reveal the unique role MBSR may have in alleviating feelings of shame and negative illness perception among individuals with SLE. These treatment effects were found in both quantitative and qualitative analysis conducted in this study. Shame is a common emotional feature of SLE. It may stem from both direct physical symptoms (e.g., facial rashes, alopecia, weight gain) as well as from the broader experience of living with a chronic disease that undermines daily functioning and affects femininity [39,40]. The decline in SLE-related shame remained stable at the 6-month follow-up assessment, thus pointing to the unique potential of MBSR in this area. As for the perception of illness, studies have shown that SLE, being a systemic, chronic condition, often exerts a massive influence on patients' lives, and may be experienced as a major focal point in their identity. Schattner and colleagues [41] has showed that SLE patients may perceive their illness as all-encompassing and extremely powerful, " . . . threatening the ties between body, mind, everyday life, and relationships". MBSR's strong emphasis on cultivating a non-judgmental stance, as well as its proved ability to promote self-compassion [42], may thus greatly contribute to SLE patients' well-being. However, we should note that while illness identity did improve between pre- and post-treatment assessments, this improvement did not seem to last when measured again at six months post-treatment. This may indicate that some aspects of SLE-related distress may require more long-term psychotherapeutic work and maintenance. One's perception of his/her identity as a person coping with a chronic illness is often multi-layered and complex. Further studies are needed to assess whether mindfulness-based therapy can serve as an add-on component used to augment other forms of interventions (e.g., cognitive-behavioral, psychodynamic) for SLE.

Another specific effect worth noting is related to pain cognitions. Pain is a highly distressing symptom for some SLE patients [43]. It is a complex sensation, involving both objective, physiological aspects, and subjective, psychological ones. Importantly, these two realms of pain were often found to affect each other, creating both positive and negative feedback loops [44]. In our study, we have shown that MBSR may cultivate a more flexible attitude towards physical pain among SLE patients. This was mostly found specifically for fusion with pain (i.e., feeling that one's pain is taking over one's body, and even life), which not only declined following treatment, but also showed stable gains after six months. Due to pain's far-reaching implications in terms of quality of life and daily functioning, this effect on SLE patients is of unique importance.

Several other effects are noteworthy. Major depression levels (i.e., percentage of those above/below clinical cutoff) showed a steady decline across the three assessments. This improvement is important, given the well-established association between SLE and negative mood [45]. Our qualitative analysis added two interesting effects. First, as would be expected from MBSR, the intervention improved patients' ability to be mindful on several aspects. In general, they reported an increased ability to observe and regulate emotions and sensations, while adopting a non-reactive and non-judgmental stance. These results were in line with another theme stemming from the interviews, which indicated decreased stress levels. Patients seemed to use MBSR to feel calmer, and to decrease psychological tension.

Interestingly, the reduction shown in this study in SLE self-reported symptoms was associated with an improvement in mental health outcomes (Quality of Life, SLE-related shame and pain cognitions). We believe that this further supports the mind-body connection in SLE, which has already been established in both quantitative [46] and qualitative [47] studies. Thus, when one's physical symptoms improve, so too do aspects of psychological distress, and vice versa. MBSR, being an inherently mind-body approach, targets both physical and psychological aspects in parallel.

This study has several limitations, most notably a modest sample size, and a reliance of self-reporting measures, which may be prone to memory or reporting bias. Thus, our findings should be considered with the adequate level of caution, as they warrant further research for support. Future studies are encouraged to employ larger samples, objective measures of physical and psychological distress, and more assessment points. Nonetheless, our findings have clinical and methodological importance. They point to the unique potential of MBSR to alleviate the distress of SLE patients, using a group intervention characterized by high cost-effective value (i.e., group setting, short time period). Methodologically, we have shown here, for the first time ever, how qualitative and quantitative methods could complement each other to assess SLE patients' response to MBSR. Finally, all of the effects discussed here should be examined in light of our attempt to offer SLE patients an adapted, disease-specific MBSR protocol. In this era of personalized medicine [48], there is a growing attempt to adapt psychotherapy protocols in general, and MBSR protocols specifically [49], to the needs and characteristics of unique patient populations. We hope that, with more research to follow the present study, this protocol can be used in multiple settings to treat individuals with SLE.

Author Contributions: Project administration and management, writing—review and editing, R.T. and D.H.; project administration and writing, N.R.; clinical management of project, I.G.; therapists, O.R. and G.S.; project and medical administration, medical consulting, writing, N.A.-L. All authors have read and agreed to the published version of the manuscript.

Funding: This research received no external funding.

Institutional Review Board Statement: his study has been reviewed by the ethics committee of Sheba Medical Center and has been performed in accordance with the ethical standards laid down in an appropriate version of the WMA Declaration of Helsinki-Ethical Principles for Medical Re-search Involving Human Subjects. Trial registration number: NCT04305418.

Informed Consent Statement: Informed consent was obtained from all subjects involved in the study. Written informed consent has been obtained from the patients to publish this paper.

Data Availability Statement: The data presented in this study are available on request from the corresponding author. The data are not publicly available due to privacy and confidentiality.

Conflicts of Interest: The authors declare no conflict of interest.

References

1. Cervera, R.; Khamashta, M.A.; Font, J.; Sebastiani, G.D.; Gil, A.; Lavilla, P.; Mejía, J.C.; Aydintug, A.O.; Chwalinska-Sadowska, H.; de Ramón, E.; et al. Morbidity and mortality in systemic lupus erythematosus during a 10-year period: A comparison of early and late manifestations in a cohort of 1000 patients. *Medicine* 2003, *82*, 299–308. [CrossRef] [PubMed]
2. Meszaros, Z.S.; Perl, A.; Faraone, S.V. Psychiatric symptoms in Systemic Lupus Erythematosus: A systemic review. *J. Clin. Psychiatry* 2012, *73*, 993–1001. [CrossRef] [PubMed]
3. Merola, J.F.; Bermas, B.; Lu, B.; Karlson, E.W.; Massarotti, E.; Schur, P.H.; Costenbader, K.H. Clinical manifestations and survival among adults with (SLE) according to age at diagnosis. *Lupus* 2014, *23*, 778–784. [CrossRef] [PubMed]
4. Adams, S.G.; Dammers, P.M.; Saia, T.L.; Brantley, P.J.; Gaydos, G.R. Stress, depression, and anxiety predict average symptom severity and daily symptom fluctuation in systemic lupus erythematosus. *J. Behav. Med.* 1994, *17*, 459–477. [CrossRef] [PubMed]
5. Wallace, D.J. The role of stress and trauma in rheumatoid arthritis and systemic lupus erythematosus *Semin. Arthritis Rheum.* 1987, *16*, 153–157. [CrossRef]
6. Pisetsky, D.S.; Clowse, M.E.; Criscione-Schreiber, L.G.; Rogers, J.L. A novel system to categorize the symptoms of systemic lupus erythematosus. *Arthritis Care Res.* 2019, *71*, 735–741. [CrossRef]
7. Kivity, S.; Agmon-Levin, N.; Zandman-Goddard, G.; Chapman, J.; Shoenfeld, Y. Neuropsychiatric lupus: A mosaic of clinical presentations. *BMC Med.* 2015, *13*, 43. [CrossRef]
8. Nishimura, K.; Omori, M.; Katsumata, Y.; Sato, E.; Kawaguchi, Y.; Harigai, M.; Yamanaka, H.; Ishigooka, J. Psychological distress in corticosteroid-naive patients with systemic lupus erythematosus: A prospective cross-sectional study. *Lupus* 2016, *25*, 463–471. [CrossRef]
9. Kozora, E.; Ellison, M.C.; West, S. Depression, fatigue, and pain in systemic lupus erythematosus (SLE): Relationship to the American College of Rheumatology SLE neuropsychological battery. *Arthritis Rheum* 2006, *55*, 628–635. [CrossRef]
10. Piga, M.; Arnaud, L. The Main Challenges in Systemic Lupus Erythematosus: Where DoWe Stand? *J. Clin. Med.* 2021, *10*, 243. [CrossRef]

11. Horesh, D.; Glick, I.; Taub, R.; Agmon-Levin, N.; Shoenfeld, Y. Mindfulness-based group therapy for systemic lupus erythematosus: A first exploration of a promising mind-body intervention. *Complement. Ther. Clin. Pract.* **2017**, *26*, 73–75. [CrossRef]
12. Kabat-Zinn, J. *Wherever You Go, There You Are: Mindfulness Meditation in Everyday Life*; Hyperion: New York, NY, USA, 1994; p. 278.
13. Langer, E.J. Minding Matters: The Consequences of Mindlessness–Mindfulness. In *Advances in Experimental Social Psychology*; Academic Press: Cambridge, MA, USA, 1989; pp. 137–173.
14. Morone, N.E.; Greco, C.M.; Weiner, D.K. Mindfulness meditation for the treatment of chronic low back pain in older adults: A randomized controlled pilot study. *Pain* **2008**, *134*, 310–319. [CrossRef]
15. Schmidt, S.; Grossman, P.; Schwarzer, B.; Jena, S.; Naumann, J.; Walach, H. Treating fibromyalgia with mindfulness-based stress reduction: Results from a 3-armed randomized controlled trial. *Pain* **2011**, *152*, 361–369. [CrossRef]
16. Bishop, S.R. What Do We Really Know About Mindfulness-Based Stress Reduction? *Psychosom. Med.* **2002**, *64*, 71–83. [CrossRef]
17. Kabat-Zinn, J. *Full Catastrophe Living: How to Cope with Stress, Pain and Illness Using Mindfulness Meditation*; Piatkus: London, UK, 2013; p. 650.
18. Lauche, R.; Cramer, H.; Dobos, G.; Langhorst, J.; Schmidt, S. A systemic review and meta-analysis of mindfulness-based stress reduction for the fibromyalgia syndrome. *J. Psychosom. Res.* **2013**, *75*, 500–510. [CrossRef]
19. Bahreini, Z.; Sanagouye-Moharer, G. The effectiveness of mindfulness-based stress reduction therapy on resilience and self-discrepancy among female patients with systemic lupus erythematosus. *Community Health* **2019**, *6*, 406–414.
20. Solati, K.; Mousavi, M. The efficacy of mindfulness-based cognitive therapy on general health in patients with Systemic Lupus Erythematosus: A randomized controlled trial. *J. Kerman Univ. Med. Sci.* **2015**, *22*, 499–509.
21. Solati, K.; Mousavi, M.; Kheiri, S.; Hasanpour-Dehkordi, A. The effectiveness of mindfulness-based cognitive therapy on psychological symptoms and quality of life in systemic lupus erythematosus patients: A randomized controlled trial. *Oman Med. J.* **2017**, *32*, 378–385. [CrossRef] [PubMed]
22. Kim, H.A.; Seo, L.; Baek, W.Y.; Jung, J.Y.; Kim, Y.W.; Lee, E.; Cho, S.M.; Suh, C.H. Mindfulness-based cognitive therapy in Korean patients with systemic lupus erythenatosus. *Complement. Ther. Clin. Pract.* **2019**, *35*, 18–21. [CrossRef] [PubMed]
23. Teasdale, J.D.; Segal, Z.V.; Williams, J.M.; Ridgewaya, V.A.; Soulsby, J.M.; Lau, M.A. Prevention of relapse/recurrence in major depression by mindfulness-based cognitive therapy. *J. Consult. Clin. Psychol* **2000**, *68*, 615–623. [CrossRef]
24. Rafie, S.; Akbari, R.; Charati, J.Y.; Elyasi, F.; Azimi-Lolaty, H. Effect of mindfulness-based metacognitive skills training on depression, Anxiety, Stress, and Well-being in Patients with systemic lupus erythematosus. *J. Maz. Univ. Med. Sci.* **2020**, *30*, 11–21.
25. Nam, S.; Toneatto, T. The Influence of attrition in evaluating the efficacy and effectiveness of mindfulness-based interventions. *Int. J. Ment. Health Addict.* **2016**, *14*, 969–981. [CrossRef]
26. Karlson, E.W.; Daltroy, L.H.; Rivest, C.; Ramsey-Goldman, R.; Wright, E.A.; Partridge, A.J.; Liang, M.H.; Fortin, P.R. Validation of a systemic lupus activity questionnaire (SLAQ) for population studies. *Lupus* **2003**, *12*, 280–286. [CrossRef] [PubMed]
27. The Whoqol Group. The World Health Organization Quality of Life Assessment (WHOQOL): Development and general psychometric properties. *Soc. Sci. Med.* **1998**, *46*, 1569–1585. [CrossRef]
28. Kroenke, K.; Spitzer, R.L. The PHQ-9: A new depression diagnostic and severity measure. *Psychiatry Ann.* **2002**, *32*, 509–515. [CrossRef]
29. Wicksell, R.K.; Lekander, M.; Sorjonen, K.; Olsson, G.L. The Psychological Inflexibility in Pain Scale (PIPS)—Statistical properties and model fit of an instrument to assess change processes in pain related disability. *Eur. J. Pain* **2010**, *14*, e1–e771. [CrossRef] [PubMed]
30. Monro, F.; Huon, G. Media-portrayed idealized images, body shame, and appearance anxiety. *Int. J. Eat. Disord.* **2005**, *38*, 85–90. [CrossRef]
31. Bae, H.; Min, B.I.; Cho, S. Efficacy of acupuncture in reducing preoperative anxiety: A meta-analysis. *Evid. Based Complement. Altern. Med.* **2014**, *37*, 1–12. [CrossRef]
32. Taylor-Powell, E.; Renner, M. Analyzing Qualitative Data. *Program Dev. Eval.* **2003**, *26*, 1–12.
33. Landis, J.R.; Koch, G.G. An application of hierarchical kappa-type statistics in the assessment of majority agreement among multiple observers. *Biometrics* **1977**, *33*, 363–374. [CrossRef]
34. Zangi, H.A.; Mowinckel, P.; Finset, A.; Eriksson, L.R.; Høystad, T.Ø.; Lunde, A.K.; Hagen, K.B. A mindfulness-based group intervention to reduce psychological distress and fatigue in patients with inflammatory rheumatic joint diseases: A randomised controlled trial. *Ann. Rheum. Dis.* **2012**, *71*, 911–917. [CrossRef] [PubMed]
35. Penberthy, J.K.; Chhabra, D.; Avitabile, N.; Penberthy, J.M.; Le, N.; Xu, Y.R.; Mainor, S.; Schiavone, N.; Katzenstein, P.; Lewis, J.E. Mindfulness based therapies for autoimmune diseases and related symptoms. *OBM Integr. Complement. Med.* **2018**, *3*, 1–11. [CrossRef]
36. Veehof, M.M.; Trompetter, H.R.; Bohlmeijer, E.T.; Schreurs, K.M. Acceptance-and mindfulness-based interventions for the treatment of chronic pain: A meta-analytic review. *Cogn. Behav. Ther.* **2016**, *45*, 5–31. [CrossRef]
37. Barbosa, F.; Mota, C.; Patrício, P.; Alcântara, C.; Ferreira, C.; Barbosa, A. Alexithymia and clinical variables in SLE patients. *Psychother. Psychosom.* **2011**, *80*, 123–124. [CrossRef]
38. Khoo, E.L.; Small, R.; Cheng, W.; Hatchard, T.; Glynn, B.; Rice, D.B.; Skidmore, B.; Kenny, S.; Hutton, B.; Poulin, P.A. Comparative evaluation of group-based mindfulness-based stress reduction and cognitive behavioural therapy for the treatment and management of chronic pain: A systematic review and network meta-analysis. *Based Ment. Health* **2019**, *22*, 26–35. [CrossRef]

39. Hale, E.D.; Treharne, G.J.; Norton, Y.; Lyons, A.C.; Douglas, K.M.; Erb, N.; Kitas, G.D. 'Concealing the evidence': The importance of appearance concerns for patients with systemic lupus erythematosus. *Lupus* **2006**, *15*, 532–540. [CrossRef]
40. Sehlo, M.G.; Bahlas, S.M. Perceived illness stigma is associated with depression in female patients with systemic lupus erythematosus. *J. Psychosom. Res.* **2013**, *74*, 248–251. [CrossRef]
41. Schattner, E.; Shahar, G.; Abu-Shakra, M. "I used to dream of lupus as some sort of creature": Chronic illness as an internal object. *Am. J. Orthopsychiatry* **2008**, *78*, 466–472. [CrossRef] [PubMed]
42. Sevel, L.S.; Finn, M.T.; Smith, R.M.; Ryden, A.M.; McKernan, L.C. Self-compassion in mindfulness-based stress reduction: An examination of prediction and mediation of intervention effects. *Stress Heal.* **2020**, *36*, 88–96. [CrossRef]
43. Waldheim, E.; Ajeganova, S.; Bergman, S.; Frostegård, J.; Welin, E. Variation in pain related to systemic lupus erythematosus (SLE): A 7-year follow-up study. *Clin. Rheumatol.* **2018**, *37*, 1825–1834. [CrossRef]
44. Granovsky, Y.; Granot, M.; Nir, R.R.; Yarnitsky, D. Objective correlate of subjective pain perception by contact heat-evoked potentials. *J. Pain* **2008**, *9*, 53–63. [CrossRef] [PubMed]
45. Palagini, L.; Mosca, M.; Tani, C.; Gemignani, A.; Mauri, M.; Bombardieri, S. Depression and systemic lupus erythematosus: A systematic review. *Lupus* **2013**, *22*, 409–416. [CrossRef] [PubMed]
46. Moraleda, V.; Prados, G.; Martínez, M.P.; Sánchez, A.I.; Sabio, J.M.; Miró, E. Sleep quality, clinical and psychological manifestations in women with systemic lupus erythematosus. *Int. J. Rheum. Dis.* **2017**, *20*, 1541–1550. [CrossRef] [PubMed]
47. Özsungur, F. The psychological effects of systemic lupus erythematosus: The imitator of aging. *Lympho Sign J.* **2020**, *7*, 37–45. [CrossRef]
48. Hamburg, M.A.; Collins, F.S. The Path to Personalized Medicine. *N. Engl. J. Med.* **2010**, *363*, 301–304. [CrossRef]
49. Moss, A.S.; Reibel, D.K.; Greeson, J.M.; Thapar, A.; Bubb, R.; Salmon, J.; Newberg, A.B. An adapted mindfulness-based stress reduction program for elders in a continuing care retirement community: Quantitative and qualitative results from a pilot randomized controlled trial. *J. Appl. Gerontol.* **2015**, *34*, 518–538. [CrossRef]

Article

Change of Renal Gallium Uptake Correlated with Change of Inflammation Activity in Renal Pathology in Lupus Nephritis Patients

Tsu-Yi Hsieh [1,2], Yi-Ching Lin [3,4], Wei-Ting Hung [1,2], Yi-Ming Chen [1,5,6,7], Mei-Chin Wen [8], Hsin-Hua Chen [1,5,6], Wan-Yu Lin [3], Chia-Wei Hsieh [1,6], Ching-Tsai Lin [1], Kuo-Lung Lai [1], Kuo-Tung Tang [1], Chih-Wei Tseng [1], Wen-Nan Huang [1,5], Yi-Hsing Chen [1,5], Shih-Chuan Tsai [3,9,*] and Yi-Da Wu [1,*]

[1] Division of Allergy, Immunology and Rheumatology, Taichung Veterans General Hospital, Taichung 40705, Taiwan; zuyihsieh@gmail.com (T.-Y.H.); wtinghung@gmail.com (W.-T.H.); blacklark@gmail.com (Y.-M.C.); shc5555@hotmail.com (H.-H.C.); chiaweih@gmail.com (C.-W.H.); chingtsia@yahoo.com.tw (C.-T.L.); kllaichiayi@yahoo.com.tw (K.-L.L.); crashbug1982@gmail.com (K.-T.T.); cwtseng@vghtc.gov.tw (C.-W.T.); gtim5555@yahoo.com (W.-N.H.); dr.yihsing@gmail.com (Y.-H.C.)
[2] Department of Medical Education, Taichung Veterans General Hospital, Taichung 40705, Taiwan
[3] Department of Nuclear Medicine, Taichung Veterans General Hospital, Taichung 40705, Taiwan; dianayjlin@gmail.com (Y.-C.L.); wy1962@gmail.com (W.-Y.L.)
[4] Department of Public Health, China Medical University, Taichung 40447, Taiwan
[5] Department of Medical Research, Taichung Veterans General Hospital, Taichung 40705, Taiwan
[6] Institute of Biomedical Science and Rong Hsing Research Center for Translational Medicine, National Chung Hsing University, Taichung 402, Taiwan
[7] Faculty of Medicine, National Yang-Ming University, Taipei 11221, Taiwan
[8] Department of Pathology and Laboratory Medicine, Taichung Veterans General Hospital, Taichung 40705, Taiwan; mewen@vghtc.gov.tw
[9] Department of Medical Imaging and Radiological Sciences, Central Taiwan University of Science and Technology, Taichung 406053, Taiwan
* Correspondence: sctsai@vghtc.gov.tw (S.-C.T.); bagidr1@hotmail.com (Y.-D.W.)

Abstract: Background: Lupus nephritis (LN) often lead to end-stage renal disease in systemic lupus erythematosus patients. This study aimed to investigate the clinical application of renal gallium-67 scans for determining renal histological parameters in LN patients. Methods: Between 2006 and 2018, 237 biopsy-proven and 35 repeat biopsies LN patients who underwent renal gallium scans before or after biopsy were included for analysis. The classification and scoring of LN were assessed according to the International Society of Nephrology/Renal Pathology Society. A delayed 48-h gallium scan was performed and interpreted by semiquantitative methods using left kidney/spine (K/S) ratio. The renal histological results were compared with gallium uptake. Results: Out of 237 participants, 180 (76%) had proliferative LN. Baseline gallium left K/S ratio was significantly higher in class IV LN as compared to class III (median (interquartile range, IQR): 1.16 (1.0–1.3), 0.95 (0.9–1.1), respectively, $p < 0.001$). Furthermore, changes in gallium uptake between two biopsies were positively correlated with changes activity index ($r = 0.357$, $p = 0.035$), endocapillary hypercellularity ($r = 0.385$, $p = 0.032$), and neutrophils infiltration ($r = 0.390$, $p = 0.030$) in renal pathology. Conclusions: Renal gallium uptake is associated with active inflammation in LN. Changes in renal gallium uptake positively correlated with changes in activity index in renal pathology.

Keywords: systemic lupus erythematosus; lupus nephritis; glomerulonephritis; gallium scan; scintigraphy; renal biopsy

1. Introduction

Lupus nephritis (LN) occurs in approximately sixty percent of patients with systemic lupus erythematosus (SLE) [1]. The goals for managing patients with lupus nephritis include early diagnosis and proper therapy, which may prevent irreversible renal damage [2]. Therefore, a kidney biopsy should be performed in LN patients who develop overt proteinuria or renal insufficiency, as it is essential in assessing disease activity and guiding treatment [3,4]. The recommendation for monitoring LN includes urinalysis, including urine protein/creatinine ratio, serum creatinine, complement 3 (C3), C4 levels, and anti-DNA levels [5]. However, some patients with the quiescent disease may develop a recurrent emergence of a new elevation in serum creatinine, and/or worsening proteinuria despite treatment. In this event, a repeat biopsy may help assess the renal inflammatory activity and chronic damage, which could help guide subsequent treatment. Renal biopsy is an invasive diagnostic procedure, and bleeding complications were significantly higher in patients with serum creatinine above 2 mg/dL (2.1 versus 0.4 percent) [6]. Therefore, detecting active disease using a non-invasive tool may ensure the levels of immunosuppressants aretailored to the disease activity.

Gallium-67 scintigraphy has been used for decades to evaluate interstitial nephritis [7,8]. After gallium injection, it may bind to lactoferrin in neutrophils, be taken up by lysosomes in mono-nuclear phagocytes, bind directly to the lymphocyte membrane, and be transported to sites of inflammatory glomeruli. Gallium-67 scintigraphy has also been described as a helpful tool in evaluating LN activity [9,10], and can also be used to monitor LN due to its relationship with disease activity, and its potential as a diagnostic alternative to renal biopsy [9–11]. Previously, our group developed a semiquantitative method for gallium renal imaging, which showed that the left kidney-to-spine ratio (K/S ratio) determined using a semiquantitative method had a better correlation with renal biopsy results than those obtained by visual grading [11]. However, no studies have evaluated the correlation between changes in renal gallium uptake and the changes in renal pathology findings.

In this hospital-based study, we aimed to investigate the clinical value of the change of renal gallium-67 scintigraphy uptake using the left K/S ratio for evaluating the change of renal histological parameters in LN patients in LN patients with repeated biopsies.

2. Materials and Methods

2.1. Participants

Between January 2006 and December 2018, a hospital-based observational study was conducted to retrospectively review 237 biopsy-proven LN patients, including 35 patients who received repeat biopsies. All patients underwent single or repeated renal gallium scans within a period of 30 days before or after the biopsy (with a median of 4 days with standard deviation of 11.97). The classification and scoring of LN and details of renal histology exams were recorded. A delayed 48-h gallium scan was performed and interpreted by semiquantitative methods. The renal histological results were compared with gallium scan parameters. This study was conducted in compliance with the Helsinki Declaration, and approval by the Institutional Review Board of Taichung Veterans General Hospital was obtained (CE18210B). As all data were de-identified before analysis, the requirement for informed consent from the participants was waived.

2.2. Clinical Parameters

Clinical data included daily urine protein, serum creatinine, estimated glomerular filtration rate (eGFR), anti-double strand DNA antibody (dsDNA Ab), C3, and C4 were collected before renal biopsy. Daily urine protein was measured by spot urine protein and creatinine ratio. Estimated GFR was calculated using the Modification of Diet in Renal Disease equations [12]. Whether or not a second kidney biopsy was deemed necessary depended on the treating clinician's decision.

2.3. Renal Histology

All patients underwent percutaneous renal biopsy, which was performed by experienced nephrologists under ultrasonic guidance. The classification and scoring of LN were assessed according to the International Society of Nephrology/Renal Pathology Society [13].

The activity index (AI) and chronicity index (CI) were calculated based on the system devised by Austin and colleagues [14]. This renal pathology grading system (AI and CI) has been widely used for several decades and has been recognized as a predictor of renal outcomes [15,16]. In this system, AI is defined as the sum of the individual scores of 6 features (glomerular cell proliferation, leukocyte exudation, fibrinoid necrosis/karyorrhexis, cellular crescents, hyaline deposits, and interstitial inflammation) considered to represent measures of active lupus nephritis. Chronicity index is defined as the sum of the individual scores of four features (glomerular sclerosis, fibrous crescents, tubular atrophy, and interstitial fibrosis), which considered to represent measures of chronic irreversible lupus nephritis. Each individual component is scored on a scale of 0 to 3+ (0, absent; 1+, mild; 2+, moderate; 3+, severe). The maximum AI value is 18 points, and the maximum CI value is 12 points. The World Health Organization classification, AI, and CI were determined by two pathologists, who were blind to the results of clinical parameters and gallium renal scans.

2.4. Gallium-67 Renal Scintigraphy

Gallium scintigraphy was performed within 30 days before or after the renal biopsy. Forty-eight hours after the injection of 111 MBq (3 mCi) of 67Ga citrate, static posterior abdominal scintigrams were obtained using a large-field-of-view camera with a medium-energy, parallel-hole collimator (ECAM; Siemens, Munich, Germany). Three 20% windows were set at 93,184 and 296 keV. Residual bowel activity is a potential source of error on the gallium image, and thus bowel preparation was performed in all patients before imaging. If the kidney image was overlapped by bowel activity at forty-eight hours, the seventy-two hours after administration of the radiotracer images were used instead. The SPECT volume session included the abdomen with an axial field of view of 40 cm, followed by a low dose CT of the same correlative territory. SPECT images were obtained with a non-circular orbit with step and shoot acquisition, obtaining 64 images of 50 s each in a 128 × 128 pixels matrix. SPECT data were reconstructed using a three-dimensional iterative algorithm. CT data information were used for attenuation correction and anatomical information. No contrast medium was injected during the examination.

2.5. Semi-Quantitative Method of Gallium Renal Scintigraphy

For semi-quantitative analysis of gallium uptake in both kidneys, regions of interest (ROIs) were drawn over both kidneys and the adjacent spine (Figure 1). To minimize subjective bias, we set each ROIs of images by the following rules. First, the ROI of kidneys should locate in the middle or inferior parts of visible renal parenchyma to avoid interference of tracer-avid organs such as liver, spleen, and bowels. Second, the average pixel size of renal ROI is 100. The ROI of spines should locate in the adjacent spines, which are longer than one vertebral height to avoid single structural or degenerative deformities and is no wider than a vertebral width to exclude the structure outside the vertebral body. The average pixel size of spine ROI is 500. Third, two experienced technicians in one workstation did all procedures. For each ROI, a value of mean counts per pixel was obtained for data analysis. The uptake ratios between ROIs were calculated and expressed as "kidney/spine ratio" (K/S ratio).

2.6. Patient and Public Involvement

We did not involve patients or the public in our work.

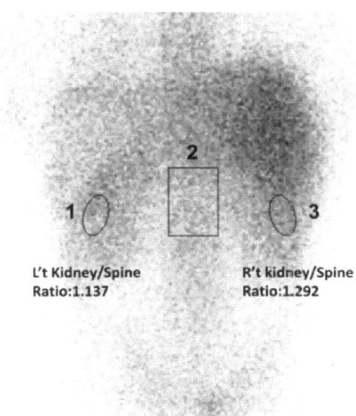

Figure 1. Semiquantitative measurement calculated by kidney/spine ratio from 67Ga renal image (posterior view) in a patient with lupus nephritis. ROIs on scintigraphy image: ROI 1: left kidney; ROI 2: spine; ROI 3: Right kidney. ROI: region of interest.

2.7. Statistical Analysis

The demographic data of continuous parameters are shown as mean ± standard deviation, and for categorical variables as the number of patients. Chi-Square test and Kruskal-Wallis test were used to perform unadjusted comparisons among patients with various classes of LN. Factors associated with renal gallium uptake were determined using multivariable linear regression. Comparisons of variables of first vs. subsequent renal biopsies were performed by Wilcoxon signed rank and McNemar test. Correlation between changes of gallium uptake between two renal biopsies and clinical/histological variables were performed by Spearman's correlation. All data were analyzed using the Statistical Package for the Social Sciences (SPSS), version 22.0. Significance was set at $p < 0.05$.

3. Results

3.1. Demographic Data of Enrolled LN Patients by Pathological Classification

A total of 237 participants (195 women, 88.6%) were included in the study. Demographic, clinical, histological features, and gallium left kidney/spine ratio (left K/S ratio) are shown in Table 1. Out of 237 participants, 170 (72%) had proliferative LN (class III and class IV). The activity index of class IV was significantly higher than class III and class V (median (inter-quartile range, IQR): 8 (5.0–10.3), 3 (1.0–3.8), 0 (0–2), respectively, $p < 0.001$). Gallium left K/S ratio was significantly higher in class IV LN as compared to class III (1.16 (1.0–1.3), and 0.95 (0.9–1.1), respectively, $p < 0.001$), but not class V.

Table 1. Basic demographic data of 237 lupus nephritis patients by histological classes.

	Class I & II ($n = 7$)	III ($n = 36$)	IV ($n = 134$)	V ($n = 60$)	p Value
Age (years)	42.0 (33.0–43.0)	31.5 (25.3–40.0)	32.0 (25.0–41.0)	31.5 (26.0–39.5)	0.586
Female gender	7 (100.0%)	30 (83.3%)	108 (80.6%)	50 (83.3%)	0.606
Laboratory data					
Daily urine protein (gram)	0.7 (0.1–1.8)	1.9 (0.9–2.4)	3.7 (2.1–5.8)	2.3 (1.1–7.0)	<0.001 **‡§∥
Creatinine (mg/dL)	0.7 (0.5–0.8)	0.9 (0.6–1.2)	1.4 (0.9–2.9)	0.8 (0.7–1.1)	<0.001 **‡∥††
eGFR (mg/mL)	97.5 (91.0–139.2)	85.1 (63.5–118.4)	51.7 (22.1–79.9)	84.3 (60.7–117.1)	<0.001 **‡∥††
Anti-dsDNA (WHO units/mL)	248.7 (166.5–477.0)	174.3 (71.2–353.0)	265.4 (125.5–464.1)	130.4 (35.6–277.6)	<0.001 **††

Table 1. Cont.

	Class I & II ($n = 7$)	III ($n = 36$)	IV ($n = 134$)	V ($n = 60$)	p Value
C3 (mg/dL)	78.2 (71.3–90.5)	77.4 (64.5–94.0)	54.6 (39.4–66.7)	63.8 (46.5–89.9)	<0.001 **∣∣††
C4 (mg/dL)	15.1 (4.1–20.9)	14.2 (10.6–22.1)	10.2 (6.3–17.6)	11.7 (6.5–23.5)	0.045 *∣∣
Renal pathology					
Activity index	0 (0–1)	3 (1.0–3.8)	8 (5.0–10.3)	0 (0–2)	<0.001 **‡∣∣††
Cellular crescents	0 (0–0)	0 (0–0)	2 (0–2)	0 (0–0)	<0.001 **‡∣∣††
Fibrinoid necrosis/ Karyorrhexis	0 (0–0)	0 (0–2)	2 (0–2)	0 (0–0)	<0.001 **‡††
Endocapillary hypercellularity	0 (0–0)	1 (0–1)	2 (2–3)	0 (0–1)	<0.001 **‡∣∣††
Subendothelial hyaline deposits	0 (0–0)	0 (0–0)	1 (0–2)	0 (0–0)	<0.001 **‡∣∣††
Leukocyte infiltration	0 (0–0)	0 (0–0)	1 (0–1)	0 (0–0)	<0.001 **∣∣††
Interstitial inflammation	0 (0–1)	0 (0–1)	1 (0–2)	0 (0–1)	<0.001 **∣∣††
Chronicity Index	0 (0–1)	3 (0–3)	1 (0–4)	1 (0–2.8)	0.159
Glomerular sclerosis	0 (0–0)	1 (0–1)	1 (0–1)	0 (0–1)	0.011 *
Tubular atrophy	0 (0–0)	1 (0–1)	0 (0–1)	0 (0–1)	0.157
Interstitial fibrosis	0 (0–1)	1 (0–1)	0 (0–1)	0 (0–1)	0.656
Fibrous crescent	0 (0–0)	0 (0–0)	0 (0–0)	0 (0–0)	0.155
Left K/S ratio	0.910 (0.8–1.2)	0.950 (0.9–1.1)	1.16 (1.0–1.3)	1.040 (1.0–1.2)	<0.001 **∣∣¶
Right K/S ratio	0.990 (0.9–1.4)	0.995 (0.9–1.2)	1.220 (1.1–1.4)	1.080 (1.0–1.2)	<0.001 **∣∣††

* $p < 0.05$, ** $p < 0.01$; Post hoc analysis. ‡ I/II vs. IV $p < 0.05$; § I/II vs. V, $p < 0.05$; ∣∣ III vs. IV, $p < 0.05$; ¶ III vs. V, $p < 0.05$; †† IV vs. V, $p < 0.05$. eGFR: estimated glomerular filtration rate, anti-dsDNA: anti-double-stranded DNA antibody, C3: complement 3, C4: complement 4, SLEDAI: systemic lupus erythematosus disease activity index, K/S ratio: kidney-to-spine ratio.

3.2. Factors Associated with Renal Gallium Uptake

The univariate and multivariate linear regression analysis in Table 2 shows the factors associated with left K/S ratio. Univariate linear regression demonstrated that daily urinary protein, eGFR, activity index, cellular crescents, fibrinoid necrosis/karyorrhexis, endocapillary hypercellularity, subendothelial hyaline deposits, leukocyte infiltration, and interstitial inflammation were significantly associated with renal gallium uptake. In multivariate analysis, daily urinary protein, activity index, endocapillary hypercellularity, and interstitial inflammation independently correlated with gallium uptake left K/S ratio. Figure 2 illustrates that the higher degree of gallium uptake calculated by left K/S ratio, the greater degree of activity index in renal histopathology.

Table 2. Linear regression of clinical and histological parameters associated with left K/S ratio.

	Univariate		Multivariate 1		Multivariate 2		Multivariate 3	
	B (95%CI)	p Value	B (95%CI)	p Value	B (95%CI)	p Value	B (95%CI)	p Value
Age (years)	−0.003 (−0.005, 0.000)	0.061						
Gender								
Female	Reference							
Male	0.004 (−0.082, 0.088)	0.941						
Laboratory data								
Daily urine protein (gram)	0.022 (0.015, 0.030)	<0.001 **	0.019 (0.011, 0.026)	<0.001 **	0.018 (0.010, 0.026)	<0.001 **	0.018 (0.010, 0.025)	<0.001 **
Creatinine (mg/dL)	0.018 (−0.001, 0.037)	0.067						
eGFR (mg/mL)	−0.001 (−0.002, 0.000)	0.016 *	0.000 (−0.001, 0.001)	0.752	0.000 (−0.001, 0.001)	0.994		
Anti-dsDNA (WHO units/mL)	0.000 (0.000, 0.000)	0.350						
C3 (mg/dL)	−0.001 (−0.002, 0.000)	0.072						
C4 (mg/dL)	−0.001 (−0.003, 0.002)	0.565						
Renal pathology								
Activity index	0.021 (0.015, 0.028)	<0.001 **	0.018 (0.010, 0.025)	<0.001 **				
Cellular crescents	0.051 (0.026, 0.070)	<0.001 **			0.008 (−0.023, 0.030)	0.618		
Fibrinoid necrosis/Karyorrhexis	0.036 (0.016, 0.057)	<0.001 **			0.017 (−0.008, 0.041)	0.185		
Endocapillary hypercellularity	0.072 (0.045, 0.098)	<0.001 **			0.025 (−0.017, 0.066)	0.241	0.041 (0.011, 0.070)	0.008 **
Subendothelial hyaline deposits	0.082 (0.046, 0.118)	<0.001 **			0.018 (−0.029, 0.065)	0.456		
Leukocyte infiltration	0.090 (0.040, 0.141)	<0.001 **			−0.014 (−0.071, 0.044)	0.643		
Interstitial inflammation	0.094 (0.059, 0.130)	<0.001 **			0.054 (0.013, 0.095)	0.010 *	0.061 (0.023, 0.100)	0.002 **
Chronicity Index	−0.002 (−0.015, 0.010)	0.694						
Glomerular sclerosis	−0.020 (−0.054, 0.014)	0.244						
Tubular atrophy	−0.009 (−0.046, 0.029)	0.648						
Interstitial fibrosis	−0.001 (−0.039, 0.036)	0.848						
Fibrous crescent	0.049 (−0.077, 0.175)	0.442						

* $p < 0.05$, ** $p < 0.01$. Multivariate 1 Adjust $R^2 = 0.217$; Multivariate 2 Adjust $R^2 = 0.219$; Multivariate 3 Adjust $R^2 = 0.225$. eGFR: estimated glomerular filtration rate; anti-dsDNA: anti-double-stranded DNA antibody; C3: complement 3; C4: complement 4; SLEDAI: systemic lupus erythematosus disease activity index; K/S ratio: kidney-to-spine ratio.

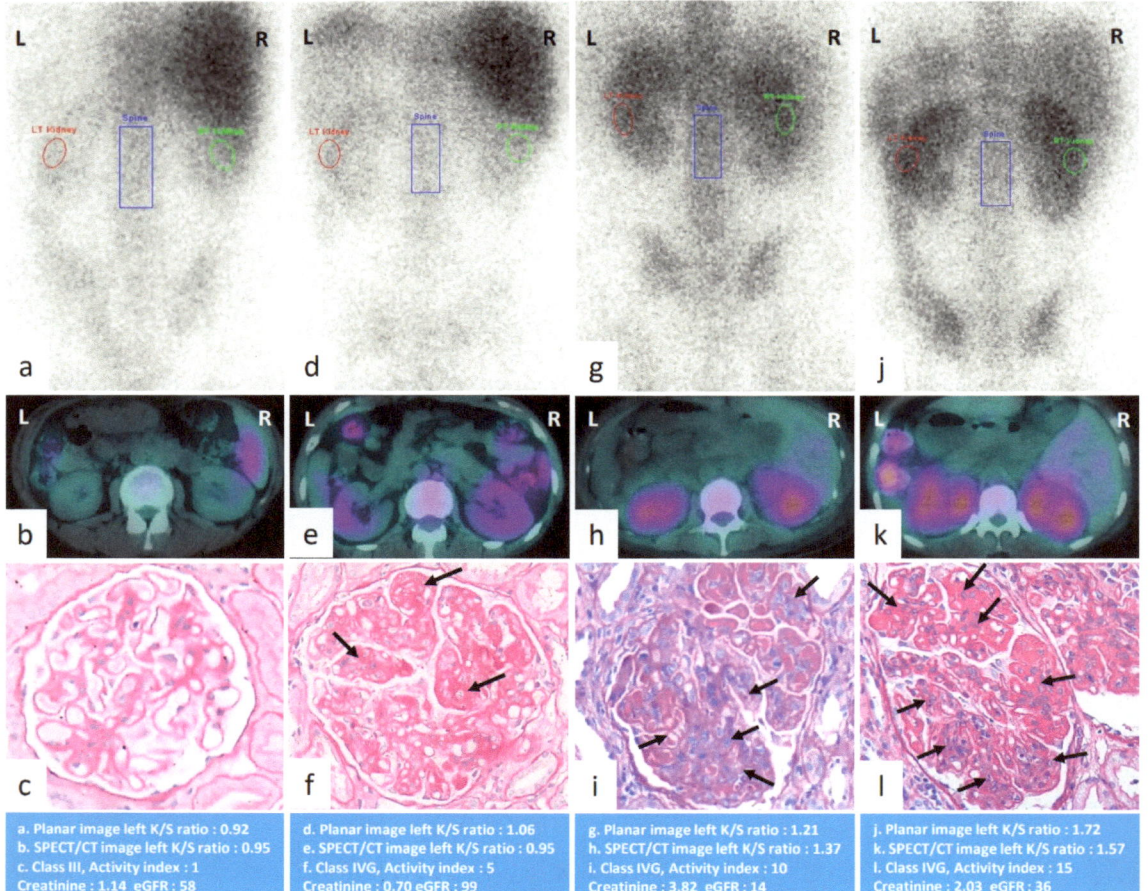

Figure 2. Renal gallium planar view (**a,d,g,j**) and SPECT/CT (**b,e,h,k**) images of four different LN patients from low to high activity index scoring in renal histopathology (**c,f,i,l**). (**a–c**) A 34-year-old LN female patient with activity index 1 in pathology, left K/S ratio 0.92 in gallium planar image; (**d,e**) A 40-year-old LN female patient with activity score 5 in pathology, left K/S ratio 1.06 in gallium planar image; (**g–i**) A 41-year-old LN female patient with activity score 10 in pathology, left K/S ratio 1.21 in gallium planar image; (**j–l**) A 14-year-old LN female patient with activity score 15 in pathology, left K/S ratio 1.72 in gallium planar image. This figure revealed that a trend of a higher degree of gallium uptake calculated by left K/S ratio, the greater degree of activity index score and endocapillary hypercellularity (arrows) L: left side; R: right side; SPECT/CT: single photon emission computed tomography; LN: lupus nephritis; K/S ratio: kidney/spine ratio.

3.3. Comparisons of Clinical Variables of LN Patients Receiving Repeat Renal Biopsies

Thirty-five patients received a second kidney biopsy and renal gallium scan (Table 3). The mean scores of activity index, fibrinoid necrosis/karyorrhexis, and endocapillary hypercellularity in the second biopsy were significantly decreased compared to the first renal biopsy. The creatinine level, C4, mean scores of chronicity index, glomerular sclerosis, tubular atrophy, and interstitial fibrosis in the second biopsy were significantly increased compared to the first renal biopsy. The K/S ratio was non-significantly decreased.

Table 3. Comparisons of clinical, pathological parameters and gallium uptake between two renal biopsies in 35 SLE patients.

	First Biopsy	Second Biopsy	p Value
Age (years)	26.0 (21.0–36.0)	30.0 (24.0–37.0)	<0.001 **
Daily urine protein (gram)	3.8 (1.8–6.7)	3.9 (1.0–5.6)	0.600
Creatinine (mg/dL)	1.0 (0.8–1.7)	1.1 (0.8–2.7)	0.013 *
eGFR (mg/mL)	74.1 (38.3–95.3)	58.1 (22.5–96.4)	0.072
Anti-dsDNA (WHO units/mL)	148.75 (95.8–409.1)	141.4 (37.0–364.7)	0.135
C3 (mg/dL)	56.9 (41.9–83.8)	70.4 (48.9–87.3)	0.109
C4 (mg/dL)	10.5 (5.7–13.5)	16.8 (6.2–22.3)	0.020 *
Lupus nephritis category			0.931
I & II	2 (5.7%)	2 (5.7%)	
III	3 (8.6%)	3 (8.6%)	
IV	22 (62.9%)	23 (65.7%)	
V	8 (22.9%)	7 (20.0%)	
Activity index	6.0 (1.0–9.0)	2.0 (0.3–6.8)	0.028 *
Cellular crescents	0 (0–2)	0 (0–0)	0.218
Fibrinoid necrosis/Karyorrhexis	2.0 (0.0–2.0)	0 (0–0)	0.028 *
Endocapillary hypercellularity	2 (0–3)	1 (0–3)	0.045 *
Subendothelial hyaline deposits	0 (0–2)	0 (0–1)	0.301
Leukocyte infiltration	0 (0–1)	0 (0–1)	0.120
Interstitial inflammation	1.0 (0.0–1.0)	1.0 (0.0–1.0)	0.655
Chronicity Index	1 (0–2)	3.0 (1.0–7.0)	<0.001 **
Glomerular sclerosis	0 (0–1)	1 (0–3)	<0.001 **
Tubular atrophy	0 (0–0)	1 (0–2)	0.001 **
Interstitial fibrosis	0 (0–1)	1 (0–2)	0.001 **
Fibrous crescent	0 (0–0)	0 (0–0)	0.317
Left K/S ratio	1.140 (1.0–1.4)	1.060 (1.0–1.3)	0.241
Right K/S ratio	1.210 (1.1–1.4)	1.120 (1.0–1.3)	0.225

* $p < 0.05$, ** $p < 0.01$. eGFR: estimated glomerular filtration rate; anti-dsDNA: anti-double-stranded DNA antibody; C3: complement 3, C4: complement 4; K/S ratio: kidney-to-spine ratio.

3.4. Correlation between Changes of Renal Gallium Uptake and Changes of Clinical Variables

To further explore the clinical significance of gallium uptake, we analyzed the change of gallium uptake and the change of variate of clinical parameters in individual patients. Table 4 shows the results of analyses performed to determine whether change of gallium uptake was sensitive to changes of clinical and pathologic parameters. A change in gallium uptake between two biopsies were positively correlated with changes of daily urine protein ($r = 0.768$, $p < 0.001$), changes of activity index scores ($r = 0.357$, $p = 0.035$), endocapillary hypercellularity ($r = 0.385$, $p = 0.032$), and leukocyte infiltration ($r = 0.390$, $p = 0.030$). Change of creatinine level and eGFR was not significantly correlated with change of left K/S ratio. Figure 3 demonstrated an example of this study that the changes in gallium uptake calculated by left K/S ratio between two biopsies were positively correlated with changes of daily urine protein and activity index score, but not chronicity index, in renal pathology. Figure 4 demonstrates an example where no significant change of renal gallium uptake between two biopsies was observed and no change in the activity index score in the renal pathology.

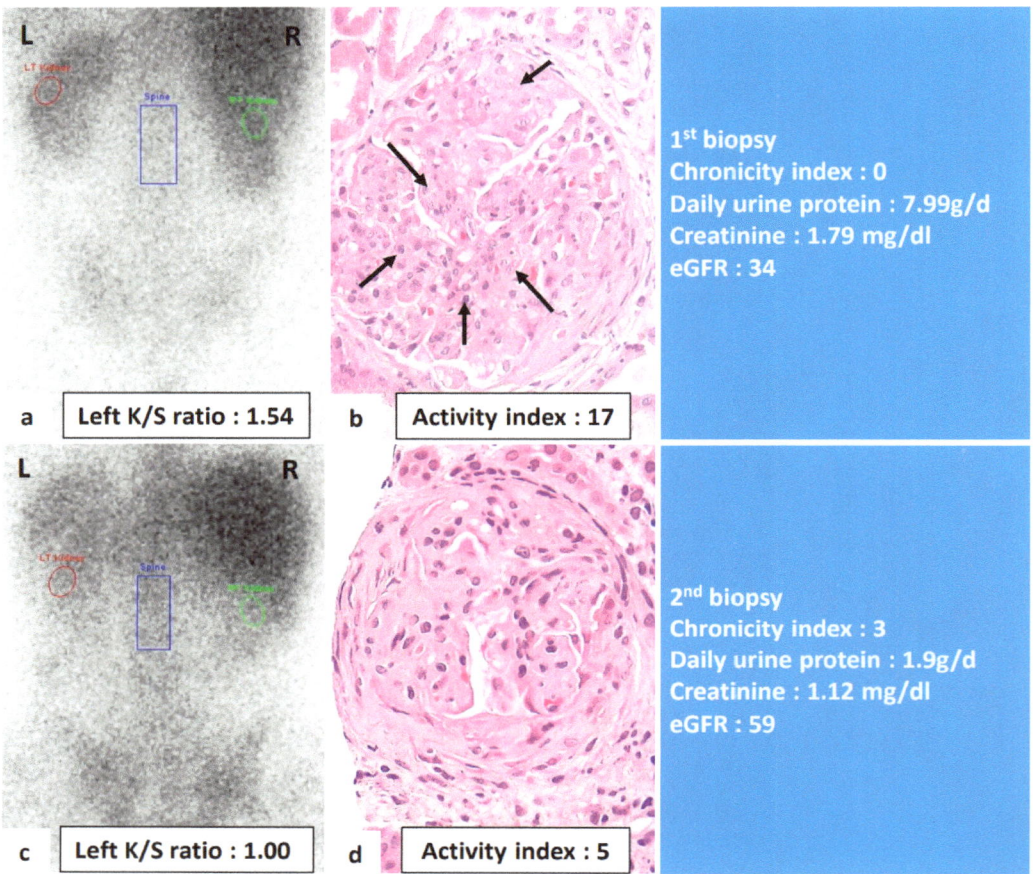

Figure 3. Renal gallium scan and renal histopathologic images in a 36-year-old female with lupus nephritis at diagnosis and one year after immunosuppressant treatment. This figure demonstrated that the change of renal gallium uptake was positively correlated with the change of the inflammatory status in renal histology and clinical proteinuria. (**a,b**) At diagnosis, renal pathology active index score was 17. The Left K/S ratio was 1.54. Daily urine protein was 7.99 g/d. (**c,d**) One year after immunosuppressant treatment, the activity index decreased to 5, left K/S ratio decreased to 1.00. Daily urine protein decreased to 1.9 g/d. L: left side; R: right side; K/S ratio: kidney/spine ratio; arrows: endocapillary hypercellularity.

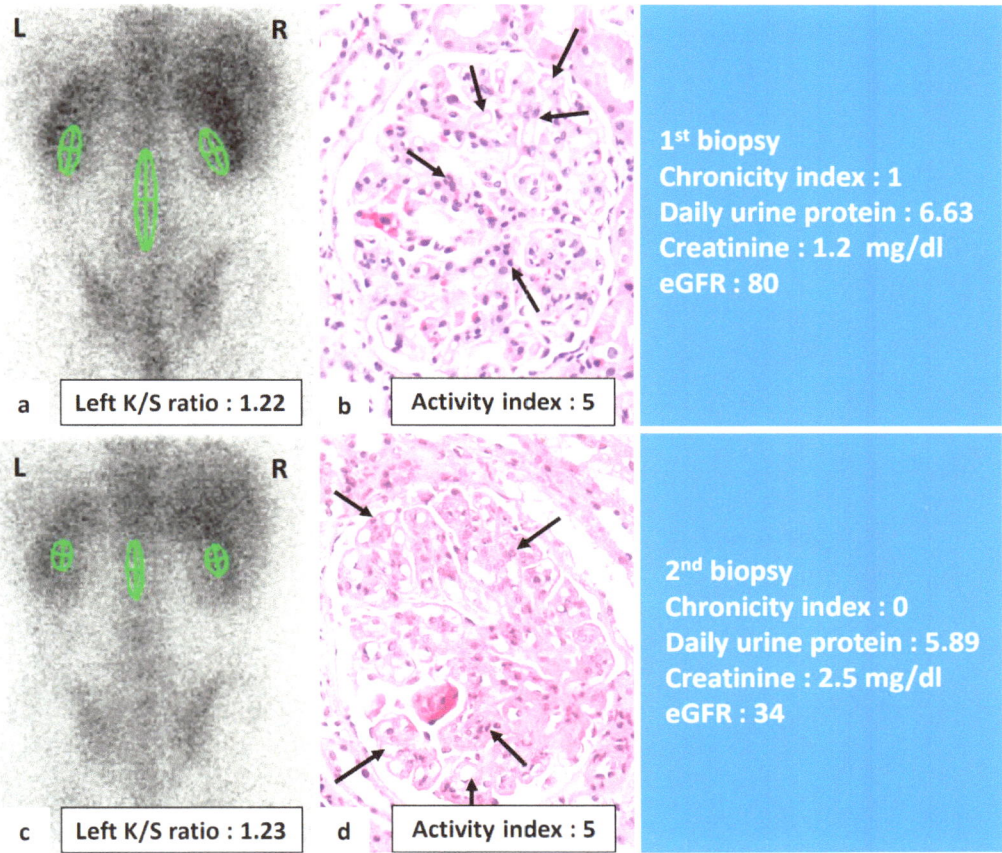

Figure 4. Renal gallium scan and renal histopathologic images of a 22-year-old male with lupus nephritis at diagnosis and two years after immunosuppressant treatment. This figure demonstrated that persistent undiminished gallium uptake was compatible with persistent active inflammation in renal histology and clinical proteinuria. (**a**,**b**) At diagnosis, renal pathologic active index score was 5. The Left K/S ratio was 1.22. Daily urine protein was 6.63 g/d. (**c**,**d**) Two years after immunosuppressant treatment, the activity index remained 5, left K/S ratio was 1.23 without diminished uptake, daily urine protein persisted at a high level of 5.89 g/d. L: left side; R: right side; K/S ratio: kidney/spine ratio; arrows: endocapillary hypercellularity.

Table 4. Correlation of changes in clinical, pathologic parameters and change of renal gallium uptake in 35 SLE patients.

Changes in Variables	Change in Left K/S Ratio	
	r_s	p Value
ΔDaily urine protein (gram)	0.768	<0.001 **
ΔCreatinine (mg/dL)	0.045	0.796
ΔeGFR (mg/mL)	−0.192	0.270
ΔAnti-dsDNA (WHO units/mL)	0.768	0.348
ΔC3 (mg/dL)	0.027	0.888
ΔC4 (mg/dL)	0.022	0.902

Table 4. Cont.

Changes in Variables	Change in Left K/S Ratio	
	r_s	p Value
ΔActivity Index	0.357	0.035 *
ΔCellular crescent	0.258	0.161
ΔFibrinoid necrosis/ Karyorrhexis	0.324	0.075
ΔEndocapillary hypercellularity	0.385	0.032 *
ΔSubendothelial hyaline deposits	0.253	0.017
ΔLeukocyte infiltration	0.390	0.030 *
ΔInterstitial inflammation	0.300	0.101
ΔChronicity Index	−0.106	0.543
ΔGlomerular sclerosis	−0.009	0.961
ΔTubular atrophy	−0.113	0.545
ΔInterstitial fibrosis	−0.070	0.707
ΔFibrous crescent	0.243	0.187

r_s: Spearman's rho coefficient. * $p < 0.05$, ** $p < 0.01$. eGFR: estimated glomerular filtration rate, anti-dsDNA: anti-double-stranded DNA antibody, C3: complement 3, C4: complement 4, K/S ratio: kidney-to-spine ratio.

4. Discussion

This work found that the degree of renal gallium uptake calculating by left K/S ratio was significantly higher in LN class IV than class III. However, not class V. Lt K/S ratio of class V is slightly significantly higher than class III. The activity index of class III was non-significantly higher than class V. From the above result, we could see a trend that renal gallium uptake is associated with active inflammation in LN, but is not sensitive, especially compared to different patients. This is a relatively small number of statistics. Another concern is that eGFR may affect the K/S ratio and reduce its sensitivity in detecting disease activity/inflammation. From Table 1, eGFR is higher in Class III and V groups than in Class IV. The K/S is correspondingly lower in Class III and V groups. Therefore, the gallium uptake and a higher K/S ratio might reflect slower renal clearance of the isotope in patients with reduced excretory renal function. From the previous studies, after administration of Ga-67, excretion of 15% to 25% of the dose occurs through the kidneys in the first 24 h, with the bowel becoming the major route of excretion after that [17]. The gallium image was used after 48 h of gallium administration to diminish the impact of renal function on gallium uptake. Besides, we did not use the absolute kidney gallium uptake value but use the spine as a reference. In theory, if a patient has a poor renal function, higher gallium accumulation in the whole body should be expected, particularly in the liver, spleen, and bones. If a patient has a higher renal inflammation, more gallium uptake is thus expected in the kidney, and this could still be demonstrated by the gallium uptake of Kidney/Spine ratio. By using the K/S ratio, the impact of renal function on gallium uptake might be minimized.

To explore whether eGFR impacts renal gallium uptake, we conducted a linear regression analysis (Table 2). From univariate linear regression analysis, eGFR is associated with left K/S ratio. In the multivariate analysis 1, the activity index is significantly associated with left K/S ratio, and eGFR is not associated with left K/S ratio.

In the pooling analysis of all 35 patients with repeated biopsy, the activity index in the second biopsy was significantly lower than the first biopsy, but the K/S ratio was non-significantly decreased. This may be associated with the increased creatinine level in the second biopsy, resulting in slightly increased gallium uptake. Besides, this was a comparison of all patients together and unable to show the difference between the two biopsies for each patient. Table 4 demonstrated that the changes in gallium uptake between the first and the second biopsies were positively correlated with the changes in histological activity index, the scores of endocapillary hypercellularity, and leukocyte infiltration. The changes in creatinine and eGFR was not correlated with change in gallium uptake. The results shed light on a novel non-invasive assessment for residual renal inflammation in LN patients that may have potential as a substitute for traditional histology exams. As discussed above, a change in creatinine may be potentially confounded by the fact that patients with higher disease activity (predominantly in first biopsy group), which may increase K/S ratio, showed lower serum creatinine (which may decrease K/S ratio).

In this study, we set smaller ROIs of kidney instead of whole kidney, which we used in our previous study in 2010 [11]. There are some reasons we considered. First, strong liver gallium uptake may physiologically mask subtle changes of kidney. Second, the renal collecting systems, such as calyces and pelvis with relative low gallium uptake might underestimate mean counts per pixel if whole kidney was included. Our limitation is the lack of validation between the data of whole kidney ROIs and smaller ROIs.

In 1978, Barry et al. reported that a SLE patient with renal biopsy-proved LN could be evaluated by renal gallium scan. Moreover, scintigraphy of kidneys showed significantly decreased inflammation after high-dose glucocorticoid therapy [18]. BAKIR et al. suggested a high correlation between gallium visualization of the kidneys and active lupus nephritis [19]. They also found that hypertension, nephrotic range proteinuria, and progressive azotemia were more frequently encountered when the gallium scan result was positive. Absolute quantitative and semi-quantitative measurements by gallium scan exhibited good correlation with the activity index of renal biopsy [20]. However, the value of the renal gallium study in evaluating LN following therapies has never been explored. To the best of our knowledge, this study is the first to evaluate the correlation of changes in renal gallium uptake with changes in pathologic parameters based on repeated renal biopsies. In our data, the mean activity index in the second biopsy was significantly decreased, and mean chronicity index was significantly increased compared to the first biopsy. However, no notable changes in class were found in our results. The above findings are compatible with the results of repeat biopsy for LN in previous reports [20–23].

Conventional laboratory markers of urine protein creatinine ratio, creatinine clearance, anti-dsDNA, and complement levels have limitation for monitoring LN, since they might be underpowered to distinguish renal inflammation activity from irreversible chronic renal damage in LN [24]. This is a critical issue, especially when LN patients develop a new onset or progressively elevated serum creatinine or proteinuria during disease monitor. In this scenario, the aggressive immunosuppressant treatment is suitable if active renal inflammation is present but may be harmful to chronic damage without inflammation process. Conventional laboratory markers could tell clinicians the worsening renal function or proteinuria severity but not correlated with active renal inflammation. We currently rely on repeated renal biopsy to differentiate these two processes. However, the renal histology exam is an invasive procedure, which makes it unsuitable for serial monitoring. In addition, there is no universal agreement regarding the indications for repeated renal biopsy in LN patients. It has been advocated that protocol biopsies could be performed at 6 months or after 1-2 years following therapies in stable patients to confirm the response to induction therapy [22,25–30] or to verify the efficacy of maintenance therapy [21,31–33]. Moreover, repeated biopsies could also provide additional valuable information in LN patients with renal flares [20,23,34–36]. Repeated renal biopsy may offer crucial information for challenging LN cases to guide the intensity of treatment in patients with quiescent LN and in those with lupus flare-up. However, due to their invasive nature, renal biopsies can also be physically painful and emotionally distressing. Furthermore, the procedure may be even more risky and challenging in LN patients whose renal function is deteriorating, and who have a thin renal cortex or severe hypertension despite medication, as there is an elevated risk of hemorrhagic complications following renal biopsy [37]. In this scenario, renal gallium scan may have value as a potential alternative to renal biopsy for interrogating the degree of renal inflammation in LN, which could, in turn, facilitate better therapeutic decisions.

A study by A. Alsuwaida et al. demonstrated that the activity index in the second renal biopsy, not the first biopsy, may predict a poor renal outcome. The 10-year renal survival rate was 100% for those with an activity index of 0; 80% for those with an activity index of 1 or 2; and 44% for those with an index of >2 on the second biopsy, regardless of remission status [31]. Similar findings were also shown by Hill GS et al. [25]. They found the rate of serum creatinine doubling was higher among LN patients with persistent active lesions, especially endocapillary proliferation and interstitial inflammation, compared to those with a resolution of active inflammation in the second biopsy. Our study found that changes in gallium uptake measured by left K/S ratio were correlated with changes in active histopathological parameters, including endocapillary proliferation and leukocyte infiltration. These findings indicate that a follow-up renal gallium scan in patients with repeated renal biopsies provided essential information related to kidney inflammation following treatment. In the LN case in our study, shown in Figure 4, the repeated renal biopsy two years after immunosuppressant treatment showed persistent active lesion, especially endocapillary hypercellularity. The repeated renal gallium uptake also remains unchanged without resolution. Finally, the patient's renal function deteriorated, and he received hemodialysis 11 years after diagnosis. Future outcome-based studies, guided by subsequent gallium scan studies, may provide more insights into the potential application of scintigraphy in clinical practice.

It remains unclear why gallium uptake in a positive renal scan was observed in active lupus nephritis patients. This study and other findings indicate that a high degree of renal gallium uptake was observed in patients with high renal activity [19]. In proliferative LN, affected glomeruli display endocapillary proliferation. These lesions are characterized by the deposition of immunoglobulins, complements, and marked influx of pro-inflammatory leukocytes, monocytes, macrophages, and suppressor/cytotoxic T cells, as well as neutrophils infiltration [38]. After gallium injection, one-fourth of the injected dose is excreted by the kidneys within 24 h [17]. Gallium-67 may bind to lactoferrin in neutrophils, are taken up by lysosomes in mononuclear phagocytes, bind directly to the lymphocyte membrane, and transported to sites of inflammatory glomeruli [39]. In this study, endocapillary proliferation and interstitial inflammation were independently positively associated with gallium uptake. The gallium-67 uptake from the proliferated endothelial cells and interstitial neutrophile cells in LN patients might explain the above phenomenon in this study. More basic research may be needed to confirm this finding.

In many areas of clinical practice, gallium scanning has been superseded by PET imaging using FDG and Tc-99 scans, which have several advantages, including a shorter delay between injection of the radioisotope and completing the imaging. However, the patient's steroids are likely to interfere with PET interpretation, especially during the high activity LN patient who received high-dose steroid. Technetium 99m (99mTc)-HMPAO is an agent that complexes avidly with polymorphonuclear leukocytes and has been used to evaluate the areas of acute inflammation. A limitation of this procedure is that 70–80 mL of blood must be drawn from the patient for this technique. This may increase the possible need for a blood transfusion in patients already experiencing anemia, especially in renal insufficiency patients under immunosuppressant agents.

Our study found that the gallium K/S ratio in the right kidney was higher than that in left side in every LN class (Table 1). This is most likely due to the high gallium radioactivity in the normal liver, which may interfere with the calculation of the right K/S ratio. In order to avoid this, we meticulously calculated the left side K/S ratio for subsequent analysis. This concept was initially explored in our previous study on renal gallium scan for evaluating lupus nephritis [11], and the findings of the present study further confirm this interference effect.

Many biomarkers based on laboratory tests have been explored as possible noninvasive methods of evaluating LN [40]. Unfortunately, very few biomarker studies have been done at the time of renal biopsy, and no studies have evaluated the correlation between the change in biomarkers and the change in repeat renal biopsy [40]. This study provides valuable image information between repeated renal biopsies in LN patients.

There were several limitations in the study. First, changes in excretory renal function have an effect on gallium uptake, which may confound some of the findings presented in this work, and limit the sensitivity of this technique in detecting small changes active inflammation. Second, subjective bias in the positioning of the ROI might lead to biased and inconsistent analysis between different patients. Third, the relatively long period of 30 days between kidney biopsy and renal gallium scan used in this study may have implications for how well the scintigraphy findings reflect the histopathological features seen on biopsy in individual patients. Fourth, this was a retrospective study with a limited sample size, and only one ethnic group (East Asians) was included. The results may not be extrapolated to other populations. Further studies using a larger cohort are needed to confirm our findings. Fifth, renal survival and patient survival were not assessed in this study. A recent study indicated that activity scores in LN histology were associated with end-stage renal disease [41]. Whether the degree of renal gallium uptake has a predicting role on renal survival in LN patients needs further study. Sixth, renal gallium uptake cannot distinguish inflammation from other conditions, such as infection (e.g., acute pyelonephritis, renal abscess) and tumor (e.g., lymphoma) [18,42,43]. Clinicians should incorporate other clinical assessments and imaging modalities to reach the final diagnosis if necessary. Finally, it remains unclear how immunosuppressants with different mechanisms of action influence gallium renal uptake. Prospective intervention studies are needed to address this issue.

5. Conclusions

This study demonstrated that renal gallium uptake is associated with pathologic active inflammation in LN but not chronicity damage lesion. The association may be impacted by renal function. Changes in renal gallium uptake positively correlated with changes in activity index in renal pathology. Currently, renal biopsy remains the standard evaluation for lupus nephritis inflammatory activity. However, as a non-invasive tool, renal gallium scan may add value to the personalized care of patients with LN, particularly those with a high risk for biopsy. More researches with large cohorts are needed for further validation.

Author Contributions: Conceptualization, T.-Y.H. and Y.-M.C.; methodology, T.-Y.H., W.-Y.L. and Y.-M.C.; software, Y.-M.C.; validation, T.-Y.H., Y.-M.C., Y.-C.L., M.-C.W. and S.-C.T.; formal analysis, T.-Y.H. and Y.-M.C.; investigation, T.-Y.H., Y.-M.C., Y.-C.L., S.-C.T. and Y.-D.W.; resources, T.-Y.H., Y.-M.C., Y.-C.L. and S.-C.T.; data curation, T.-Y.H., Y.-C.L., W.-T.H., Y.-M.C., M.-C.W., H.-H.C., C.-W.H., C.-T.L., K.-L.L., K.-T.T., C.-W.T., W-N.H., Y.-H.C., S.-C.T. and Y.-D.W.; writing—original and draft preparation, T.-Y.H. Y.-C.L., W.-T.H. and Y.-D.W.; writing—review and editing, T.-Y.H. and Y.-D.W.; visualization, T.-Y.H.; supervision, T.-Y.H.; project administration, T.-Y.H.; funding acquisition, T.-Y.H. All authors have read and agreed to the published version of the manuscript.

Funding: This research received no external funding.

Institutional Review Board Statement: This study was conducted in compliance with the Helsinki Declaration and approval by the Institutional Review Board of Taichung Veterans General Hospital was obtained (CE18210B).

Informed Consent Statement: Because all data were de-identified prior to analysis, the requirement for informed consent from the participants was waived.

Data Availability Statement: Raw data are available from the corresponding author on reasonable request.

Acknowledgments: We would like to thank the Biostatistics Task Force of Taichung Veterans General Hospital for their assistance in performing the statistical analysis.

Conflicts of Interest: The authors declare that they have no competing interests.

References

1. Almaani, S.; Meara, A.; Rovin, B.H. Update on Lupus Nephritis. *Clin. J. Am. Soc. Nephrol.* **2017**, *12*, 825–835. [CrossRef]
2. Houssiau, F.A.; Vasconcelos, C.; D'Cruz, D.; Sebastiani, G.D.; Garrido, E.D.R.; Danieli, M.G.; Abramovicz, D.; Blockmans, D.; Mathieu, A.; Direskeneli, H.; et al. Early response to immunosuppressive therapy predicts good renal outcome in lupus nephritis: Lessons from long-term followup of patients in the Euro-Lupus Nephritis Trial. *Arthritis Rheum.* **2004**, *50*, 3934–3940. [CrossRef] [PubMed]

3. Gladman, D.D.; Urowitz, M.B.; Cole, E.; Ritchie, S.; Chang, C.H.; Churg, J. Kidney Biopsy in SLE. I. A Clinical-Morphologic Evaluation. *QJM Int. J. Med.* **1989**, *73*, 1125–1133.
4. Nossent, J.C.; Henzen-Logmans, S.C.; Vroom, T.M.; Huysen, V.; Berden, J.H.; Swaak, A.J. Relation between serological data at the time of biopsy and renal histology in lupus nephritis. *Rheumatol. Int.* **1991**, *11*, 77–82. [CrossRef] [PubMed]
5. Hahn, B.H.; McMahon, M.A.; Wilkinson, A.; Wallace, W.D.; Daikh, D.I.; FitzGerald, J.; Karpouzas, G.A.; Merrill, J.T.; Wallace, D.J.; Yazdany, J.; et al. American College of Rheumatology guidelines for screening, treatment, and management of lupus nephritis. *Arthritis Rheum.* **2012**, *64*, 797–808. [CrossRef] [PubMed]
6. Corapi, K.M.; Chen, J.L.; Balk, E.M.; Gordon, C.E. Bleeding complications of native kidney biopsy: A systematic review and meta-analysis. *Am. J. Kidney Dis.* **2012**, *60*, 62–73. [CrossRef] [PubMed]
7. Yasuda, K.; Sasaki, K.; Yamato, M.; Rakugi, H.; Isaka, Y.; Hayashi, T. Tubulointerstitial nephritis and uveitis syndrome with transient hyperthyroidism in an elderly patient. *Clin. Exp. Nephrol.* **2011**, *15*, 927–932. [CrossRef] [PubMed]
8. Joaquim, A.I.; Mendes, G.E.; Ribeiro, P.F.; Baptista, M.A.; Burdmann, E.A. Ga-67 scintigraphy in the differential diagnosis between acute interstitial nephritis and acute tubular necrosis: An experimental study. *Nephrol. Dial. Transplant.* **2010**, *25*, 3277–3282. [CrossRef] [PubMed]
9. Lin, W.Y.; Lan, J.L.; Wang, S.J. Gallium-67 scintigraphy to predict response to therapy in active lupus nephritis. *J. Nucl. Med.* **1998**, *39*, 2137–2141.
10. Lin, W.Y.; Lan, J.L.; Cheng, K.Y.; Wang, S.J. Value of gallium-67 scintigraphy in monitoring the renal activity in lupus nephritis. *Scand. J. Rheumatol.* **1998**, *27*, 42–45.
11. Lin, W.Y.; Hsieh, J.F.; Tsai, S.C.; Lan, J.L.; Cheng, K.Y.; Wang, S.J. Semi-quantitative evaluation of gallium-67 scintigraphy in lupus nephritis. *Eur. J. Nucl. Med.* **2000**, *27*, 1626–1631. [CrossRef]
12. Levey, A.S.; Bosch, J.P.; Lewis, J.B.; Greene, T.; Rogers, N.; Roth, D. A more accurate method to estimate glomerular filtration rate from serum creatinine: A new prediction equation. Modification of Diet in Renal Disease Study Group. *Ann. Intern. Med.* **1999**, *130*, 461–470. [CrossRef]
13. Weening, J.J.; D'Agati, V.D.; Schwartz, M.M.; Seshan, S.V.; Alpers, C.E.; Appel, G.B.; Balow, J.E.; Bruijn, J.A.; Cook, T.; Ferrario, F.; et al. The classification of glomerulonephritis in systemic lupus erythematosus revisited. *J. Am. Soc. Nephrol.* **2004**, *15*, 241–250. [CrossRef]
14. Austin, H.A., 3rd; Boumpas, D.T.; Vaughan, E.M.; Balow, J.E. Predicting renal outcomes in severe lupus nephritis: Contributions of clinical and histologic data. *Kidney Int.* **1994**, *45*, 544–550. [CrossRef]
15. Contreras, G.; Pardo, V.; Cely, C.; Borja, E.; Hurtado, A.; De La Cuesta, C.; Iqbal, K.; Lenz, O.; Asif, A.; Nahar, N.; et al. Factors associated with poor outcomes in patients with lupus nephritis. *Lupus* **2005**, *14*, 890–895. [CrossRef]
16. Zappitelli, M.; Duffy, C.M.; Bernard, C.; Gupta, I.R. Evaluation of activity, chronicity and tubulointerstitial indices for childhood lupus nephritis. *Pediatr. Nephrol.* **2008**, *23*, 83–91. [CrossRef] [PubMed]
17. Seabold, J.E.; Palestro, C.J.; Brown, M.L.; Datz, F.L.; Forstrom, L.A.; Greenspan, B.S.; McAfee, J.G.; Schauwecker, D.S.; Royal, H.D. Procedure guideline for gallium scintigraphy in inflammation. Society of Nuclear Medicine. *J. Nucl. Med.* **1997**, *38*, 994–997. [PubMed]
18. Wood, B.C.; Sharma, J.N.; Germann, D.R.; Wood, W.G.; Crouch, T.T. Gallium citrate Ga 67 imaging in noninfectious interstitial nephritis. *Arch. Intern. Med.* **1978**, *138*, 1665–1666. [CrossRef] [PubMed]
19. Bakir, A.A.; Lopez-Majano, V.; Hryhorczuk, D.O.; Rhee, H.L.; Dunea, G. Appraisal of lupus nephritis by renal imaging with gallium-67. *Am. J. Med.* **1985**, *79*, 175–182. [CrossRef]
20. Daleboudt, G.M.; Bajema, I.M.; Goemaere, N.N.; van Laar, J.M.; Bruijn, J.A.; Berger, S.P. The clinical relevance of a repeat biopsy in lupus nephritis flares. *Nephrol. Dial. Transplant.* **2009**, *24*, 3712–3717. [CrossRef]
21. Esdaile, J.M.; Joseph, L.; MacKenzie, T.; Kashgarian, M.; Hayslett, J.P. The pathogenesis and prognosis of lupus nephritis: Information from repeat renal biopsy. *Semin. Arthritis Rheum.* **1993**, *23*, 135–148. [CrossRef]
22. Zickert, A.; Sundelin, B.; Svenungsson, E.; Gunnarsson, I. Role of early repeated renal biopsies in lupus nephritis. *Lupus Sci. Med.* **2014**, *1*, e000018. [CrossRef]
23. Bajaj, S.; Albert, L.; Gladman, D.D.; Urowitz, M.B.; Hallett, D.C.; Ritchie, S. Serial renal biopsy in systemic lupus erythematosus. *J. Rheumatol.* **2000**, *27*, 2822–2826. [PubMed]
24. Mok, C.C. Biomarkers for lupus nephritis: A critical appraisal. *J. Biomed. Biotechnol.* **2010**, *2010*, 638413. [CrossRef] [PubMed]
25. Hill, G.S.; Delahousse, M.; Nochy, D.; Remy, P.; Mignon, F.; Mery, J.P.; Bariéty, J. Predictive power of the second renal biopsy in lupus nephritis: Significance of macrophages. *Kidney Int.* **2001**, *59*, 304–316. [CrossRef] [PubMed]
26. Gunnarsson, I.; Sundelin, B.; Heimburger, M.; Forslid, J.; van Vollenhoven, R.; Lundberg, I.; Jacobson, S.H. Repeated renal biopsy in proliferative lupus nephritis—predictive role of serum C1q and albuminuria. *J. Rheumatol.* **2002**, *29*, 693–699.
27. Askenazi, D.; Myones, B.; Kamdar, A.; Warren, R.; Perez, M.; De Guzman, M.; Minta, A.; Hicks, M.J.; Kale, A. Outcomes of children with proliferative lupus nephritis: The role of protocol renal biopsy. *Pediatr. Nephrol.* **2007**, *22*, 981–986. [CrossRef]
28. Alvarado, A.; Malvar, A.; Lococo, B.; Alberton, V.; Toniolo, F.; Nagaraja, H.; Rovin, B. The value of repeat kidney biopsy in quiescent Argentinian lupus nephritis patients. *Lupus* **2014**, *23*, 840–847. [CrossRef]
29. Singh, A.; Ghosh, R.; Kaur, P.; Golay, V.; Pandey, R.; Roychowdhury, A. Protocol renal biopsy in patients with lupus nephritis: A single center experience. *Saudi J. Kidney Dis. Transpl.* **2014**, *25*, 801–807. [CrossRef]

30. Malvar, A.; Pirruccio, P.; Alberton, V.; Lococo, B.; Recalde, C.; Fazini, B.; Nagaraja, H.; Indrakanti, D.; Rovin, B.H. Histologic versus clinical remission in proliferative lupus nephritis. *Nephrol. Dial. Transplant.* **2017**, *32*, 1338–1344. [CrossRef]
31. Alsuwaida, A.; Husain, S.; Alghonaim, M.; AlOudah, N.; Alwakeel, J.; Ullah, A.; Kfoury, H. Strategy for second kidney biopsy in patients with lupus nephritis. *Nephrol. Dial. Transplant.* **2011**, *27*, 1472–1478. [CrossRef] [PubMed]
32. Stoenoiu, M.S.; Aydin, S.; Tektonidou, M.; Ravelingien, I.; le Guern, V.; Fiehn, C.; Remy, P.; Delahousse, M.; Petera, P.; Quémeneur, T.; et al. Repeat kidney biopsies fail to detect differences between azathioprine and mycophenolate mofetil maintenance therapy for lupus nephritis: Data from the MAINTAIN Nephritis Trial. *Nephrol. Dial. Transplant.* **2012**, *27*, 1924–1930. [CrossRef]
33. Grootscholten, C.; Bajema, I.M.; Florquin, S.; Steenbergen, E.J.; Peutz-Kootstra, C.J.; Goldschmeding, R.; Bijl, M.; Hagen, E.C.; van Houwelingen, H.C.; Derksen, R.H.W.M.; et al. Treatment with cyclophosphamide delays the progression of chronic lesions more effectively than does treatment with azathioprine plus methylprednisolone in patients with proliferative lupus nephritis. *Arthritis Rheum.* **2007**, *56*, 924–937. [CrossRef]
34. Moroni, G.; Pasquali, S.; Quaglini, S.; Banfi, G.; Casanova, S.; Maccario, M.; Zucchelli, P.; Ponticelli, C. Clinical and prognostic value of serial renal biopsies in lupus nephritis. *Am. J. Kidney Dis.* **1999**, *34*, 530–539. [CrossRef]
35. Wang, G.B.; Xu, Z.J.; Liu, H.F.; Zhou, Q.G.; Zhou, Z.M.; Jia, N. Changes in pathological pattern and treatment regimens based on repeat renal biopsy in lupus nephritis. *Chin. Med. J.* **2012**, *125*, 2890–2894. [PubMed]
36. Greloni, G.; Scolnik, M.; Marin, J.; Lancioni, E.; Quiroz, C.; Zacariaz, J.; Niveyro, P.D.L.I.; Christiansen, S.; Pierangelo, A.M.; Varela, C.F.; et al. Value of repeat biopsy in lupus nephritis flares. *Lupus Sci. Med.* **2014**, *1*, e000004. [CrossRef] [PubMed]
37. Moroni, G.; Depetri, F.; Ponticelli, C. Lupus nephritis: When and how often to biopsy and what does it mean? *J. Autoimmun.* **2016**, *74*, 27–40. [CrossRef] [PubMed]
38. Akashi, Y.; Oshima, S.; Takeuchi, A.; Kubota, T.; Shimizu, J.; Shimizu, E.; Ishida, A.; Nakabayashi, I.; Nishiyama, J.; Tazawa, K.; et al. Identification and analysis of immune cells infiltrating into the glomerulus and interstitium in lupus nephritis. *Nihon Rinsho Meneki Gakkai Kaishi.* **1995**, *18*, 545–551. [CrossRef] [PubMed]
39. Tsan, M.F. Mechanism of gallium-67 accumulation in inflammatory lesions. *J. Nucl. Med.* **1985**, *26*, 88–92. [PubMed]
40. Soliman, S.; Mohan, C. Lupus nephritis biomarkers. *Clin. Immunol.* **2017**, *185*, 10–20. [CrossRef]
41. Chen, Y.-M.; Hung, W.T.; Liao, Y.W.; Hsu, C.Y.; Hsieh, T.-Y.; Chen, H.H.; Hsieh, C.W.; Lin, C.T.; Lai, K.L.; Tang, K.T.; et al. Combination immunosuppressant therapy and lupus nephritis outcome: A hospital-based study. *Lupus* **2019**, *28*, 658–666. [CrossRef] [PubMed]
42. Yen, T.C.; Tzen, K.Y.; Chen, W.P.; Lin, C.Y. The value of Ga-67 renal SPECT in diagnosing and monitoring complete and incomplete treatment in children with acute pyelonephritis. *Clin. Nucl. Med.* **1999**, *24*, 669–673. [CrossRef] [PubMed]
43. Taniguchi, M.; Higashi, K.; Ohguchi, M.; Okimura, T.; Yamamoto, I. Gallium-67-citrate scintigraphy of primary renal lymphoma. *Ann. Nucl. Med.* **1998**, *12*, 51–53. [CrossRef] [PubMed]

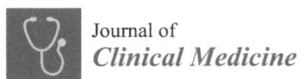

Article

Lack of Association between Serum Interleukin-23 and Interleukin-27 Levels and Disease Activity in Patients with Active Systemic Lupus Erythematosus

Katarzyna Pawlak-Buś [1,2,*], Wiktor Schmidt [1,2] and Piotr Leszczyński [1,2]

[1] Department of Rheumatology, Rehabilitation and Internal Medicine, Poznań University of Medical Sciences, 61-701 Poznań, Poland; wiktorpawelschmidt@gmail.com (W.S.); piotr_leszczynski@wp.pl (P.L.)
[2] Department of Rheumatology and Osteoporosis, J. Struś Municipal Hospital in Poznań, 61-285 Poznań, Poland
* Correspondence: k.bus@makabu.net

Abstract: Systemic lupus erythematosus (SLE) is a chronic systemic autoimmune disease characterized by the production of multiple autoantibodies, resulting in tissue and organ damage. Recent studies have revealed that interleukin-23 (IL-23) and interleukin-27 (IL-27) may be therapeutically relevant in selected SLE manifestations. This study aimed to identify associations between serum IL-27 and IL-23 levels and disease activity in Polish patients with different manifestations of SLE: neuropsychiatric lupus (NPSLE), and lupus nephritis (LN). Associations between interleukin levels and oligo-specific antibodies against double-stranded DNA (dsDNA), dose of glucocorticoids, and type of treatment were also analyzed. An enzyme-linked immunosorbent assay was used to assess anti-dsDNA antibodies and analyze the serum concentration of IL-27 and IL-23 from 72 patients aged 19–74 years with confirmed active SLE. Disease activity was measured using the Systemic Lupus Erythematosus Disease Activity Index 2000 (SLEDAI 2-K). No significant correlations between interleukin levels and SLEDAI score, anti-dsDNA, corticosteroid dose, or type of treatment were noted. Patients with NPSLE and LN presented the highest median scores of SLEDAI.

Keywords: systemic lupus erythematosus; neuropsychiatric lupus; interleukin-23; interleukin-27; SLEDAI

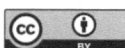

1. Introduction

Systemic lupus erythematosus (SLE) is a complex autoimmune disease with unclear pathogenesis that causes systemic inflammation [1]. Dysfunction of the immune system involves the production of multiple autoantibodies and the formation and deposition of immune complexes. This contributes to damage to various organs [2], including the kidneys and both the central and peripheral nervous systems [3]. Consequently, two common SLE manifestations are neuropsychiatric lupus (NPSLE) and lupus nephritis (LN). Lupus nephritis, observed in ~30% of SLE patients [4], is the primary SLE complication [5]. The prevalence of NPSLE varies widely, as it is estimated that it may affect between 37% and 95% of SLE patients [6]. Up to 75% of adult and pediatric patients with SLE will experience various disabling effects of NPSLE that impact their quality of life and prognosis [7]. In Poland, the population of treated SLE patients is highly stable, at ~20,000 per year [8].

In recent years, an increasing number of authors have analyzed the role of cytokines in the pathogenesis of SLE [9–14]. It has been shown that crucial features of SLE's pathogenesis and progression include aberrations in the T-lymphocyte compartment and abnormal cytokine production [15]. Interleukin-23 (IL-23) and interleukin-27 (IL-27) regulate T helper 1 (Th1)-cell responses. IL-23 plays an important role in autoimmune inflammation by stimulating a unique T-cell subset to produce interleukin-17 (IL-17) [16,17]. In contrast, IL-27 is responsible for the reduction in the intensity and duration of adaptive immune responses [18,19]. Some studies have shown that IL-27 controls the development of T helper 17 (Th17) cells, which are implicated in the pathogenesis of SLE [20]. Moreover, the elevated gene expression of IL-27 was found in immune cells from SLE patients with a high type I interferon (I-IFN) signature, which further confirms the importance of IL-27 in SLE [21].

The role of both interleukins in the pathogenesis of SLE, their association with disease activity, and their therapeutic potential have been analyzed over the past decade; however, these studies were based on small sample sizes, and provided inconsistent results [20,22–28]. In patients with SLE, it was shown that serum IL-23 concentration is higher [24–27] and IL-27 concentration is lower when compared to healthy controls [20,23]. Most authors found a positive correlation between IL-23 concentration and disease activity [24,28], and a lack of correlation between IL-27 levels and disease activity [20]. Higher levels of IL-23 were also associated with LN [24,25,27]. Vukelic et al. found that increased IL-23 levels are characteristic of patients with LN, but also patients with non-renal lupus. Furthermore, they observed the correlation between increased levels of IL-23 and positive anti-dsDNA antibodies and/or low C3 levels [28]. Interestingly, Xia et al. showed that both IL-23 and IL-27 urine levels were significantly correlated with the renal SLE Disease Activity Index (SLEDAI) [26]. On the other hand, Li et al. and Gaber et al. reported a negative association of IL-27 levels and the occurrence of LN [20,23]. These results suggest that the concentration of both interleukins may be more significantly associated with disease activity in patients with LN. To the best of our knowledge, there are no similar analyses for patients with NPSLE.

The primary aim of this study was to identify associations between serum IL-27 and IL-23 levels and disease activity in Polish patients with different manifestations of SLE (LN and NPSLE). We also assessed the association between interleukin levels and oligo-specific antibodies against double-stranded DNA (dsDNA), the dose of glucocorticoids (GCs), and the type of treatment in the analyzed groups of patients.

2. Materials and Methods

2.1. Diagnostic Criteria

Patients were considered eligible for the study if they fulfilled the criteria of the American College of Rheumatology (ACR) classification for SLE [29], and if they were diagnosed as having clinically active SLE qualifying for treatment. According to the ACR and the European League Against Rheumatism (EULAR) [30], one of the criteria of SLE is positive antinuclear antibodies (ANAs) at a titer of 1:80 or greater [31]. Another biomarker of SLE is the presence of oligo-specific antibodies against dsDNA at a nominal value of 100 units/ampoule (WHO Reference Reagent for lupus) [32].

The diagnostics included the profile of autoantibodies determined via indirect immunofluorescence assay (IIFA) and sandwich enzyme-linked immunosorbent assay (ELISA).

Lupus nephritis was confirmed via kidney involvement (proteinuria, active urine sediment) and/or kidney biopsy; NPSLE was confirmed via neuropsychiatric manifestations under the 1999 ACR nomenclature [33].

2.2. Methodology

This is a retrospective, cross-sectional study. Clinical information was assessed with the application of a questionnaire that included:

- Demographic data (age, sex);
- Medical history/clinical data;
- Current treatment;
- Laboratory results (titer and profile of ANAs [31], anti-dsDNA [34], complement components C3 and C4 concentrations, and serum IL-23 and IL-27 concentrations);
- Measurements (morphology, biochemistry, urinalysis, daily proteinuria);
- Disease activity measured with the Systemic Lupus Erythematosus Disease Activity Index 2000 (SLEDAI 2-K) [35,36], Physician Global Assessment (PGA) [37], and

organ damage determined using the Systemic Lupus International Collaborating Clinics/American College of Rheumatology (SLICC/ACR) Damage Index (SDI) [38].

The SLEDAI is a global index for the assessment of lupus disease activity in the previous 10 days; it consists of 24 weighted clinical and laboratory variables of 9 organ systems. The scores of the descriptors range from 1 to 8, and the total possible score for all 24 descriptors is 105 [36].

The PGA is a visual analogue score, recommended in the recent European League Against Rheumatism (EULAR) guidelines [39], for evaluating disease activity, treatment response, and remission in SLE [37].

The SLICC/ACR DI was used to measure damage—defined as irreversible organ dysfunction, present for 6 months or longer, regardless of etiology—in all organ systems. The SLICC/ACR DI was calculated based on organ damage accumulated since the onset of SLE up until the last visit [38].

2.3. Immunoassays

Blood samples were collected from patients during their admission to the hospital due to SLE activity, and immediately frozen at a temperature below 70 °C, then thawed and measured without repeated freeze/thawing. All of these activities were performed under standardized conditions to enable direct comparison of the results.

IgG ANAs were assessed in the HEp-2 cell line using the IIFA technique. Anti-dsDNA antibodies were assessed via monospecific sandwich ELISA tests. Concentrations of serum interleukins were measured via ELISA, using the Human IL-23 Quantikine ELISA Kit (R&D Systems) and Invitrogen™ eBioscience™ Human IL-27 Platinum ELISA Kit according to their respective manuals. The reaction results were measured using an EPOCH BioTek plate reader spectrophotometer at 450 nm, and calculated as pg/mL.

2.4. Statistics

Data distribution was checked using the Shapiro–Wilk test. Data with normal distribution were presented as mean ± SD, and non-parametrical data were presented as median and range. Differences in selected parameters between two groups of patients were assessed using Student's *t*-test or the Mann–Whitney test. One-way analysis of variance or the Kruskal–Wallis test were used to determine whether there were significant differences in the analyzed parameters between patients with different SLE manifestations. Spearman's correlation was applied to assess associations between measures. Logistic regression was used to calculate the odds ratios (ORs) and 95% confidence intervals (CIs) for selected determinants concerning disease activity in the whole group of patients, and in selected groups of patients with LN and NPSLE. STATISTICA 12 (StatSoft Inc., Tulsa, OK, USA) and R 4.0.2 (R Statistics) software were used.

2.5. Ethics

This study obtained approval from the Bioethical Committee of the Poznań University of Medical Sciences (no. 107/21).

3. Results

3.1. Patient Characteristics

A total of 144 Caucasian patients from the Department of Rheumatology and Osteoporosis, Józef Struś Specialist Municipal Hospital, Poznań, Poland were screened. Results of 72 patients aged 19–74 years with confirmed active SLE (NPSLE—29%; LN—22%; NPSLE + LN—7%; non-LN and non-NPSLE—42%) were included in the statistical analysis. Details concerning clinical characteristics are presented in Table 1. Patients were treated with chloroquine (CQ, $n = 47$, 65%), hydroxychloroquine (HCQ, $n = 13$, 18%), glucocorticoids (GCs, $n = 59$, 82%) (<7.5 mg, $n = 28$, 7.5–10 mg, $n = 13$, >10 mg, $n = 16$), and the following immunosuppressant medications (IS, $n = 58$, 81%): cyclophosphamide (CTX, $n = 10$, 14%), mycophenolate mofetil (MMF, $n = 16$, 22%), methotrexate (MTX, $n = 6$, 8%), azathioprine (AZA, n = 21, 29%), and cyclosporine A (CsA, n = 5, 7%). Among 21 patients with LN (16 with LN, 5 with LN and NPSLE), 7 had renal biopsy (n = 3, class III nephritis; and n = 4, class IV nephritis). Antiphospholipid syndrome was confirmed in 6 (8%) patients, whereas antiphospholipid antibodies were confirmed in 11 (15%).

Table 1. Clinical characteristics of the study group and neuropsychiatric lupus/lupus nephritis subgroups.

Variables	All Patients	Non-LN and Non-NPSLE	NPSLE	LN	NPSLE + LN	p
n	72	30	21	16	5	-
Sex (♂/♀)	4/68	2/28	2/19	0/16	0/5	0.39
Age (mean ± SD) (years)	42.9 ± 13.3	47.7 ± 12.2	38.3 ± 11.4	42.1 ± 14.6	36.4 ± 16.9	<0.05
Age at disease onset (mean ± SD) (years)	36.5 ± 12.6	41.9 ± 10.8	32.5 ± 10.7	33.6 ± 14.4	29.4 ± 14.8	<0.05
Disease duration (median, min–max) (years)	5, 1–20	5, 1–12	4, 1–15	5, 1–20	7, 1–12	0.78
Fever (yes/no)	4/68	0/30	1/20	2/14	1/4	0.12
Lupus rash (yes/no)	53/19	22/8	5/16	4/12	2/3	0.91
Alopecia (yes/no)	45/27	19/11	12/9	12/4	2/3	0.49
Mucosal ulcers (yes/no)	5/67	0/30	2/19	2/14	1/4	0.11
Arthritis (yes/no)	53/19	21/9	15/6	13/3	4/1	0.83
Myositis (yes/no)	0/72	0/30	0/21	0/16	0/5	-
Psychosis (yes/no)	4/68	0/30	4/17	0/16	5/0	<0.05
Organic brain syndrome (yes/no)	25/47	0/30	21/0	0/16	4/1	<0.001
Cranial nerves disorder (yes/no)	1/71	0/30	1/20	0/16	0/5	0.48
Vision disturbances (yes/no)	1/71	0/30	1/20	0/16	0/5	0.48
Lupus headache (yes/no)	6/66	0/30	5/16	0/16	1/4	<0.01
Cerebrovascular accident (yes/no)	2/70	0/30	1/20	0/16	1/4	0.16
Vasculitis (yes/no)	11/61	2/28	4/17	3/13	2/3	0.24
Pleuritis (yes/no)	4/68	0/30	2/19	0/16	2/3	<0.05
Pericarditis (yes/no)	2/70	0/30	0/21	1/15	1/4	0.12
Active urinary sediment (yes/no)	3/69	0/30	0/21	1/15	2/3	<0.05
Hematuria (yes/no)	2/70	0/30	0/21	0/16	2/3	<0.01
Proteinuria (yes/no)	18/54	0/30	0/21	13/3	5/0	<0.001
Leukocyturia (yes/no)	7/65	0/30	0/21	5/11	2/3	<0.001
Leukopenia (yes/no)	11/61	4/26	5/16	1/15	1/4	0.48
Thrombocytopenia (yes/no)	9/63	4/26	1/20	2/14	2/3	0.28

NPSLE: neuropsychiatric lupus; LN: lupus nephritis.

3.2. Disease Activity and Laboratory Test Results

Table 2 presents the analysis of variance for disease assessment, laboratory results, and interleukin levels in the whole study group and in the NPSLE/LN subgroups. There were significant differences in SLEDAI and PGA scores between patients with different manifestations, i.e., patients with NPSLE and LN presented the highest median scores of SLEDAI and PGA. There were no significant differences in the other measured variables.

Table 2. Disease assessment, laboratory test results, and interleukin levels in the study group and neuropsychiatric lupus/lupus nephritis subgroups.

Variables	All Patients	Non-LN and Non-NPSLE	NPSLE	LN	NPSLE + LN	p
SLEDAI (median, min–max) (points)	14, 2–55	8, 2–20	24, 12–36	15, 8–27	32, 26–55	<0.001
PGA (median, min–max) (points)	1, 0–3	1, 0–3	2, 0–3	1, 0–3	3, 0–3	<0.05
SDI (yes/no)	30/42	11/19	8/13	9/7	2/3	0.61
Low C3/C4 (yes/no)	36/36	13/17	11/10	11/5	1/4	0.19
Elevated anti-dsDNA (yes/no)	49/23	16/14	16/5	12/4	5/0	0.05
Elevated anti-dsDNA and low C3/C4 (yes/no)	33/39	11/19	10/11	10/6	2/3	0.41
IL-23 (median, min–max) (pg/mL)	1.18, 0.11–3.28	1.16, 0.11–2.67	1.23, 0.16–3.19	1.06, 0.14–3.28	0.96, 0.46–3.15	0.70
IL-27 (median, min–max) (pg/mL)	0.09, 0.07–0.26	0.09, 0.07–0.16	0.09, 0.08–0.26	0.09, 0.07–0.14	0.10, 0.08–0.12	0.47

NPSLE: neuropsychiatric lupus; LN: lupus nephritis; SLEDAI: Systemic Lupus Erythematosus Disease Activity Index; PGA: Physician Global Assessment; SDI: Systemic Lupus International Collaborating Clinics/American College of Rheumatology (SLICC/ACR) Damage Index; anti-dsDNA: autoantibodies against double-stranded DNA; IL: interleukin.

3.3. Determinants of Disease Activity and Different Disease Manifestations

The independent variables that were associated with SLEDAI scores in the whole group of patients were age at disease onset, decreased C3/C4, and anti-dsDNA (Table 3).

Table 3. Determinants of disease activity in the whole group of patients.

		SLEDAI Score (Points)		Odds Ratio		
Determinant	n	1–11, n = 27 n (%)	≥12, n = 45 n (%)	OR	95% CI	p
Disease duration (years)	72					0.33
[1, 4]		9 (33%)	23 (51%)	—	—	
(4, 7.57]		7 (26%)	9 (20%)	0.50	0.14, 1.78	
(7.57, 20]		11 (41%)	13 (29%)	0.46	0.15, 1.40	
Age at disease onset (years) median (IQR)	72	42 (39, 50)	35 (22, 43)	0.94	0.90, 0.98	<0.01
IL-27 (pg/mL)	72					0.29
[0.067, 0.0837]		12 (44%)	12 (27%)	—	—	
(0.0837, 0.0983]		7 (26%)	17 (38%)	2.43	0.75, 8.31	
(0.0983, 0.255]		8 (30%)	16 (36%)	2.00	0.63, 6.62	
IL-23 (pg/mL)	72					0.10
[0.112, 0.776]		13 (48%)	11 (24%)	—	—	
(0.776, 1.55]		6 (22%)	18 (40%)	3.55	1.08, 12.8	
(1.55, 3.28]		8 (30%)	16 (36%)	2.36	0.75, 7.87	
Decreased C3/C4	72					<0.01
No		19 (70%)	17 (38%)	—	—	
Yes		8 (30%)	28 (62%)	3.91	1.45, 11.4	
Anti-dsDNA	72					<0.001
No		15 (56%)	8 (18%)	—	—	
Yes		12 (44%)	37 (82%)	5.78	2.03, 17.8	

SLEDAI: Systemic Lupus Erythematosus Disease Activity Index; OR: odds ratio; CI: confidence interval; anti-dsDNA: autoantibodies against double-stranded DNA; IL: interleukin.

A total of 24 patients (NPSLE = 7; LN = 7; NPSLE and LN = 1; non-LN and non-NPSLE = 9) presented cutaneous and musculoskeletal manifestations. The SLEDAI score (median, range) in this group was 17.5 (8.0–36.0), and in selected subgroups, was as follows: NPSLE = 26.0 (17.0–36.0); LN = 16.0 (12.0–27.0); non-LN and non-NPSLE = 12.0 (8.0–20.0).

There were no significant independent variables associated with the presence of LN (Table 4). Age at disease onset was the only significant determinant associated with the presence of NPSLE (Table 5).

Table 4. Determinants of disease activity in a group of LN patients.

Determinant	n	LN		Odds Ratio		
		0, n = 51 n (%)	1, n = 21 n (%)	OR	95% CI	p
Disease duration (years)	72					0.84
[1, 4]		23 (45%)	9 (43%)	—	—	
(4, 7.57]		12 (24%)	4 (19%)	0.85	0.20, 3.23	
(7.57, 20]		16 (31%)	8 (38%)	1.28	0.40, 4.06	
Age at disease onset (years) median (IQR)	72	40 (31, 44)	28 (21, 45)	0.97	0.92, 1.01	0.09
IL-27 (pg/mL)	72					0.82
[0.067, 0.0837]		18 (35%)	6 (29%)	—	—	
(0.0837, 0.0983]		17 (33%)	7 (33%)	1.24	0.34, 4.56	
(0.0983, 0.255]		16 (31%)	8 (38%)	1.50	0.43, 5.46	
IL-23 (pg/mL)	72					0.82
[0.112, 0.776]		17 (33%)	7 (33%)	—	—	
(0.776, 1.55]		16 (31%)	8 (38%)	1.21	0.36, 4.22	
(1.55, 3.28]		18 (35%)	6 (29%)	0.81	0.22, 2.92	
Decreased C3/C4	72					0.44
No		27 (53%)	9 (43%)	—	—	
Yes		24 (47%)	12 (57%)	1.50	0.54, 4.27	
Anti-dsDNA	72					0.12
No		19 (37%)	4 (19%)	—	—	
Yes		32 (63%)	17 (81%)	2.52	0.79, 9.76	

OR: odds ratio; CI: confidence interval; anti-dsDNA: autoantibodies against double-stranded DNA; IL: interleukin, 0 = patients without LN, 1 = patients with LN.

Table 5. Determinants of disease activity in a group of NPSLE patients.

Determinant	n	NPSLE		Odds Ratio		
		0, n = 46 n (%)	1, n = 26 n (%)	OR	95% CI	p
Disease duration (years)	72					0.55
[1, 4]		19 (41%)	13 (50%)	—	—	
(4, 7.57]		12 (26%)	4 (15%)	0.49	0.12, 1.76	
(7.57, 20]		15 (33%)	9 (35%)	0.88	0.29, 2.59	

Table 5. Cont.

Determinant	n	NPSLE		Odds Ratio		
		0, n = 46 n (%)	1, n = 26 n (%)	OR	95% CI	p
Age at disease onset (years) median (IQR)	72	42 (31, 48)	32 (22, 39)	0.95	0.91, 0.99	<0.05
IL-27 (pg/mL)	72					0.31
[0.067, 0.0837]		18 (39%)	6 (23%)	—	—	
(0.0837, 0.0983]		13 (28%)	11 (42%)	2.54	0.76, 9.09	
(0.0983, 0.255]		15 (33%)	9 (35%)	1.80	0.53, 6.49	
IL-23 (pg/mL)	72					0.37
[0.112, 0.776]		18 (39%)	6 (23%)	—	—	
(0.776, 1.55]		14 (30%)	10 (38%)	2.14	0.64, 7.69	
(1.55, 3.28]		14 (30%)	10 (38%)	2.14	0.64, 7.69	
Decreased C3/C4	72					0.62
No		22 (48%)	14 (54%)	—	—	
Yes		24 (52%)	12 (46%)	0.79	0.30, 2.06	
Anti-dsDNA	72					0.08
No		18 (39%)	5 (19%)	—	—	
Yes		28 (61%)	21 (81%)	2.70	0.91, 9.24	

OR: odds ratio, CI: confidence interval; 0 = patients without NPSLE, 1 = patients with NPSLE.

3.4. Association between IL-23/IL-27 Levels and Disease Activity

Figures 1 and 2 present associations between serum IL-23 and IL-27 levels, respectively, and disease activity in the whole group of patients, as well as in selected subgroups with different SLE manifestations. There were no significant correlations between interleukin levels and SLEDAI scores in the whole group, nor in the subgroups.

To employ multiple tools of disease activity measurement, we checked the associations between serum IL-23 and IL-27 levels and SLEDAI scores in patients with PGA > 0. We found no correlation—R was 0.04 ($p = 0.79$) for IL-23, and R was 0.13 ($p = 0.352$) for IL-27.

Furthermore, there was no significant correlation between interleukin levels and anti-dsDNA (Supplementary Materials, Figure S1).

3.5. Associatiosn between IL-23 Levels, IL-27 Levels, dsDNA, and Complement C3/C4 Components

There were no associations between elevated anti-dsDNA and low C3/C4, IL-23, or IL-27 (Table 6).

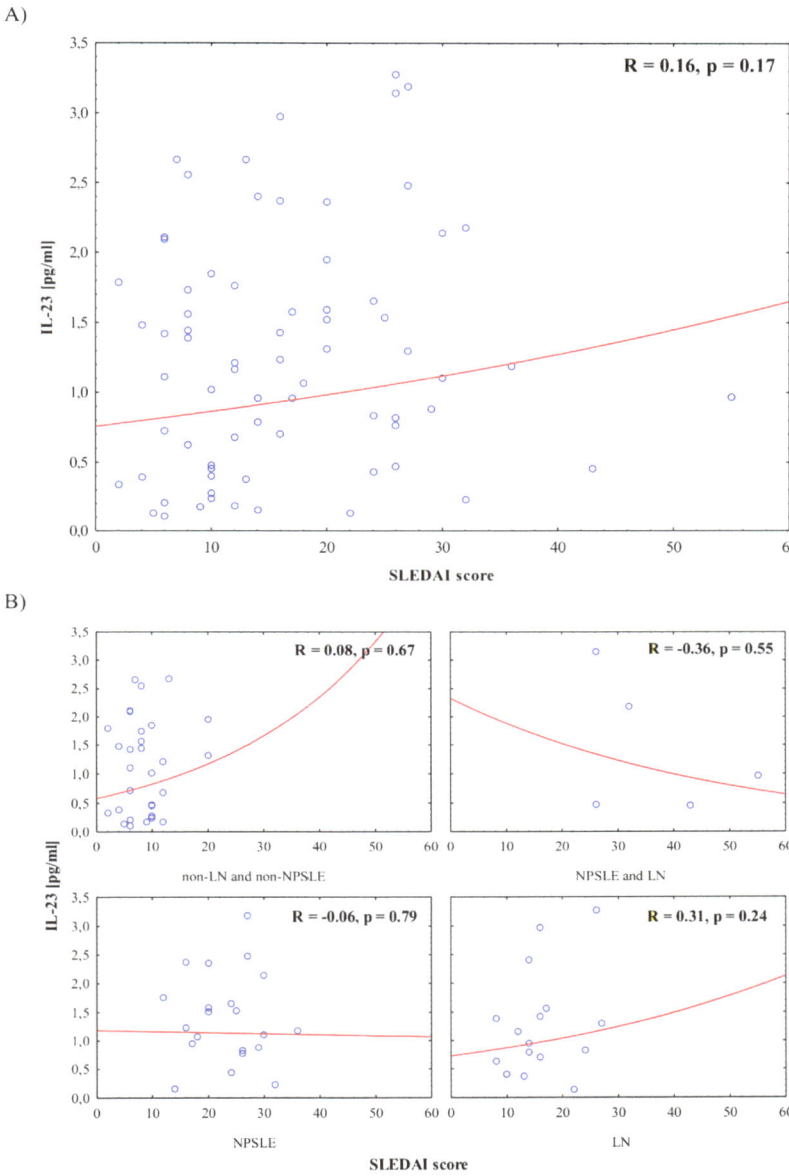

Figure 1. Association between serum IL-23 levels and disease activity in the whole group of patients (**A**), and in selected groups of patients (**B**).

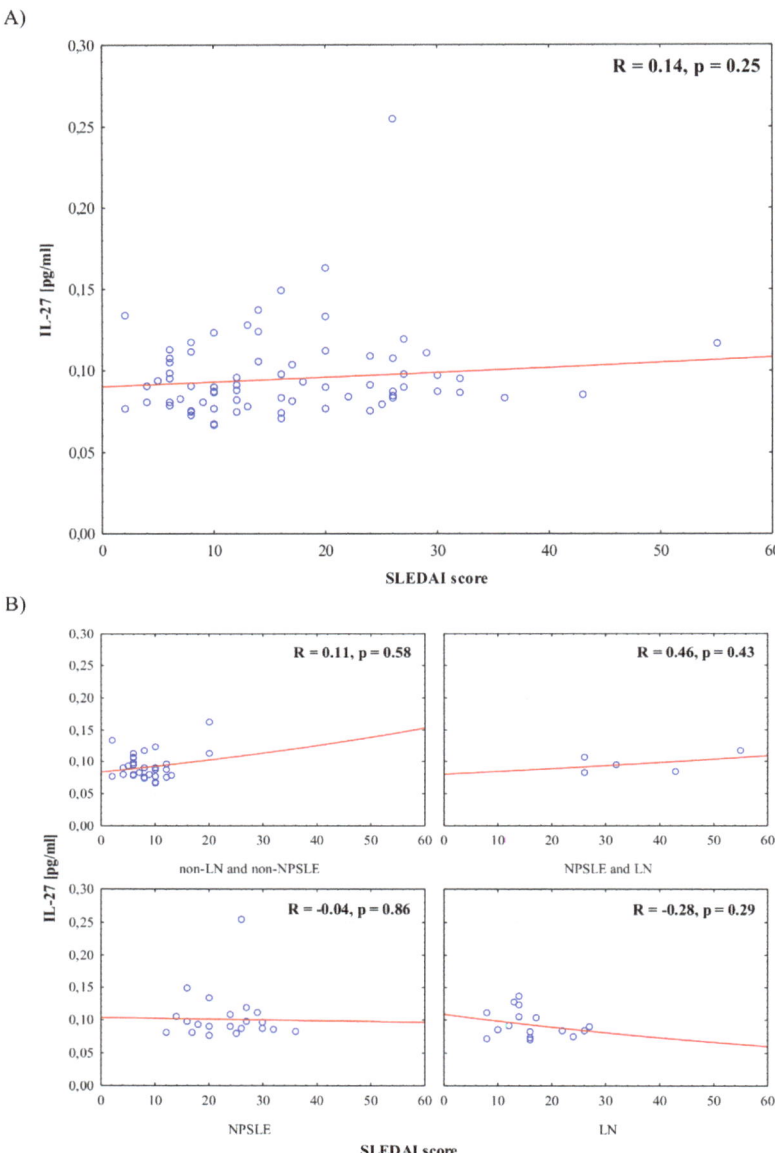

Figure 2. Association between serum IL-27 levels and disease activity in the whole group of patients (**A**), and in selected groups of patients (**B**).

Table 6. Differences in IL-23 and IL-27 (median, min–max) between patients with and without elevated anti-dsDNA and decreased C3/C4.

	Elevated Anti-dsDNA and Low C3/C4 No (n = 39)	Elevated Anti-dsDNA and Low C3/C4 Yes (n = 33)	p
IL-23 (pg/mL)	0.96, 0.11–3.28	1.30, 0.14–3.19	0.31
IL-27 (pg/mL)	0.09, 0.07–0.16	0.09, 0.07–0.26	0.63

dsDNA: double-stranded DNA.

3.6. Association between IL-23/IL-27 Levels and SLE Treatment

There was no significant correlation between interleukin levels and corticosteroid dose (Supplementary Materials, Figure S2), or between interleukin levels and type of treatment (Supplementary Materials, Figure S3).

4. Discussion

In the present study, we analyzed associations between IL-23 and IL-27 levels and disease activity in patients with SLE. We decided to stratify patients according to renal and neurological involvement in order to investigate IL-23 and IL-27 in the patients with the highest SLE activity in the respective organs, thereby identifying the highest risk of damage. We found a lack of correlation between serum IL-23 and IL-27 levels and disease activity measured with the SLEDAI in both the whole group and the selected subgroups of patients with different manifestations of the disease. Nevertheless, one can notice that patients with NPSLE and LN presented the highest SLEDAI and PGA scores. Nominally, the highest median value of IL-23 concentration was observed in patients with NPSLE. Additionally, we found that in the whole group of patients, there was no significant association between interleukin levels and anti-dsDNA, dose of GCs, or type of treatment. Moreover, there were no significant differences in interleukin levels between patients with and without immunologically active disease.

In recent years, an increasing number of studies have been published analyzing the possible role of IL-23 and IL-27 (members of the IL-12 family) in the pathogenesis of SLE, and their potential contribution to immune imbalance [9,20–28]. Differences in both IL-23 and IL-27 levels between patients with SLE and healthy controls were shown. Several authors showed that the IL-27 levels were significantly lower, whereas the IL-23 levels were significantly higher, in SLE patients in comparison to healthy controls [20,23–25,27]. Contrary to our results, Hegab et al. [24] and, more recently, Vukelic et al. [28] found a positive correlation between IL-23 levels and disease activity measured with the SLEDAI. On the other hand, our results are consistent with data presented by Li et al. [20], showing no correlation between IL-27 levels and disease activity.

We also evaluated interleukin levels in patients with various manifestations of SLE. We found that, in patients with LN and NPSLE + LN, IL-23 levels were nominally (but not significantly) lower, while IL-27 levels were similar to other subgroups of patients with different manifestations of SLE. However, there was no association between interleukin levels and disease activity in these subgroups (LN subgroup and NPSLE + LN subgroup). Several authors found high levels of IL-23 in patients with LN in comparison to healthy controls [24,25,27], and a negative association between IL-27 levels and LN occurrence [20,23]. In other research, IL-23 and IL-27 levels were positively and negatively associated with the renal SLEDAI, respectively [26]. To the best of our knowledge, there have been no studies on the association between IL-23 and/or IL-27 levels and disease activity in patients with NPSLE.

In our study, an association between interleukin levels and anti-dsDNA antibodies was not confirmed for IL-23 or IL-27. However, interleukin levels in immunologically active patients were nominally higher. Immunologically active patients and patients with high SLEDAI were treated with immunosuppressants and GCs, which could have a significant impact on the pro-inflammatory effect of IL-23. In 2020, Vukelic et al. showed a strong correlation between IL-23 levels and anti-dsDNA antibodies [28]. In an animal model of lupus, deletion of the IL-23 receptor blocks the interleukin signaling [40] and, consequently, decreases the production of anti-dsDNA antibodies [28]. However, there are some differences between our study and the Vukelic et al. study. Our group consisted of Caucasian patients who presented a median SLEDAI value of 14, whereas in Vukelic et al.'s study, the mean SLEDAI value in patients of different ethnicities was 6.7 [28].

In the present study, GC doses were not associated with the levels of either interleukin in patients with active SLE, i.e., patients with higher doses of medications did not present lower values of IL-23 or IL-27. These results are, to some extent, consistent with those presented in 2020 by Vukelic et al., who showed that immunomodulatory medications used for mild or severe LN did not affect IL-23 levels [28]; the authors suggested that drugs commonly used in patients with SLE may not be effective in shutting down the IL-23/IL-17 axis [28]. However, some authors found that six months of immunosuppressive treatment (GCs together with CTX or MMF) may decrease urine IL-23 concentrations in patients with a complete response, supporting the potential role of IL-23 in the pathogenesis of LN [26].

In our study, patients with NPSLE presented the highest serum concentrations of IL-23. This group of patients may be predisposed to IL-23 blockade treatment response [22]. IL-23 has pro-inflammatory and inhibitory functions; it is produced in response to microbial pathogens, and is essential for the differentiation of naïve CD4 T cells [41]. Anti-IL-23 therapy is intended to inhibit multiple inflammatory pathways critical for driving autoimmune inflammation [24,42,43]. Recent data suggest that IL-23 inhibitors offer safe and effective treatment of autoimmune inflammatory diseases. Ustekinumab, the first agent of this pharmacological class—also targeting IL-12/IL-23p40—has been approved for Crohn's disease, ulcerative colitis, plaque psoriasis, and psoriatic arthritis treatment. However, despite the initially promising phase II trial results, Janssen recently announced the discontinuation of the phase III LOTUS study evaluating ustekinumab (STELARA®) in patients with SLE, due to lack of efficacy [44].

Risankizumab has been approved for the treatment of moderate-to-severe plaque psoriasis and, in Japan, also for psoriasis vulgaris, generalized pustular psoriasis, erythrodermic psoriasis, and psoriatic arthritis [41,45–50].

Another IL-23 blocker, guselkumab, approved for the treatment of plaque psoriasis and psoriatic arthritis, also has the potential to treat patients with Crohn's disease [47,50–54] and ulcerative colitis [50,55–57].

Some reports suggest that patients with positive anti-dsDNA antibodies and/or low C3 levels are more likely to have elevated levels of IL-23 [28] and, due to immunological disease activity and lack of full disease remission, are in a high-risk group for "immune-mediated" and "treatment-mediated" tissue damage. In our study, patients with positive anti-dsDNA antibodies and low C3/C4 presented higher serum concentrations of IL-23 than those with negative anti-dsDNA antibodies; however, the difference was not statistically significant. Patients with clinically and immunologically active SLE require more aggressive therapy, which significantly modifies cytokine activity [58].

An increase in IL-27 serum concentration is a protective response to pathogenic factors, preventing the impairment of tissues and organs due to the promotion of specific Treg cell subsets, and inhibition of Th1, Th2, Th17, and antigen-presenting cells [59]. In our study, levels of both interleukins were not related to the type of treatment in the whole group of patients. Xia et al. showed that IL-27 levels can be successfully increased after six months of treatment with GCs together with CTX or MMF in patients with LN [26]. The discrepancies between the abovementioned studies may result from differences in the immunological and clinical activity of SLE, the degree of the therapy aggressiveness, the heterogeneity of the disease, and small sample sizes.

Due to scarce and inconsistent data that hinder the drawing of unambiguous conclusions, the exact roles of IL-27 and IL-23 in the pathogenesis of SLE should be verified in future studies.

The heterogeneous group of patients, lack of a control group, and the retrospective nature of our work should be mentioned here as limitations of our study.

5. Conclusions

Our findings suggest a lack of correlation between serum IL-23 and IL-27 levels and disease activity measured with the SLEDAI in a group of patients with different manifestations of SLE disease. We additionally found no significant associations between interleukin levels and anti-dsDNA, dose of GCs, or type of treatment. Moreover, no significant differences in interleukin levels between patients with and without immunologically active disease were observed.

Supplementary Materials: The following are available online at https://www.mdpi.com/article/10.3390/jcm10204788/s1: Figure S1: Association between serum IL-27 and IL-23 levels and anti-dsDNA; Figure S2: Association between corticosteroid dose and IL-23 and IL-27 levels. Corticosteroid doses expressed as prednisolone equivalents were classified as follows: 1: ≤ 7.5 mg; 2: 7.6–10 mg; 3: >10 mg; 4: high intravenous corticosteroid doses; Figure S3: Association between IL-23 and IL-27 levels and type of treatment. CS: corticosteroids; IS: immunosuppressant medications; whiskers: min–max, inside box corresponds to the median, outside box boundaries correspond to 25% and 75%.

Author Contributions: All authors were involved in project design and collection and analysis of data. All authors edited and approved the final version of the manuscript. All authors have read and agreed to the published version of the manuscript.

Funding: This research received no external funding.

Institutional Review Board Statement: This study was approved by the Bioethical Committee of the Poznań University of Medical Sciences (no. 107/21).

Informed Consent Statement: Patient consent was waived due to the retrospective design of the study.

Data Availability Statement: Restrictions apply to the availability of these data. Data were obtained from J. Struś Municipal Hospital in Poznań, Poland, and are available from the corresponding author with the permission of the hospital authorities.

Acknowledgments: The authors would like to thank Jakub Żurawski for his assistance in conducting serological examinations, and Proper Medical Writing for their support in preparation of this manuscript.

Conflicts of Interest: The authors declare no conflict of interest.

References

1. Bertsias, G.K.; Pamfil, C.; Fanouriakis, A.; Boumpas, D.T. Diagnostic criteria for systemic lupus erythematosus: Has the time come? *Nat. Rev. Rheumatol.* **2013**, *9*, 687–694. [CrossRef]
2. Tsokos, G.C. Systemic lupus erythematosus. *N. Engl. J. Med.* **2011**, *365*, 2110–2121. [CrossRef] [PubMed]
3. Kaul, A.; Gordon, C.; Crow, M.K.; Touma, Z.; Urowitz, M.B.; van Vollenhoven, R.; Ruiz-Irastorza, G.; Hughes, G. Systemic lupus erythematosus. *Nat. Rev. Dis. Primers* **2016**, *2*, 16039. [CrossRef] [PubMed]
4. Furst, D.E.; Clarke, A.; Fernandes, A.W.; Bancroft, T.; Gajria, K.; Greth, W.; Iorga, Ş.R. Medical costs and healthcare resource use in patients with lupus nephritis and neuropsychiatric lupus in an insured population. *J. Med. Econ.* **2013**, *16*, 500–509. [CrossRef]
5. Parikh, S.V.; Almaani, S.; Brodsky, S.; Rovin, B.H. Update on Lupus Nephritis: Core Curriculum 2020. *Am. J. Kidney Dis.* **2020**, *76*, 265–281. [CrossRef] [PubMed]
6. Carrión-Barberà, I.; Salman-Monte, T.C.; Vílchez-Oya, F.; Monfort, J. Neuropsychiatric involvement in systemic lupus erythematosus: A review. *Autoimmun. Rev.* **2021**, *20*, 102780. [CrossRef]
7. Jeltsch-David, H.; Muller, S. Neuropsychiatric systemic lupus erythematosus: Pathogenesis and biomarkers. *Nat. Rev. Neurol.* **2014**, *10*, 579–596. [CrossRef]
8. Śliwczyński, A.; Brzozowska, M.; Iltchev, P.; Czeleko, T.; Teter, Z.; Tłustochowicz, W.; Marczak, M.; Tłustochowicz, M. Changes in the morbidity and costs of systemic lupus erythematosus in Poland in the years 2008–2012. *Reumatologia* **2015**, *53*, 79–86. [CrossRef]
9. Lourenço, E.V.; La Cava, A. Cytokines in systemic lupus erythematosus. *Curr. Mol. Med.* **2009**, *9*, 242–254. [CrossRef]
10. Yap, D.Y.; Lai, K.N. Cytokines and their roles in the pathogenesis of systemic lupus erythematosus: From basics to recent advances. *J. Biomed. Biotechnol.* **2010**, *2010*, 365083. [CrossRef]

11. Mikita, N.; Ikeda, T.; Ishiguro, M.; Furukawa, F. Recent advances in cytokines in cutaneous and systemic lupus erythematosus. *J. Dermatol.* **2011**, *38*, 839–849. [CrossRef] [PubMed]
12. Moulton, V.R.; Suárez-Fueyo, A.; Meidan, E.; Li, H.; Mizui, M.; Tsokos, G.C. Pathogenesis of Human Systemic Lupus Erythematosus: A Cellular Perspective. *Trends Mol. Med.* **2017**, *23*, 615–635. [CrossRef] [PubMed]
13. Xu, W.; Su, L.; Liu, X.; Wang, J.; Yuan, Z.; Qin, Z.; Zhou, X.; Huang, A. IL-38: A novel cytokine in systemic lupus erythematosus pathogenesis. *J. Cell. Mol. Med.* **2020**, *24*, 12379–12389. [CrossRef] [PubMed]
14. Muhammad Yusoff, F.; Wong, K.K.; Mohd Redzwan, N. Th1, Th2, and Th17 cytokines in systemic lupus erythematosus. *Autoimmunity* **2020**, *53*, 8–20. [CrossRef] [PubMed]
15. Puwipirom, H.; Hirankarn, N.; Sodsai, P.; Avihingsanon, Y.; Wongpiyabovorn, J.; Palaga, T. Increased interleukin-23 receptor+ T cells in peripheral blood mononuclear cells of patients with systemic lupus erythematosus. *Arthritis Res. Ther.* **2010**, *12*, R215. [CrossRef]
16. Curtis, M.M.; Way, S.S.; Wilson, C.B. IL-23 promotes the production of IL-17 by antigen-specific CD8 T cells in the absence of IL-12 and type-I interferons. *J. Immunol.* **2009**, *183*, 381–387. [CrossRef]
17. Sutton, C.E.; Lalor, S.J.; Sweeney, C.M.; Brereton, C.F.; Lavelle, E.C.; Mills, K.H. Interleukin-1 and IL-23 induce innate IL-17 production from gammadelta T cells, amplifying Th17 responses and autoimmunity. *Immunity* **2009**, *31*, 331–341. [CrossRef]
18. Cao, Y.; Doodes, P.D.; Glant, T.T.; Finnegan, A. IL-27 induces a Th1 immune response and susceptibility to experimental arthritis. *J. Immunol.* **2008**, *180*, 922–930. [CrossRef]
19. Su, Y.; Yao, H.; Wang, H.; Xu, F.; Li, D.; Li, D.; Zhang, X.; Yin, Y.; Cao, J. IL-27 enhances innate immunity of human pulmonary fibroblasts and epithelial cells through upregulation of TLR4 expression. *Am. J. Physiol. Lung Cell. Mol. Physiol.* **2016**, *310*, L133–L141. [CrossRef]
20. Li, T.-T.; Zhang, T.; Chen, G.-M.; Zhu, Q.-Q.; Tao, J.-H.; Pan, H.-F.; Ye, D.-Q. Low level of serum interleukin 27 in patients with systemic lupus erythematosus. *J. Investig. Med.* **2010**, *58*, 737–739. [CrossRef]
21. Lee, M.H.; Gallo, P.M.; Hooper, K.M.; Corradetti, C.; Ganea, D.; Caricchio, R.; Gallucci, S. The cytokine network Type I Interferon, IL-27 and IL-10 is augmented in murine and human lupus. *J. Leukoc. Biol.* **2019**, *106*, 967–975. [CrossRef]
22. Leng, R.-X.; Pan, H.-F.; Chen, G.-M.; Wang, C.; Qin, W.-Z.; Chen, L.-L.; Tao, J.-H.; Ye, D.-Q. IL-23: A Promising Therapeutic Target for Systemic Lupus Erythematosus. *Arch. Med. Res.* **2010**, *41*, 221–225. [CrossRef]
23. Gaber, W.; Sayed, S.; Rady, H.M.; Mohey, A.M. Interleukin-27 and its relation to disease parameters in SLE patients. *Egypt. Rheumatol.* **2012**, *34*, 99–105. [CrossRef]
24. Hegab, D.S.; Saudi, W.M.; Ammo, D.E.A.; El Bedewy, M.M.; Elhabian, N.F.; Gamei, M.M. Role of interleukin-23 in the immunopathogenesis of systemic lupus erythematosus. *Egypt. J. Dermatol. Venerol.* **2014**, *34*, 120. [CrossRef]
25. Du, J.; Li, Z.; Shi, J.; Bi, L. Associations between serum interleukin-23 levels and clinical characteristics in patients with systemic lupus erythematosus. *J. Int. Med. Res.* **2014**, *42*, 1123–1130. [CrossRef] [PubMed]
26. Xia, L.P.; Li, B.F.; Shen, H.; Lu, J. Interleukin-27 and interleukin-23 in patients with systemic lupus erythematosus: Possible role in lupus nephritis. *Scand. J. Rheumatol.* **2015**, *44*, 200–205. [CrossRef] [PubMed]
27. Fischer, K.; Przepiera-Bedzak, H.; Sawicki, M.; Walecka, A.; Brzosko, I.; Brzosko, M. Serum Interleukin-23 in Polish Patients with Systemic Lupus Erythematosus: Association with Lupus Nephritis, Obesity, and Peripheral Vascular Disease. *Mediat. Inflamm.* **2017**, *2017*, 9401432. [CrossRef]
28. Vukelic, M.; Laloo, A.; Kyttaris, V.C. Interleukin 23 is elevated in the serum of patients with SLE. *Lupus* **2020**, *29*, 1943–1947. [CrossRef] [PubMed]
29. Hochberg, M.C. Updating the American College of Rheumatology revised criteria for the classification of systemic lupus erythematosus. *Arthritis Rheum.* **1997**, *40*, 1725. [CrossRef]
30. Aringer, M.; Costenbader, K.; Daikh, D.; Brinks, R.; Mosca, M.; Ramsey-Goldman, R.; Smolen, J.S.; Wofsy, D.; Boumpas, D.T.; Kamen, D.L.; et al. 2019 EULAR/ACR classification criteria for systemic lupus erythematosus. *Ann. Rheum. Dis.* **2019**, *78*, 1151–1159. [CrossRef]
31. Leuchten, N.; Hoyer, A.; Brinks, R.; Schoels, M.; Schneider, M.; Smolen, J.; Johnson, S.R.; Daikh, D.; Dörner, T.; Aringer, M.; et al. Performance of Antinuclear Antibodies for Classifying Systemic Lupus Erythematosus: A Systematic Literature Review and Meta-Regression of Diagnostic Data. *Arthritis Rheum.* **2018**, *70*, 428–438. [CrossRef] [PubMed]
32. Fox, B.J.; Hockley, J.; Rigsby, P.; Dolman, C.; Meroni, P.L.; Rönnelid, J. A WHO Reference Reagent for lupus (anti-dsDNA) antibodies: International collaborative study to evaluate a candidate preparation. *Ann. Rheum. Dis.* **2019**, *78*, 1677–1680. [CrossRef]
33. Liang, M.H.; Corzillius, M.; Bae, S.C.; Lew, R.A.; Fortin, P.R.; Gordon, C.; Isenberg, D.; Alarcón, G.S.; Straaton, K.V.; Denburg, J.; et al. The American College of Rheumatology nomenclature and case definitions for neuropsychiatric lupus syndromes. *Arthritis Rheum.* **1999**, *42*, 599–608.
34. Rekvig, O.P. Anti-dsDNA antibodies as a classification criterion and a diagnostic marker for systemic lupus erythematosus: Critical remarks. *Clin. Exp. Immunol.* **2015**, *179*, 5–10. [CrossRef]
35. Gladman, D.D.; Ibañez, D.; Urowitz, M.B. Systemic lupus erythematosus disease activity index 2000. *J. Rheumatol.* **2002**, *29*, 288–291.
36. Mikdashi, J.; Nived, O. Measuring disease activity in adults with systemic lupus erythematosus: The challenges of administrative burden and responsiveness to patient concerns in clinical research. *Arthritis Res. Ther.* **2015**, *17*, 183. [CrossRef]

37. Chessa, E.; Piga, M.; Floris, A.; Devilliers, H.; Cauli, A.; Arnaud, L. Use of Physician Global Assessment in systemic lupus erythematosus: A systematic review of its psychometric properties. *Rheumatology* **2020**, *59*, 3622–3632. [CrossRef]
38. Gladman, D.D.; Urowitz, M.B. The SLICC/ACR damage index: Progress report and experience in the field. *Lupus* **1999**, *8*, 632–637. [CrossRef]
39. Fanouriakis, A.; Kostopoulou, M.; Alunno, A.; Aringer, M.; Bajema, I.; Boletis, J.N.; Cervera, R.; Doria, A.; Gordon, C.; Govoni, M.; et al. 2019 update of the EULAR recommendations for the management of systemic lupus erythematosus. *Ann. Rheum. Dis.* **2019**, *78*, 736–745. [CrossRef] [PubMed]
40. Zhang, Z.; Kyttaris, V.C.; Tsokos, G.C. The role of IL-23/IL-17 axis in lupus nephritis. *J. Immunol.* **2009**, *183*, 3160–3169. [CrossRef] [PubMed]
41. Argollo, M.C.; Allocca, M.; Furfaro, F.; Peyrin-Biroulet, L.; Danese, S. Interleukin-23 Blockers: Born to be First-line Biologic Agents in Inflammatory Bowel Disease? *Curr. Pharm. Des.* **2019**, *25*, 25–31. [CrossRef]
42. Chen, Y.; Langrish, C.L.; McKenzie, B.; Joyce-Shaikh, B.; Stumhofer, J.S.; McClanahan, T.; Blumenschein, W.; Churakovsa, T.; Low, J.; Presta, L. Anti–IL-23 therapy inhibits multiple inflammatory pathways and ameliorates autoimmune encephalomyelitis. *J. Clin. Investig.* **2006**, *116*, 1317–1326. [CrossRef]
43. Kyttaris, V.C.; Kampagianni, O.; Tsokos, G.C. Treatment with anti-interleukin 23 antibody ameliorates disease in lupus-prone mice. *BioMed Res. Int.* **2013**, *2013*, 861028. [CrossRef]
44. Janssen Announces Discontinuation of Phase 3 LOTUS Study Evaluating Ustekinumab in Systemic Lupus Erythematosus. Available online: https://www.janssen.com/janssen-announces-discontinuation-phase-3-lotus-study-evaluating-ustekinumab-systemic-lupus (accessed on 12 October 2021).
45. Sbidian, E.; Chaimani, A.; Garcia-Doval, I.; Do, G.; Hua, C.; Mazaud, C.; Droitcourt, C.; Hughes, C.; Ingram, J.R.; Naldi, L.; et al. Systemic pharmacological treatments for chronic plaque psoriasis: A network meta-analysis. *Cochrane Database Syst. Rev.* **2017**, *12*, CD011535. [CrossRef]
46. Youn, S.W.; Tsai, T.-F.; Theng, C.; Choon, S.-E.; Wiryadi, B.E.; Pires, A.; Tan, W.; Lee, M.-G.; MARCOPOLO Investigators. The MARCOPOLO Study of Ustekinumab Utilization and Efficacy in a Real-World Setting: Treatment of Patients with Plaque Psoriasis in Asia-Pacific Countries. *Ann. Dermatol.* **2016**, *28*, 222–231. [CrossRef] [PubMed]
47. Biemans, V.B.C.; Van Der Woude, C.J.; Dijkstra, G.; Jong, A.E.V.D.M.-D.; Löwenberg, M.; de Boer, N.; Oldenburg, B.; Srivastava, N.; Jansen, J.M.; Bodelier, A.G.L.; et al. Ustekinumab is associated with superior effectiveness outcomes compared to vedolizumab in Crohn's disease patients with prior failure to anti-TNF treatment. *Aliment. Pharmacol. Ther.* **2020**, *52*, 123–134. [CrossRef]
48. Blauvelt, A.; Leonardi, C.L.; Gooderham, M.; Papp, K.A.; Philipp, S.; Wu, J.J.; Igarashi, A.; Flack, M.; Geng, Z.; Wu, T.; et al. Efficacy and Safety of Continuous Risankizumab Therapy vs Treatment Withdrawal in Patients with Moderate to Severe Plaque Psoriasis: A Phase 3 Randomized Clinical Trial. *JAMA Dermatol.* **2020**, *156*, 649–658. [CrossRef] [PubMed]
49. Papp, K.A.; de Vente, S.; Zeng, J.; Flack, M.; Padilla, B.; Tyring, S.K. Long-Term Safety and Efficacy of Risankizumab in Patients with Moderate-to-Severe Chronic Plaque Psoriasis: Results from a Phase 2 Open-Label Extension Trial. *Dermatol. Ther.* **2021**, *11*, 487–497. [CrossRef] [PubMed]
50. McKeage, K.; Duggan, S. Risankizumab: First Global Approval. *Drugs* **2019**, *79*, 893–900. [CrossRef] [PubMed]
51. Khorrami, S.; Ginard, D.; Marín-Jiménez, I.; Chaparro, M.; Sierra, M.; Aguas, M.; Sicilia, B.; García-Sánchez, V.; Suarez, C.; Villoria, A.; et al. Ustekinumab for the Treatment of Refractory Crohn's Disease: The Spanish Experience in a Large Multicentre Open-label Cohort. *Inflamm. Bowel Dis.* **2016**, *22*, 1662–1669. [CrossRef] [PubMed]
52. Macaluso, F.S.; Orlando, A.; Cottone, M. Anti-interleukin-12 and anti-interleukin-23 in Crohn's disease. *Expert Opin. Biol. Ther.* **2019**, *19*, 89–98. [CrossRef]
53. Berman, H.S.; Villa, N.M.; Shi, V.Y.; Hsiao, J.L. Guselkumab in the treatment of concomitant hidradenitis suppurativa, psoriasis, and Crohn's disease. *J. Dermatol. Treat.* **2021**, *32*, 261–263. [CrossRef]
54. Jørgensen, A.R.; Holm, J.G.; Thomsen, S.F. Guselkumab for hidradenitis suppurativa in a patient with concomitant Crohn's disease: Report and systematic literature review of effectiveness and safety. *Clin. Case Rep.* **2020**, *8*, 2874–2877. [CrossRef]
55. Fiorino, G.; Allocca, M.; Correale, C.; Roda, G.; Furfaro, F.; Loy, L.; Zilli, A.; Peyrin-Biroulet, L.; Danese, S. Positioning ustekinumab in moderate-to-severe ulcerative colitis: New kid on the block. *Expert Opin. Biol. Ther.* **2020**, *20*, 421–427. [CrossRef]
56. Hanžel, J.; D'Haens, G.R. Anti-interleukin-23 agents for the treatment of ulcerative colitis. *Expert Opin. Biol. Ther.* **2020**, *20*, 399–406. [CrossRef]
57. Chiricozzi, A.; Costanzo, A.; Fargnoli, M.C.; Malagoli, P.; Piaserico, S.; Amerio, P.; Argenziano, G.; Balato, N.; Bardazzi, F.; Bianchi, L.; et al. Guselkumab: An anti-IL-23 antibody for the treatment of moderate-to-severe plaque psoriasis. *Eur. J. Dermatol.* **2021**, *31*, 3–16.
58. Leszczyński, P.; Pawlak-Buś, K. New treatment strategy including biological agents in patients with systemic lupus erythematosus. *Pol. Arch. Med. Wewn* **2013**, *123*, 482–490. [CrossRef]
59. Murugaiyan, G.; Mittal, A.; Lopez-Diego, R.; Maier, L.M.; Anderson, D.E.; Weiner, H.L. IL-27 Is a Key Regulator of IL-10 and IL-17 Production by Human CD4+ T Cells. *J. Immunol.* **2009**, *183*, 2435–2443. [CrossRef]

Article

Association of microRNA-34a rs2666433 (A/G) Variant with Systemic Lupus Erythematosus in Female Patients: A Case-Control Study

Nesreen M. Ismail [1], Eman A. Toraih [2,3,*], Mai H. S. Mohammad [4], Eida M. Alshammari [5] and Manal S. Fawzy [6,7,*]

1. Department of Rheumatology and Rehabilitation, Faculty of Medicine, Suez Canal University, Ismailia 41522, Egypt; tasneemge@yahoo.com
2. Department of Surgery, Tulane University School of Medicine, New Orleans, LA 70112, USA
3. Genetics Unit, Department of Histology and Cell Biology, Suez Canal University, Ismailia 41522, Egypt
4. Department of Clinical Pathology, Faculty of Medicine, Suez Canal University, Ismailia 41522, Egypt; maii81hs@hotmail.com
5. Department of Chemistry, College of Science, University of Ha'il, Ha'il 2440, Saudi Arabia; eida.alshammari@uoh.edu.sa
6. Department of Medical Biochemistry and Molecular Biology, Faculty of Medicine, Suez Canal University, Ismailia 41522, Egypt
7. Department of Biochemistry, Faculty of Medicine, Northern Border University, Arar 1321, Saudi Arabia
* Correspondence: etoraih@tulane.edu (E.A.T.); manal_mohamed@med.suez.edu.eg (M.S.F.); Tel.: +1-346-907-4237 (E.A.T.); +20-1008584720 (M.S.F.)

Abstract: Several microRNAs (miRNAs) are associated with autoimmune disease susceptibility and phenotype, including systemic lupus erythematosus (SLE). We aimed to explore for the first time the role of the miRNA-34a gene (MIR34A) rs2666433A > G variant in SLE risk and severity. A total of 163 adult patients with SLE and matched controls were recruited. Real-Time allelic discrimination PCR was applied for genotyping. Correlation with disease activity and clinic-laboratory data was done. The rs2666433 variant conferred protection against SLE development under heterozygous [A/G vs. G/G; OR = 0.57, 95%CI = 0.34–0.95], homozygous [A/A vs. G/G; OR = 0.52, 95%CI = 0.29–0.94], dominant [A/G + A/A vs. GG; OR = 0.55, 95%CI = 0.35–0.88], and log-additive [OR = 0.71, 95%CI = 0.53–0.95] models. Data stratification by sex revealed a significant association with SLE development in female participants under heterozygous/homozygous models (p-interaction = 0.004). There was no clear demarcation between SLE patients carrying different genotypes regarding the disease activity index or patients stratified according to lupus nephritis. Enrichment analysis confirmed the implication of MIR34A in the SLE pathway by targeting several genes related to SLE etiopathology. In conclusion, although the MIR34A rs2666433 variant conferred protection against developing SLE disease in the study population, it showed no association with disease activity. Replication studies in other populations are warranted.

Keywords: MIR34A; lupus nephritis; single nucleotide polymorphism; SLE

1. Introduction

The systemic lupus erythematosus (SLE) (OMIM: 152700) is a complex autoimmune disease characterized by a loss of tolerance against nuclear autoantigens and complex dysfunction of innate and adaptive immunity [1]. The worldwide overall incidence rates of SLE range from 1 to 10 per 100,000 person-years, affecting predominantly females (the female/male ratio is 9:1) of a reproductive age [2]. The major pathogenic mechanisms of SLE include an inappropriate immune response to the nucleic acid-containing cellular particles, which impact different organ systems [3,4]. Clinical and epidemiological studies suggest genetic factors, in addition to environmental insults, play an important role in SLE pathogenesis [5–8].

MicroRNAs are small non-coding RNAs that predominantly bind to the 3′-untranslated region (3′-UTR) of target messenger RNAs (mRNAs) and then promote mRNAs degradation or inhibit translation [9]. Emerging studies have shown that they play important roles in various immunological and autoimmune disorders, including SLE [10–12].

The miR-34a gene (MIR34A), located at the chromosome 1p36 locus, is an essential modulator of the immune system [13,14]. It is widely expressed in immune cells, including B cells and T cells, regulating their function, development, and survival [14]. By targeting the Forkhead "Foxp1" transcription factor, miR-34a could inhibit B cell development at the "pro-B cell" to "pre-B cell" transition, leading to a decline in mature B cells [13]. Furthermore, it was implicated with other microRNAs in modulating the "T cell responses" process [14]. For example, miR-34a can directly target the diacylglycerol kinase zeta, and in turn, through this signal pathway, lead to enhance T cell activity [15]. Moreover, targeting five members of the protein kinase C family, miR-34a can regulate T cell migration and control cell signaling via the immunological synapses downstream of the "T cell receptors" [16]. By modulating the nuclear factor kappa B signaling in T cells, miR-34a can regulate T cell functions and control several aspects of innate/adaptive immune functions [17].

The deregulated expression of miR-34a was observed in several autoimmune disorders like multiple sclerosis [18] and rheumatoid arthritis (RA) [19], among others [14]. A recent study by Xie and colleagues reported that miR-34a derived from peripheral blood mononuclear cells of SLE patients could play a putative role in disease activity, and its gene expression levels were directly correlated with several disease indices, such as "erythrocyte sedimentation rate, anti-streptolysin antibody, rheumatoid factor, and C-reactive protein" [20]. Furthermore, by targeting Foxp3, miR-34a could limit Tregs differentiation with subsequent Tregs/Th17 cells imbalance and immune tolerance breakdown [20,21]. This suggests that miR-34a could be a potential biomarker or a new potential target for SLE disease.

Single nucleotide polymorphisms (SNPs) are ubiquitous genetic variations at certain nucleotide positions of the genome, implicated in several human disorders, including immunological diseases [22]. Further, miRNAs expression can be affected by SNPs locating in their coding genes with a subsequent change in several biological functions [23]. Earlier studies have shown that individuals' susceptibility to human diseases may be modified by SNPs of the MIR34A gene, such as type 2 diabetes [24], ischemic stroke [25], and colon cancer [26], among others. However, the association between MIR34A variants and SLE susceptibility has not been reported before. In this sense, a common SNP in MIR34A (rs2666433: A > G) was selected based on location, minor allele frequency, and previous supporting reports. In the current case-control study, the authors aimed to investigate the association of this specified variant with SLE susceptibility and severity. The identification and characterization of such associations may highlight this variant's role in disease susceptibility and help develop novel genetic risk stratification for targeted screening and management in the near future.

2. Materials and Methods

2.1. Study Subjects

A total of 326 adult participants (163 SLE patients and 163 controls) were recruited in this case-control study. The consecutive SLE cases were enrolled from the "Rheumatology and Nephrology Departments at the Suez Canal University (SCU) Hospitals, Ismailia, Egypt". Based on the updated SLE classification criteria specified by the 2019 European League Against Rheumatism (EULAR)/American College of Rheumatology (ACR) classification criteria for SLE [27], cases were diagnosed by experienced clinical Rheumatologist. Patients with a history of other chronic/autoimmune disorders and cancers were excluded from the study; the control group included 163 age- and sex-matched healthy blood donors attending the blood bank in the same period with no history of chronic disorders, including autoimmune diseases. Helsinki declarations were followed during work execution, and the ethical committee of the Faculty of Medicine, SCU, approved the study (approval no. 4268). Informed written consent was obtained from all participants before taking part in the study.

2.2. Clinical Assessment

The demographic, clinical, and laboratory data were collected from all patients. According to disease activity, patients were classified into four groups, from mild to very high activity based on the "SLE Disease Activity Index (SLEDAI) score" that classifies SLE patients into i—No activity (SLEDAI = 0), ii—Mild activity (SLEDAI = 1:5), iii—Moderate activity (SLEDAI = 6:10), iv—High activity (SLEDAI = 11:19), and v—Very high activity (SLEDAI $\geq$ 20) [28]. According to the ACR criteria of lupus nephritis [27], patients were divided into 93 patients with lupus nephritis and 70 SLE with no renal involvement.

2.3. Blood Sampling and Laboratory Evaluations

A total of five milliliters of peripheral venous blood was withdrawn from all participants under aseptic condition and divided into two aliquots; 2 mL were collected on EDTA tubes for hematological and genetic assessment, and 3 mL blood was collected on serum separator tubes, which were subjected to centrifugation to separate serum for the biochemical and immunological evaluations.

An automated hematology analyzer CELL-DYN 1700 (Abbott Diagnostics, Abbott Park, IL, USA) was applied to evaluate the complete blood count (CBC) and complemented by microscopic differential count examination. An automated biochemical analyzer Cobas c501 (Roche Diagnostics, Manheim, Germany), was applied for liver and kidney function evaluation as well as C-reactive protein (CRP) and complement proteins (C3 and C4) estimations. The advanced Westergren method was run for erythrocyte sedimentation rate (ESR) calculation. Anti-nuclear antibodies (ANA) and anti-double-stranded DNA antibodies (Anti-dsDNA) were quantified using Bio-Rad technology through indirect immunofluorescence assay (Bio-Rad Laboratories, Hercules, CA, USA). All the laboratory tests and the quality control measurements were run according to the supplier protocols and the local laboratory guidelines.

2.4. DNA Extraction and Purification

Genomic DNA was extracted and processed from the buffy coat of whole blood using the QIAamp DNA extraction Mini kit for blood samples (Qiagen; Catalog #: 51104) according to the manufacturer's protocols. The concentration and purity of genomic DNA were evaluated utilizing NanoDrop™ ND-1000 spectrophotometer (NanoDrop Technologies, Inc., Wilmington, DE, USA).

2.5. Genotyping of MIR34A rs2666433 A > G Variant

Real-Time TaqMan allelic discrimination polymerase chain reaction (PCR) assay (C_2800266_10) was run for detection of the specified study variant, as explained in detail in our previous work (2020). Negative controls were run in each PCR experiment to ensure the absence of amplicon contamination. A StepOne Real-Time PCR System (Applied Biosystems) was programmed as follows: an initial hold for 10 min (95 °C) followed by a 40-cycle two-step PCR (denaturation for 15 s at 95 °C and annealing/extension for 1 min at 60 °C). The SDS software version 1.3.1 (Applied Biosystems, Foster City, CA, USA) was used for allelic discrimination data recall. Genotyping was performed by two persons independently blinded to case/control status. Ten percent of the randomly selected samples were re-genotyped in separate runs to exclude the possibility of false genotype calls, with a 100% concordance rate for the results.

2.6. Functional Role of miRNA-34a in SLE Disease

The microRNAs involved in Systemic lupus erythematosus l hsa05322 pathway were determined from mirPath v.3, a microRNA pathway analysis webserver (DIANA TOOLS-mirPath v.3 (grnet.gr)); hsa-miR-34a-5p was the second after hsa-miR-16–5p that are highly enriched in the SLE pathway. Next, microRNA gene targets were identified from TarBase v7.0 (DIANA TOOLS-TarBase v7.0 (Athena-innovation.gr)). Their gene ontology and function were explored in STRING v11.0 (STRING interaction network (string-db.org)) (last accessed on 23 May 2021).

Validation of the role of miR-34a in SLE was screened in high-throughput experiments stored in online data repositories. Data were retrieved for similar experiments on SLE from the Gene Expression Omnibus (GEO) (Home-GEO-NCBI (nih.gov)) (last accessed on 23 May 2021) with microRNA seq analysis. Two datasets were available [GSE80183 and GSE72509], and raw data were analyzed using GEO RNA-seq Experiments Interactive Navigator (GREIN (ilincs.org)) (last accessed on 23 May 2021). and the comprehensive network visual analytics platform for gene expression analysis NetworkAnalyst (www.networkanalyst.ca) (last accessed on 23 May 2021). In the first experiment, 117 RNA-seq of SLE whole blood and healthy controls and patients were stratified according to their autoantibody status. In the second experiment, 12 SLE patients were segregated into three groups based on the presence of autoantibodies against (i) dsDNA only (ii) ENA (extractable nuclear antigens) only, or (iii) both compared to 4 control samples.

2.7. Selection of the Study Genetic Variant of MIR34A Gene

MIR34A gene encodes for a single primary transcript with one exon that encloses 32 variant alleles. However, they were very rare (<0.001). In dbSNP version 135, we identified a common SNP rs2666433 caused due to point mutation substituting A with G. The minor allele frequency (MAF) was 0.259 (according to 1000Genome project), 0.191 (according to TOPMED project), and 0.30 (according to HapMap). The rs2666433 polymorphism is located at 1:9213177 (chromosome 1p36.22) 2KB upstream to the MIR34A gene and overlaps the first intron of the MIR34A host gene (MIR34AHG) (position 28889 of 30171: −1283 upstream to the splicing site). Despite being predicted to be a benign variant, it was previously reported to be associated with human diseases [25,26].

2.8. Statistical Analysis

Statistical analysis was performed by GraphPad Prism v9.0 and Statistical Package for Social Science (version 27.0). The Shapiro–Wilk test was applied to assess the normality of continuous variables, then analyzed by the Kruskal-Wallis or Mann–Whitney U tests (if non-parametric) or the One-Way ANOVA or Student's t-test (if parametric). Genotype and allele frequencies were estimated as previously described, and SNPstats software was applied [29]. Genotypes and alleles distribution of rs2666433 in different populations were compared from the Ensemble database (ensemble.org) (last accessed on 23 May 2021). Hardy–Weinberg equilibrium (HWE) testing and categorical variables comparison were preceded by a two-sided Chi-Square test. Logistic regression was used for evaluating the association between miR-34a polymorphisms and SLE disease risk, and odds ratio (OR), 95% confidence interval (CI), and p-values were adjusted by age and sex; $p < 0.05$ indicated statistical significance. The principal component analysis was plotted using R packages. The power calculation was performed by the G*Power version 3.1.9.2. Under the parameters of α error probability = 0.05, total sample size (326; each case/control subgroup = 163), and calculated effect size = 0.288, the study has 99% statistical power to identify a convincing association between the rs2666433 variant and SLE risk.

3. Results

3.1. Characteristics of the Study Population

This case-control study included 163 SLE patients (147 females and 16 males) and 163 controls (148 females and 15 males). Their mean age was 35.6 ± 9.6 years for patients and 35.8 ± 9.9 years for controls. The characteristics of the study population are demonstrated in Table 1. Females represented 90% of the SLE population. Positive family history (history of rheumatic diseases and/or autoimmune diseases as SLE, RA, autoimmune thyroid disease, diabetes mellitus type 1, inflammatory bowel disease, and psoriasis) was identified in 35% of patients. Almost 49% of patients presented with arthritis/arthralgia symptoms, CNS manifestations (25%), and peripheral neuropathy (42%). According to the

SLEDAI score, patients were divided into four groups: 7.4% Grade 1, 30% Grade 2, 34% Grade 3, and 23% Grade 4.

Table 1. Baseline characteristics of SLE patients.

Characteristics		$n = 163$
Demographics		
Sex	Male	16 (9.8)
	Female	147 (90.2)
Family history	Negative	105 (64.4)
	Positive	58 (35.6)
Clinical manifestations		
Organ involvement	Malar rash	109 (66.9)
	Discoid rash	77 (47.2)
	Photosensitivity	61 (37.4)
	Hair loss	129 (79.1)
	Oral ulcer	46 (28.2)
	Arthritis	81 (49.7)
	Ecchymosis	19 (11.7)
	Fever	30 (18.4)
	Infection	26 (16)
	Dyspnea	68 (41.7)
	Chest pain	35 (21.5)
	Cough	35 (21.5)
	CNS	41 (25.2)
	Peripheral neuropathy	70 (42.9)
	Lupus nephritis	98 (60.1)
	Hematuria	56 (34.4)
	Weight loss *	76 (46.6)
Severity		
SLEDAI score	Mean ± SD	15.97 ± 9.82
	Grade 1	12 (7.4)
	Grade 2	50 (30.7)
	Grade 3	56 (34.4)
	Grade 4	45 (27.6)
Markers for severity and kidney damage	Hypocomplementemia	47 (28.8)
	Elevated inflammatory markers	67 (41.1)
	High S. creatinine	72 (44.2)
	Casts in urine	29 (17.8)
	Proteinuria	92 (56.4)
	Thrombocytopenia	5 (3.1)
Laboratory data		
Autoantibodies	Positive dsDNA	147 (90.2)
	Positive ANA titer	162 (99.4)
Biochemical tests	Hemoglobin (g/dL)	11.66 ± 2.89
	RBC ($\times 10^6$ per mm^3)	4.09 ± 0.74
	HCT (%)	38.18 ± 6.05
	MCV (fl)	81.42 ± 6.36
	Platelet count ($\times 10^3$/mm^3)	264.51 ± 77.59
	WBC ($\times 10^3$/uL)	6.58 ± 2.22
	Neutrophil (%)	63.30 ± 10.46
	Lymphocyte (%)	30.01 ± 9.66
	C3 (mg/dL)	95.52 ± 47.86
	C4 (mg/dL)	27.94 ± 15.62
	CRP (mg/L)	2.95 ± 2.89
	ESR 1st h	26.84 ± 13.58
	ALT (U/L)	26.61 ± 9.62
	AST (U/L)	26.50 ± 8.48
	Serum creatinine (mg/dL)	1.18 ± 1.19
	Blood urea (mg/dL)	35.11 ± 11.86

Values are shown as number (%) or mean and standard deviation. Positive family history: history of rheumatic diseases and/or autoimmune diseases as SLE, RA, autoimmune thyroid disease, diabetes mellitus type 1, inflammatory bowel disease, and psoriasis), *: "Unintentional weight loss of >5% of body weight over 6–12 months" [8]. CNS: the central nervous system; SLEDAI: Systemic Lupus Erythematosus Disease Activity index; dsDNA: Double-stranded deoxyribonucleic acid; ANA: Anti-nuclear antibody; RBC: red blood cell; HCT: hematocrit; MCV: mean cell volume; WBC: white blood cell; C3/4, complement 3/4; CRP: C—reactive protein; ALT: alanine transaminase; AST: aspartate transaminase.

Comparison between patients with different disease activities is illustrated in Table 2. As expected, oral ulcers presented in 44% of patients within grade 4 ($p = 0.043$), while lupus nephritis was more prevalent in patients within grades 3 and 4 (60% and 82%, respectively) ($p < 0.001$). In addition, significant differences regarding casts in urine and proteinuria were evident ($p > 0.001$).

Table 2. Characteristics of SLE patients according to their disease activity.

Characteristics		Grade 1 ($n = 12$)	Grade 2 ($n = 50$)	Grade 3 ($n = 56$)	Grade 4 ($n = 45$)	p-Value
Demographics						
Age, years	Median (quartiles)	27.5 (26–38)	35 (30–43.5)	36 (29.8–43.3)	36 (30.3–42.8)	0.43
Sex	Male	1 (8.3)	4 (8)	5 (8.9)	6 (13.3)	0.82
	Female	11 (91.7)	46 (92)	51 (91.1)	39 (86.7)	
Family history	Negative	6 (50)	36 (72)	36 (64.3)	27 (60)	0.43
	Positive	6 (50)	14 (28)	20 (35.7)	18 (40)	
Clinical manifestations						
Organ involvement	Malar rash	10 (83.3)	35 (70)	38 (67.9)	25 (57.8)	0.33
	Discoid rash	5 (41.7)	21 (42)	28 (50)	23 (51.1)	0.77
	Photosensitivity	5 (41.7)	18 (36)	20 (35.7)	18 (40)	0.95
	Hair loss	11 (91.7)	39 (78)	49 (87.5)	30 (66.7)	0.05
	Oral ulcer	3 (25)	11 (22)	12 (21.4)	20 (44.4)	**0.043**
	Arthritis	5 (41.7)	23 (46)	33 (58.9)	20 (44.4)	0.39
	Ecchymosis	1 (8.3)	6 (12)	10 (17.9)	2 (4.4)	0.21
	Fever	1 (8.3)	15 (30)	9 (16.1)	5 (11.1)	0.07
	Infection	2 (16.7)	8 (16)	9 (16.1)	7 (15.6)	1.00
	Dyspnea	8 (66.7)	20 (40)	22 (39.3)	18 (40)	0.34
	Chest pain	2 (16.7)	7 (14)	20 (35.7)	6 (13.3)	**0.016**
	Cough	6 (50)	8 (16)	16 (28.6)	5 (11.1)	**0.011**
	CNS	4 (33.3)	13 (26)	15 (26.8)	9 (20)	0.76
	Peripheral neuropathy	7 (58.3)	20 (40)	25 (44.6)	18 (40)	0.67
	Lupus nephritis	3 (25)	24 (48)	34 (60.7)	37 (82.2)	**<0.001**
	Hematuria	5 (41.7)	17 (34)	20 (35.7)	14 (31.1)	0.91
	Weight loss *	6 (50)	25 (50)	24 (42.9)	21 (46.7)	0.90
Severity						
Markers for severity and Kidney damge	Hypocomplementemia	3 (25)	15 (30)	13 (23.2)	16 (35.6)	0.58
	Elevated Inflammatory markers	7 (58.3)	23 (46)	21 (37.5)	16 (35.6)	0.42
	High S. creatinine	1 (8.3)	18 (36)	28 (50)	25 (55.6)	**0.013**
	Casts in urine	1 (8.3)	1 (2)	10 (17.9)	17 (37.8)	**<0.001**
	Proteinuria	1 (8.3)	21 (42)	34 (60.7)	36 (80)	**<0.001**
	Thrombocytopenia	1 (8.3)	1 (2)	1 (1.8)	2 (4.4)	0.59
Laboratory data						
Autoantibodies	Positive dsDNA	8 (66.7)	41 (82)	54 (96.4)	44 (97.8)	0.001
	Positive ANA titer	12 (100)	49 (98)	56 (100)	45 (100)	0.52
Biochemical tests	Hemoglobin (g/dL)	11.5 (10.6–13.1)	11.2 (10.4–12.1)	11.4 (10.7–12.3)	11.2 (10.4–12.9)	0.87
	RBC ($\times 10^6$ per mm^3)	3.9 (3.6–4.3)	4 (3.6–4.5)	4.2 (3.8–4.6)	4.1 (3.7–4.5)	0.42
	HCT (%)	39 (30.5–41)	38 (34–41)	39 (33–42)	39 (36.3–42)	0.52
	MCV (fl)	81.8 (77–89.3)	80 (76–88)	82 (80.3–87)	79.5 (77–87)	0.56
	Platelet count ($\times 10^3$ per mm^3)	227 (179.5–261)	248 (211.5–321)	239.5 (212–325)	268.5 (201–320)	0.50
	WBC (x10^3 /uL)	6.4 (4.1–7.6)	6.5 (5.3–7.7)	7 (5–7.9)	6.1 (5.3–7.7)	0.62
	Neutrophil (%)	70.5 (57–71)	66 (56–71)	66 (54.8–70)	65 (59–70.8)	0.86
	Lymphocyte (%)	27 (23–35)	29 (22–35.5)	31.5 (22–39)	30 (26–34.5)	0.65
	C3 (mg/dL)	89.5 (83–120.3)	88 (50–123)	91.5 (50–123)	122 (93–138)	**0.003**
	C4 (mg/dL)	35 (27–41.5)	25 (9–37)	32.5 (8.8–42.3)	37 (23–43)	**0.028**
	CRP (mg/L)	2.9 (1.5–3.9)	2.1 (1.7–3.4)	2.8 (1.4–3.7)	2.5 (1.8–3.2)	0.81
	ESR 1st h	26 (20.8–33)	23 (16.5–36)	23 (19–33)	21 (15.3–30)	0.31
	ALT (U/L)	28.5 (22.3–30)	28 (19.5–33)	29 (19–33.5)	27.5 (17.3–33)	0.99
	AST (U/L)	25 (23.3–33.8)	28 (22–34)	27 (19.8–33)	24 (15.3–33)	0.26
	Serum creatinine (mg/dL)	1 (0.8–1.2)	1.1 (0.9–1.2)	0.9 (0.7–1.1)	1 (0.8–1.3)	**0.022**
	Blood urea (mg/dL)	36 (29–41.8)	33 (29–39)	33 (29–42)	33 (28–40)	0.80

Values are shown as number (%) or median quartiles. Chi-square and Student t-tests were used. Positive family history: history of rheumatic diseases and/or autoimmune diseases as SLE, RA, autoimmune thyroid disease, diabetes mellitus type 1, inflammatory bowel disease, and psoriasis), *: "Unintentional weight loss of >5% of body weight over 6–12 months" [8]. Bold values indicate statistically significant p-value < 0.05. CNS: central nervous system; dsDNA: Double-stranded deoxyribonucleic acid; ANA: Anti-nuclear antibody; RBC: red blood cell; HCT: hematocrit; MCV: mean cell volume; WBC: white blood cell; C3/4, complement 3/4; CRP: C—reactive protein; ESR: erythrocyte sedimentation rate; ALT: alanine transaminase; AST: aspartate transaminase.

3.2. Role of miRNA-34a in SLE Disease

As depicted in Figure 1A, miR-34a-5p has 27 experimentally validated gene targets in SLE KEGG pathway (hsa05322 | Adj p-value = 2.4×10^{-7}, including several histone variants, RNA-binding proteins, and immune response-related genes (Table S1). Validation of miR-34a expression in two independent SLE cohorts from online GEO datasets revealed microRNA upregulation in patients compared to controls (Figure 1B). In GSE80183, miR-34a was upregulated in patients with anti-dsDNA (FC = 1.04, p = 0.017), anti-ENA (FC = 1.133, p = 0.015), and both anti-dsDNA and anti-ENA (FC = 1.016, p = 0.039) in comparison with healthy individuals. In GSE72509, relative expression was 0.579 ($p = 11.7 \times 10^{-7}$) and 0.538 ($p = 18.6 \times 10^{-6}$) in patients with high anti-Ro and moderate anti-Ro, and 0.514 ($p = 11.8 \times 10^{-8}$) in patients with high Interferon Signature Metric (ISM) compared to controls.

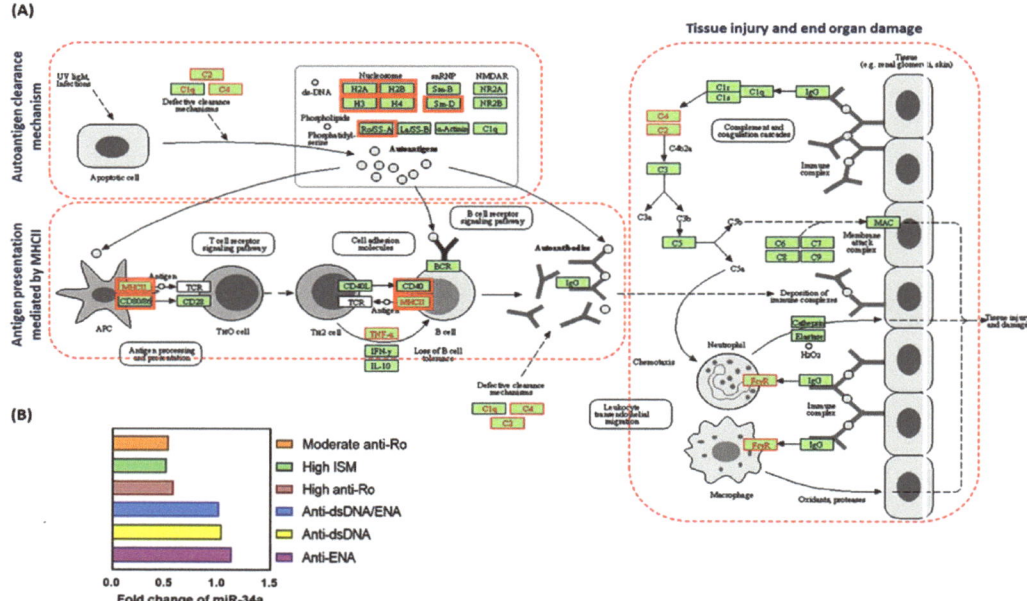

Figure 1. SLE is an autoimmune disease characterized by augmented self-antigen specific auto-antibodied production that contribute to a pleotropic clinical presentation. (**A**) MicroRNA-34a is significantly enriched in the SLE pathway. Gene targets of miR-34a were labeled in red bold-colored boxes in the SLE KEGG pathway (hsa05322) [30]. MiR-34a target genes code for different histone family members (i.e., H2A, H2B, H3, and H4) that are implicated in tolerance mechanism/autoantigen clearance and the "major histocompatibility complex class II (MHCII)", which plays an essential role in antigen presentation [31]. All the stages of antigen processing and autoantibodies generation lead to tissue injury and end-organ damage (left panel) [32]. More detail for gene names and functions are provided in Table S1. Data source: Diana Lab tools (DIANA TOOLS-Reverse Mirpath (grnet.gr) (last accessed on 25 May 2021). (**B**) The expression level of the MIR34A gene in SLE patients in independent cohorts from Gene Expression Omnibus datasets (GSE80183 and GSE72509), Anti-Ro: a type of RNA-binding proteins; ISM: Interferon Signature Metric; dsDNA: double-stranded DNA; ENA: extractable nuclear antigens (RNAassociated proteins) [33,34].

3.3. MIR34A rs2666433 Genotype and Allelic Frequencies

The HWE among controls was in line with observed equilibrium (p = 0.21). The A allele of the rs2666433 variant was 0.39 among patients with SLE compared to 0.49 among controls, while the G allele frequency was 0.61 among patients vs. 0.51 in healthy controls (p = 0.014) (Figure 2B). The most predominant genotype among patients with SLE was G/G genotype (42%), while the most frequent genotype among controls was the G/A genotype (45%) (Figure 2C).

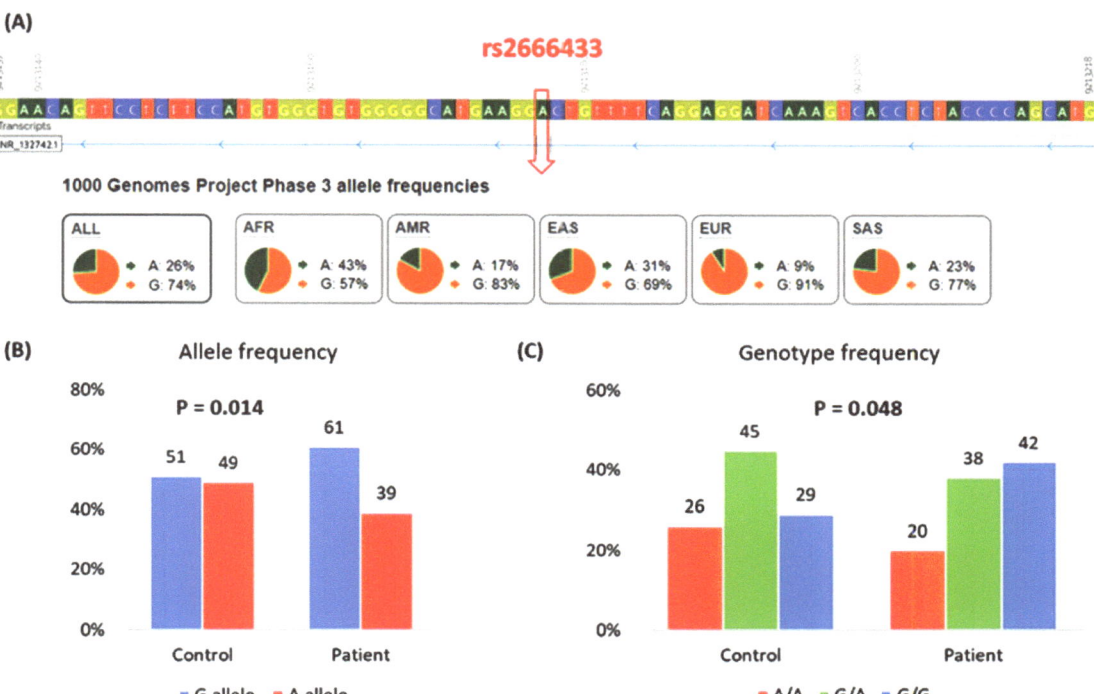

Figure 2. Genotype and allele frequencies of MIR34A rs2666433 (A/G) polymorphism. (**A**) Genomic location and allele frequencies of rs2666433 variant. Data source: (Ensembl.org) last accessed on 25 May 2021). (**B**) Allele frequency in the current study. (**C**) Genotype frequency in the current study. Values are shown as a percentage. A Chi-square test was used. *p*-value < 0.05 was considered as statistically significant. The *p*-value for Hardy–Weinberg equilibrium is 0.21.

3.4. Association of MIR34A rs2666433 Variant with SLE Development

Upon adjusting the covariates; age and sex, the MIR34A rs2666433 polymorphism conferred a protection against developing SLE under several genetic models, including heterozygous [A/G versus G/G; OR = 0.57, 95%CI =0.34–0.95], homozygous [A/A vs. G/G; OR = 0.52, 95%CI = 0.29–0.94], dominant [A/G + A/A vs. GG; OR = 0.55, 95%CI = 0.35–0.88], and log-additive [OR = 0.71, 95%CI = 0.53–0.95] models (Table 3). When genotyping data stratified by sex, the study variant showed significant association with SLE development in female participants compared to males under heterozygous model (OR = 0.45, 95%CI = 0.26–0.77) and homozygous model (OR = 0.39, 95%CI = 0.21–0.74) (*p*-interaction was 0.004) (Table 4).

3.5. Association of MIR34A rs2666433 Variant with Clinic-Laboratory Variables

Table 5 indicates that among A/A carriers there were a higher proportion of photosensitive patients ($p = 0.002$), experiencing weight loss ($p = 0.011$), anemia ($p = 0.005$), lymphopenia ($p = 0.048$), and raising blood urea ($p = 0.034$), in comparison to A/G and G/G carriers.

Table 3. Risk of systemic lupus erythematosus by genetic association models of miR-34a rs2666433 (A/G) genotypes.

Model	Genotype	Controls (n = 163)	Cases (n = 163)	Adjusted OR (95% CI)	p-Value
Codominant	G/G	47 (28.8%)	68 (41.7%)	1.00	**0.041**
	A/G	73 (44.8%)	62 (38%)	**0.57 (0.34–0.95)**	
	A/A	43 (26.4%)	33 (20.2%)	**0.52 (0.29–0.94)**	
Dominant	G/G	47 (28.8%)	68 (41.7%)	1.00	**0.012**
	A/G-A/A	116 (71.2%)	95 (58.3%)	**0.55 (0.35–0.88)**	
Recessive	G/G-A/G	120 (73.6%)	130 (79.8%)	1.00	0.18
	A/A	43 (26.4%)	33 (20.2%)	0.70 (0.42–1.18)	
Over dominant	G/G-A/A	90 (55.2%)	101 (62%)	1.00	0.21
	A/G	73 (44.8%)	62 (38%)	0.75 (0.48–1.17)	
Log-additive	—	—	—	**0.71 (0.53–0.95)**	**0.02**

Values are shown as numbers (%). A chi-square test was used. OR (95% CI), odds ratio, and 95% confidence interval. Bold values indicate statistically significant p-value < 0.05. Adjusted covariates were age and sex.

Table 4. Stratified analysis by sex for genotype frequencies between cases and controls.

SNP	Females			Males		
	Controls n	Cases n	Adjusted OR (95% CI)	Controls n	Cases n	Adjusted OR (95% CI)
G/G	38	65	1.00	9	3	1.00
A/G	69	54	**0.45 (0.26–0.77)**	4	8	5.85 (0.99–34.62)
A/A	41	28	**0.39 (0.21–0.74)**	2	5	7.19 (0.88–58.93)

Values are shown as numbers (N). Chi-square and Fisher exact tests were applied. OR (95% CI): odds ratio and confidence interval. Bold values indicate statistically significant p-value < 0.05. Adjusted OR with age. p-interaction was 0.004.

Table 5. Association between miR-34a rs2666433 (A/G) genotypes and the clinic-laboratory variables.

	Total	A/A	A/G	G/G	p-Value
Total number	163	33	62	68	
Early onset	112	20 (60.6)	41 (66.1)	51 (75)	0.29
Female	147	28 (84.8)	54 (87.1)	65 (95.6)	0.13
Positive FH	58	7 (21.2)	31 (50)	20 (29.4)	**0.008**
Severe stage	44	10 (30.3)	15 (24.2)	19 (27.9)	0.79
Organ involvement					
Malar rash	109	18 (54.5)	41 (66.1)	50 (73.5)	0.16
Discoid rash	77	12 (36.4)	26 (41.9)	39 (57.4)	0.08
Photosensitivity	61	21 (63.6)	19 (30.6)	21 (30.9)	**0.002**
Hair loss	129	27 (81.8)	48 (77.4)	54 (79.4)	0.87
Oral ulcer	46	9 (27.3)	19 (30.6)	18 (26.5)	0.86
Arthritis	81	9 (27.3)	37 (59.7)	35 (51.5)	**0.010**
Ecchymosis	19	4 (12.1)	9 (14.5)	6 (8.8)	0.59
Fever	30	3 (9.1)	12 (19.4)	15 (22.1)	0.28
Infection	26	4 (12.1)	9 (14.5)	13 (19.1)	0.61
Dyspnea	68	18 (54.5)	27 (43.5)	23 (33.8)	0.13
Chest pain	35	7 (21.2)	15 (24.2)	13 (19.1)	0.78
Cough	35	4 (12.1)	15 (24.2)	16 (23.5)	0.34
CNS	41	12 (36.4)	12 (19.4)	17 (25)	0.19
Peripheral neuropathy	70	18 (54.5)	27 (43.5)	25 (36.8)	0.23
Hematuria	56	9 (27.3)	17 (27.4)	30 (44.1)	0.08
Renal injury	93	22 (66.7)	32 (51.6)	39 (57.4)	0.36
Weight loss *	76	23 (69.7)	24 (38.7)	29 (42.6)	**0.011**
Laboratory test					
Hemoglobin (g/dL)		10.97 ± 2.08	12.54 ± 4.03	11.08 ± 1.33	**0.005**

Table 5. Cont.

	Total	A/A	A/G	G/G	p-Value
RBC ($\times 10^6$/mm^3)		3.81 ± 1.25	4.31 ± 0.62	3.94 ± 0.60	**0.004**
HCT (%)		38.21 ± 7.01	39.15 ± 5.69	37.01 ± 5.76	0.13
MCV (fl)		80.85 ± 6.20	82.63 ± 5.82	80.78 ± 6.79	0.20
Platelet count ($\times 10^3$ per mm^3)		292.21 ± 94.31	255.84 ± 69.54	257.40 ± 72.93	0.06
WBC ($\times 10^3$ /uL)		6.99 ± 2.06	6.35 ± 1.94	6.51 ± 2.52	0.41
Neutrophil (%)		66.42 ± 10.49	62.35 ± 10.70	63.00 ± 9.89	0.17
Lymphocyte (%)		26.61 ± 10.45	31.87 ± 10.41	30.44 ± 9.03	**0.048**
C3 (mg/dL)		100.63 ± 56.09	94.31 ± 39.65	94.69 ± 52.05	0.81
C4 (mg/dL)		24.63 ± 16.29	28.22 ± 13.50	29.44 ± 16.64	0.33
CRP (mg/L)		2.48 ± 1.14	2.56 ± 1.27	3.43 ± 4.16	0.14
ALT (U/L)		25.09 ± 10.88	28.11 ± 9.83	25.93 ± 8.57	0.26
AST (U/L)		24.30 ± 8.60	29.02 ± 8.99	26.18 ± 8.33	**0.030**
Serum creatinine (mg/dL)		1.39 ± 1.85	1.07 ± 0.73	1.15 ± 1.11	0.44
Blood urea (mg/dL)		39.01 ± 19.71	35.40 ± 10.30	32.58 ± 6.63	**0.034**

Early onset: Age at diagnosis <40 years, severe Stage: SLEDAI score > 6. A chi-square test was used for frequency comparison. Analysis of variance (ANOVA) test is applied for data presented as mean ± SD between different subgroups. *: "Unintentional weight loss of >5% of body weight over 6–12 months" [8]. Bold values indicate statistically significant p-value < 0.05. Positive family history: family history of rheumatic diseases and/or autoimmune diseases as SLE, RA, autoimmune thyroid disease, diabetes mellitus type 1, inflammatory bowel disease, and psoriasis); CNS: the central nervous system; RBC: red blood cell; HCT: hematocrit; MCV: mean cell volume; WBC: white blood cell; C3/4, complement 3/4; CRP: C—reactive protein; ALT: alanine transaminase; AST: aspartate transaminase.

3.6. Impact of MIR34A rs2666433 Variant on the Disease Activity Index

The principal component analysis for data exploration showed no clear demarcation between SLE patients carrying different genotypes regarding the disease activity index (Figure 3A). Moreover, the study variant genotypes showed no significant association with SLEDAI upon stratifying patients according to the presence or absence of lupus nephritis (p = 0.29 and = 0.55, respectively) (Figure 3B).

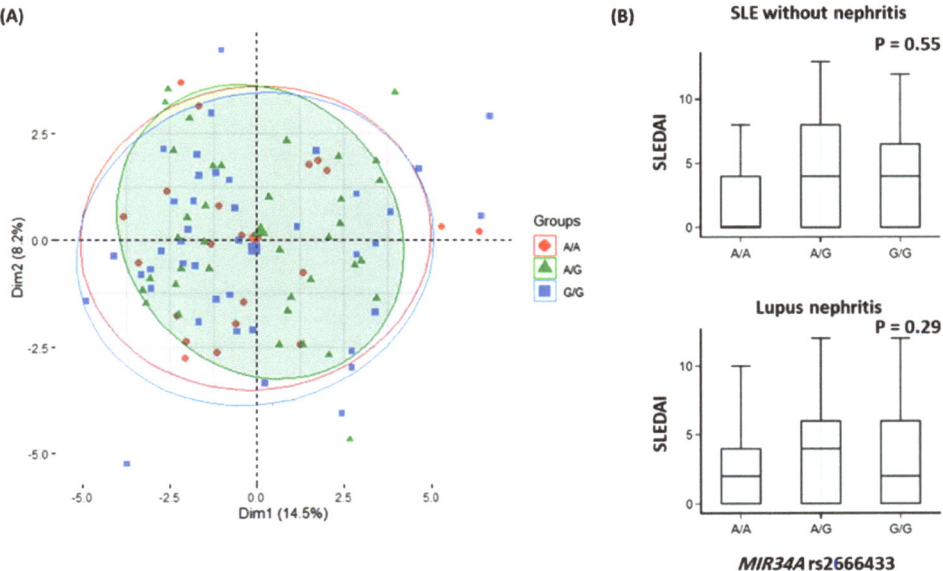

Figure 3. Impact of MIR34A rs2666433 (A/G) variant on disease activity index. (**A**) The principal component analysis for data exploration showed no clear demarcation between patients with different genotypes. (**B**) Box plots in SLE with and without nephritis show no significant difference in SLE disease activity index (SLEDAI).

4. Discussion

Accumulating evidence indicates that a "dose-dependent combination" of susceptibility genes, estrogenic hormones, immunological and environmental factors are involved in lupus etiopathology [35–37]. Unraveling the genetic/epigenetic contribution to SLE pathogenesis will pave the road to personalized medicine [38].

The microRNA family of non-coding RNAs has been implicated in immune system homeostasis, and its genetic variants and gene signature deregulation are associated with several immunological disorders, including SLE [32,39–42]. The present study identified for the first time that MIR34A rs2666433 A/A and A/G genotypes are less likely to develop SLE in the study population. On searching the national library of medicine (https://www.ncbi.nlm.nih.gov/snp/?term=rs2666433) (last accessed on 23 May 2021), there are only two rs2666433-related studies; one relates this specified variant with ischemic stroke in the Chinese population [25], and another publication explored the impact of this variant on CRC risk [26]. Sun and colleagues reported that this variant might impact the binding of several transcription factors to promoter elements of this gene [24] that results in a change of the type of activated/suppressed gene targets. Indeed, Wei and colleagues reported that "patients with ischemic stroke carrying A/A genotype had a higher level of transcript levels than carriers of G/G and G/A genotypes" [25], suggesting that this variant may impact gene expression level. The exact molecular mechanism(s) by which the rs2666433 variant implicated in SLE pathogenesis will need further functional analyses to unleash the relation of this SNP to SLE risk.

On searching "HaploReg V4.1: an online tool for exploring annotations of the non-coding genome (https://pubs.broadinstitute.org/mammals/haploreg/haploreg.php) (last accessed on 27 May 2021) [43] to predict the impact of rs2666433 SNP, we found that it is in linkage disequilibrium ($r^2 \geq 0.8$) with other variants present in chromosome 1 (i.e., rs34196792, rs113390912, rs34174278, and rs34619897), and can influence the Ets, peroxisome proliferator-activated receptor (PPAR), and the paired box-4 (Pax-4) DNA motifs (Table S2). Dysregulation of the specified transcriptional factors and/or their binding to these motifs was associated with autoimmune disorders in previous reports, including SLE susceptibility and pathogenesis [44–46]. For example, Ets1 has been reported to regulate lymphocyte/plasma cell differentiation, B cell tolerance to self-antigens, and autoantibodies/cytokine production [44], PPARγ was implicated in the regulation of the inflammatory signal initiated by CD40/CD40L activation [44], and PAX4 expression signature was identified in the differentially expressed significant probes of peripheral cells samples in patients with SLE and/or vasculitis [47].

Furthermore, our in silico analysis confirmed the implication of miR-34a in the SLE pathway (Figure 1 and Table S1) by targeting several genes coding for different histone family proteins, RNA-binding proteins, including the spliceosome small nuclear ribonucleoproteins, and several immune response-related proteins as CD86, CD40, and HLA class II histocompatibility antigen; DM alpha chain (Table S1). The functional roles of these target genes could support the significant association of the studied variant with SLE development and other phenotypic features observed in the present study.

Interestingly, when genotyping data stratified by sex, the rs2666433 variant showed significant association with SLE development in female participants compared to males under heterozygous and homozygous genetic models. Apart of the predominance of female gender among SLE participants in the present study and previous ones [8,48], estrogen has been reported to stimulate the secretion of pro-inflammatory cytokines such as "interleukin-17 and interferon-α", which are implicated in SLE etiopathology, either through "the modification of key transcription factors in inflammation or through the regulation of miRNA expression" [49]. Several microRNAs were identified to be dysregulated in SLE under the influence of estrogen, such as miR-146a, miR-155, miR-125a, miR-181a/b, and miR-21 [49–52]. Future in vivo and in vitro studies are recommended to investigate whether miR-34a gene signature/variants in SLE could be influenced by estrogen to confirm the current finding.

Although overall analysis and stratified analysis by presence/absence of lupus nephritis demonstrated an insignificant association of the rs2666433 variant with disease severity, it showed significant association with some clinical features, including arthritis. Interestingly, Kurowska–Stolarska et al reported that miR-34a could be an "epigenetic regulator" of the dendritic cells-mediated arthritis in patients with RA through tyrosine kinase receptor (AXL) downregulation and auto-reactive T cells activation [19]. Moreover, in vitro study has implicated miR34a in osteoarthritis synovial cell apoptosis via regulation of TGIF2 [53]. Furthermore, Zhang et al. uncovered the essential role of the long non-coding RNA "UFC1" in the osteoarthritis-associated chondrocyte survival through miR-34a sponging [54]. In addition, MiR-34a was reported to promote "Fas-mediated cartilage endplate chondrocyte apoptosis" by targeting Bcl-2 [55]. Taken together, all these studies highlight the important role of miR-34a could play in several types of arthritis, and hence the miR-34a-related variant could be associated with arthritis and other phenotypic features (such as photosensitivity and weight loss) according to the type of miR-34a target genes/molecular pathways dysregulated.

Regarding the laboratory variables, we found that among A/A carriers there were a higher proportion of patients experiencing anemia, lymphopenia and raising blood urea, in comparison to A/G and G/G carriers. As mentioned above, allele A substitution to allele G has been found to disrupt several transcriptional factor-binding DNA motifs with subsequent change in the type of deregulated genes. In this sense, the presence of double dose of allele "A" as an AA genotype might promote and impact the expression of gene set which differs from that expressed or affected by AG and/or GG genotypes.

It is worth noting that besides the current gene variant, additional contributing genetic/epigenetic and environmental factors play essential roles in SLE etiopathology. Furthermore, this study is limited by the relatively small sample size from which an association conclusion could be drawn. The exploratory nature of the study design also lacks the follow-up of patients and inability to unravel the molecular mechanism(s) by which the current variant could impact the disease. In this sense, future longitudinal confirmatory studies in large-scale cohorts, including functional experiments are required to decipher the biological significance of the MIR34A (rs266643 A > G) variant in SLE.

5. Conclusions

The present study revealed higher occurrence of MIR34A (rs266643) GG genotype carriers in SLE cohort of the present population rather than the AG/AA genotypes. Further large-scale studies supported by functional analyses on different ethnicities are highly recommended to explore the genotype-phenotype association details of this variant.

Supplementary Materials: The following are available online at https://www.mdpi.com/article/10.3390/jcm10215095/s1, Table S1: Gene targets for microRNA-34a-5p in the SLE KEGG pathway (hsa05322) and their structural and functional role in the cell. Table S2: Impact and linkage disequilibrium of MIR34A rs2666433 variant with other SNPs ($r^2 \geq 0.8$) predicted by HaploReg V4.1.

Author Contributions: Conceptualization, E.A.T. and M.S.F.; data curation, N.M.I., M.H.S.M. and E.M.A.; formal analysis, E.A.T. and M.S.F.; investigation, N.M.I., E.A.T., M.H.S.M. and M.S.F.; methodology, N.M.I., E.A.T., M.H.S.M., E.M.A. and M.S.F.; resources, N.M.I., E.A.T., M.H.S.M. and E.M.A.; software, E.A.T. and M.S.F.; validation, E.A.T.; visualization, E.A.T. and M.S.F.; writing—original draft, N.M.I., E.A.T., M.H.S.M., E.M.A. and M.S.F.; writing—review and editing, N.M.I. All authors have read and agreed to the published version of the manuscript.

Funding: This research received no external funding.

Institutional Review Board Statement: The study was conducted according to the guidelines of the Declaration of Helsinki and approved by the Ethics Committee of the Faculty of Medicine, Suez Canal University (approval no. 4268).

Informed Consent Statement: Informed consent was obtained from all subjects involved in the study.

Data Availability Statement: All generated data in this study are included in the article and supplementary material.

Acknowledgments: The authors thank all the participants who agree to join the study.

Conflicts of Interest: The authors declare no conflict of interest.

References

1. Pan, L.; Lu, M.P.; Wang, J.H.; Xu, M.; Yang, S.R. Immunological pathogenesis and treatment of systemic lupus erythematosus. *World J. Pediatr.* **2020**, *16*, 19–30. [CrossRef]
2. Stojan, G.; Petri, M. Epidemiology of systemic lupus erythematosus: An update. *Curr. Opin. Rheumatol.* **2018**, *30*, 144–150. [CrossRef] [PubMed]
3. Kaul, A.; Gordon, C.; Crow, M.K.; Touma, Z.; Urowitz, M.B.; van Vollenhoven, R.; Ruiz-Irastorza, G.; Hughes, G. Systemic lupus erythematosus. *Nat. Rev. Dis. Primers* **2016**, *2*, 16039. [CrossRef]
4. Phuti, A.; Schneider, M.; Tikly, M.; Hodkinson, B. Living with systemic lupus erythematosus in the developing world. *Rheumatol. Int.* **2018**, *38*, 1601–1613. [CrossRef] [PubMed]
5. Ramos, P.S.; Brown, E.E.; Kimberly, R.P.; Langefeld, C.D. Genetic factors predisposing to systemic lupus erythematosus and lupus nephritis. *Semin. Nephrol.* **2010**, *30*, 164–176. [CrossRef]
6. Tiffin, N.; Adeyemo, A.; Okpechi, I. A diverse array of genetic factors contribute to the pathogenesis of systemic lupus erythematosus. *Orphanet J. Rare Dis.* **2013**, *8*, 2. [CrossRef] [PubMed]
7. Kamen, D.L. Environmental influences on systemic lupus erythematosus expression. *Rheum. Dis. Clin. N. Am.* **2014**, *40*, 401–412. [CrossRef] [PubMed]
8. El Hadidi, K.T.; Medhat, B.M.; Abdel Baki, N.M.; Abdel Kafy, H.; Abdelrahaman, W.; Yousri, A.Y.; Attia, D.H.; Eissa, M.; El Dessouki, D.; Elgazzar, I.; et al. Characteristics of systemic lupus erythematosus in a sample of the Egyptian population: A retrospective cohort of 1109 patients from a single center. *Lupus* **2018**, *27*, 1030–1038. [CrossRef] [PubMed]
9. O'Brien, J.; Hayder, H.; Zayed, Y.; Peng, C. Overview of MicroRNA Biogenesis, Mechanisms of Actions, and Circulation. *Front. Endocrinol.* **2018**, *9*, 402. [CrossRef] [PubMed]
10. Zhang, C. MicroRNomics: A newly emerging approach for disease biology. *Physiol. Genom.* **2008**, *33*, 139–147. [CrossRef]
11. Pauley, K.M.; Chan, E.K. MicroRNAs and their emerging roles in immunology. *Ann. N. Y. Acad. Sci.* **2008**, *1143*, 226–239. [CrossRef]
12. Tsokos, G.C.; Lo, M.S.; Costa Reis, P.; Sullivan, K.E. New insights into the immunopathogenesis of systemic lupus erythematosus. *Nat. Rev. Rheumatol.* **2016**, *12*, 716–730. [CrossRef]
13. Rao, D.S.; O'Connell, R.M.; Chaudhuri, A.A.; Garcia-Flores, Y.; Geiger, T.L.; Baltimore, D. MicroRNA-34a perturbs B lymphocyte development by repressing the forkhead box transcription factor Foxp1. *Immunity* **2010**, *33*, 48–59. [CrossRef]
14. Taheri, F.; Ebrahimi, S.O.; Shareef, S.; Reiisi, S. Regulatory and immunomodulatory role of miR-34a in T cell immunity. *Life Sci.* **2020**, *262*, 118209. [CrossRef]
15. Shin, J.; Xie, D.; Zhong, X.P. MicroRNA-34a enhances T cell activation by targeting diacylglycerol kinase ζ. *PLoS ONE* **2013**, *8*, e77983. [CrossRef]
16. Hart, M.; Rheinheimer, S.; Leidinger, P.; Backes, C.; Menegatti, J.; Fehlmann, T.; Grässer, F.; Keller, A.; Meese, E. Identification of miR-34a-target interactions by a combined network based and experimental approach. *Oncotarget* **2016**, *7*, 34288–34299. [CrossRef] [PubMed]
17. Hart, M.; Walch-Rückheim, B.; Friedmann, K.S.; Rheinheimer, S.; Tänzer, T.; Glombitza, B.; Sester, M.; Lenhof, H.P.; Hoth, M.; Schwarz, E.C.; et al. miR-34a: A new player in the regulation of T cell function by modulation of NF-κB signaling. *Cell Death Dis.* **2019**, *10*, 46. [CrossRef]
18. Ghadiri, N.; Emamnia, N.; Ganjalikhani-Hakemi, M.; Ghaedi, K.; Etemadifar, M.; Salehi, M.; Shirzad, H.; Nasr-Esfahani, M.H. Analysis of the expression of mir-34a, mir-199a, mir-30c and mir-19a in peripheral blood CD4+T lymphocytes of relapsing-remitting multiple sclerosis patients. *Gene* **2018**, *659*, 109–117. [CrossRef]
19. Kurowska-Stolarska, M.; Alivernini, S.; Melchor, E.G.; Elmesmari, A.; Tolusso, B.; Tange, C.; Petricca, L.; Gilchrist, D.S.; Di Sante, G.; Keijzer, C.; et al. MicroRNA-34a dependent regulation of AXL controls the activation of dendritic cells in inflammatory arthritis. *Nat. Commun.* **2017**, *8*, 15877. [CrossRef] [PubMed]
20. Xie, M.; Wang, J.; Gong, W.; Xu, H.; Pan, X.; Chen, Y.; Ru, S.; Wang, H.; Chen, X.; Zhao, Y.; et al. NF-κB-driven miR-34a impairs Treg/Th17 balance via targeting Foxp3. *J. Autoimmun.* **2019**, *102*, 96–113. [CrossRef] [PubMed]
21. Chi, M.; Ma, K.; Li, Y.; Quan, M.; Han, Z.; Ding, Z.; Liang, X.; Zhang, Q.; Song, L.; Liu, C. Immunological Involvement of MicroRNAs in the Key Events of Systemic Lupus Erythematosus. *Front. Immunol.* **2021**, *12*, 699684. [CrossRef] [PubMed]
22. Lazarus, R.; Vercelli, D.; Palmer, L.J.; Klimecki, W.J.; Silverman, E.K.; Richter, B.; Riva, A.; Ramoni, M.; Martinez, F.D.; Weiss, S.T.; et al. Single nucleotide polymorphisms in innate immunity genes: Abundant variation and potential role in complex human disease. *Immunol. Rev.* **2002**, *190*, 9–25. [CrossRef]
23. Kim, Y.; Choi, G.H.; Ko, K.H.; Kim, J.O.; Oh, S.H.; Park, Y.S.; Kim, O.J.; Kim, N.K. Association of the Single Nucleotide Polymorphisms in microRNAs 130b, 200b, and 495 with Ischemic Stroke Susceptibility and Post-Stroke Mortality. *PLoS ONE* **2016**, *11*, e0162519. [CrossRef]

24. Sun, Y.; Peng, R.; Li, A.; Zhang, L.; Liu, H.; Peng, H.; Zhang, Z. Sequence variation in microRNA-34a is associated with diabetes mellitus susceptibility in a southwest Chinese Han population. *Int. J. Clin. Exp. Pathol.* **2018**, *11*, 1637–1644. [PubMed]
25. Wei, G.J.; Yuan, M.Q.; Jiang, L.H.; Lu, Y.L.; Liu, C.H.; Luo, H.C.; Huang, H.T.; Qi, Z.Q.; Wei, Y.S. A Genetic Variant of miR-34a Contributes to Susceptibility of Ischemic Stroke Among Chinese Population. *Front. Physiol.* **2019**, *10*, 432. [CrossRef]
26. Fawzy, M.S.; Ibrahiem, A.T.; AlSel, B.T.A.; Alghamdi, S.A.; Toraih, E.A. Analysis of microRNA-34a expression profile and rs2666433 variant in colorectal cancer: A pilot study. *Sci. Rep.* **2020**, *10*, 16940. [CrossRef] [PubMed]
27. Aringer, M.; Costenbader, K.; Daikh, D.; Brinks, R.; Mosca, M.; Ramsey-Goldman, R.; Smolen, J.S.; Wofsy, D.; Boumpas, D.T.; Kamen, D.L.; et al. 2019 European League Against Rheumatism/American College of Rheumatology Classification Criteria for Systemic Lupus Erythematosus. *Arthritis Rheumatol.* **2019**, *71*, 1400–1412. [CrossRef] [PubMed]
28. Bombardier, C.; Gladman, D.D.; Urowitz, M.B.; Caron, D.; Chang, C.H. Derivation of the SLEDAI. A disease activity index for lupus patients. The Committee on Prognosis Studies in SLE. *Arthritis Rheum.* **1992**, *35*, 630–640. [CrossRef] [PubMed]
29. Solé, X.; Guinó, E.; Valls, J.; Iniesta, R.; Moreno, V. SNPStats: A web tool for the analysis of association studies. *Bioinformatics* **2006**, *22*, 1928–1929. [CrossRef]
30. Kanehisa, M.; Goto, S. KEGG: Kyoto encyclopedia of genes and genomes. *Nucleic Acids Res* **2000**, *28*, 27–30. [CrossRef] [PubMed]
31. Malekina, S.; Salehi, Z.; Rezaei Tabar, V.; Sharifi-Zarchi, A.; Kavousi, K. An integrative Bayesian network approach to highlight key drivers in systemic lupus erythematosus. *Arthritis Res. Ther.* **2020**, *22*, 156. [CrossRef]
32. Abdel-Gawad, A.R.; Shaheen, S.; Babteen, N.A.; Toraih, E.A.; Elshazli, R.M.; Fawzy, M.S.; Gouda, N.S. Association of microRNA 17 host gene variant (rs4284505) with susceptibility and severity of systemic lupus erythematosus. *Immun. Inflamm. Dis.* **2020**, *8*, 595–604. [CrossRef] [PubMed]
33. Rai, R.; Chauhan, S.K.; Singh, V.V.; Rai, M.; Rai, G. RNA-seq Analysis Reveals Unique Transcriptome Signatures in Systemic Lupus Erythematosus Patients with Distinct Autoantibody Specificities. *PLoS ONE* **2016**, *11*, e0166312. [CrossRef]
34. Hung, T.; Pratt, G.A.; Sundararaman, B.; Townsend, M.J.; Chaivorapol, C.; Bhangale, T.; Graham, R.R.; Ortmann, W.; Criswell, L.A.; Yeo, G.W.; et al. The Ro60 autoantigen binds endogenous retroelements and regulates inflammatory gene expression. *Science* **2015**, *350*, 455–459. [CrossRef]
35. Somers, E.C.; Richardson, B.C. Environmental exposures, epigenetic changes and the risk of lupus. *Lupus* **2014**, *23*, 568–576. [CrossRef] [PubMed]
36. Chen, L.; Wang, Y.F.; Liu, L.; Bielowka, A.; Ahmed, R.; Zhang, H.; Tombleson, P.; Roberts, A.L.; Odhams, C.A.; Cunninghame Graham, D.S.; et al. Genome-wide assessment of genetic risk for systemic lupus erythematosus and disease severity. *Hum. Mol. Genet.* **2020**, *29*, 1745–1756. [CrossRef]
37. Demirkaya, E.; Sahin, S.; Romano, M.; Zhou, Q.; Aksentijevich, I. New Horizons in the Genetic Etiology of Systemic Lupus Erythematosus and Lupus-Like Disease: Monogenic Lupus and Beyond. *J. Clin. Med.* **2020**, *9*, 712. [CrossRef] [PubMed]
38. Lever, E.; Alves, M.R.; Isenberg, D.A. Towards Precision Medicine in Systemic Lupus Erythematosus. *Pharm. Pers. Med.* **2020**, *13*, 39–49. [CrossRef]
39. Le, X.; Yu, X.; Shen, N. Novel insights of microRNAs in the development of systemic lupus erythematosus. *Curr. Opin. Rheumatol.* **2017**, *29*, 450–457. [CrossRef] [PubMed]
40. Eissa, E.; Morcos, B.; Abdelkawy, R.F.M.; Ahmed, H.H.; Kholoussi, N.M. Association of microRNA-125a with the clinical features, disease activity and inflammatory cytokines of juvenile-onset lupus patients. *Lupus* **2021**, *30*, 1180–1187. [CrossRef] [PubMed]
41. Omidi, F.; Hosseini, S.A.; Ahmadi, A.; Hassanzadeh, K.; Rajaei, S.; Cesaire, H.M.; Hosseini, V. Discovering the signature of a lupus-related microRNA profile in the Gene Expression Omnibus repository. *Lupus* **2020**, *29*, 1321–1335. [CrossRef]
42. Xu, H.; Chen, W.; Zheng, F.; Tang, D.; Liu, D.; Wang, G.; Xu, Y.; Yin, L.; Zhang, X.; Dai, Y. Reconstruction and analysis of the aberrant lncRNA-miRNA-mRNA network in systemic lupus erythematosus. *Lupus* **2020**, *29*, 398–406. [CrossRef]
43. Ward, L.D.; Kellis, M. HaploReg: A resource for exploring chromatin states, conservation, and regulatory motif alterations within sets of genetically linked variants. *Nucleic Acids Res.* **2012**, *40*, D930–D934. [CrossRef] [PubMed]
44. Garrett-Sinha, L.A.; Kearly, A.; Satterthwaite, A.B. The Role of the Transcription Factor Ets1 in Lupus and Other Autoimmune Diseases. *Crit. Rev. Immunol.* **2016**, *36*, 485–510. [CrossRef]
45. Oxer, D.S.; Godoy, L.C.; Borba, E.; Lima-Salgado, T.; Passos, L.A.; Laurindo, I.; Kubo, S.; Barbeiro, D.F.; Fernandes, D.; Laurindo, F.R.; et al. PPARγ expression is increased in systemic lupus erythematosus patients and represses CD40/CD40L signaling pathway. *Lupus* **2011**, *20*, 575–587. [CrossRef] [PubMed]
46. Jo, W.; Endo, M.; Ishizu, K.; Nakamura, A.; Tajima, T. A novel PAX4 mutation in a Japanese patient with maturity-onset diabetes of the young. *Tohoku J. Exp. Med.* **2011**, *223*, 113–118. [CrossRef] [PubMed]
47. Lyons, P.A.; McKinney, E.F.; Rayner, T.F.; Hatton, A.; Woffendin, H.B.; Koukoulaki, M.; Freeman, T.C.; Jayne, D.R.; Chaudhry, A.N.; Smith, K.G. Novel expression signatures identified by transcriptional analysis of separated leucocyte subsets in systemic lupus erythematosus and vasculitis. *Ann. Rheum. Dis.* **2010**, *69*, 1208–1213. [CrossRef] [PubMed]
48. Weckerle, C.E.; Niewold, T.B. The unexplained female predominance of systemic lupus erythematosus: Clues from genetic and cytokine studies. *Clin. Rev. Allergy Immunol.* **2011**, *40*, 42–49. [CrossRef]
49. Zan, H.; Tat, C.; Casali, P. MicroRNAs in lupus. *Autoimmunity* **2014**, *47*, 272–285. [CrossRef] [PubMed]
50. Leivonen, S.K.; Mäkelä, R.; Ostling, P.; Kohonen, P.; Haapa-Paananen, S.; Kleivi, K.; Enerly, E.; Aakula, A.; Hellström, K.; Sahlberg, N.; et al. Protein lysate microarray analysis to identify microRNAs regulating estrogen receptor signaling in breast cancer cell lines. *Oncogene* **2009**, *28*, 3926–3936. [CrossRef]

51. Lu, Z.; Liu, M.; Stribinskis, V.; Klinge, C.M.; Ramos, K.S.; Colburn, N.H.; Li, Y. MicroRNA-21 promotes cell transformation by targeting the programmed cell death 4 gene. *Oncogene* **2008**, *27*, 4373–4379. [CrossRef] [PubMed]
52. Dai, R.; Phillips, R.A.; Zhang, Y.; Khan, D.; Crasta, O.; Ahmed, S.A. Suppression of LPS-induced Interferon-gamma and nitric oxide in splenic lymphocytes by select estrogen-regulated microRNAs: A novel mechanism of immune modulation. *Blood* **2008**, *112*, 4591–4597. [CrossRef]
53. Luo, C.; Liang, J.S.; Gong, J.; Zhang, H.L.; Feng, Z.J.; Yang, H.T.; Zhang, H.B.; Kong, Q.H. The function of microRNA-34a in osteoarthritis. *Bratisl. Lek. Listy* **2019**, *120*, 386–391. [CrossRef] [PubMed]
54. Zhang, G.; Wu, Y.; Xu, D.; Yan, X. Long Noncoding RNA UFC1 Promotes Proliferation of Chondrocyte in Osteoarthritis by Acting as a Sponge for miR-34a. *DNA Cell Biol.* **2016**, *35*, 691–695. [CrossRef]
55. Chen, H.; Wang, J.; Hu, B.; Wu, X.; Chen, Y.; Li, R.; Yuan, W. MiR-34a promotes Fas-mediated cartilage endplate chondrocyte apoptosis by targeting Bcl-2. *Mol. Cell. Biochem.* **2015**, *406*, 21–30. [CrossRef] [PubMed]

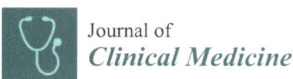 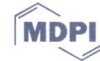

Review

Patient-Reported Outcomes in Systemic Lupus Erythematosus. Can Lupus Patients Take the Driver's Seat in Their Disease Monitoring?

Ioannis Parodis [1,2,*] and Paul Studenic [1,3]

1. Division of Rheumatology, Department of Medicine Solna, Karolinska Institutet and Karolinska University Hospital, 171 76 Stockholm, Sweden; paul.studenic@ki.se
2. Department of Rheumatology, Faculty of Medicine and Health, Örebro University, 701 82 Örebro, Sweden
3. Division of Rheumatology, Department of Internal Medicine 3, Medical University of Vienna, 1090 Vienna, Austria
* Correspondence: ioannis.parodis@ki.se; Tel.: +46-722321322

Abstract: Systemic lupus erythematosus (SLE) is a chronic autoimmune disorder that has detrimental effects on patient's health-related quality of life (HRQoL). Owing to its immense heterogeneity of symptoms and its complexity regarding comorbidity burden, management of SLE necessitates interdisciplinary care, with the goal being the best possible HRQoL and long-term outcomes. Current definitions of remission, low disease activity, and response to treatment do not incorporate self-reported patient evaluation, while it has been argued that the physician's global assessment should capture the patient's perspective. However, even the judgment of a very well-trained physician might not replace a patient-reported outcome measure (PROM), not only owing to the multidimensionality of self-perceived health experience but also since this notion would constitute a direct contradiction to the definition of PROMs. The proper use of PROMs is not only an important conceptual issue but also an opportunity to build bridges in the partnership between patients and physicians. These points of consideration adhere to the overall framework that there will seldom be one single best marker that helps interpret the activity, severity, and impact of SLE at the same time. For optimal outcomes, we not only stress the importance of the use of PROMs but also emphasize the urgency of adoption of the conception of forming alliances with patients and facilitating patient participation in surveillance and management processes. Nevertheless, this should not be misinterpreted as a transfer of responsibility from healthcare professionals to patients but rather a step towards shared decision-making.

Keywords: systemic lupus erythematosus; patient-reported outcomes; patient perspective; health-related quality of life; shared decision; person-centred care

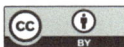

1. Introduction

Systemic lupus erythematosus (SLE) is a chronic autoimmune disorder that has detrimental effects on a patient's health-related quality of life (HRQoL) [1]. It is widely known that SLE is a rheumatic condition that is challenging to diagnose and treat, mainly owing to its immense heterogeneity of clinical symptoms and complexity with regard to comorbidity burden, often necessitating interdisciplinary care, with the goal being the best possible quality of life and long-term outcomes [2,3]. With the premise that preventing is better than restoring, early diagnosis and treatment initiation is imperative [4], a need of particular urgency given that up to 10% of SLE patients develop life-threatening conditions or complications, such as end-stage kidney disease [5,6]. Patient-reported outcome measures (PROMs) receive increasing attention within the lupus research community, especially PROMs addressing HRQoL [7] Even though this signifies a shift of the current paradigm towards increasing patient participation in their care, more distance has to be bridged before PROMs are an integral part of the evaluation in clinical practice.

2. PROMs in the Treat-to-Target Context

Remission of systemic symptoms and organ manifestations was identified by the treat-to-target for SLE initiative (T2T/SLE) as one of the most important targets in the management of patients with SLE [8]. Several definitions of remission were used in clinical trials and observational studies of SLE [9]. The Definitions Of Remission In SLE (DORIS) is an international task force consisting of expert rheumatologists, nephrologists, dermatologists, clinical immunologists, and patient representatives, who jointly proposed a set of remission definitions in response to the T2T/SLE research agenda [10]. Later, the group decided on one prevailing remission definition that incorporated a physician-reported global assessment (PhGA), the SLE Disease Activity Index 2000 (SLEDAI-2K) [11] after suppression of the serological descriptors (anti-double-stranded (ds)DNA and complement levels), the current daily glucocorticoid dose, and restrictions regarding medication allowance. Practically, however, some patients' individual situations make it hard for them to achieve this stringent target. In such cases, one should aim for low disease activity (LDA). Again, several definitions of LDA have been proposed in the literature, with the Lupus Low Disease Activity State (LLDAS) [12] being the most commonly used.

In addition, several recent clinical trials of SLE have used composite indices to define response to treatment, e.g., the SLEDAI Responder Index (SRI) [13] or the British Isles Lupus Assessment Group (BILAG)-based Combined Lupus Assessment (BICLA) [14]. Notably, none of the proposed definitions of remission, LDA, or response to treatment incorporate self-reported patient evaluation, which may constitute a pitfall of the definitions. Indeed, the DORIS task force discussed the issue of the non-inclusion of a PROM and partwise argued that the PhGA should incorporate the patient's perspective by paying careful attention to the patient's symptoms and experience [15]. However, even the judgment of a very well-trained physician might not replace a PROM, not only owing to the multidimensionality of patient-perceived health experience (Figure 1), but also since this notion would constitute a direct contradiction to the definition of a PROM; patient-reported outcomes are directly recorded by patients, without interpretation by their clinicians, and are additional markers in the assessment of treatment impact [16,17]. In the definition of remission in rheumatoid arthritis (RA), the patient's global assessment (PtGA) was chosen as one of the four Boolean criteria because of its ability to show a large sensitivity to change and its discriminatory validity between active drug and placebo in clinical trials [15]. However, it is not easy to address the question of whether PtGA is an ideal PROM to complement the current definition of remission. In fact, a debate has been ongoing for a decade with regard to the appropriateness of PtGA to be included in the remission definition in RA, at least with the currently used cut-offs, since substantial proportions of patients score their disease activity higher than their rheumatologists [18–20]. Due to the lack of evidence-based alternatives to PtGA, a summary report of an Outcome Measures in Rheumatology (OMERACT) interest group recently stated that currently, no better tools for representing the patients' perspective are available, thus the definition should be kept as is [21]. It is, however, worth noting that the differences in heterogeneity and complexity between SLE and RA are also reflected in discrepant longitudinal patterns of self-reported health experience [22] and direct comparisons or extrapolations of psychometric properties of PROMs between the two diseases may be misleading.

The issue of imperfect agreement in the perception of disease severity between patients and physicians was also addressed in the field of SLE. While LDA is coupled with an overall favorable HRQoL experience, at least when assessed with the LLDAS [23], results from other investigations are conflicting. One study used a Systemic Lupus Activity Questionnaire (SLAQ) score < 6 as the cut-off for LDA as perceived by the patients and found that only one-quarter of patients who were classified as being in LLDAS fulfilled the definition of SLAQ score < 6 [24]. In the same study, Medical Outcomes Survey Short Form 36 (SF-36) component summary scores and Functional Assessment of Chronic Illness Therapy Fatigue scale (FACIT-F) scores were higher among patients in LLDAS who reported SLAQ scores < 6 than among patients in LLDAS who reported SLAQ scores ≥ 6 [24].

This not only underscores that the physician's perspective does not entirely represent the patient's perception of HRQoL, but also highlights that LLDAS alone may not be a sufficient target in the management of people with SLE. The inclusion of HRQoL measures in treatment evaluation processes was supported by the T2T statements and received additional weight through findings indicating that poor HRQoL is associated with increased mortality [8,25]. To this end, it is important to clarify that this discussion is not intended to devalue the PhGA or the rheumatologists' ability to perform adequate clinical judgment; in fact, PhGA scores have shown good correlates with mental health, overall disease activity, and flares [26].

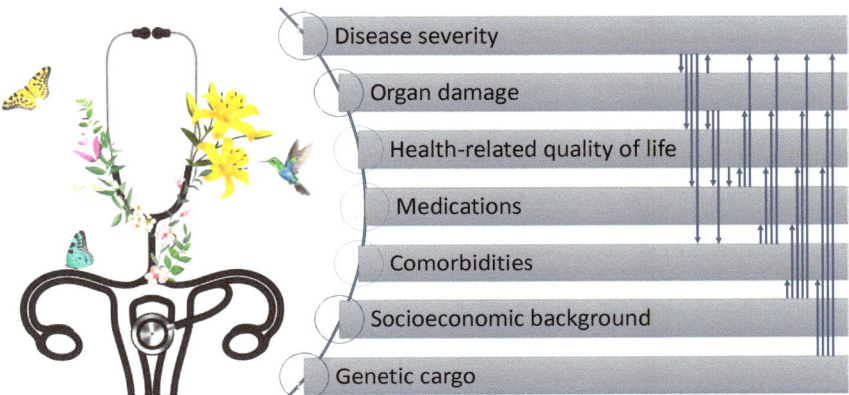

Figure 1. Illustration of the multilateral impact across disease facets and health-related quality of life in people living with systemic lupus erythematosus.

3. The Matter of Not Only Optimal Choice but Also Optimal Use of PROMs

The OMERACT IV consensus conference [27] propounded disease activity, HRQoL, medication side-effects, and organ damage as the four core outcomes for SLE clinical trials in that priority order. In light of accumulating evidence of the discordance in perceptions of disease activity between physicians and patients with SLE [28], PROMs are increasingly used in SLE clinical trials [7]. The SF-36 [29] and FACIT-F [30] were reviewed for their psychometric properties with regard to the extent to which they comply with the US Food and Drug Administration (FDA) guidance [31] and were suggested as secondary endpoints to support the labeling of novel therapies for SLE [32]. Changes in scores in various SF-36 domains and FACIT-F have shown an ability to discriminate between verum drug (belimumab) and placebo in the BLISS-52 and BLISS-76 clinical trials [33]. In the same analysis, changes in EQ-5D utility index scores [34] did not exhibit discriminative ability. However, in light of satisfactory psychometric properties of EQ-5D for SLE patients, particularly in terms of validity and reliability [35], a recent study investigated the discriminative ability and known-group validity of EQ-5D full health state (FHS), i.e., a utility index score of 1, and found a remarkably robust ability of EQ-5D FHS to discriminate between drug and placebo, and between responders and non-responders in the BLISS-52 and BLISS-76 clinical trials [36]. This not only illustrates the need for determining optimal PROMs in SLE but also supports the notion that optimal use of the currently available ones may be even more important. For example, the differential ability of PROMs to capture changes in the different SLE disease patterns, i.e., persistently quiescent, persistently relapsing-remitting, and persistently active disease [37], comprises one of the many questions framing the future research agenda.

4. Can Lupus Patients Take the Driver's Seat in Their Disease Monitoring?

Several questions regarding the validity of PROMs for people with SLE were clarified over the past decades [38,39]. We outlined their value in the interpretation of trial data for therapies that are potentially beneficial in the management of SLE. It is apparent that treatment cannot be narrowed down to the pharmacological component only, when the goal is remission on the one hand and a state of good or acceptable HRQoL for people living with SLE on the other. Knowing that SLE influences multiple domains of life, the use of generic and disease-specific measures in structured evaluation processes is justified. In this regard, it is worth noting that mainly generic PROMs have been used in randomized clinical trials of SLE, particularly the SF-36, while instruments with the ability to discriminate across clinically distinct groups are found to be more responsive to change, lending support for broader use of disease-specific PROMs [40]. The SLE-specific SLAQ is designed to capture self-reported symptoms that are usually evaluated by the rheumatologist [41] and is based on the Systemic Lupus Activity Measure [42]. While it shows adequate reliability and correlates with SF-36, it is not always congruous with traditional clinical parameters [43]. The Lupus Patient-Reported Outcome tool (LupusPRO) entails several domains of HRQoL and additionally prompts patients to reflect on support, medications, satisfaction, and cognition [44]. The LupusPRO correlates with the SF-36 and shows responsiveness in relation to the physician-reported activity index BILAG [45]. However, a systematic comparison across available PROMs in relation to generic domains of HRQoL and SLE-specific symptoms to determine the best correlates with traditional physician-reported disease features has yet to be conducted.

Assessments and interventions need to be tailored to the individual patient and decided upon together with the patient. In fact, shared decision-making constitutes a primary overarching principle of the T2T/SLE task force recommendations [8]. For some people with SLE, the impact of the disease acts as a negative spiral, in particular with regard to mental health, whereas high pain and global disease burden are coupled with negative future outcomes [46]. Physical or functional domains of HRQoL may still be contracted in considerable proportions of patients irrespective of their overall response to treatment, which has been shown to be more prominent in patients with established organ damage, and furthermore, dependent on ethnicity [47]. PROMs are scored worse in people with lower health literacy, which is not necessarily related to lower income or education, albeit resources of people with lower socioeconomic backgrounds are under stronger constraints [48,49]. It is also important to bear in mind that comorbidities may have an impact on how patients score their HRQoL, e.g., depressive or other disorders causing chronic mental distress may impact on pain, fatigue, or PtGA scores [46,50]. Thus, persistently high scores or persistent discordance between patient's and physician's assessments should intrinsically prompt further investigation for potential comorbid conditions as underlying causes and, if needed, the commencement of suitable adjunct therapy. Nevertheless, the considerable variability of PhGA scoring across assessors highlights the need to adopt optimal tools and determine the optimal timing for the assessment, as well as integrate multiple items, including the patient perspective, with the ultimate goal being a holistic apprehension of the disease status [51,52].

The proper use of PROMs is not only an important conceptual issue but also an opportunity to build bridges in the partnership between patients and physicians. These points of consideration adhere to the overall framework that there will seldom be one single best marker that helps us to interpret the activity, severity, and impact of SLE at the same time. By contrast, in clinical practice, there is a battery of tests and assessment instruments that the healthcare team may choose from, based on what is relevant to the respective patient and the respective condition. However, harmonization and integration of different tests in surveillance and overall patient management should be supported by data and strive for optimization, taking environmental, personal, and disease-specific conditions into account.

5. Conclusions

As a concluding remark, for optimal outcomes, we not only stress the importance of the use of PROMs but also emphasize the urgency to adopt the concept of forming alliances with each individual patient and facilitating active patient participation in surveillance and management processes as an integral part within the clinical consultations, and continuously during the disease course. The positive impact of this mindset on patients' lives has been explored more in-depth for people with inflammatory arthritis [53,54]; being a considerably more complex condition, it would be counterintuitive to anticipate holistic pertinence in the management of SLE without active patient involvement in all steps. Nevertheless, this should not be misinterpreted as a transfer of responsibility from healthcare professionals to patients, but should rather be considered a step towards shared decision-making, which in fact should impose responsibility to healthcare to ensure adequate patient education and confidence in patients in understanding the need and the options. Thus, while time becomes more mature for patients with SLE to take the driver's seat in their disease monitoring and management, healthcare professionals should not release themselves from responsibility but retain the seat of the navigator and inspirer.

Author Contributions: Conceptualization, I.P. and P.S.; investigation, I.P. and P.S.; resources, I.P. and P.S.; writing—original draft preparation, I.P. and P.S.; writing—review and editing, I.P. and P.S.; visualization, I.P. and P.S.; funding acquisition, I.P. and P.S. All authors have read and agreed to the published version of the manuscript.

Funding: I.P. is supported by the Swedish Rheumatism Association (R-941095), King Gustaf V's 80-year Foundation (FAI-2020-0741), Professor Nanna Svartz Foundation (2020-00368), Ulla and Roland Gustafsson Foundation (2021-26), Region Stockholm (FoUI-955483) and Karolinska Institutet. P.S. is supported by the FOREUM research fellowship grant.

Institutional Review Board Statement: Not applicable.

Informed Consent Statement: Not applicable.

Acknowledgments: The authors would like to express their gratitude to Yvonne Enman and Gunilla von Perner, both representatives of the Swedish lupus patient community, for reviewing the manuscript and providing useful patient insights and perspectives. We also thank Sarai Llamas (http://saraillamas.com; Accessed on 11 January 2022) for kindly providing the artistic illustration used to create the figure.

Conflicts of Interest: The authors declare no conflict of interest related to this work.

References

1. Jolly, M. How does quality of life of patients with systemic lupus erythematosus compare with that of other common chronic illnesses? *J. Rheumatol.* **2005**, *32*, 1706–1708.
2. Piga, M.; Arnaud, L. The Main Challenges in Systemic Lupus Erythematosus: Where Do We Stand? *J. Clin. Med.* **2021**, *10*, 243. [CrossRef] [PubMed]
3. Kaul, A.; Gordon, C.; Crow, M.K.; Touma, Z.; Urowitz, M.; Van Vollenhoven, R.; Ruiz-Irastorza, G.; Hughes, G. Systemic lupus erythematosus. *Nat. Rev. Dis. Prim.* **2016**, *2*, 16039. [CrossRef]
4. Kernder, A.; Richter, J.G.; Fischer-Betz, R.; Winkler-Rohlfing, B.; Brinks, R.; Aringer, M.; Schneider, M.; Chehab, G. Delayed diagnosis adversely affects outcome in systemic lupus erythematosus: Cross sectional analysis of the LuLa cohort. *Lupus* **2021**, *30*, 431–438. [CrossRef] [PubMed]
5. Moe, S.R.; Haukeland, H.; Molberg, Ø.; Lerang, K. Long-Term Outcome in Systemic Lupus Erythematosus; Knowledge from Population-Based Cohorts. *J. Clin. Med.* **2021**, *10*, 4306. [CrossRef]
6. Anders, H.-J.; Saxena, R.; Zhao, M.-H.; Parodis, I.; Salmon, J.E.; Mohan, C. Lupus nephritis. *Nat. Rev. Dis. Prim.* **2020**, *6*, 1–25. [CrossRef]
7. Annapureddy, N.; Devilliers, H.; Jolly, M. Patient-reported outcomes in lupus clinical trials with biologics. *Lupus* **2016**, *25*, 1111–1121. [CrossRef] [PubMed]
8. Van Vollenhoven, R.F.; Mosca, M.; Bertsias, G.; Isenberg, D.; Kuhn, A.; Lerstrøm, K.; Aringer, M.; Bootsma, H.; Boumpas, D.; Bruce, I.N.; et al. Treat-to-target in systemic lupus erythematosus: Recommendations from an international task force. *Ann. Rheum. Dis.* **2014**, *73*, 958–967. [CrossRef]

9. Steiman, A.J.; Urowitz, M.B.; Ibanez, D.; Papneja, A.; Gladman, D.D. Prolonged clinical remission in patients with systemic lupus erythematosus. *J. Rheumatol.* **2014**, *41*, 1808–1816. [CrossRef] [PubMed]
10. Van Vollenhoven, R.; Voskuyl, A.; Bertsias, G.; Aranow, C.; Aringer, M.; Arnaud, L.; Askanase, A.; Balážová, P.; Bonfa, E.; Bootsma, H.; et al. A framework for remission in SLE: Consensus findings from a large international task force on definitions of remission in SLE (DORIS). *Ann. Rheum. Dis.* **2016**, *76*, 554–561. [CrossRef]
11. Gladman, D.D.; Ibañez, D.; Urowitz, M.B. Systemic lupus erythematosus disease activity index 2000. *J. Rheumatol.* **2002**, *29*, 288–291.
12. Franklyn, K.; Lau, C.S.; Navarra, S.V.; Louthrenoo, W.; Lateef, A.; Hamijoyo, L.; Wahono, C.S.; Chen, S.L.; Jin, O.; Morton, S.; et al. Definition and initial validation of a Lupus Low Disease Activity State (LLDAS). *Ann. Rheum. Dis.* **2015**, *75*, 1615–1621. [CrossRef] [PubMed]
13. Luijten, K.; Tekstra, J.; Bijlsma, J.; Bijl, M. The Systemic Lupus Erythematosus Responder Index (SRI); A new SLE disease activity assessment. *Autoimmun. Rev.* **2012**, *11*, 326–329. [CrossRef]
14. Wallace, D.J.; Kalunian, K.; Petri, M.A.; Strand, V.; Houssiau, F.A.; Pike, M.; Kilgallen, B.; Bongardt, S.; Barry, A.; Kelley, L.; et al. Efficacy and safety of epratuzumab in patients with moderate/severe active systemic lupus erythematosus: Results from EMBLEM, a phase IIb, randomised, double-blind, placebo-controlled, multicentre study. *Ann. Rheum. Dis.* **2013**, *73*, 183–190. [CrossRef]
15. Felson, D.; Smolen, J.S.; Wells, G.; Zhang, Y.; van Tuyl, L.; Funovits, J.; Aletaha, D.; Allaart, C.F.; Bathon, J.; Bombardieri, S.; et al. American College of Rheumatology/European League Against Rheumatism Provisional Definition of Remission in Rheumatoid Arthritis for Clinical Trials. *Ann. Rheum. Dis.* **2011**, *70*, 404–413. [CrossRef] [PubMed]
16. EULAR. Outcome Measures Library. Available online: http://oml.eular.org/ (accessed on 9 April 2020).
17. Weldring, T.; Smith, S.M. Article Commentary: Patient-Reported Outcomes (PROs) and Patient-Reported Outcome Measures (PROMs). *Health Serv. Insights* **2013**, *6*, HSI.S11093–68. [CrossRef]
18. Studenic, P.; Radner, H.; Smolen, J.S.; Aletaha, D. Discrepancies between patients and physicians in their perceptions of rheumatoid arthritis disease activity. *Arthritis Care Res.* **2012**, *64*, 2814–2823. [CrossRef]
19. Studenic, P.; Smolen, J.S.; Aletaha, D. Near misses of ACR/EULAR criteria for remission: Effects of patient global assessment in Boolean and index-based definitions. *Ann. Rheum. Dis.* **2012**, *71*, 1702–1705. [CrossRef]
20. Studenic, P.; Felson, D.; De Wit, M.; Alasti, F.; Stamm, T.A.; Smolen, J.S.; Aletaha, D. Testing different thresholds for patient global assessment in defining remission for rheumatoid arthritis: Are the current ACR/EULAR Boolean criteria optimal? *Ann. Rheum. Dis.* **2020**, *79*, 445–452. [CrossRef]
21. Jones, B.; Flurey, C.A.; Proudman, S.; Ferreira, R.J.; Voshaar, M.; Hoogland, W.; Chaplin, H.; Goel, N.; Hetland, M.L.; Hill, C.; et al. Considerations and priorities for incorporating the patient perspective on remission in rheumatoid arthritis: An OMERACT 2020 special interest group report. *Semin. Arthritis Rheum.* **2021**, *51*, 1108–1112. [CrossRef] [PubMed]
22. Heijke, R.; Björk, M.; Thyberg, I.; Kastbom, A.; McDonald, L.; Sjöwall, C. Comparing longitudinal patient-reported outcome measures between Swedish patients with recent-onset systemic lupus erythematosus and early rheumatoid arthritis. *Clin. Rheumatol.* **2021**, 1–8. [CrossRef] [PubMed]
23. Golder, V.; Kandane-Rathnayake, R.; Hoi, A.Y.-B.; Huq, M.; Louthrenoo, W.; An, Y.; Li, Z.G.; Luo, S.F.; Sockalingam, S.; Lau, C.S.; et al. Association of the lupus low disease activity state (LLDAS) with health-related quality of life in a multinational prospective study. *Arthritis Res. Ther.* **2017**, *19*, 1–11. [CrossRef] [PubMed]
24. Elefante, E.; Tani, C.; Stagnaro, C.; Signorini, V.; Parma, A.; Carli, L.; Zucchi, D.; Ferro, F.; Mosca, M. Articular involvement, steroid treatment and fibromyalgia are the main determinants of patient-physician discordance in systemic lupus erythematosus. *Arthritis Res.* **2020**, *22*, 1–8. [CrossRef]
25. Azizoddin, D.R.; Jolly, M.; Arora, S.; Yelin, E.; Katz, P. Patient-Reported Outcomes Predict Mortality in Lupus. *Arthritis Rheum.* **2018**, *71*, 1028–1035. [CrossRef] [PubMed]
26. Louthrenoo, W.; Kasitanon, N.; Morand, E.; Kandane-Rathnayake, R. Associations between physicians' global assessment of disease activity and patient-reported outcomes in patients with systemic lupus erythematosus: A longitudinal study. *Lupus* **2021**, *30*, 1586–1595. [CrossRef] [PubMed]
27. Strand, V.; Gladman, D.; Isenberg, D.; Petri, M.; Smolen, J.; Tugwell, P. Endpoints: Consensus recommendations from OMERACT IV. *Lupus* **2000**, *9*, 322–327. [CrossRef] [PubMed]
28. Yen, J.C.; Neville, C.; Fortin, P.R. Discordance between patients and their physicians in the assessment of lupus disease activity: Relevance for clinical trials. *Lupus* **1999**, *8*, 660–670. [CrossRef] [PubMed]
29. Ware, J.E., Jr.; Sherbourne, C.D. The MOS 36-item short-form health survey (SF-36). I. Conceptual framework and item selection. *Med. Care* **1992**, *30*, 473–483. [CrossRef] [PubMed]
30. Yellen, S.B.; Cella, D.F.; Webster, K.; Blendowski, C.; Kaplan, E. Measuring fatigue and other anemia-related symptoms with the Functional Assessment of Cancer Therapy (FACT) measurement system. *J. Pain Symptom Manag.* **1997**, *13*, 63–74. [CrossRef]
31. U.S. Department of Health and Human Services FDA Center for Drug Evaluation and Research; U.S. Department of Health and Human Services FDA Center for Biologics Evaluation and Research; U.S. Department of Health and Human Services FDA Center for Devices and Radiological Health. Guidance for industry: Patient-reported outcome measures: Use in medical product development to support labeling claims: Draft guidance. *Health Qual. Life Outcomes* **2006**, *4*, 1–79. [CrossRef] [PubMed]

32. Strand, V.; Simon, L.S.; Meara, A.S.; Touma, Z. Measurement properties of selected patient-reported outcome measures for use in randomised controlled trials in patients with systemic lupus erythematosus: A systematic review. *Lupus Sci. Med.* **2020**, *7*, e000373. [CrossRef] [PubMed]
33. Strand, V.; Levy, R.A.; Cervera, R.; Petri, M.A.; Birch, H.; Freimuth, W.W.; Zhong, Z.J.; Clarke, A.E. Improvements in health-related quality of life with belimumab, a B-lymphocyte stimulator-specific inhibitor, in patients with autoantibody-positive systemic lupus erythematosus from the randomised controlled BLISS trials. *Ann. Rheum. Dis.* **2013**, *73*, 838–844. [CrossRef] [PubMed]
34. The EuroQol Group. EuroQol-a new facility for the measurement of health-related quality of life. *Health Policy* **1990**, *16*, 199–208. [CrossRef]
35. Aggarwal, R.; Wilke, C.T.; Pickard, A.S.; Vats, V.; Mikolaitis, R.; Fogg, L.; Block, J.A.; Jolly, M. Psychometric Properties of the EuroQol-5D and Short Form-6D in Patients with Systemic Lupus Erythematosus. *J. Rheumatol.* **2009**, *36*, 1209–1216. [CrossRef]
36. Lindblom, J.; Gomez, A.; Borg, A.; Emamikia, S.; Ladakis, D.; Matilla, J.; Pehr, M.; Cobar, F.; Enman, Y.; Heintz, E.; et al. EQ-5D-3L full health state discriminates between drug and placebo in clinical trials of systemic lupus erythematosus. *Rheumatology* **2021**, *60*, 4703–4716. [CrossRef] [PubMed]
37. Györi, N.; Giannakou, I.; Chatzidionysiou, K.; Magder, L.; Van Vollenhoven, R.F.; Petri, M. Disease activity patterns over time in patients with SLE: Analysis of the Hopkins Lupus Cohort. *Lupus Sci. Med.* **2017**, *4*, e000192. [CrossRef]
38. Izadi, Z. Health-Related Quality of Life Measures in Adult Systemic Lupus Erythematosus. *Arthritis Rheum.* **2020**, *72*, 577–592. [CrossRef] [PubMed]
39. Holloway, L.; Humphrey, L.; Heron, L.; Pilling, C.; Kitchen, H.; Højbjerre, L.; Strandberg-Larsen, M.; Hansen, B.B. Patient-reported outcome measures for systemic lupus erythematosus clinical trials: A review of content validity, face validity and psychometric performance. *Health Qual. Life Outcomes* **2014**, *12*, 116. [CrossRef]
40. Izadi, Z.; Gandrup, J.D.F.; Katz, P.P.; Yazdany, J. Patient-reported outcome measures for use in clinical trials of SLE: A review. *Lupus Sci. Med.* **2018**, *5*, e000279. [CrossRef] [PubMed]
41. Karlson, E.W.; Daltroy, L.H.; Rivest, C.; Ramsey-Goldman, R.; Wright, E.A.; Partridge, A.J.; Liang, M.H.; Fortin, P.R. Validation of a systemic lupus activity questionnaire (SLAQ) for population studies. *Lupus* **2003**, *12*, 280–286. [CrossRef]
42. Bae, S.C.; Koh, H.K.; Chang, D.K.; Kim, M.H.; Park, J.K.; Kim, S.Y. Reliability and validity of systemic lupus activity measure-revised (SLAM-R) for measuring clinical disease activity in systemic lupus erythematosus. *Lupus* **2001**, *10*, 405–409. [CrossRef] [PubMed]
43. Yazdany, J.; Yelin, E.H.; Panopalis, P.; Trupin, L.; Julian, L.; Katz, P.P. Validation of the systemic lupus erythematosus activity questionnaire in a large observational cohort. *Arthritis Care Res.* **2007**, *59*, 136–143. [CrossRef] [PubMed]
44. Azizoddin, D.R.; Weinberg, S.; Gandhi, N.; Arora, S.; Block, J.; Sequeira, W.; Jolly, M. Validation of the LupusPRO version 1.8: An update to a disease-specific patient-reported outcome tool for systemic lupus erythematosus. *Lupus* **2017**, *27*, 728–737. [CrossRef] [PubMed]
45. Jolly, M.; Pickard, A.S.; Block, J.; Kumar, R.B.; Mikolaitis, R.A.; Wilke, C.T.; Rodby, R.A.; Fogg, L.; Sequeira, W.; Utset, T.O.; et al. Disease-Specific Patient Reported Outcome Tools for Systemic Lupus Erythematosus. *Semin. Arthritis Rheum.* **2012**, *42*, 56–65. [CrossRef]
46. Parperis, K.; Psarelis, S.; Chatzittofis, A.; Michaelides, M.; Nikiforou, D.; Antoniade, E.; Bhattarai, B. Association of clinical characteristics, disease activity and health-related quality of life in SLE patients with major depressive disorder. *Rheumatology* **2021**, *60*, 5369–5378. [CrossRef] [PubMed]
47. Gomez, A.; Qiu, V.; Cederlund, A.; Borg, A.; Lindblom, J.; Emamikia, S.; Enman, Y.; Lampa, J.; Parodis, I. Adverse Health-Related Quality of Life Outcome Despite Adequate Clinical Response to Treatment in Systemic Lupus Erythematosus. *Front. Med.* **2021**, *8*. [CrossRef] [PubMed]
48. Katz, P.; Dall'Era, M.; Trupin, L.; Rush, S.; Murphy, L.B.; Lanata, C.; Criswell, L.A.; Yazdany, J. Impact of Limited Health Literacy on Patient-Reported Outcomes in Systemic Lupus Erythematosus. *Arthritis Rheum.* **2020**, *73*, 110–119. [CrossRef] [PubMed]
49. DeQuattro, K.; Yelin, E. Socioeconomic Status, Health Care, and Outcomes in Systemic Lupus Erythematosus. *Rheum. Dis. Clin. N. Am.* **2020**, *46*, 639–649. [CrossRef] [PubMed]
50. Dey, M.; Parodis, I.; Nikiphorou, E. Fatigue in Systemic Lupus Erythematosus and Rheumatoid Arthritis: A Comparison of Mechanisms, Measures and Management. *J. Clin. Med.* **2021**, *10*, 3566. [CrossRef] [PubMed]
51. Chessa, E.; Piga, M.; Floris, A.; Devilliers, H.; Cauli, A.; Arnaud, L. Use of Physician Global Assessment in systemic lupus erythematosus: A systematic review of its psychometric properties. *Rheumatology* **2020**, *59*, 3622–3632. [CrossRef] [PubMed]
52. Aranow, C. A pilot study to determine the optimal timing of the Physician Global Assessment (PGA) in patients with systemic lupus erythematosus. *Immunol. Res.* **2015**, *63*, 167–169. [CrossRef] [PubMed]
53. Nikiphorou, E.; Santos, E.J.F.; Marques, A.; Böhm, P.; Bijlsma, J.W.; Daien, C.I.; Esbensen, B.A.; Ferreira, R.J.O.; Fragoulis, G.E.; Holmes, P.; et al. 2021 EULAR recommendations for the implementation of self-management strategies in patients with inflammatory arthritis. *Ann. Rheum. Dis.* **2021**, *80*, 1278–1285. [CrossRef]
54. Rn, I.L.; Bremander, A.; Andersson, M. Patient Empowerment and Associations with Disease Activity and Pain-Related and Lifestyle Factors in Patients With Rheumatoid Arthritis. *ACR Open Rheumatol.* **2021**, *3*, 842–849. [CrossRef]

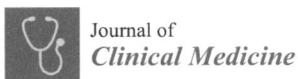

Review

Rapid Response of Refractory Systemic Lupus Erythematosus Skin Manifestations to Anifrolumab—A Case-Based Review of Clinical Trial Data Suggesting a Domain-Based Therapeutic Approach

Marlene Plüß [1], Silvia Piantoni [2], Chris Wincup [3] and Peter Korsten [1,*]

1 Department of Nephrology and Rheumatology, University Medical Center Göttingen, 37075 Göttingen, Germany; marlene.pluess@med.uni-goettingen.de
2 Rheumatology and Clinical Immunology Unit, Department of Clinical and Experimental Sciences, ASST Spedali Civili and University of Brescia, 25121 Brescia, Italy; slv.piantoni@gmail.com
3 Department of Rheumatology, King's College Hospital, London SE5 9RS, UK; c.wincup@ucl.ac.uk
* Correspondence: peter.korsten@med.uni-goettingen.de; Tel.: +49-551-396-0400

Abstract: Systemic lupus erythematosus (SLE) is a clinically heterogeneous autoimmune disease, and organ manifestations, such as lupus nephritis (LN) or skin disease, may be refractory to standard treatment. Therefore, new agents are required to allow for a more personalized therapeutic approach. Recently, several new therapies have been approved internationally, including voclosporine for LN and anifrolumab for moderately to severely active SLE. Here, we report a case of SLE with a predominant and refractory cutaneous manifestation despite combination treatment with glucocorticoids, hydroxychloroquine, mycophenolate mofetil, and belimumab, which had been present for more than 12 months. Belimumab was switched to anifrolumab, and the patient responded quickly after two infusions (eight weeks) with a reduction in the Cutaneous Lupus Assessment and Severity Index (CLASI) from 17 to 7. In addition, we review the available clinical trial data for anifrolumab with a focus on cutaneous outcomes. Based on phase II and III clinical trials investigating the intravenous administration, a consistent CLASI improvement was observed at 12 weeks. Interestingly, in a phase II trial of subcutaneous anifrolumab application, CLASI response was not different from placebo at 12 weeks but numerically different at 24 and 52 weeks, respectively. Thus, anifrolumab emerges as an attractive new therapeutic option suggesting a possible domain-based approach.

Keywords: systemic lupus erythematosus; anifrolumab; interferon; cutaneous lupus erythematosus

1. Introduction

Anifrolumab (ANI), a fully human monoclonal antibody directed against the type I interferon (IFN) receptor subunit 1, has recently been approved as add-on therapy for moderately to severely active systemic lupus erythematosus (SLE) based on the results of two phase III trials (TULIP-1 and TULIP-2) [1,2]. There is limited experience in clinical practice outside of a trial setting, but an early access program was available in Germany until March 2022. Here, we report the first use of ANI in an SLE patient with refractory cutaneous manifestations outside a clinical trial setting and review the data of ANI clinical trials focusing on the cutaneous domain.

2. Case Description

The patient is a 30-year-old female with a 13-year history of SLE based on acute cutaneous lupus, polyarthritis, positivity for antinuclear antibodies (abs), anti-double-stranded DNA, anti-Ro/SSA, anti-U1-snRNP abs, and complement consumption. Over the years, additional findings included photosensitivity, class II lupus nephritis (LN), and positive anti-phospholipid abs.

She presented in October 2021 to her routine visit and complained of worsening skin lesions and joint pain over the preceding three months (Figure 1A–C).

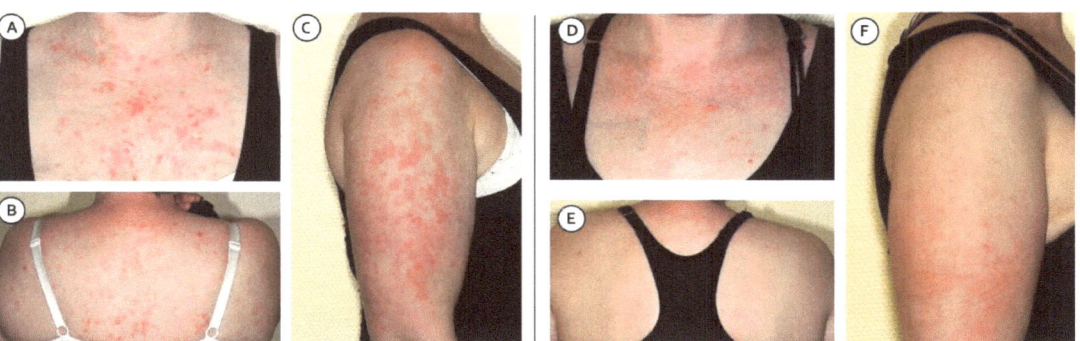

Figure 1. Cutaneous manifestations of the patient before (**A–C**) and eight weeks after the initiation of anifrolumab treatment (**D–F**).

Her skin lesions consisted of non-pruritic erythematous lesions distributed symmetrically over the upper trunk and back, as well as the face, arms, and hands. There were no areas of scarring. Her skin rash was most consistent with subacute cutaneous lupus erythematosus (SCLE). The Cutaneous Lupus Erythematosus Disease Area and Severity Index (CLASI) was determined with a score of 17.

The metacarpophalangeal II to V and proximal interphalangeal joints II to V were slightly swollen and tender to palpation. Anti-dsDNA abs were elevated at 114 IU/mL (normal range [NR] <15 IU/mL), C3 was 0.71 g/L (NR 0.82–1.93 g/L), and C4 was 0.08 g/L (NR 0.15–0.57 g/L). The Systemic Lupus Erythematosus Disease Activity Index 2000 (SLEDAI-2K) was calculated as 10.

Previous therapy included hydroxychloroquine (200 mg/day), azathioprine, and varying doses of prednisolone. Three courses of medium to high oral prednisolone doses (0.5–1 mg/kg of body weight) to control her skin disease and flares of polyarthritis were given over the previous six months.

Her current SLE treatment included hydroxychloroquine (200 mg/day), low-dose prednisolone (5 mg/day), mycophenolate mofetil (500 mg twice daily, higher doses not tolerated), and subcutaneous belimumab (BEL) (200 mg/week), which had been started more than 12 months before. In this refractory patient with active cutaneous and joint disease, BEL was switched to ANI.

Anifrolumab treatment was initiated in January 2022. Eight weeks later, after receiving two intravenous infusions of 300 mg four weeks apart, the skin lesions had improved significantly (Figure 1D–F).

In addition, her complement levels and anti-dsDNA antibody titer improved moderately (Figure 2A,B). The CLASI improved from 17 to 7 (Figure 2C). Joint pain and swelling also improved with treatment. No side effects or infusion reactions occurred, and the patient has lowered her prednisolone dose to 2 mg/day. After four infusions, the patient reduced her dose of mycophenolate mofetil to 500 mg/day. Follow-up is ongoing.

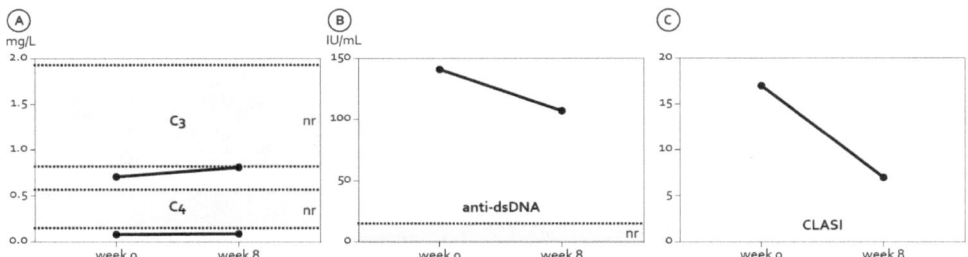

Figure 2. Changes in serologic parameters and the disease activity at baseline and after eight weeks. (**A**) Complement factors C3 and C4. (**B**) Anti-double stranded (ds) DNA levels. (**C**) Cutaneous lupus activity and severity index (CLASI).

3. Review of Anifrolumab Mechanism of Action and Clinical Trials

3.1. Development and Mechanism of Action of Anifrolumab

The pathogenesis of SLE, which is considered a prototypic autoimmune disease, is complex and involves a myriad of immune mechanisms and various cell types [3] (Figure 3). In brief, environmental (e.g., ultraviolet radiation), viral (e.g., Ebstein–Barr virus), and hormonal triggers lead to an increased rate of apoptosis in an (epi)genetically susceptible individual [3,4]. Autoreactive B and T cells process this increased number of antigens, leading to autoantibody and immune complex formation [4]. As a result, there is an increased production of type 1 interferons (IFNs) by plasmacytoid dendritic cells (pDCs), which is a central pathogenic process [5,6]. Type 1 interferons maintain an increased autoantibody production through an autocrine loop, further activating B cells, which undergo class switching [4].

Recently, an increasing number of clinical trials, including the TULIP trials, stratified patients according to their IFN gene expression status (high vs. low) [7]. However, this has not been adopted for routine clinical practice. In view of IFNs as a key mediator in SLE pathogenesis, targeting IFNs by monoclonal antibodies (mAbs) is an appealing approach. Sifalimumab and rontalizumab, two other mAbs targeting IFN alpha, have yielded mixed results in phase II trials [8,9], and have not been developed and tested in phase III trials.

Anifrolumab is a fully human, effector-null monoclonal antibody directed against the type I interferon (IFN) receptor subunit 1 (IFNAR1) [10]. It was engineered with mutations inserted in the heavy chain with the aim of reducing Fcγ receptor (FcγR)-mediated effector functions, such as antibody-dependent cell-mediated cytotoxicity and complement-dependent cytotoxicity [11], ultimately improving efficacy and reducing resistance through internalization by FcR [12].

Further, it has been shown that ANI promotes IFNAR1 internalization, thus blocking downstream signaling, such as signal transducers and activators of transcription 1 (STAT1) phosphorylation [10]. Finally, ANI reduces the type I IFN autoamplificaton loop sustained by pDCs [10,13].

The mechanism of action of ANI in the context of a proposed model of SLE pathogenesis is shown in Figure 3.

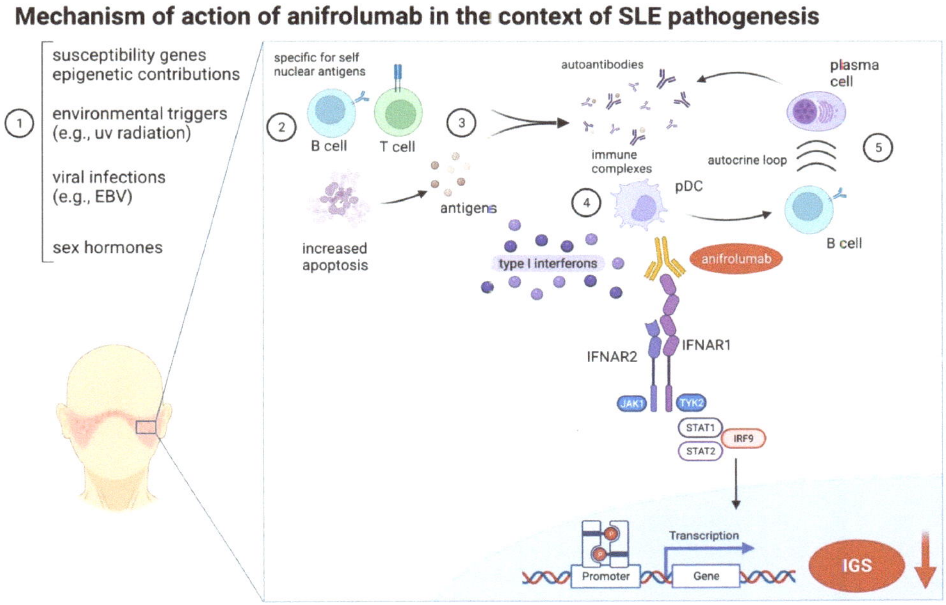

Figure 3. Mechanism of action of anifrolumab in the context of the hypothesized systemic lupus erythematosus (SLE) pathogenesis [3,4,6]. Genetic, epigenetic, environmental, and hormonal factors (**1**) lead to an increased rate of apoptosis. Autoreactive B and T cells specific for self-nuclear antigens recognize and process these antigens (**2**), which, in turn, leads to autoantibody and immune complex generation (**3**). Toll-like receptor signaling in B cells and pDCs (not shown) results in increased levels of type 1 interferons, mainly produced by pDCs (**4**). Type 1 interferons further stimulate B cells in an autocrine loop, and B cells exhibit class switching, which leads to a persistent production of autoantibodies (**5**). Anifrolumab binds to IFNAR1, thus inhibiting dimerization and subsequent intracellular signaling mechanisms mediated by STAT1/2 and IRF9. The net result is a decreased transcription of proinflammatory genes (the so-called interferon-gene signature, IGS) in cells of both the innate and adaptive immune systems [10]. Created with biorender.com. EBV, Ebstein–Barr virus; IFNAR, interferon receptor subunit; IGS, interferon gene signature; IRF9, interferon regulatory factor 9; JAK, Janus kinase; pDC, plasmacytoid dendritic cells; STAT, signal transducers and activators of transcription; TYK, tyrosine kinase; UV, ultraviolet.

3.2. Clinical Trial Data

In this section, we will review the available clinical trial data from phase I–III clinical trials of ANI, which resulted in the approval for the treatment of moderately-to-severely active SLE in addition to standard therapy. Figure 4 shows a timeline of major clinical trials and approval dates of ANI in non-renal SLE. Of note, a phase II clinical trial in LN has been published [14]. However, we will not further analyze this trial since the focus of this review is the cutaneous domain.

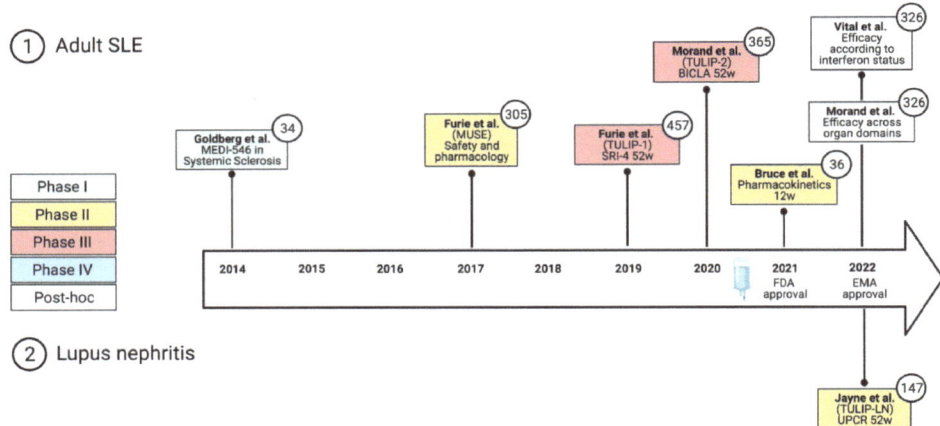

Figure 4. Timeline of major clinical trials, primary outcome measures, and authorization of anifrolumab [1–8]. BICLA, British Isles Lupus Assessment Group-based composite lupus assessment; EMA, European Medicines Agency; FDA, Federal Drug Agency; SC, subcutaneous; SRI-4, systemic lupus erythematosus responder index-4; UPCR, urine protein–creatinine ratio; w, weeks. Numbers in circles denote the number of participants. Created with biorender.com.

3.2.1. Early Phase I and Phase II Trials

Interestingly, ANI, then termed MEDI-546, was first tested in a phase I clinical trial in Systemic Sclerosis (SSc) patients [15]. In this phase I trial, 34 subjects received MEDI-546 in a dose-escalation fashion for 12 weeks. A total of 68.9% of subjects experienced mild adverse events (AEs), and 27.7% experienced moderate AEs. In addition, there were four serious AEs (skin ulcer, osteomyelitis, vertigo, and chronic myelogenous leukemia). Only the latter was judged as possibly treatment-related [15].

Since interferon signaling pathways involved in the pathogenesis of SSc and SLE share similarities [16], MEDI-546, later renamed ANI, was further investigated in a phase IIb trial in non-renal SLE [17]. In this trial, 305 participants with moderate-to-severely active SLE were randomized to receive one of two doses of ANI (300 vs. 1000 mg every four weeks for 48 weeks) or a placebo (PBO). Patients were randomized based on disease activity (SLE disease activity index-2000 [SLEDAI-2K] >10 vs. <10), glucocorticoid (GC) dose (>10 vs. ≤10 mg/day), and type I interferon gene expression (high vs. low). The SRI4 endpoint was met by more patients treated with ANI (34.3% of 99 patients for 300 mg and 28.8% of 104 for 1000 mg) compared to PBO (17.6% of 102 patients) (Table 1). With these encouraging results, two phase III trials were performed subsequently.

3.2.2. Phase III Trials—TULIP-1 and TULIP-2

In the phase III trial TULIP-1, ANI 150 mg or 300 mg were compared to PBO. TULIP-1 randomized 457 patients; the primary endpoint systemic lupus erythematosus responder index-4 (SRI-4) was assessed at 52 weeks. There were no statistically significant differences in patients receiving 300 mg of ANI compared to PBO regarding this outcome measure (36% vs. 40%, respectively). Since the primary endpoint was not met, no statistical testing was performed as per the prespecified study analysis plan. However, the British Isles Lupus Assessment Group-based composite lupus assessment (BICLA), another robust outcome measure used for SLE, was numerically different (37% vs. 27% responders for ANI 300 mg vs. PBO) [2].

Therefore, the TULIP-2 clinical trial used the BICLA as the primary outcome measure [1]. TULIP-2 randomized 365 patients to ANI 300 mg or PBO. At 52 weeks, there was a statistically significant difference in the BICLA response in favor of ANI 300 mg (47.8% vs. 31.5%). These results finally led to ANI's approval by the Federal Drug Administration

(FDA) in 2021 and the European Medicines Agency (EMA) in early 2022. The different results of TULIP-1 and TULIP-2 regarding their primary efficacy measures have been discussed widely [18–20]. Table 1 gives an overview of the main published clinical trials and the primary outcomes.

Table 1. Overview of clinical trials of anifrolumab in non-renal Systemic Lupus erythematosus.

First Author, Year	Trial Acronym	Phase	N of Participants	Primary Endpoint Assessment	Outcome Measures (% Responders) § (Anifrolumab 300 mg/Placebo)		
					SRI-4	BICLA	CLASI
Intravenous administration							
Furie, 2017 [17]	MUSE	IIb	305	24 weeks	**34.3/17.6**	53.5/25.7	63/30.8
Furie, 2019 [2]	TULIP-1	III	457	52 weeks	**36/40**	37/27	42/25 *
Morand, 2020 [1]	TULIP-2	III	365	52 weeks	55.5/37.3	**47.8/31.5**	49/25 *
Subcutaneous administration							
Bruce, 2021 [21]	-	II	36	12 weeks	-/-	-/-	45/44 *

§ Bold indicates the primary outcome measure. Outcome measures: BICLA, British Isles Lupus Assessment Group-based composite lupus assessment; CLASI, cutaneous lupus erythematosus disease area and severity index; SRI-4, systemic lupus erythematosus responder index-4. * at 12 weeks.

4. Discussion

To our knowledge, this is the first description of therapy with ANI for refractory cutaneous manifestations outside a clinical trial, demonstrating very quick clinical efficacy. It is unclear which primary outcome measure is best for trials in SLE [19]. Both SRI, used in TULIP-1 [2], and the BICLA, used in TULIP-2 [1], are robust measures of treatment response. They consist of different domains and give more weight to the SLEDAI response (SRI), or BILAG domains (BICLA), respectively. Both measures do not allow for any domain to worsen. In TULIP-1, there was no difference in the CLASI between ANI and PBO; in TULIP-2, a statistically significant difference was found at week 12 [1]. A post-hoc analysis of pooled data in patients with CLASI ≥ 10 at baseline confirmed these results [22].

In all published phase II and III clinical trials, the Cutaneous Lupus erythematosus disease area and severity index (CLASI) was used to assess changes in skin manifestations. The CLASI aims to distinguish between activity and damage [23]. In the activity domain, erythema is graded from 0 (absent) to 3 (dark red; purple/violaceous/crusted/hemorrhagic) in different body areas. Likewise, scales/hypertrophy are judged from 0 (absent) to 2 (verrucous/hypertrophic). Further, lesions of the mucous membranes are searched for. Lastly, alopecia is assessed as present or absent. If present, the scalp is divided into four quadrants and scored, ranging from 0 (absent) to 3 (focal or patchy in more than one quadrant). To analyze the damage, various lesions are scored: First, dyspigmentation is documented as 0 (absent) or 1 (present). Next, scarring/atrophy/panniculitis is scored, ranging from 0 (absent) to 2 (severely atrophic scarring or panniculitis). Then, the duration of dyspigmentation is considered (more or less than 12 months). Finally, scarring of the scalp is scored as 0 (absent), 3 (present in one quadrant), 4 (present in two quadrants), 5 (three quadrants), or 6 (affects the whole skull). The overall score ranges from 0 to 70, and higher scores indicate more severe skin disease.

It must be noted that the CLASI response was defined as an improvement of at least 50% in participants with a minimum score ≥ 10. In the MUSE phase IIb trial, 77 (25%) of patients fulfilled this definition [17]. The percentage of CLASI responders at 24 weeks was 63% for 300 mg of ANI vs. PBO (30.8%), and responses were seen early on (around 50% at eight weeks) with a plateau of 60–65% response rates around week 20. In TULIP-1, the CLASI response followed the same definition, and there were 42% vs. 25% of responders favoring ANI 300 mg at 12 weeks [2]. However, the difference between ANI and PBO evened out at the end of the trial. Finally, TULIP-2 reported a CLASI responder rate of 49% vs. 25% at 12 weeks, which was maintained through 52 weeks [1].

Lastly, a phase II of subcutaneous administration of ANI in 36 patients showed no numerical differences in the CLASI response at 12 weeks (45% vs. 44%) [21]. Nevertheless, unlike the TULIP trials, the response rates steadily increased from 82% vs. 50% at 24 weeks to 91% vs. 44% at 52 weeks. The number of subjects was small, and this phase II trial was also not designed to assess any differences in the CLASI response. One possible explanation for the steadier increase compared to the rapid rise in response rates with the intravenous administration may be the slower absorption and biological efficacy following a subcutaneous application.

Furthermore, it has been shown that IFN signaling has a central role in SLE skin pathology as the IFN signature correlates with cutaneous disease activity in SLE [24], and IFN pathways contribute to enhancing apoptosis of skin cells interfering with the protective Langerhans cell–keratinocytes axis [25]. More recently, these processes have been shown to be mediated by keratinocytes and dendritic cells in non-lesional skin lesions [26].

The available clinical trial data regarding musculoskeletal manifestations demonstrate an improvement in the phase IIb trial MUSE [17]. Of those patients with ≥ 8 tender and swollen joints, the percentual difference at 24 weeks of ANI responders (n = 46) was 8.9% ($p = 0.351$) compared to PBO (n = 37) at a dose of 300 mg. However, at 52 weeks, 48.6% (PBO) vs. 69.6% (ANI 300 mg) of patients responded (percentual difference of 21%, $p = 0.038$) [17]. In the TULIP-1 trial, 22/68 (32%) PBO-treated patients versus 33/70 (47%) ANI-treated patients had a ≥ 50% reduction in active joints at 52 weeks [2]. Lastly, in the TULIP-2 trial, 42.4% of ANI-treated patients with ≥ 6 swollen or tender joints had a non-statistically significant response compared to PBO (37.5%, $p = 0.55$) [1].

Taken together, numerically more patients with at least six swollen or tender joints treated with ANI had a 50% or greater reduction from baseline to 52 weeks in the swollen joint count (57% vs. 46%, $p = 0.027$), and a 50% vs. 43% reduction in the tender joint count ($p = 0.095$). Thus, ANI seems to lead to an improvement of joint manifestations in a relevant proportion of patients after 52 weeks.

5. Conclusions

Overall, biological therapies with different mechanisms of action are sparse in SLE, and ANI is only the second approved biological therapy after BEL. There is vast experience with BEL as an add-on therapy for non-renal and, more recently, also LN [27]. Anifrolumab's place in therapeutic algorithms has not been determined as of yet. However, our early clinical experience and review of the available clinical trial data show promising and rapid results for (refractory) cutaneous and joint manifestations in SLE, suggesting a potential domain-based approach in the near future.

Author Contributions: Conceptualization, S.P. and P.K.; methodology, P.K.; software, P.K.; validation, M.P., S.P., C.W. and P.K.; formal analysis, M.P., S.P., C.W. and P.K.; investigation, M.P., S.P., C.W. and P.K.; resources, P.K.; data curation, M.P., S.P., C.W. and P.K.; writing—original draft preparation, P.K.; writing—review and editing, M.P., S.P. and C.W.; visualization, P.K.; supervision, P.K.; project administration, P.K. All authors have read and agreed to the published version of the manuscript.

Funding: The APC was supported by the Open Access funds of the Georg-August University Göttingen.

Institutional Review Board Statement: The study was conducted in accordance with the Declaration of Helsinki. As per local legislation, no formal ethics approval was required to use routine clinical data.

Informed Consent Statement: Written informed consent has been obtained from the patient to publish this paper.

Data Availability Statement: Not applicable.

Acknowledgments: The authors are grateful for AstraZeneca's early access program, which allowed the patient to receive anifrolumab before its commercial availability.

Conflicts of Interest: M.P. has no conflict of interest. S.P. has received honoraria or travel support from Abbvie, AstraZeneca, Bristol-Myers-Squibb, Galapagos, Janssen-Cilag, and Pfizer, all unrelated to this paper. C.W. has received travel support from Abbvie, unrelated to this paper. P.K. has received honoraria or travel support from Abbvie, AstraZeneca, Boehringer Ingelheim, Bristol-Myers-Squibb, Chugai, EUSA Pharma, Gilead, GlaxoSmithKline, Janssen-Cilag, Lilly, Pfizer, and

Sanofi-Aventis, all unrelated to this paper. P.K. received research grants from GlaxoSmithKline and Diamed Medizintechnik GmbH, outside this work.

References

1. Morand, E.F.; Furie, R.; Tanaka, Y.; Bruce, I.N.; Askanase, A.D.; Richez, C.; Bae, S.-C.; Brohawn, P.Z.; Pineda, L.; Berglind, A.; et al. Trial of Anifrolumab in Active Systemic Lupus Erythematosus. *N. Engl. J. Med.* **2020**, *382*, 211–221. [CrossRef] [PubMed]
2. Furie, R.A.; Morand, E.F.; Bruce, I.N.; Manzi, S.; Kalunian, K.C.; Vital, E.M.; Ford, T.L.; Gupta, R.; Hiepe, F.; Santiago, M.; et al. Type I Interferon Inhibitor Anifrolumab in Active Systemic Lupus Erythematosus (TULIP-1): A Randomised, Controlled, Phase 3 Trial. *Lancet Rheumatol.* **2019**, *1*, e208–e219. [CrossRef]
3. Tsokos, G.C.; Lo, M.S.; Costa Reis, P.; Sullivan, K.E. New Insights into the Immunopathogenesis of Systemic Lupus Erythematosus. *Nat. Rev. Rheumatol.* **2016**, *12*, 716–730. [CrossRef] [PubMed]
4. Kaul, A.; Gordon, C.; Crow, M.K.; Touma, Z.; Urowitz, M.B.; van Vollenhoven, R.; Ruiz-Irastorza, G.; Hughes, G. Systemic Lupus Erythematosus. *Nat. Rev. Dis. Primers* **2016**, *2*, 1–21. [CrossRef] [PubMed]
5. Niewold, T.B. Interferon Alpha as a Primary Pathogenic Factor in Human Lupus. *J. Interferon Cytokine Res.* **2011**, *31*, 887–892. [CrossRef]
6. Rönnblom, L.; Leonard, D. Interferon Pathway in SLE: One Key to Unlocking the Mystery of the Disease. *Lupus Sci. Med.* **2019**, *6*, e000270. [CrossRef]
7. Cooles, F.A.H.; Isaacs, J.D. The Interferon Gene Signature as a Clinically Relevant Biomarker in Autoimmune Rheumatic Disease. *Lancet Rheumatol.* **2022**, *4*, e61–e72. [CrossRef]
8. Khamashta, M.; Merrill, J.T.; Werth, V.P.; Furie, R.; Kalunian, K.; Illei, G.G.; Drappa, J.; Wang, L.; Greth, W. Sifalimumab, an Anti-Interferon-α Monoclonal Antibody, in Moderate to Severe Systemic Lupus Erythematosus: A Randomised, Double-Blind, Placebo-Controlled Study. *Ann. Rheum. Dis.* **2016**, *75*, 1909–1916. [CrossRef]
9. Kalunian, K.C.; Merrill, J.T.; Maciuca, R.; McBride, J.M.; Townsend, M.J.; Wei, X.; Davis, J.C.; Kennedy, W.P. A Phase II Study of the Efficacy and Safety of Rontalizumab (RhuMAb Interferon-α) in Patients with Systemic Lupus Erythematosus (ROSE). *Ann. Rheum. Dis.* **2016**, *75*, 196–202. [CrossRef]
10. Riggs, J.M.; Hanna, R.N.; Rajan, B.; Zerrouki, K.; Karnell, J.L.; Sagar, D.; Vainshtein, I.; Farmer, E.; Rosenthal, K.; Morehouse, C.; et al. Characterisation of Anifrolumab, a Fully Human Anti-Interferon Receptor Antagonist Antibody for the Treatment of Systemic Lupus Erythematosus. *Lupus Sci. Med.* **2018**, *5*, e000261. [CrossRef]
11. Oganesyan, V.; Gao, C.; Shirinian, L.; Wu, H.; Dall'Acqua, W.F. Structural Characterization of a Human Fc Fragment Engineered for Lack of Effector Functions. *Acta Cryst. D Biol. Cryst.* **2008**, *64*, 700–704. [CrossRef] [PubMed]
12. Lee, D.S.W.; Rojas, O.L.; Gommerman, J.L. B Cell Depletion Therapies in Autoimmune Disease: Advances and Mechanistic Insights. *Nat. Rev. Drug Discov.* **2021**, *20*, 179–199. [CrossRef] [PubMed]
13. Chasset, F.; Dayer, J.-M.; Chizzolini, C. Type I Interferons in Systemic Autoimmune Diseases: Distinguishing Between Afferent and Efferent Functions for Precision Medicine and Individualized Treatment. *Front. Pharmacol.* **2021**, *12*, 633821. [CrossRef] [PubMed]
14. Jayne, D.; Rovin, B.; Mysler, E.F.; Furie, R.A.; Houssiau, F.A.; Trasieva, T.; Knagenhjelm, J.; Schwetje, E.; Chia, Y.L.; Tummala, R.; et al. Phase II Randomised Trial of Type I Interferon Inhibitor Anifrolumab in Patients with Active Lupus Nephritis. *Ann. Rheum. Dis.* **2022**, *81*, 496–506. [CrossRef] [PubMed]
15. Goldberg, A.; Geppert, T.; Schiopu, E.; Frech, T.; Hsu, V.; Simms, R.W.; Peng, S.L.; Yao, Y.; Elgeioushi, N.; Chang, L.; et al. Dose-Escalation of Human Anti-Interferon-α Receptor Monoclonal Antibody MEDI-546 in Subjects with Systemic Sclerosis: A Phase 1, Multicenter, Open Label Study. *Arthritis Res. Ther.* **2014**, *16*, R57. [CrossRef]
16. Muskardin, T.L.W.; Niewold, T.B. Type I Interferon in Rheumatic Diseases. *Nat. Rev. Rheumatol.* **2018**, *14*, 214–228. [CrossRef]
17. Furie, R.; Khamashta, M.; Merrill, J.T.; Werth, V.P.; Kalunian, K.; Brohawn, P.; Illei, G.G.; Drappa, J.; Wang, L.; Yoo, S.; et al. Anifrolumab, an Anti-Interferon-α Receptor Monoclonal Antibody, in Moderate-to-Severe Systemic Lupus Erythematosus. *Arthritis Rheumatol.* **2017**, *69*, 376–386. [CrossRef]
18. Salmon, J.E.; Niewold, T.B. A Successful Trial for Lupus—How Good Is Good Enough? *N. Engl. J. Med.* **2020**, *382*, 287–288. [CrossRef]
19. Ohmura, K. Which Is the Best SLE Activity Index for Clinical Trials? *Mod. Rheumatol.* **2021**, *31*, 20–28. [CrossRef]
20. Merrill, J.T. For Lupus Trials, the Answer Might Depend on the Question. *Lancet Rheumatol.* **2019**, *1*, e196–e197. [CrossRef]
21. Bruce, I.N.; Nami, A.; Schwetje, E.; Pierson, M.E.; Rouse, T.; Chia, Y.L.; Kuruvilla, D.; Abreu, G.; Tummala, R.; Lindholm, C. Pharmacokinetics, Pharmacodynamics, and Safety of Subcutaneous Anifrolumab in Patients with Systemic Lupus Erythematosus, Active Skin Disease, and High Type I Interferon Gene Signature: A Multicentre, Randomised, Double-Blind, Placebo-Controlled, Phase 2 Study. *Lancet Rheumatol.* **2021**, *3*, e101–e110. [CrossRef]
22. Morand, E.F.; Furie, R.A.; Bruce, I.N.; Vital, E.M.; Dall'Era, M.; Maho, E.; Pineda, L.; Tummala, R. Efficacy of Anifrolumab across Organ Domains in Patients with Moderate-to-Severe Systemic Lupus Erythematosus: A Post-Hoc Analysis of Pooled Data from the TULIP-1 and TULIP-2 Trials. *Lancet Rheumatol.* **2022**, *4*, e282–e292. [CrossRef]
23. Klein, R.; Moghadam-Kia, S.; LoMonico, J.; Okawa, J.; Coley, C.; Taylor, L.; Troxel, A.B.; Werth, V.P. Development of the CLASI as a Tool to Measure Disease Severity and Responsiveness to Therapy in Cutaneous Lupus Erythematosus. *Arch. Dermatol.* **2011**, *147*, 203–208. [CrossRef] [PubMed]

24. Braunstein, I.; Klein, R.; Okawa, J.; Werth, V.P. The Interferon-Regulated Gene Signature Is Elevated in Subacute Cutaneous Lupus Erythematosus and Discoid Lupus Erythematosus and Correlates with the Cutaneous Lupus Area and Severity Index Score. *Br. J. Derm.* **2012**, *166*, 971–975. [CrossRef] [PubMed]
25. Shipman, W.D.; Chyou, S.; Ramanathan, A.; Izmirly, P.M.; Sharma, S.; Pannellini, T.; Dasoveanu, D.C.; Qing, X.; Magro, C.M.; Granstein, R.D.; et al. A Protective Langerhans Cell-Keratinocyte Axis That Is Dysfunctional in Photosensitivity. *Sci. Transl. Med.* **2018**, *10*, eaap9527. [CrossRef]
26. Billi, A.C.; Ma, F.; Plazyo, O.; Gharaee-Kermani, M.; Wasikowski, R.; Hile, G.A.; Xing, X.; Yee, C.M.; Rizvi, S.M.; Maz, M.P.; et al. Nonlesional Lupus Skin Contributes to Inflammatory Education of Myeloid Cells and Primes for Cutaneous Inflammation. *Sci. Transl. Med.* **2022**, *14*, eabn2263. [CrossRef]
27. Plüß, M.; Piantoni, S.; Tampe, B.; Kim, A.; Korsten, P. Product Review: Belimumab for Systemic Lupus Erythematosus–Focus on Lupus Nephritis. *Hum. Vaccines Immunother.* **2022**, 2072143. [CrossRef]

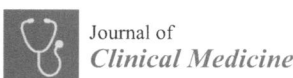

Review

Progress in the Pathogenesis and Treatment of Neuropsychiatric Systemic Lupus Erythematosus

Minhui Wang [†], Ziqian Wang [†], Shangzhu Zhang *, Yang Wu, Li Zhang, Jiuliang Zhao, Qian Wang, Xinping Tian, Mengtao Li * and Xiaofeng Zeng

Department of Rheumatology and Clinical Immunology, Chinese Academy of Medical Sciences and Peking Union Medical College, National Clinical Research Center for Dermatologic and Immunologic Diseases (NCRC-DID), Ministry of Science and Technology, State Key Laboratory of Complex Severe and Rare Diseases, Peking Union Medical College Hospital (PUMCH), Key Laboratory of Rheumatology and Clinical Immunology, Ministry of Education, Beijing 100730, China
* Correspondence: irenezhangpumch@163.com (S.Z.); mengtao.li@cstar.org.cn (M.L.)
† These authors contributed equally to this work.

Abstract: Neuropsychiatric systemic lupus erythematosus (NPSLE) has a broad spectrum of subtypes with diverse severities and prognoses. Ischemic and inflammatory mechanisms, including autoantibodies and cytokine-mediated pathological processes, are key components of the pathogenesis of NPSLE. Additional brain-intrinsic elements (such as the brain barrier and resident microglia) are also important facilitators of NPSLE. An improving understanding of NPSLE may provide further options for managing this disease. The attenuation of neuropsychiatric disease in mouse models demonstrates the potential for novel targeted therapies. Conventional therapeutic algorithms include symptomatic, anti-thrombotic, and immunosuppressive agents that are only supported by observational cohort studies, therefore performing controlled clinical trials to guide further management is essential and urgent. In this review, we aimed to present the latest pathogenetic mechanisms of NPSLE and discuss the progress in its management.

Keywords: systemic lupus erythematosus; neuropsychiatric lupus erythematosus; pathogenesis; management; novel targeted therapies

1. Introduction

Systemic lupus erythematosus (SLE) is an autoimmune disease that may affect almost every organ [1,2]. SLE with nervous system involvement is known as neuropsychiatric systemic lupus erythematosus (NPSLE). NPSLE is a major contributor to morbidity and mortality in SLE patients. The American College of Rheumatology (ACR) defined 19 neuropsychiatric syndromes, ranging from central neurologic and psychiatric disorders to peripheral neuropathy [3–5]. The challenge now is that the underlying pathogenesis remains ambiguous [6–8], due to the limited access to nerve tissue, the complex nature of clinical manifestations, and overlap with non-lupus-associated neuropsychiatric events. These difficulties limit the optimization of NPSLE management.

In this review, we discuss the latest pathogenic mechanisms of NPSLE and explore new ideas and directions for the management of this complicated disease.

2. Pathogenesis of NPSLE

The exact immunopathogenesis of NPSLE is complex and unclear. Ischemic and autoimmune-mediated neuroinflammatory pathways are now considered two main, and probably complementary, pathogenetic mechanisms leading to NPSLE (Figure 1).

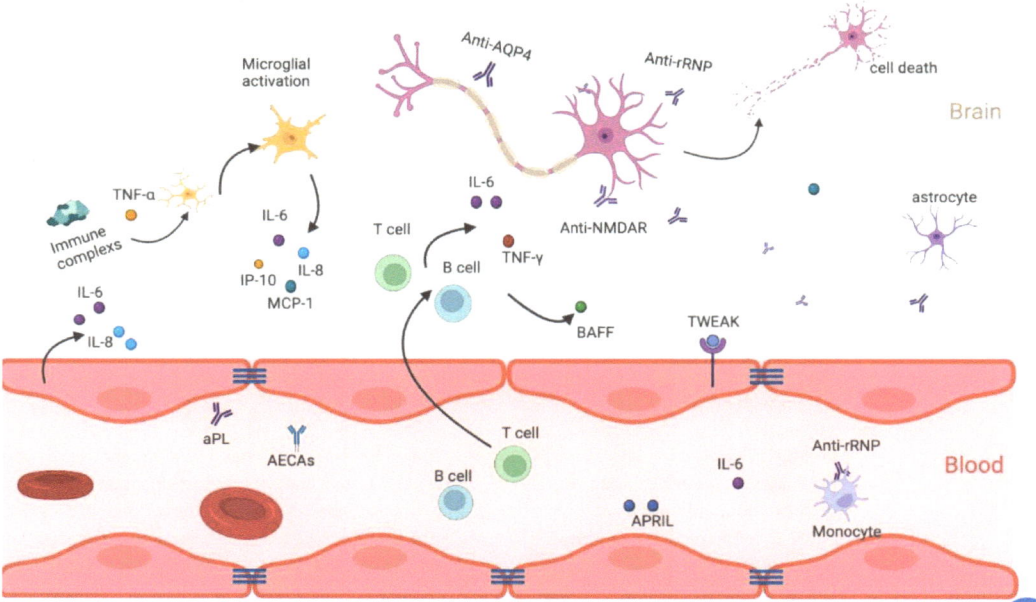

Figure 1. Pathogenetic mechanisms in diffuse NPSLE.

2.1. Ischemic Pathway

Ischemic injury to large- and small- blood vessels, mediated by antiphospholipid (aPL) antibodies, immune complexes, and complement activation leads to focal (e.g., stroke) and diffuse (e.g., cognitive dysfunction) neuropsychiatric events. Among these, aPL antibodies play a predominant role in the intravascular thrombosis [9]. Some studies have reported that SLE patients positive for aPL antibodies are approximately twice as likely to develop NPSLE than aPL-negative patients. aPL antibodies may also increase the risk of subclinical atherosclerosis, leading to a propensity for cerebral ischemia. The central nervous system is more susceptible than most tissues to thrombus formation, which accounts for the increased risk of stroke and transient ischemic attack seen in aPL antibody-positive patients [10]. Apart from thrombosis, aPL antibody positivity has also been correlated with other NPSLE manifestations, such as seizures, chorea, cognitive dysfunction, and myelopathy [11–13], especially psychosis [14–16]. Recent evidence suggests that aPL antibodies are also linked to direct neuronal damage by inducing oxidative stress and damage to neuronal cell membranes via the β2-glycoprotein. In an in vitro study, aPL antibodies bound to neurons and other CNS cells, and the intracerebroventricular injection of aPL induced a hyperactive behavior in animal models [17], thereby supporting a direct effect of these antibodies on the brain.

The aPL-mediated procoagulant state has traditionally been considered noninflammatory. However, a recent study found that mice deficient in C3 and C5 complement components were resistant to aPL-induced thrombosis and endothelial activation [18]. Thus, complement activation is associated with focal NPSLE, psychosis, and cognitive dysfunction, suggesting an additional inflammatory pathogenic component in NPSLE [19].

2.2. Neuroinflammatory Pathway

Autoimmune-mediated neuroinflammatory pathways with complement activation, enhanced the permeability of the blood–brain barrier (BBB), the intrathecal migration of neuronal autoantibodies, and the local production of pro-inflammatory cytokines, and other inflammatory mediators are associated with mostly diffuse neuropsychiatric manifestations, such as psychosis, mood disorders, and cognitive dysfunction [8,18,20,21].

2.2.1. Enhanced Permeability of Brain Barrier

BBB disruption was the first pathophysiological mechanism proposed to play an imperative role in the development of NPSLE [22]. It establishes a structural and functional interface between the brain and general circulation to prevent the passive transfer of immune mediators from the blood to the central nervous system (CNS). Excessive levels of neurotransmitters, cytokines, chemokines, and peripheral hormones may influence BBB permeability [23].

Moreover, animal models of NPSLE have shown that increased BBB permeability is essential for autoantibodies to enter the brain [20,21] and then bind to neurons, which may lead to apoptosis [24]. However, the evidence for persistent BBB dysfunction is controversial [25].

Aside from BBB, the blood–cerebrospinal fluid barrier (BCSFB)—located at choroid plexus epithelial cells—is the natural 'dam' between the systemic circulation and the cerebrospinal fluid (CSF). It is a secretory epithelial structure surrounding a highly vascularized capillary plexus that produces cerebrospinal fluid (CSF) [26]. An increasing number of studies have focused on BCSFB in animal models, demonstrating that the choroid plexus epithelium has been identified as a route of entry into the CSF for pathogenic autoantibodies and leukocytes and as a primary site of neuropathology [27–29]. Additionally, some studies have implicated that in the absence of BBB dysfunction, the BCSFB could still be disrupted, supporting BCSFB dysfunction as a possible causative factor for immune mediators penetrating the brain [28].

Furthermore, the meningeal barrier and glymphatic system have also been proposed as potential sites of neuroimmune interactions, but their exact pathogenic roles await further validation in future studies [30,31].

2.2.2. Autoantibody-Induced Inflammation

A typical feature of SLE is the formation of various autoantibodies, several of which are involved in NPSLE development. Here we will illustrate the identified autoantibodies that have been linked to NPSLE and their potential role in its pathogenesis.

Anti-NMDAR Antibodies

N-methyl D-aspartate receptors (NMDARs) are receptors for the neurotransmitter glutamate, which is a major excitatory neurotransmitter that is important for many brain functions [32]. It has been reported that anti-NMDAR antibodies are related to the psychiatric manifestations of NPSLE [33–35].

Anti-NMDAR antibodies became important upon the observation that some anti-DNA antibodies might cross-react with NMDARs subunits on neurons [36]. These cross-reactive anti-NMDAR antibodies occur in SLE patients and are frequently associated with NPSLE [37–39].

The CSF titers of these antibodies are higher in patients with active diffuse NPSLE than in those with focal NPSLE or non-inflammatory CNS diseases [34,40]. In vitro studies have shown that anti-NMDARs may damage the BBB and penetrate the CNS [41]. Furthermore, the effect of anti-NMDARs is dose-dependent, as at low concentrations they seem to impair synaptic transmission, whereas at high concentrations they may cause neuronal apoptosis [32,33].

Nevertheless, these antibodies may also be present in SLE patients without neuropsychiatric involvement [42,43]. Thus, further research is needed to investigate the effect of anti-NMDARs on the pathogenesis of NPSLE development.

Anti-RP Antibodies

Antibodies targeting the ubiquitous ribosomal P (RP) proteins have been associated with NPSLE, especially when manifested as psychosis and depression [42,44,45]. Anti-RP antibodies were predominantly detected in patients with SLE and were not detected in the control population [21]. The levels of anti-RP were higher in the serum/CSF of NPSLE patients with psychosis, depression, and asymptomatic cranial involvement [46], suggesting a potential role of anti-RP in the pathogenesis of NPSLE. Despite the above findings, some clinical studies that examined whether serum anti-RP antibodies correlated with psychosis have yielded inconsistent results [22]. Moreover, serum anti-RP antibodies are significantly associated with a worse prognosis in patients with diffuse NPSLE [47].

Importantly, the injection of anti-RP antibodies through the nervous system or peripheral circulation leads to cognitive impairment and depression in mice [21,48]. In vitro studies have shown that anti-RP antibodies could induce concentration-dependent neuronal dysfunction or apoptosis by increasing intracellular calcium release and disrupting protein synthesis [9,49].

Above all, anti-RP antibodies may be a relatively strong marker associated with psychiatric NPSLE.

AECAs

Anti-endothelial cell antibodies (AECAs) mediate the expression of adhesion molecules in endothelial cells. They are found in more than half of patients with NPSLE and are also correlated with psychosis and depression manifestations [50,51]. The activation of endothelial cells by AECAs might contribute to cerebral vasculopathy, which, in turn, induces the neuropsychiatric symptoms of SLE [8].

Anti-Ganglioside Antibodies

Gangliosides, spread across neurons' surfaces, are crucial for signal transition [52]. One study reported that positivity for anti-ganglioside antibodies is frequent in lupus patients with PNS involvement [53]. However, this finding needs further investigation to achieve a consistent result [54].

Endothelial cells connected by tight junctions form the blood–brain barrier (BBB). After the BBB is compromised, antibodies gain access to the CSF while activated endothelial cells secrete pro-inflammatory cytokines, including interleukin-6 (IL-6) and interleukin-8 (IL-8). The associated signaling pathways involve the cytokine tumor necrosis factor-like weak inducer of apoptosis (TWEAK) to promote BBB disruption through the induction of inflammatory cytokines. Cytokines and chemokines, such as IL-6 and a proliferation-inducing ligand (APRIL), enhance B-cell activation and survival.

Immune complexes could induce interferon-α (IFN-α) production. IFN-α could activates microglial engulfment of neurons and directly damages them. Microglial activation further propagates local cytokine and chemokine signaling cascades. Furthermore, IFN-α enhances microglial cytokine and chemokine (IL-6, IL-8, MCP-1, IP-10) production. Finally, several neuropathic autoantibodies have been implicated in NPSLE. Autoantibodies, such as anti-NMDAR and anti-RP, directly bind to neurons and lead to neuronal dysfunction or apoptosis. Following neuronal cell damage, antibodies form immune complexes with neuronal antigens, contributing to the diffuse neuronal damage/dysfunction in the brain. Created with biorender.com.

2.2.3. Cytokines-Mediated Inflammation

In CNS, cytokines are expressed at low levels by neurons, astrocytes, microglia, and oligodendrocytes. The expression of genes encoding cytokines and their receptors in the brain suggests that cytokines contribute to the normal physiological functions of CNS. Cytokines and other immune factors are important for the modulation of brain development and affect adult neuronal plasticity, leading to cognitive and mood disorders [55]. Below, we will discuss the cytokines that potentially participate in the pathogenesis of NPSLE.

TWEAK/Fn14

The tumor necrosis factor-like weak inducer of apoptosis (TWEAK), a member of the tumor necrosis factor (TNF) superfamily of cytokines, promotes the activation of NF-kB and mitogen-activated protein kinase (MAPK) by binding to fibroblast growth factor-inducible 14 (Fn14), a 14 kDa member of the TNF receptor superfamily. Fn14 is expressed in a variety of cells and tissue types, including fibroblasts, endothelial cells, and epithelial cells [56].

TWEAK plays an important role in BBB disruption and the development of NPSLE [57]. Fn14 exhibited upregulation within the cerebral cortex of lupus-prone mice. In addition, the severe depression-like behavior observed in MRL/lpr mice was significantly reduced in Fn14-deficient mice, indicating that Fn14 improved depression and cognitive function [58]. Moreover, the intracerebroventricular injection of TWEAK in wild-type mice induced cognitive dysfunction and depression-like behavior through increased BBB permeability and accelerated neuronal apoptosis [59]. However, this cytokine seems to be elevated in the CSF of SLE patients, regardless of the presence or absence of neuropsychiatric symptoms.

IL-6

Interleukin-6 (IL-6) is thought to have the strongest positive association with NPSLE [60]. The elevated intrathecal levels of IL-6 have been found in patients with diffuse NPSLE, such as those experiencing an acute confusional state or psychosis [61]. In addition, the positive correlation between IL-6 levels and the levels of the neuronal degradation product denominated neurofilament light chains (NFL), which indicates that IL-6 exerts destructive effect on nerve cells [62]. Nevertheless, research on the correlation between serum IL-6 and psychiatric NPSLE provided inconclusive results [63]. This difference needs to be further explored.

IFN-α

An animal models have demonstrated a significant association between IFN-α in the CSF and NPSLE, identifying a novel IFN-α-dependent mechanism for NPSLE. IFN-α has been proposed to cause damage by activating microglia in the CSF and stimulating the microglial engulfment of neuronal cells [64]. IFN-α may also impair brain function by altering the levels of neurotransmitters and generating damage by the secondary release of cytokines and chemokines, such as IL-6- and interferon-gamma-inducible protein-10 (IP-10) [65].

Additionally, neuropsychiatric manifestations observed in lupus-prone animal models were reversible with IFN-α inhibition, indicating that IFN-α is imperative in the pathogenesis of NPSLE [64].

BAFF and APRIL

The TNF family ligands B-cell activating factor of the TNF family (BAFF) and APRIL are crucial in the survival, differentiation, and isotype switching of B lymphocytes [66].

One study found a close relationship between APRIL in the CSF and NPSLE but not between BAFF in the CSF and NPSLE [67]. To date, there have been few studies regarding their exact role in the pathogenesis of NPSLE.

2.2.4. Brain-Resident and Infiltrating Cells

Apart from structural changes, autoantibodies and cytokines, alterations in brain-resident cells in the CNS may be instrumental in the development of NPSLE.

Microglia, the resident macrophage cells of the brain, are the main antigen-presenting cells (APCs) in the CNS. They play a fundamental role in regulating BBB function and shaping the brain circuits. They could also secrete various cytokines, chemokines, prostaglandins, and reactive oxygen species [68].

Increasing evidence supports an active role for microglial cells in the pathogenesis of NPSLE. Activated microglia are a feature of several models of the lupus-prone mouse [69,70]. MLR/lpr mice lacking estrogen receptor alpha experienced a significant neuropsychiatric disorder, which correlated with a decreased number of activated microglial cells and an accompanying reduction in CNS inflammation [71].

The intrathecal synthesis of cytokines as a potential mechanism of damage, and neural damage may develop in NPSLE without the involvement of factors derived from blood [72]. Although the cellular origin of these cytokines production in the brain remains unknown, macrophages and endothelial cells (ECs), as well as brain-derived microglia and astrocytes, are probable sources of these cytokines. Microglial depletion by colony-stimulating factor-1 receptor (CSF1R) inhibitors resulted in preserved neuronal integrity in an inducible mouse model (NMDAR peptide immunized BALB/c mice). Interestingly, another study showed that the administration of captopril (an angiotensin-converting enzyme (ACE)) inhibitor significantly reversed the activation of microglia and improved the cognitive function of mice [73].

Large clusters of leukocytes infiltrate the choroid plexus in vitro. The analysis of the choroid plexus indicated a tertiary lymphoid structure formation, with evidence of APC-lymphocyte interactions, cytokine production, and in situ somatic hypermutation [74].

3. Current Management of NPSLE

The management of NPSLE can be challenging, because of the complexity of its pathogenesis, difficulty in its accurate diagnosis, and a lack of clinical trials in NPSLE. Current treatment options for NPSLE are usually derived from observational studies and refer to the experience of treatment of other SLE subtypes, such as lupus nephritis and similar neuropsychiatric disorders [8,75].

Initially, it is crucial to develop pragmatic therapeutic strategies to determine the attribution of nervous system disease to SLE, non-SLE causes, or both. Confounders and mimics should be ruled out and the symptoms should be initially attributable to SLE at the beginning. The goal of management of NPSLE is to meet two criteria. First, symptomatic therapy is necessary: anti-epileptics for seizures, and anxiolytics, antidepressants, mood-stabilizers, or antipsychotics should be administered as appropriate. Neurotrophic and neuroleptic agents were generally adopted in case with peripheral nervous system involvement [4]. The treatment of the underlying SLE process should be undertaken based on whether the pathogenesis is primarily related to an inflammatory or ischemic disease pathway (Figure 2).

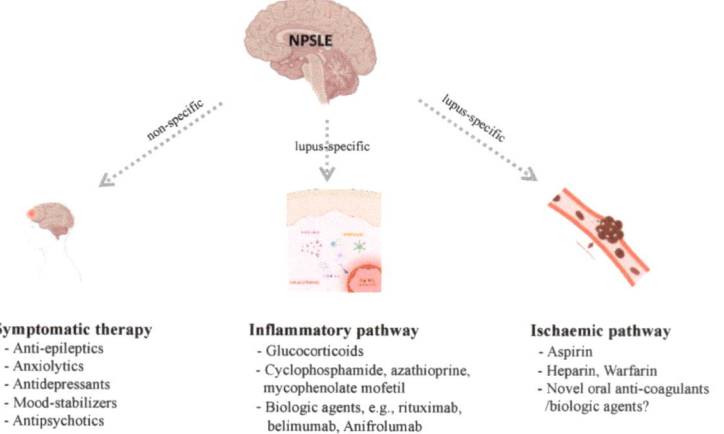

Figure 2. Management for patients with neuropsychiatric systemic lupus erythematosus (NPSLE). Created with biorender.com.

3.1. Inflammatory Pathway Therapies

Glucocorticoids have been a cornerstone in the treatment of various manifestations of NPSLE, especially in those associated with an immune-inflammatory pathogenesis [76,77]. High-dose glucocorticoids, alone or in combination with cyclophosphamide, azathioprine, and mycophenolate mofetil, are reported to be effective, but their use is mainly based on patient's clinical experience of disease severity and their clinician's preference. Given the evidence linking glucocorticoids use to cumulative organ damage in SLE [78] and its associated psychiatric symptoms [79,80], alternative therapeutic strategies are essential.

Unfortunately, high-level clinical evidence regarding the optimization of NPSLE treatment is lacking. Only two of these agents (oral prednisone and intravenous cyclophosphamide) have been subjected to clinical trials for NPSLE [76], and both had positive outcomes. In addition, a regimen of oral cyclophosphamide for 6 months followed by azathioprine maintenance therapy was effective for the treatment of lupus psychosis [81].

The examination of biological agents in NPSLE is limited to uncontrolled studies. Open studies on B-lymphocyte depletion with rituximab used alone or in combination with conventional immunosuppressive agents, including cyclophosphamide, have reported favorable results in children [82] and adults [83] with NPSLE; however, this requires further study. Perhaps of relevance is the observation that rituximab can be beneficial in other inflammatory neurological conditions, such as neuromyelitis optica, anti-NMDAR encephalitis, and opsoclonus–myoclonus syndrome [84,85]. Studies of belimumab suggested a beneficial response to belimumab in SLE, but patients with severe NPSLE were excluded from these clinical trials [86].

3.2. Ischemic Pathway Therapies

Cerebral ischemia attributed to NPSLE, such as transient ischemic attacks and stroke attributed to NPSLE events and is thought to be correlated with aPL antibodies. Thus, the primary prevention of cerebral ischemia in NPSLE is linked to a reduction in prothrombotic risk.

Low-dose aspirin is recommended for patients with cardiovascular risk factors [87]. However, a previous review of primary prevention in antiphospholipid syndrome (APS) concluded that the current evidence does not support either the use of low-dose aspirin or warfarin [88]. The optimal target international normalized ratio (INR) in such cases is inconsistent [87] and the recommended INR target in patients with APS is 2.5–3.0. In patients with recurrent thrombosis despite optimal warfarin therapy, the INR should be kept at 3.0–4.0. Nevertheless, there is no obvious difference between low-intensity (target INR 2.0–3.0] and high-intensity (target INR > 3.0) warfarin in the prevention of recurrent thrombosis in controlled trials with APS patients [89,90]. Therefore, well-designed clinical trials are needed to address this issue. Currently, the data are insufficient to recommend the use of direct novel oral anti-coagulants to prevent aPL antibody-mediated thromboembolic events [91].

Potential adjunctive therapies, especially in patients with arterial thrombosis and recurrent venous thrombosis, include antimalarials and statins [87]. Statins can prevent endothelial cell activation secondary to aPL antibodies [92], while antimalarial agents are protective against thrombosis in patients with SLE [93].

4. Promising Targeted Therapies

Due to the lack of understanding of the exact pathogenic mechanisms behind this condition as well as its diverse neuropsychiatric manifestations, we have limited experience in targeted therapies for patients with NPSLE. The attenuation of neuropsychiatric diseases in related animal models demonstrates the potential for targeted therapies, which are based on a current understanding of the pathogenesis of NPSLE (Table 1).

Table 1. Promising targeted therapies in NPSLE.

Promising Targeted Therapies	Underlying Mechanisms and Clinical Findings	Experimental Arrangement	Potential Drugs
Complement inhibitors	Complement signaling promotes the loss of BBB integrity. Blocking the complement cascades relieved the symptoms of NPSLE. Complement deposits were present in most of patients with NPSLE.	Human brain autopsies	Eculizumab
BBB-targeted therapy	BBB disruption is essential in the neuronal damage process. Restoration of normal BBB function may reduce the development of neuropsychiatric manifestations	Human and mouse cells; C57 BL/6J mice, respectively	GW0742, a peroxisome proliferator-activated receptor β/δ agonist; KD025, a rho kinase inhibitor.
MMPs inhibitors	There is an association between CSF/serum levels of MMP-9, psychiatric NPSLE, and markers for neuronal/astrocytic damage. MMP-9 may contribute to the pathogenesis of psychiatric NPSLE by stimulating T-cell migration	-	-
IFN-α/β receptor antagonists	IFN receptor inhibition decreased microglia-related synaptic loss and attenuated anxiety-like behavior and cognitive deficits in animal models.	564Igi lupus-prone mice	Anifrolumab
BTK inhibitors	Use of BI-BTK-1 (an inhibitor of BTK) in MRL/lpr mice, decreased the infiltration of macrophages, T cells, and B cells in the choroid plexus, and improved cognitive function.	MRL/lpr mice	Ibrutinib; Evobrutinib
S1P receptor modulator	S1P receptor modulators decreased proinflammatory cytokine secretion by microglia and significantly improved spatial memory and depression-like behavior. Fingolimod (a S1P receptor modulator) treatment attenuated neuropsychiatric manifestations, reversed the entry of immune components, and decreased BBB leakage. Fingolimod-treated microglia revealed down- regulated of multiple immune-mediated pathways, including NF-kB signaling and the IFN response with the negative regulation of type I IFN-mediated signaling.	MRL/lpr mice	Fingolimod
ACE inhibitors	ACE inhibitors treatment suppressed microglial activation and promoted cognitive status.	BALB/c mice	Captopril; Perindopril
CSF1R inhibitors	CSF1R is essential in both macrophage and microglia function. Inhibition of CSF1R signaling in MRL/lpr mice reduced the brain expression of proinflammatory cytokines and attenuated depression performance.	MRL/lpr mice	GW2580, a small CSF-1R kinase inhibitor; depletion of microglia
Nogo-a/NgR1 antagonists	Nogo-a/NgR1 in the CSF is significantly increased in NPSLE. Nogo-a/NgR1 antagonists improved cognitive function, decreased the expression of pro-inflammatory components, and reduced axonal degeneration and demyelination.	MRL/lpr mice	Nogo-66
JAK inhibitors	JAK inhibitors penetrate the BBB and reduce the production of several cytokines, including type I IFNs.	-	Tofacitinib

4.1. Complement Inhibitors

A study devoted to the role of the complement protein C5a in the brain vasculature indicated that the C5a/C5aR signaling plays a key role in disrupting the BBB integrity [94]. C5aR was blocked the complement cascades and retained their protective functions, which relieved the symptoms of NPSLE. Thus, C5aR may be a potentially important therapeutic target for NPSLE [95]. In addition, the presence of C5b-9 deposits in most patients with NPSLE is important in the interaction between circulating autoantibodies and thrombo-ischemic lesions observed in NPSLE. Therefore, the complement inhibitor eculizumab may have novel therapeutic potential for NPSLE [68,96]. However, the efficacy of such treatment in NPSLE remains to be further investigated.

4.2. BBB-Targeted Therapies

BBB dysfunction exposes the brain to components of the blood that are normally excluded. Decreasing the permeability of the BBB could be advantageous for a patient with NPSLE. This could prevent autoantibodies, cytokines, and non-immune proteins from causing inflammation, neuronal hyperexcitability, and degeneration [97].

The restoration of normal BBB function is a potential therapeutic strategy. Two compounds that reduce BBB permeability (GW0742, a peroxisome proliferator-activated receptor β/δ agonist [98], and KD025, a Rho kinase inhibitor [99]) have been studied in experimental systems and may be considered as therapies.

4.3. MMPs Inhibitors

Matrix metalloproteinases (MMPs) are proteolytic enzymes that could degrade basement membranes, disrupt inter-endothelial tight junctions, and activate membrane-bound proinflammatory molecules. Among those, MMP-9 induces the production of cytokines and leukocyte adhesion molecules by endothelial cells, facilitating the entry of leukocytes and proteins into the CSF [100,101].

Studies have demonstrated an association between CSF/serum levels of MMP-9, psychiatric NPSLE, and the markers of neuronal/astrocytic damage [102]. MMP-9 may contribute to the pathogenesis of psychiatric NPSLE by stimulating T-cell migration. Therefore, the inhibition of MMPs, especially MMP-9 [103], could introduce a novel biological agent and may be beneficial in NPSLE.

4.4. IFN-α/β Receptor Antagonists

Anifrolumab, a type I interferon receptor antagonist that binds to the IFN-α/β receptor, has been successfully used in phase III clinical trials for SLE treatment [104]. The adoption of anifrolumab leads to a substantial reduction in moderate-to-severe active SLE; however, patients with severe NPSLE were not involved in these trials [105]. Therefore, the results may not support the efficacy of this drug in the treatment of NPSLE. However, as mentioned before, the type I interferon receptor inhibition decreases microglia related synaptic loss and attenuates anxiety-like behavior and cognitive deficits in lupus-prone mice [38]. This implies that type I interferon inhibition may be an option for the treatment of NPSLE in the future [106], especially in patients with a strong type I interferon signature.

4.5. BTK Inhibitors

Bruton's tyrosine kinase (BTK) is essential for B cell function, including B cell development and survival; for crystallizable fragment (Fc) receptor and toll-like receptor (TLR) signaling in macrophages; and for macrophage polarization [107–109].

The inhibition of this pathway using of a specific inhibitor (BI-BTK-1) in MRL/lpr mice resulted in the decreased infiltration of macrophages, T cells, and B cells in the choroid plexus and improved cognitive function [110].

Ibrutinib, a selective BTK inhibitor, could potentially prove useful in the treatment of neuropsychiatric disease, such as SLE [111]. This inhibitor has already have already been approved for clinical use in hematological indications [112] and results from ongoing early phase clinical trials of BTK inhibitors in patients with SLE are eagerly awaited.

4.6. S1P Receptor Modulator

Fingolimod, a sphingosine-1-phosphate (S1P) receptor modulator, was shown to decrease macrophage infiltration and proinflammatory cytokine secretion by microglia, resulting in improved spatial memory and reduced depression-like behavior in MRL/lpr mice [113]. Fingolimod administration attenuated neuropsychiatric manifestations, reversed the entry of immune components, and decreased BBB leakage in the above studies [114].

In addition to the possible mechanisms mentioned above, fingolimod-treated microglia revealed the downregulation of multiple immune-mediated pathways, including NF-kB signaling and the IFN response, with the negative regulation of type I IFN-mediated signaling [113].

In line with the approved use of fingolimod in relapsing–remitting multiple sclerosis, these studies may support the potential use of fingolimod as a therapeutic strategy for NPSLE patients.

4.7. ACE Inhibitors

ACE inhibitors, such as captopril and perindopril, improve cognitive status and neuronal functions in lupus-prone mice [73].

Additionally, ACE inhibitors treatment in a lupus-prone model suppressed microglial activation, which in turn preserved dendritic complexity in hippocampal neurons. Further analysis is needed to explore the specific pathogenesis, but this therapeutic regimen may also be considered in the future to treat cognitive impairment in NPSLE patients.

4.8. CSF1R Inhibitors

Macrophage colony stimulating factor 1 receptor (CSF1R) is an important regulator of both macrophage and microglial functions. It plays a pivotal role in macrophage and microglia development, survival, and activation [115].

In a mouse model, the inhibition of CSF1R signaling reduced the brain expression of pro-inflammatory cytokines and attenuated depression performance [116], indicating that CSF1R is a potential target for treating NPSLE in the future.

4.9. Nogo-a/NgR1 Antagonists

Neurite outgrowth inhibitor-A (Nogo-a) with its respective receptor, NgR1, forms a signaling pathway that mediates the inhibition of neuron generation. Patients with NPSLE have significantly increased levels of Nogo-a/NgR1 in the CSF, compared to other neurological diseases. It has also been demonstrated in MLR/lpr mice that the administration of Nogo-66 [117], an antagonist of Nogo-a, improved cognitive function, decreased the expression of pro-inflammatory components, and reduced axonal degeneration and demyelination, implying that Nogo-a is a potential therapeutic target for cognitive impairment in NPSLE.

4.10. JAK Inhibitors

JAK inhibitors, which interfere with the JAK-STAT signaling pathway, are small molecules that penetrate the BBB [118] and reduce the production of several cytokines, including type I IFNs. Tofacitinib, a JAK1/JAK3 inhibitor is currently in phase II studies for SLE treatment and is worthy of consideration in this regard [119]. However, whether it is effective for NPSLE still requires further research.

5. Conclusions

Neuropsychiatric events in SLE patients are common and tend to be heterogeneous, and many knowledge gaps remain in our basic understanding of NPSLE and its clinical management. Current available therapies are largely empirical, and most evidence is derived from studies in animal models, which do not manifest the full spectrum of human NPSLE.

Advances remain to be made in enhancing the understanding of the pathogenesis, and optimizing our ability to diagnose, prognosticate, and treat NPSLE. Innovative strategies targeting the brain structural barrier, specifically autoantibodies, cytokines, and brain-resident cells, are worthy of exploration and further study.

We anticipate that some of these pathways could serve as targets for the development of a new therapeutic strategies. Promising research efforts into novel targeted therapies and improved diagnostic tools are ongoing; however, much work remains to be done to optimize our ability to diagnose, prognosticate, and treat NPSLE.

Author Contributions: M.L., M.W., Z.W. and S.Z. designed the review; Y.W., L.Z., J.Z., Q.W., X.T. and X.Z. performed the literature search; M.W., Z.W. and M.L. drafted the manuscript, critically revised, and approved the final version of the manuscript. All authors have read and agreed to the published version of the manuscript.

Funding: This study was supported by the Chinese National Key Technology R&D Program, Ministry of Science and Technology (2021YFC2501301-5, 2017YFC0907601-3), Beijing Municipal Science and Technology Commission (No. Z201100005520022,23,25–27), CAMS Innovation Fund for Medical Sciences (CIFMS) (2021-I2M-1-005), National High Level Hospital Clinical Research Funding (2022-PUMCH-A-229).

Institutional Review Board Statement: Not applicable.

Informed Consent Statement: Not applicable.

Data Availability Statement: Not applicable.

Conflicts of Interest: The authors declare no conflict of interest.

References

1. Li, M.; Wang, Y.; Zhao, J.; Wang, Q.; Wang, Z.; Tian, X.; Zeng, X. Chinese SLE Treatment and Research group (CSTAR) registry 2009–2019: Major clinical characteristics of Chinese patients with systemic lupus erythematosus. *Rheumatol. Immunol. Res.* **2021**, *2*, 43–47. [CrossRef]
2. Wang, Z.; Li, M.; Ye, Z.; Li, C.; Li, Z.; Li, X.; Wu, L.; Liu, S.; Zuo, X.; Zhu, P.; et al. Long-term outcomes of patients with systemic lupus erythematosus: A Multicenter Cohort Study from CSTAR registry. *Rheumatol. Immunol. Res.* **2021**, *2*, 195–202. [CrossRef]
3. Liang, M.H.; Corzillius, M.; Bae, S.C.; Lew, R.A.; Fortin, P.R.; Gordon, C.; Isenberg, D.; Alarcón, G.S.; Straaton, K.V.; Denburg, J.; et al. The American College of Rheumatology nomenclature and case definitions for neuropsychiatric lupus syndromes. *Arthritis Rheum.* **1999**, *42*, 599–608. [CrossRef]
4. Bortoluzzi, A.; Piga, M.; Silvagni, E.; Chessa, E.; Mathieu, A.; Govoni, M. Peripheral nervous system involvement in systemic lupus erythematosus: A retrospective study on prevalence, associated factors and outcome. *Lupus* **2019**, *28*, 465–474. [CrossRef]
5. Hanly, J.G.; Li, Q.; Su, L.; Urowitz, M.B.; Gordon, C.; Bae, S.C.; Romero-Diaz, J.; Sanchez-Guerrero, J.; Bernatsky, S.; Clarke, A.E.; et al. Peripheral Nervous System Disease in Systemic Lupus Erythematosus: Results From an International Inception Cohort Study. *Arthritis Rheumatol.* **2020**, *72*, 67–77. [CrossRef] [PubMed]
6. Moore, E.; Huang, M.W.; Putterman, C. Advances in the diagnosis, pathogenesis and treatment of neuropsychiatric systemic lupus erythematosus. *Curr. Opin. Rheumatol.* **2020**, *32*, 152–158. [CrossRef]
7. Govoni, M.; Hanly, J.G. The management of neuropsychiatric lupus in the 21st century: Still so many unmet needs? *Rheumatology* **2020**, *59* (Suppl. S5), v52–v62. [CrossRef]
8. Schwartz, N.; Stock, A.D.; Putterman, C. Neuropsychiatric lupus: New mechanistic insights and future treatment directions. *Nat. Rev. Rheumatol.* **2019**, *15*, 137–152. [CrossRef]
9. Ho, R.C.; Thiaghu, C.; Ong, H.; Lu, Y.; Ho, C.S.; Tam, W.W.; Zhang, M.W. A meta-analysis of serum and cerebrospinal fluid autoantibodies in neuropsychiatric systemic lupus erythematosus. *Autoimmun. Rev.* **2016**, *15*, 124–138. [CrossRef]
10. Ben Salem, C. The pathogenesis of the antiphospholipid syndrome. *N. Engl. J. Med.* **2013**, *368*, 2334. [CrossRef]
11. Mikdashi, J.; Handwerger, B. Predictors of neuropsychiatric damage in systemic lupus erythematosus: Data from the Maryland lupus cohort. *Rheumatology* **2004**, *43*, 1555–1560. [CrossRef] [PubMed]
12. Andrade, R.M.; Alarcón, G.S.; González, L.A.; Fernández, M.; Apte, M.; Vilá, L.M.; McGwin, G., Jr.; Reveille, J.D. Seizures in patients with systemic lupus erythematosus: Data from LUMINA, a multiethnic cohort (LUMINA LIV). *Ann. Rheum. Dis.* **2008**, *67*, 829–834. [CrossRef] [PubMed]

13. Tomietto, P.; Annese, V.; D'Agostini, S.; Venturini, P.; La Torre, G.; De Vita, S.; Ferraccioli, G.F. General and specific factors associated with severity of cognitive impairment in systemic lupus erythematosus. *Arthritis Rheum.* **2007**, *57*, 1461–1472. [CrossRef]
14. Shoenfeld, Y.; Nahum, A.; Korczyn, A.D.; Dano, M.; Rabinowitz, R.; Beilin, O.; Pick, C.G.; Leider-Trejo, L.; Kalashnikova, L.; Blank, M.; et al. Neuronal-binding antibodies from patients with antiphospholipid syndrome induce cognitive deficits following intrathecal passive transfer. *Lupus* **2003**, *12*, 436–442. [CrossRef] [PubMed]
15. Caronti, B.; Calderaro, C.; Alessandri, C.; Conti, F.; Tinghino, R.; Pini, C.; Palladini, G.; Valesini, G. Serum anti-beta2-glycoprotein I antibodies from patients with antiphospholipid antibody syndrome bind central nervous system cells. *J. Autoimmun.* **1998**, *11*, 425–429. [CrossRef]
16. Chapman, J.; Cohen-Armon, M.; Shoenfeld, Y.; Korczyn, A.D. Antiphospholipid antibodies permeabilize and depolarize brain synaptoneurosomes. *Lupus* **1999**, *8*, 127–133. [CrossRef]
17. Katzav, A.; Ben-Ziv, T.; Blank, M.; Pick, C.G.; Shoenfeld, Y.; Chapman, J. Antibody-specific behavioral effects: Intracerebroventricular injection of antiphospholipid antibodies induces hyperactive behavior while anti-ribosomal-P antibodies induces depression and smell deficits in mice. *J. Neuroimmunol.* **2014**, *272*, 10–15. [CrossRef]
18. Hanly, J.G.; Kozora, E.; Beyea, S.D.; Birnbaum, J. Review: Nervous System Disease in Systemic Lupus Erythematosus: Current Status and Future Directions. *Arthritis Rheumatol.* **2019**, *71*, 33–42. [CrossRef]
19. Magro-Checa, C.; Schaarenburg, R.A.; Beaart, H.J.; Huizinga, T.W.; Steup-Beekman, G.M.; Trouw, L.A. Complement levels and anti-C1q autoantibodies in patients with neuropsychiatric systemic lupus erythematosus. *Lupus* **2016**, *25*, 878–888. [CrossRef]
20. Kowal, C.; DeGiorgio, L.A.; Nakaoka, T.; Hetherington, H.; Huerta, P.T.; Diamond, B.; Volpe, B.T. Cognition and immunity; antibody impairs memory. *Immunity* **2004**, *21*, 179–188. [CrossRef]
21. Bravo-Zehnder, M.; Toledo, E.M.; Segovia-Miranda, F.; Serrano, F.G.; Benito, M.J.; Metz, C.; Retamal, C.; Álvarez, A.; Massardo, L.; Inestrosa, N.C.; et al. Anti-ribosomal P protein autoantibodies from patients with neuropsychiatric lupus impair memory in mice. *Arthritis Rheumatol.* **2015**, *67*, 204–214. [CrossRef] [PubMed]
22. Nikolopoulos, D.; Fanouriakis, A.; Boumpas, D.T. Update on the pathogenesis of central nervous system lupus. *Curr. Opin. Rheumatol.* **2019**, *31*, 669–677. [CrossRef] [PubMed]
23. de Boer, A.G.; Gaillard, P.J. Blood-brain barrier dysfunction and recovery. *J. Neural. Transm.* **2006**, *113*, 455–462. [CrossRef] [PubMed]
24. Lauvsnes, M.B.; Omdal, R. Systemic lupus erythematosus, the brain, and anti-NR2 antibodies. *J. Neurol.* **2012**, *259*, 622–629. [CrossRef]
25. Duarte-Delgado, N.P.; Vásquez, G.; Ortiz-Reyes, B.L. Blood-brain barrier disruption and neuroinflammation as pathophysiological mechanisms of the diffuse manifestations of neuropsychiatric systemic lupus erythematosus. *Autoimmun. Rev.* **2019**, *18*, 426–432. [CrossRef]
26. Tumani, H.; Huss, A.; Bachhuber, F. The cerebrospinal fluid and barriers—Anatomic and physiologic considerations. *Handb. Clin. Neurol.* **2017**, *146*, 21–32. [CrossRef]
27. James, W.G.; Hutchinson, P.; Bullard, D.C.; Hickey, M.J. Cerebral leucocyte infiltration in lupus-prone MRL/MpJ-fas lpr mice—Roles of intercellular adhesion molecule-1 and P-selectin. *Clin. Exp. Immunol.* **2006**, *144*, 299–308. [CrossRef]
28. Gelb, S.; Stock, A.D.; Anzi, S.; Putterman, C.; Ben-Zvi, A. Mechanisms of neuropsychiatric lupus: The relative roles of the blood-cerebrospinal fluid barrier versus blood-brain barrier. *J. Autoimmun.* **2018**, *91*, 34–44. [CrossRef]
29. Ballok, D.A.; Ma, X.; Denburg, J.A.; Arsenault, L.; Sakic, B. Ibuprofen fails to prevent brain pathology in a model of neuropsychiatric lupus. *J. Rheumatol.* **2006**, *33*, 2199–2213.
30. Verheggen, I.C.M.; Van Boxtel, M.P.J.; Verhey, F.R.J.; Jansen, J.F.A.; Backes, W.H. Interaction between blood-brain barrier and glymphatic system in solute clearance. *Neurosci. Biobehav. Rev.* **2018**, *90*, 26–33. [CrossRef]
31. Brøchner, C.B.; Holst, C.B.; Møllgård, K. Outer brain barriers in rat and human development. *Front. Neurosci.* **2015**, *9*, 75. [CrossRef] [PubMed]
32. Aranow, C.; Diamond, B.; Mackay, M. Glutamate receptor biology and its clinical significance in neuropsychiatric systemic lupus erythematosus. *Rheum. Dis. Clin. N. Am.* **2010**, *36*, 187–201. [CrossRef] [PubMed]
33. Hirohata, S.; Arinuma, Y.; Yanagida, T.; Yoshio, T. Blood-brain barrier damages and intrathecal synthesis of anti-N-methyl-D-aspartate receptor NR2 antibodies in diffuse psychiatric/neuropsychological syndromes in systemic lupus erythematosus. *Arthritis Res. Ther.* **2014**, *16*, R77. [CrossRef] [PubMed]
34. Arinuma, Y.; Yanagida, T.; Hirohata, S. Association of cerebrospinal fluid anti-NR2 glutamate receptor antibodies with diffuse neuropsychiatric systemic lupus erythematosus. *Arthritis Rheum.* **2008**, *58*, 1130–1135. [CrossRef] [PubMed]
35. Steup-Beekman, G.; Steens, S.; van Buchem, M.; Huizinga, T. Anti-NMDA receptor autoantibodies in patients with systemic lupus erythematosus and their first-degree relatives. *Lupus* **2007**, *16*, 329–334. [CrossRef]
36. Diamond, B.; Volpe, B.T. A model for lupus brain disease. *Immunol. Rev.* **2012**, *248*, 56–67. [CrossRef]
37. Omdal, R.; Brokstad, K.; Waterloo, K.; Koldingsnes, W.; Jonsson, R.; Mellgren, S.I. Neuropsychiatric disturbances in SLE are associated with antibodies against NMDA receptors. *Eur. J. Neurol.* **2005**, *12*, 392–398. [CrossRef]
38. Lapteva, L.; Nowak, M.; Yarboro, C.H.; Takada, K.; Roebuck-Spencer, T.; Weickert, T.; Bleiberg, J.; Rosenstein, D.; Pao, M.; Patronas, N.; et al. Anti-N-methyl-D-aspartate receptor antibodies, cognitive dysfunction, and depression in systemic lupus erythematosus. *Arthritis Rheum.* **2006**, *54*, 2505–2514. [CrossRef]

39. Gao, H.X.; Campbell, S.R.; Cui, M.H.; Zong, P.; Hee-Hwang, J.; Gulinello, M.; Putterman, C. Depression is an early disease manifestation in lupus-prone MRL/lpr mice. *J. Neuroimmunol.* **2009**, *207*, 45–56. [CrossRef]
40. Brimberg, L.; Mader, S.; Fujieda, Y.; Arinuma, Y.; Kowal, C.; Volpe, B.T.; Diamond, B. Antibodies as Mediators of Brain Pathology. *Trends Immunol.* **2015**, *36*, 709–724. [CrossRef]
41. Wang, J.Y.; Zhao, Y.H.; Zhang, J.H.; Lei, H.W. Anti-N-Methyl-D-Aspartic Acid Receptor 2 (Anti-NR2) Antibody in Neuropsychiatric Lupus Serum Damages the Blood-Brain Barrier and Enters the Brain. *Med. Sci. Monit.* **2019**, *25*, 532–539. [CrossRef] [PubMed]
42. Karassa, F.B.; Afeltra, A.; Ambrozic, A.; Chang, D.M.; De Keyser, F.; Doria, A.; Galeazzi, M.; Hirohata, S.; Hoffman, I.E.; Inanc, M.; et al. Accuracy of anti-ribosomal P protein antibody testing for the diagnosis of neuropsychiatric systemic lupus erythematosus: An international meta-analysis. *Arthritis Rheum.* **2006**, *54*, 312–324. [CrossRef] [PubMed]
43. Husebye, E.S.; Sthoeger, Z.M.; Dayan, M.; Zinger, H.; Elbirt, D.; Levite, M.; Mozes, E. Autoantibodies to a NR2A peptide of the glutamate/NMDA receptor in sera of patients with systemic lupus erythematosus. *Ann. Rheum. Dis.* **2005**, *64*, 1210–1213. [CrossRef] [PubMed]
44. Isshi, K.; Hirohata, S. Association of anti-ribosomal P protein antibodies with neuropsychiatric systemic lupus erythematosus. *Arthritis Rheum.* **1996**, *39*, 1483–1490. [CrossRef]
45. Choi, M.Y.; FitzPatrick, R.D.; Buhler, K.; Mahler, M.; Fritzler, M.J. A review and meta-analysis of anti-ribosomal P autoantibodies in systemic lupus erythematosus. *Autoimmun. Rev.* **2020**, *19*, 102463. [CrossRef]
46. Gaber, W.; Ezzat, Y.; El Fayoumy, N.M.; Helmy, H.; Mohey, A.M. Detection of asymptomatic cranial neuropathies in patients with systemic lupus erythematosus and their relation to antiribosomal P antibody levels and disease activity. *Clin. Rheumatol.* **2014**, *33*, 1459–1466. [CrossRef]
47. Arinuma, Y.; Kikuchi, H.; Hirohata, S. Anti-ribosomal P protein antibodies influence mortality of patients with diffuse psychiatric/neuropsychological syndromes in systemic lupus erythematous involving a severe form of the disease. *Mod. Rheumatol.* **2019**, *29*, 612–618. [CrossRef]
48. Katzav, A.; Solodeev, I.; Brodsky, O.; Chapman, J.; Pick, C.G.; Blank, M.; Zhang, W.; Reichlin, M.; Shoenfeld, Y. Induction of autoimmune depression in mice by anti-ribosomal P antibodies via the limbic system. *Arthritis Rheum.* **2007**, *56*, 938–948. [CrossRef]
49. Matus, S.; Burgos, P.V.; Bravo-Zehnder, M.; Kraft, R.; Porras, O.H.; Farías, P.; Barros, L.F.; Torrealba, F.; Massardo, L.; Jacobelli, S.; et al. Antiribosomal-P autoantibodies from psychiatric lupus target a novel neuronal surface protein causing calcium influx and apoptosis. *J. Exp. Med.* **2007**, *204*, 3221–3234. [CrossRef]
50. Song, J.; Park, Y.B.; Lee, W.K.; Lee, K.H.; Lee, S.K. Clinical associations of anti-endothelial cell antibodies in patients with systemic lupus erythematosus. *Rheumatol. Int.* **2000**, *20*, 1–7. [CrossRef]
51. Conti, F.; Alessandri, C.; Bompane, D.; Bombardieri, M.; Spinelli, F.R.; Rusconi, A.C.; Valesini, G. Autoantibody profile in systemic lupus erythematosus with psychiatric manifestations: A role for anti-endothelial-cell antibodies. *Arthritis Res. Ther.* **2004**, *6*, R366–R372. [CrossRef] [PubMed]
52. Lubarski, K.; Mania, A.; Michalak, S.; Osztynowicz, K.; Mazur-Melewska, K.; Figlerowicz, M. The Clinical Spectrum of Autoimmune-Mediated Neurological Diseases in Paediatric Population. *Brain Sci.* **2022**, *12*, 584. [CrossRef] [PubMed]
53. Bortoluzzi, A.; Silvagni, E.; Furini, F.; Piga, M.; Govoni, M. Peripheral nervous system involvement in systemic lupus erythematosus: A review of the evidence. *Clin. Exp. Rheumatol.* **2019**, *37*, 146–155.
54. Labrador-Horrillo, M.; Martinez-Valle, F.; Gallardo, E.; Rojas-Garcia, R.; Ordi-Ros, J.; Vilardell, M. Anti-ganglioside antibodies in patients with systemic lupus erythematosus and neurological manifestations. *Lupus* **2012**, *21*, 611–615. [CrossRef] [PubMed]
55. Loftis, J.M.; Huckans, M.; Morasco, B.J. Neuroimmune mechanisms of cytokine-induced depression: Current theories and novel treatment strategies. *Neurobiol. Dis.* **2010**, *37*, 519–533. [CrossRef]
56. Yepes, M. TWEAK and Fn14 in the Neurovascular Unit. *Front. Immunol.* **2013**, *4*, 367. [CrossRef]
57. Stock, A.D.; Wen, J.; Putterman, C. Neuropsychiatric Lupus, the Blood Brain Barrier, and the TWEAK/Fn14 Pathway. *Front. Immunol.* **2013**, *4*, 484. [CrossRef]
58. Wen, J.; Xia, Y.; Stock, A.; Michaelson, J.S.; Burkly, L.C.; Gulinello, M.; Putterman, C. Neuropsychiatric disease in murine lupus is dependent on the TWEAK/Fn14 pathway. *J. Autoimmun.* **2013**, *43*, 44–54. [CrossRef]
59. Wen, J.; Chen, C.H.; Stock, A.; Doerner, J.; Gulinello, M.; Putterman, C. Intracerebroventricular administration of TNF-like weak inducer of apoptosis induces depression-like behavior and cognitive dysfunction in non-autoimmune mice. *Brain Behav. Immun.* **2016**, *54*, 27–37. [CrossRef]
60. Hirohata, S.; Kanai, Y.; Mitsuo, A.; Tokano, Y.; Hashimoto, H. Accuracy of cerebrospinal fluid IL-6 testing for diagnosis of lupus psychosis. A multicenter retrospective study. *Clin. Rheumatol.* **2009**, *28*, 1319–1323. [CrossRef]
61. Katsumata, Y.; Harigai, M.; Kawaguchi, Y.; Fukasawa, C.; Soejima, M.; Takagi, K.; Tanaka, M.; Ichida, H.; Tochimoto, A.; Kanno, T.; et al. Diagnostic reliability of cerebral spinal fluid tests for acute confusional state (delirium) in patients with systemic lupus erythematosus: Interleukin 6 (IL-6), IL-8, interferon-alpha, IgG index, and Q-albumin. *J. Rheumatol.* **2007**, *34*, 2010–2017. [PubMed]
62. Trysberg, E.; Nylen, K.; Rosengren, L.E.; Tarkowski, A. Neuronal and astrocytic damage in systemic lupus erythematosus patients with central nervous system involvement. *Arthritis Rheum.* **2003**, *48*, 2881–2887. [CrossRef] [PubMed]

63. Dellalibera-Joviliano, R.; Dos Reis, M.L.; Cunha Fde, Q.; Donadi, E.A. Kinins and cytokines in plasma and cerebrospinal fluid of patients with neuropsychiatric lupus. *J. Rheumatol.* **2003**, *30*, 485–492. [PubMed]
64. Bialas, A.R.; Presumey, J.; Das, A.; van der Poel, C.E.; Lapchak, P.H.; Mesin, L.; Victora, G.; Tsokos, G.C.; Mawrin, C.; Herbst, R.; et al. Retraction Note: Microglia-dependent synapse loss in type I interferon-mediated lupus. *Nature* **2020**, *578*, 177. [CrossRef] [PubMed]
65. Santer, D.M.; Yoshio, T.; Minota, S.; Möller, T.; Elkon, K.B. Potent induction of IFN-alpha and chemokines by autoantibodies in the cerebrospinal fluid of patients with neuropsychiatric lupus. *J. Immunol.* **2009**, *182*, 1192–1201. [CrossRef] [PubMed]
66. Okamoto, H.; Kobayashi, A.; Yamanaka, H. Cytokines and chemokines in neuropsychiatric syndromes of systemic lupus erythematosus. *J. Biomed. Biotechnol.* **2010**, *2010*, 268436. [CrossRef]
67. George-Chandy, A.; Trysberg, E.; Eriksson, K. Raised intrathecal levels of APRIL and BAFF in patients with systemic lupus erythematosus: Relationship to neuropsychiatric symptoms. *Arthritis Res. Ther.* **2008**, *10*, R97. [CrossRef]
68. Lenz, K.M.; Nelson, L.H. Microglia and Beyond: Innate Immune Cells As Regulators of Brain Development and Behavioral Function. *Front. Immunol.* **2018**, *9*, 698. [CrossRef]
69. Wen, J.; Doerner, J.; Weidenheim, K.; Xia, Y.; Stock, A.; Michaelson, J.S.; Baruch, K.; Deczkowska, A.; Gulinello, M.; Schwartz, M.; et al. TNF-like weak inducer of apoptosis promotes blood brain barrier disruption and increases neuronal cell death in MRL/lpr mice. *J. Autoimmun.* **2015**, *60*, 40–50. [CrossRef]
70. Crupi, R.; Cambiaghi, M.; Spatz, L.; Hen, R.; Thorn, M.; Friedman, E.; Vita, G.; Battaglia, F. Reduced adult neurogenesis and altered emotional behaviors in autoimmune-prone B-cell activating factor transgenic mice. *Biol. Psychiatry* **2010**, *67*, 558–566. [CrossRef]
71. Cunningham, M.A.; Wirth, J.R.; Freeman, L.R.; Boger, H.A.; Granholm, A.C.; Gilkeson, G.S. Estrogen receptor alpha deficiency protects against development of cognitive impairment in murine lupus. *J. Neuroinflamm.* **2014**, *11*, 171. [CrossRef] [PubMed]
72. Fragoso-Loyo, H.; Richaud-Patin, Y.; Orozco-Narváez, A.; Dávila-Maldonado, L.; Atisha-Fregoso, Y.; Llorente, L.; Sánchez-Guerrero, J. Interleukin-6 and chemokines in the neuropsychiatric manifestations of systemic lupus erythematosus. *Arthritis Rheum.* **2007**, *56*, 1242–1250. [CrossRef] [PubMed]
73. Nestor, J.; Arinuma, Y.; Huerta, T.S.; Kowal, C.; Nasiri, E.; Kello, N.; Fujieda, Y.; Bialas, A.; Hammond, T.; Sriram, U.; et al. Lupus antibodies induce behavioral changes mediated by microglia and blocked by ACE inhibitors. *J. Exp. Med.* **2018**, *215*, 2554–2566. [CrossRef]
74. Stock, A.D.; Der, E.; Gelb, S.; Huang, M.; Weidenheim, K.; Ben-Zvi, A.; Putterman, C. Tertiary lymphoid structures in the choroid plexus in neuropsychiatric lupus. *JCI Insight* **2019**, *4*, e124203. [CrossRef] [PubMed]
75. Li, M.; Zhao, Y.; Zhang, Z.; Huang, C.; Liu, Y.; Gu, J.; Zhang, X.; Xu, H.; Li, X.; Wu, L.; et al. 2020 Chinese guidelines for the diagnosis and treatment of systemic lupus erythematosus. *Rheumatol. Immunol. Res.* **2020**, *1*, 5–23. [CrossRef]
76. Barile-Fabris, L.; Ariza-Andraca, R.; Olguín-Ortega, L.; Jara, L.J.; Fraga-Mouret, A.; Miranda-Limón, J.M.; Fuentes de la Mata, J.; Clark, P.; Vargas, F.; Alocer-Varela, J. Controlled clinical trial of IV cyclophosphamide versus IV methylprednisolone in severe neurological manifestations in systemic lupus erythematosus. *Ann. Rheum. Dis.* **2005**, *64*, 620–625. [CrossRef]
77. Denburg, S.D.; Carbotte, R.M.; Denburg, J.A. Corticosteroids and neuropsychological functioning in patients with systemic lupus erythematosus. *Arthritis Rheum.* **1994**, *37*, 1311–1320. [CrossRef]
78. Ruiz-Arruza, I.; Lozano, J.; Cabezas-Rodriguez, I.; Medina, J.A.; Ugarte, A.; Erdozain, J.G.; Ruiz-Irastorza, G. Restrictive Use of Oral Glucocorticoids in Systemic Lupus Erythematosus and Prevention of Damage Without Worsening Long-Term Disease Control: An Observational Study. *Arthritis Care Res.* **2018**, *70*, 582–591. [CrossRef]
79. Bolanos, S.H.; Khan, D.A.; Hanczyc, M.; Bauer, M.S.; Dhanani, N.; Brown, E.S. Assessment of mood states in patients receiving long-term corticosteroid therapy and in controls with patient-rated and clinician-rated scales. *Ann. Allergy Asthma Immunol.* **2004**, *92*, 500–505. [CrossRef]
80. Lewis, D.A.; Smith, R.E. Steroid-induced psychiatric syndromes. A report of 14 cases and a review of the literature. *J. Affect. Disord.* **1983**, *5*, 319–332. [CrossRef]
81. Mok, C.C.; Lau, C.S.; Wong, R.W. Treatment of lupus psychosis with oral cyclophosphamide followed by azathioprine maintenance: An open-label study. *Am. J. Med.* **2003**, *115*, 59–62. [CrossRef]
82. Dale, R.C.; Brilot, F.; Duffy, L.V.; Twilt, M.; Waldman, A.T.; Narula, S.; Muscal, E.; Deiva, K.; Andersen, E.; Eyre, M.R.; et al. Utility and safety of rituximab in pediatric autoimmune and inflammatory CNS disease. *Neurology* **2014**, *83*, 142–150. [CrossRef] [PubMed]
83. Narváez, J.; Ríos-Rodriguez, V.; de la Fuente, D.; Estrada, P.; López-Vives, L.; Gómez-Vaquero, C.; Nolla, J.M. Rituximab therapy in refractory neuropsychiatric lupus: Current clinical evidence. *Semin. Arthritis Rheum.* **2011**, *41*, 364–372. [CrossRef]
84. Pranzatelli, M.R.; Tate, E.D.; Travelstead, A.L.; Barbosa, J.; Bergamini, R.A.; Civitello, L.; Franz, D.N.; Greffe, B.S.; Hanson, R.D.; Hurwitz, C.A.; et al. Rituximab (anti-CD20) adjunctive therapy for opsoclonus-myoclonus syndrome. *J. Pediatr. Hematol. Oncol.* **2006**, *28*, 585–593. [CrossRef]
85. Jacob, A.; Weinshenker, B.G.; Violich, I.; McLinskey, N.; Krupp, L.; Fox, R.J.; Wingerchuk, D.M.; Boggild, M.; Constantinescu, C.S.; Miller, A.; et al. Treatment of neuromyelitis optica with rituximab: Retrospective analysis of 25 patients. *Arch. Neurol.* **2008**, *65*, 1443–1448. [CrossRef] [PubMed]

86. Manzi, S.; Sánchez-Guerrero, J.; Merrill, J.T.; Furie, R.; Gladman, D.; Navarra, S.V.; Ginzler, E.M.; D'Cruz, D.P.; Doria, A.; Cooper, S.; et al. Effects of belimumab, a B lymphocyte stimulator-specific inhibitor, on disease activity across multiple organ domains in patients with systemic lupus erythematosus: Combined results from two phase III trials. *Ann. Rheum. Dis.* **2012**, *71*, 1833–1838. [CrossRef]
87. de Amorim, L.C.; Maia, F.M.; Rodrigues, C.E. Stroke in systemic lupus erythematosus and antiphospholipid syndrome: Risk factors, clinical manifestations, neuroimaging, and treatment. *Lupus* **2017**, *26*, 529–536. [CrossRef]
88. Vadgama, T.S.; Smith, A.; Bertolaccini, M.L. Treatment in thrombotic antiphospholipid syndrome: A review. *Lupus* **2019**, *28*, 1181–1188. [CrossRef]
89. Finazzi, G.; Marchioli, R.; Brancaccio, V.; Schinco, P.; Wisloff, F.; Musial, J.; Baudo, F.; Berrettini, M.; Testa, S.; D'Angelo, A.; et al. A randomized clinical trial of high-intensity warfarin vs. conventional antithrombotic therapy for the prevention of recurrent thrombosis in patients with the antiphospholipid syndrome (WAPS). *J. Thromb. Haemost.* **2005**, *3*, 848–853. [CrossRef]
90. Crowther, M.A.; Ginsberg, J.S.; Julian, J.; Denburg, J.; Hirsh, J.; Douketis, J.; Laskin, C.; Fortin, P.; Anderson, D.; Kearon, C.; et al. A comparison of two intensities of warfarin for the prevention of recurrent thrombosis in patients with the antiphospholipid antibody syndrome. *N. Engl. J. Med.* **2003**, *349*, 1133–1138. [CrossRef]
91. Dobrowolski, C.; Erkan, D. Treatment of antiphospholipid syndrome beyond anticoagulation. *Clin. Immunol.* **2019**, *206*, 53–62. [CrossRef] [PubMed]
92. Meroni, P.L.; Raschi, E.; Testoni, C.; Tincani, A.; Balestrieri, G.; Molteni, R.; Khamashta, M.A.; Tremoli, E.; Camera, M. Statins prevent endothelial cell activation induced by antiphospholipid (anti-beta2-glycoprotein I) antibodies: Effect on the proadhesive and proinflammatory phenotype. *Arthritis Rheum.* **2001**, *44*, 2870–2878. [CrossRef]
93. Jung, H.; Bobba, R.; Su, J.; Shariati-Sarabi, Z.; Gladman, D.D.; Urowitz, M.; Lou, W.; Fortin, P.R. The protective effect of antimalarial drugs on thrombovascular events in systemic lupus erythematosus. *Arthritis Rheum.* **2010**, *62*, 863–868. [CrossRef]
94. Jacob, A.; Hack, B.; Chiang, E.; Garcia, J.G.; Quigg, R.J.; Alexander, J.J. C5a alters blood-brain barrier integrity in experimental lupus. *FASEB J.* **2010**, *24*, 1682–1688. [CrossRef] [PubMed]
95. Mahajan, S.D.; Parikh, N.U.; Woodruff, T.M.; Jarvis, J.N.; Lopez, M.; Hennon, T.; Cunningham, P.; Quigg, R.J.; Schwartz, S.A.; Alexander, J.J. C5a alters blood-brain barrier integrity in a human in vitro model of systemic lupus erythematosus. *Immunology* **2015**, *146*, 130–143. [CrossRef]
96. Di Minno, M.N.D.; Emmi, G.; Ambrosino, P.; Scalera, A.; Tufano, A.; Cafaro, G.; Peluso, R.; Bettiol, A.; Di Scala, G.; Silvestri, E.; et al. Subclinical atherosclerosis in asymptomatic carriers of persistent antiphospholipid antibodies positivity: A cross-sectional study. *Int. J. Cardiol.* **2019**, *274*, 1–6. [CrossRef]
97. De Luca, C.; Virtuoso, A.; Maggio, N.; Papa, M. Neuro-Coagulopathy: Blood Coagulation Factors in Central Nervous System Diseases. *Int. J. Mol. Sci.* **2017**, *18*, 2128. [CrossRef]
98. Chehaibi, K.; le Maire, L.; Bradoni, S.; Escola, J.C.; Blanco-Vaca, F.; Slimane, M.N. Effect of PPAR-β/δ agonist GW0742 treatment in the acute phase response and blood-brain barrier permeability following brain injury. *Transl. Res.* **2017**, *182*, 27–48. [CrossRef]
99. Niego, B.; Lee, N.; Larsson, P.; De Silva, T.M.; Au, A.E.; McCutcheon, F.; Medcalf, R.L. Selective inhibition of brain endothelial Rho-kinase-2 provides optimal protection of an in vitro blood-brain barrier from tissue-type plasminogen activator and plasmin. *PLoS ONE* **2017**, *12*, e0177332. [CrossRef]
100. Lu, X.Y.; Zhu, C.Q.; Qian, J.; Chen, X.X.; Ye, S.; Gu, Y.Y. Intrathecal cytokine and chemokine profiling in neuropsychiatric lupus or lupus complicated with central nervous system infection. *Lupus* **2010**, *19*, 689–695. [CrossRef]
101. Klein-Gitelman, M.; Brunner, H.I. The impact and implications of neuropsychiatric systemic lupus erythematosus in adolescents. *Curr. Rheumatol. Rep.* **2009**, *11*, 212–217. [CrossRef] [PubMed]
102. Ainiala, H.; Hietaharju, A.; Dastidar, P.; Loukkola, J.; Lehtimäki, T.; Peltola, J.; Korpela, M.; Heinonen, T.; Nikkari, S.T. Increased serum matrix metalloproteinase 9 levels in systemic lupus erythematosus patients with neuropsychiatric manifestations and brain magnetic resonance imaging abnormalities. *Arthritis Rheum.* **2004**, *50*, 858–865. [CrossRef] [PubMed]
103. Trysberg, E.; Blennow, K.; Zachrisson, O.; Tarkowski, A. Intrathecal levels of matrix metalloproteinases in systemic lupus erythematosus with central nervous system engagement. *Arthritis Res. Ther.* **2004**, *6*, R551–R556. [CrossRef] [PubMed]
104. Morand, E.F.; Furie, R.; Tanaka, Y.; Bruce, I.N.; Askanase, A.D.; Richez, C.; Bae, S.C.; Brohawn, P.Z.; Pineda, L.; Berglind, A.; et al. Trial of Anifrolumab in Active Systemic Lupus Erythematosus. *N. Engl. J. Med.* **2020**, *382*, 211–221. [CrossRef] [PubMed]
105. Furie, R.; Khamashta, M.; Merrill, J.T.; Werth, V.P.; Kalunian, K.; Brohawn, P.; Illei, G.G.; Drappa, J.; Wang, L.; Yoo, S. Anifrolumab, an Anti-Interferon-α Receptor Monoclonal Antibody, in Moderate-to-Severe Systemic Lupus Erythematosus. *Arthritis Rheumatol.* **2017**, *69*, 376–386. [CrossRef]
106. Mok, C.C. The dawn of a new era of therapies in systemic lupus erythematosus. *Rheumatol. Immunol. Res.* **2020**, *1*, 31–37. [CrossRef]
107. Hendriks, R.W. Drug discovery: New Btk inhibitor holds promise. *Nat. Chem. Biol.* **2011**, *7*, 4–5. [CrossRef]
108. Jongstra-Bilen, J.; Puig Cano, A.; Hasija, M.; Xiao, H.; Smith, C.I.; Cybulsky, M.I. Dual functions of Bruton's tyrosine kinase and Tec kinase during Fcgamma receptor-induced signaling and phagocytosis. *J. Immunol.* **2008**, *181*, 288–298. [CrossRef]
109. Gabhann-Dromgoole, J.N.; Hams, E.; Smith, S.; Wynne, C.; Byrne, J.C.; Brennan, K.; Spence, S.; Kissenpfennig, A.; Johnston, J.A.; Fallon, P.G.; et al. Btk regulates macrophage polarization in response to lipopolysaccharide. *PLoS ONE* **2014**, *9*, e85834. [CrossRef]

110. Chalmers, S.A.; Wen, J.; Doerner, J.; Stock, A.; Cuda, C.M.; Makinde, H.M.; Perlman, H.; Bosanac, T.; Webb, D.; Nabozny, G.; et al. Highly selective inhibition of Bruton's tyrosine kinase attenuates skin and brain disease in murine lupus. *Arthritis Res. Ther.* **2018**, *20*, 10. [CrossRef]
111. Werth, V.P.; Merrill, J.T. A double-blind, randomized, placebo-controlled, phase II trial of baricitinib for systemic lupus erythematosus: How to optimize lupus trials to examine effects on cutaneous lupus erythematosus. *Br. J. Dermatol.* **2019**, *180*, 964–965. [CrossRef] [PubMed]
112. Byrd, J.C.; Furman, R.R.; Coutre, S.E.; Flinn, I.W.; Burger, J.A.; Blum, K.A.; Grant, B.; Sharman, J.P.; Coleman, M.; Wierda, W.G.; et al. Targeting BTK with ibrutinib in relapsed chronic lymphocytic leukemia. *N. Engl. J. Med.* **2013**, *369*, 32–42. [CrossRef] [PubMed]
113. Mike, E.V.; Makinde, H.M.; Der, E.; Stock, A.; Gulinello, M.; Gadhvi, G.T.; Winter, D.R.; Cuda, C.M.; Putterman, C. Neuropsychiatric Systemic Lupus Erythematosus Is Dependent on Sphingosine-1-Phosphate Signaling. *Front. Immunol.* **2018**, *9*, 2189. [CrossRef] [PubMed]
114. Shi, D.; Tian, T.; Yao, S.; Cao, K.; Zhu, X.; Zhang, M.; Wen, S.; Li, L.; Shi, M.; Zhou, H. FTY720 attenuates behavioral deficits in a murine model of systemic lupus erythematosus. *Brain Behav. Immun.* **2018**, *70*, 293–304. [CrossRef] [PubMed]
115. Chitu, V.; Stanley, E.R. Colony-stimulating factor-1 in immunity and inflammation. *Curr. Opin. Immunol.* **2006**, *18*, 39–48. [CrossRef]
116. Chalmers, S.A.; Wen, J.; Shum, J.; Doerner, J.; Herlitz, L.; Putterman, C. CSF-1R inhibition attenuates renal and neuropsychiatric disease in murine lupus. *Clin. Immunol.* **2017**, *185*, 100–108. [CrossRef]
117. Chi, O.Z.; Hunter, C.; Liu, X.; Weiss, H.R. Effects of exogenous excitatory amino acid neurotransmitters on blood-brain barrier disruption in focal cerebral ischemia. *Neurochem. Res.* **2009**, *34*, 1249–1254. [CrossRef]
118. Fukuyama, T.; Tschernig, T.; Qi, Y.; Volmer, D.A.; Bäumer, W. Aggression behaviour induced by oral administration of the Janus-kinase inhibitor tofacitinib, but not oclacitinib, under stressful conditions. *Eur. J. Pharmacol.* **2015**, *764*, 278–282. [CrossRef]
119. Hasni, S.A.; Gupta, S.; Davis, M.; Poncio, E.; Temesgen-Oyelakin, Y.; Carlucci, P.M.; Wang, X.; Naqi, M.; Playford, M.P.; Goel, R.R.; et al. Phase 1 double-blind randomized safety trial of the Janus kinase inhibitor tofacitinib in systemic lupus erythematosus. *Nat. Commun.* **2021**, *12*, 3391. [CrossRef]

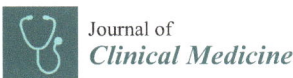
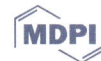

Article

Predictors of Early Response, Flares, and Long-Term Adverse Renal Outcomes in Proliferative Lupus Nephritis: A 100-Month Median Follow-Up of an Inception Cohort

Eleni Kapsia [1], Smaragdi Marinaki [1], Ioannis Michelakis [2], George Liapis [3], Petros P. Sfikakis [4], John Boletis [1] and Maria G. Tektonidou [4],*

[1] Department of Nephrology and Renal Transplantation, Laiko Hospital, Medical School, National & Kapodistrian University of Athens, 11527 Athens, Greece
[2] Department of Hygiene, Epidemiology and Medical Statistics, Medical School, National & Kapodistrian University of Athens, 11527 Athens, Greece
[3] Department of Pathology, Medical School, National & Kapodistrian University of Athens, 11527 Athens, Greece
[4] Rheumatology Unit, First Department of Propaedeutic Internal Medicine, Joint Academic Rheumatology Program, Laiko Hospital, Medical School, National & Kapodistrian University of Athens, 11527 Athens, Greece
* Correspondence: mtektonidou@gmail.com; Tel.: +30-2107462710

Citation: Kapsia, E.; Marinaki, S.; Michelakis, I.; Liapis, G.; Sfikakis, P.P.; Boletis, J.; Tektonidou, M.G. Predictors of Early Response, Flares, and Long-Term Adverse Renal Outcomes in Proliferative Lupus Nephritis: A 100-Month Median Follow-Up of an Inception Cohort. *J. Clin. Med.* **2022**, *11*, 5017. https://doi.org/10.3390/jcm11175017

Academic Editors: Matteo Piga and Christopher Sjöwall

Received: 27 July 2022
Accepted: 22 August 2022
Published: 26 August 2022

Publisher's Note: MDPI stays neutral with regard to jurisdictional claims in published maps and institutional affiliations.

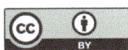

Copyright: © 2022 by the authors. Licensee MDPI, Basel, Switzerland. This article is an open access article distributed under the terms and conditions of the Creative Commons Attribution (CC BY) license (https://creativecommons.org/licenses/by/4.0/).

Abstract: Objective: To define predictors of response, time to response, flares, and long-term renal outcome in an inception cohort of proliferative lupus nephritis (PLN). **Methods:** We included 100 patients (80% female; mean age 31 ± 13 years) with biopsy-proven PLN (III, IV, III/IV + V). Clinical, laboratory, histological and therapeutical parameters were recorded at baseline, 6, 9, 12, 18, 24, 36, 72 months, time of flare, and last follow-up visit. Logistic and Cox-regression models were applied. **Results:** After induction treatment (69% received cyclophosphamide (CYC) and 27% mycophenolic acid (MPA)), partial (PR) or complete (CR) response was achieved in 59% (26% CR, 33% PR) and 67% (43% CR, 24% PR) of patients at 3 and 6 months, respectively; median time to PR was 3 months (IQR 5) and median time to CR was 6 months (IQR 9). Baseline proteinuria <1.5 g/day correlated with a shorter time to CR (HR 1.77) and with CR at 3, 6, and 9 months (OR 9.4, OR 5.3 and OR 3.7, respectively). During 100-month median follow-up, 33% of patients had ≥1 renal flares (median time: 38 months). Proteinuria >0.8 g/day at 12 months was associated with a higher risk of flares (OR 4.12), while MPA and mixed classes with lower risk (OR 0.14 and OR 0.13, respectively). Baseline proteinuria >2 g/day and 12-month proteinuria >0.8 g/day correlated with a shorter time to flare (HR 2.56 and HR 2.57, respectively). At the end of follow-up, 10% developed stage 3–4 chronic kidney disease (CKD), and 12% end-stage renal disease (ESRD). Twelve-month proteinuria >0.8 g/day (OR 10.8) and interstitial fibrosis/tubular atrophy >25% (OR 7.7) predicted CKD or ESRD at last visit. **Conclusions:** Baseline proteinuria <1.5 g/day predicted time to CR. Twelve-month proteinuria >0.8 g/day correlated with flares (ever) and time to flare and, along with baseline interstitial fibrosis/tubular atrophy >25%, predicted CKD or ESRD at the last visit.

Keywords: lupus nephritis; renal response; renal survival; twelve-month proteinuria; interstitial fibrosis/tubular atrophy

1. Introduction

In systemic lupus erythematosus (SLE), renal involvement is the most common severe complication of the disease affecting approximately 20–60% of patients [1] and conferring a high morbidity and mortality risk [2–4]. End-stage renal disease (ESRD) still occurs at varying rates among different cohorts of patients with lupus nephritis (LN), despite the revolutionary changes in LN treatment over the past fifty years [5,6]. A wide range of demographic, socioeconomic and disease-related parameters have been associated with LN's short- and long-term outcomes. Histological class is a major determinant of renal survival in LN, with the proliferative classes having the worst prognosis compared to other classes [5,7].

The main therapeutic goal in patients with LN is the long-term preservation of renal function, preventing and managing comorbidities, and improving disease-related quality of life [8]. These goals can be achieved by inducing and maintaining disease remission and by preventing and timely treating disease flares [9,10]. In this context, recognizing early predictors of renal response, flare and long-term renal survival is paramount in guiding the therapeutic management of LN patients.

The aim of the present study is (a) to examine the response to treatment and short- and long-term renal outcomes in an inception cohort of patients with proliferative LN; (b) to define predictors of response, time to response, flares and long-term adverse renal outcomes.

2. Patients and Methods

2.1. Study Population

We examined an inception cohort of 100 patients with proliferative LN diagnosed between 1992 and 2021 and followed up at our joint academic center (Nephrology and Rheumatology Units) at Laiko General Hospital of Athens until April 2022. All patients fulfilled the 2019 classification criteria for SLE and had a biopsy-proven diagnosis of proliferative LN (class III, IV, III/IV + V), classified according to the International Society of Nephrology/ Renal Pathology Society (ISN/RPS) 2003 lupus nephritis classification system. Among 100 patients identified with PLN, 28% (28/100) had class III, 47% (47/100) class IV, 9% (9/100) mixed class III + V and 16% (16/100) mixed class IV + V.

2.2. Data Collection

We retrospectively reviewed medical charts of patients and recorded clinical, laboratory, histological and therapeutical parameters at the following time points: time of histological diagnosis of LN; 3, 6, 9, 12, 18, 24, 36, 72 months after the diagnosis; time of renal flare (with or without a repeat biopsy), and at last follow-up visit. Patients with inadequate data and less than 6 months of follow-up were excluded.

Data collected included demographic parameters, time from SLE diagnosis to LN onset, disease activity (assessed by Systemic Lupus Erythematosus Disease Activity Index 2000, SLEDAI-2K score) [11], anti-ds DNA titers, C3 and C4 levels, serum urea (Ur), creatinine (Cr) and albumin, eGFR (based on the CKD-EPI formula), 24-h proteinuria, urine sediment, renal biopsy histological parameters (LN class, activity index (AI), chronicity index (CI), crescents, interstitial fibrosis/tubular atrophy (IF/TA)), and treatment regimens.

All data (demographic, clinical, laboratory and histological) were extracted from our anonymized cohort dataset. No individualized or identifiable data are presented in this study. The study was approved by the Institutional Review Board (protocol number 1725/14-12-2017) of Laiko General Hospital of Athens.

2.3. Patient and Public Involvement

Patients and/or the public were not involved in this research's design, conduct, reporting or dissemination plans.

2.4. Definitions

Response and flares were defined according to the 2012 EULAR/ERA-EDTA [8] and the 2012 KDIGO recommendations [12] as follows: Active urine sediment: the presence of >5 RBCs/hpf or ≥1 red cell casts. Complete response (CR): proteinuria <500 mg/24 h and serum creatinine within 10% of baseline values. Partial response (PR): ≥50% reduction in proteinuria to subnephrotic levels and serum creatinine within 10% of baseline values. Nephritic flare: increase in glomerular haematuria by ≥10 RBCs/hpf with or without a decrease in eGFR by ≥10%, irrespective of changes in proteinuria. Nephrotic flare: reproducible doubling of proteinuria to >1000 mg/24 h if a complete response had been previously achieved or reproducible doubling of proteinuria to ≥2000 mg/24 h if a partial response has been previously achieved. Stage 3–4 chronic kidney disease (CKD): eGFR 15–60 mL/min/1.73 m^2 for more than 3 months, and end-stage renal disease (ESRD) as eGFR < 15 mL/min/1.73 m^2 or initiation of renal replacement therapy [13].

2.5. Statistical Analysis

Continuous variables were expressed as the mean value and standard deviation or median value and interquartile range (IQR), whereas categorical variables as frequencies and percentages. To investigate the differences in baseline parameters between patients with different therapeutical schemes, the t-test and Mann–Whitney U test for independent samples for continuous variables and the χ^2 and Fisher exact test for categorical variables were applied. Univariate logistic regression analyses were performed to estimate the prognostic effect of various variables on the risk of renal flare and adverse renal outcomes. Cox regression analyses investigated the association between patients' variables and time to response or response at specific time points. Variables found to be significant in the univariate analyses were included in the multivariate models. In the models identifying predictors of flare and adverse renal outcome, due to a small number of events, selected independent variables were included in the multivariate analyses after multicollinearity was examined. Multicollinearity issues were assessed with appropriate tests (χ^2, Cramer's V coefficient (V), analysis of variants (ANOVA), Spearman correlation coefficient (r_s) and Mann–Whitney U test) before performing multivariate analyses. Strong correlation among specific variables excluded some parameters from the multivariate models. Significance was set at $\alpha = 0.05$. The estimated odds ratios (ORs) and hazard ratios (HRs) of both the univariate and multivariate models and the related p-values are presented. Data were analyzed using Stata 13.0 software (Stata Corporation, College Station, TX). All tests proceeded as two-tailed.

3. Results

3.1. Baseline Characteristics

We studied 100 patients with biopsy-proven proliferative LN. The baseline demographic, clinical, laboratory and histological characteristics and the therapeutic regimens applied are shown in Table 1. All biopsies contained ≥ 10 glomeruli, and those performed before 2003 were reassessed based on ISN/RPS 2003 classification system. The median follow-up time was 100 months (IQR = 108).

Table 1. Baseline demographic, clinical, laboratory and histological characteristics and immunosuppressive treatment regimens.

Baseline Characteristics	Mean $\pm$ SD, Median(IQR), N/%
Age (yr) mean $\pm$ SD	31 $\pm$ 13
Sex (M-F) N/%	20/20–80/80
Race (Caucasian-Other) N/%	96/96–4/4
Time from SLE diagnosis to LN (years)median(IQR)	()
LN as first presentation of SLE N/%	51/51
SLEDAI score median(IQR)	12(4)
Low C3 N/% [1]	65/77.5
Low C4 N/% [1]	55/65.5

Table 1. Cont.

Baseline Characteristics	Mean ± SD, Median(IQR), N/%
Positive anti-dsDNA antibodies N/% [2]	63/78.5
Proteinuria (g/24 h) median (IQR)	2.6(4)
• Proteinuria >3 g/d N/%	48/48
• Proteinuria 1–3 g/d N/%	31/31
• Proteinuria <1 g/d N/%	21/21
Active urine sediment N/%	92/92
Hypertension N/%	28/28
Serum albumin (g/dL) mean ± SD	3.1 ± 0.8
Serum Cr (mg/dL) median(IQR)	0.8(0.5)
eGFR (mL/min/1.73 m^2) median(IQR)	94.5(50)
• eGFR >60 N/%	75/75
• eGFR 30–60 N/%	14/14
• eGFR <30 N/%	11/11
LN class	
• III N/%	28/28
• IV N/%	47/47
• III + V N/%	9/9
• IV + V N/%	16/16
Number of crescents median(IQR)	2(4)
Activity Index median(IQR)	10(6)
Chronicity Index median(IQR)	2(2)
Interstitial fibrosis/tubular atrophy *,[3]	
• <25% N/%	85/87
• >25% N/%	13/13
Induction Treatment	
• mycophenolic acid N/%	27/27
• cyclophosphamide N/%	69/69
• other	3/3
• none N/%	1/1
Maintenance Treatment	
• mycophenolic acid N/%	77/77
• azathioprine N/%	8/8
• cyclophosphamide N/%	5/5
• none N/%	10/10
Duration of total treatment (months)median(IQR)	39(38)

eGFR: estimated glomerular filtration rate using the CKD-EPI formula, SLEDAI: systemic lupus erythematosus disease activity index, anti-ds DNA: antibodies against double-stranded DNA. * refers to the percentage of the renal cortex involved by interstitial fibrosis and tubular atrophy. [1] data available for 84/100 patients, [2] data available for 80/100 patients, [3] data available for 98/100 patients.

3.2. Immunosuppressive Regimens

Induction treatment consisted of cyclophosphamide (CYC) in 69% (69/100) of patients (in combination with rituximab (RTX) in 12/69), mycophenolic acid (MPA) in 27% (27/100, in combination with RTX in 4/27) and RTX alone in 2 patients. All the above patients received corticosteroids. One patient was treated only with corticosteroids due to non-compliance, while one patient did not receive any immunosuppressive treatment due to progression to ESRD soon after LN diagnosis (Table 1). CYC was given in all 69 patients intravenously, following the NIH regimen in 96% and the ELNT regimen in 4% of cases.

Patients treated with CYC differed significantly in several baseline parameters compared to those treated with MPA (Supplemental Table S1). Although baseline eGFR did not differ between the two treatment groups, all patients with eGFR <30 mL/min/1.73 m^2 were treated with CYC. Half of the patients with class III were treated with CYC and half with MPA (13/26 vs. 13/26). CYC was more often preferred over MPA for patients with class IV (87% (40/46) vs. 13% (6/46)) and for patients with class IV + V (88% (14/16) versus 12% (2/16)). Patients with class III + V received more often MPA than CYC (75% (6/8) versus 25% (2/8)) (data not shown).

Maintenance treatment consisted of MPA in 77% (77/100) of patients, azathioprine (AZA) in 8% (8/100) and CYC in 5% (5/100). Ten patients (10/100, 10%) did not receive any immunosuppressive maintenance treatment (Table 1); 5/10 due to early progression to ESRD, 2/10 who received RTX as induction continued with steroids only, 1/10 due to non-compliance, and 2/10 were lost to follow-up after completing the 6-month induction treatment.

The median duration of treatment was 39 months (IQR = 38) and did not differ between the CYC and MPA groups. Additionally, 76% (76/100) of patients received hydroxychloroquine and 65% (65/100) an ACEi or ARB.

3.3. Renal Response and Determinants of Response

For up to 72 months, 59% of patients achieved complete (CR) or partial (PR) response at 3 months (26% CR, 33% PR), 67% at 6 months (43% CR, 24% PR), 75% at 9 months (45% CR, 30% PR), 88% at 12 months (69% CR, 19% PR), and 86% at 18 months (71% CR, 15% PR), with similar percentages at all the following time points (Figure 1).

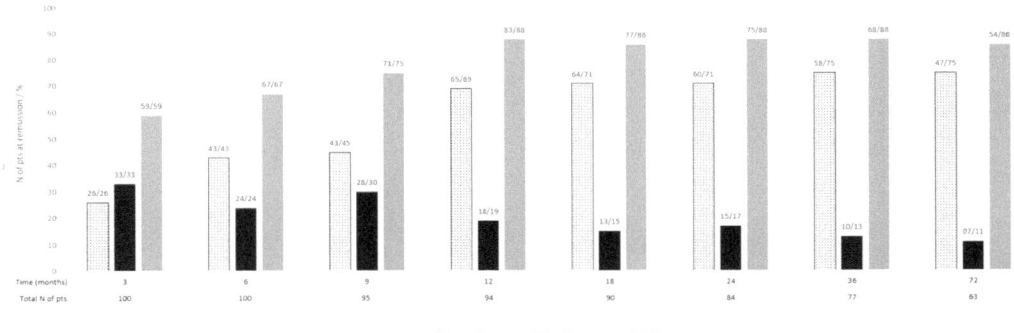

Figure 1. Patients with a renal response at different time points during follow-up.

The median time to PR and CR was 3 months (IQR = 5) and 6 months (IQR = 9), respectively. Time to CR was significantly shorter in patients with class III (median/IQR 3/4) compared to patients with class IV (median/IQR 10/13, p <0.001) and those with mixed classes (median/IQR 10/11, p = 0.006) in the 6, 9, 12 and 18-month time points (p for log-rank = 0.49, p for Wilcoxon = 0.02) (Supplemental Figure S1). There was no difference in time to CR between class IV and mixed classes (p = 0.94). Time to response between the two treatment groups (CYC versus MPA) did not differ significantly (Supplemental Figure S1). Median time to CR was 6 months (IQR = 7.5) in the MPA group and 7 months (IQR = 15) in the CYC group (p = 0.09).

Moreover, 7% of patients (7/100) of the cohort did not ever respond to treatment, 6 of whom progressed to ESRD, while one patient had a preserved renal function at 7 months but was lost to follow-up afterward. Two nonresponders, who progressed to ESRD after 4 and 5 months, died at 6 and 7 months, respectively, after LN diagnosis.

In Cox regression analysis, proteinuria <1.5 g/day at LN diagnosis was the only parameter that significantly correlated with a shorter time to complete response (HR 1.77, $p = 0.01$) (Table 2). The two treatment groups were compared when they were used alone or in combination with RTX.

Table 2. Predictors of time to complete response.

Variables	Univariate Models		Multivariate Model	
	HR	95% Cis (p-Value)	HR	95% Cis (p-Value)
Age (years)	1.01	0.98, 1.02 (0.53)		
Sex				
• Male	Reference Group			
• Female	1.29	0.73, 2.29 (0.36)		
Time from SLE diagnosis to LN (years)	0.98	0.94, 1.03 (0.6)		
Hypertension				
• No	Reference Group			
• Yes	0.7	0.43, 1.16 (0.18)		
Low C3				
• Yes	Reference Group			
• No	0.73	0.40, 1.33 (0.31)		
Low C4				
• Yes	Reference Group			
• No	0.68	0.4, 1.15 (0.15)		
Anti-dsDNA antibodies				
• Negative	Reference Group			
• Positive	1.26	0.7, 2.32 (0.44)		
eGFR at diagnosis (mL/min/1.73 m^2)				
• >60	Reference Group			
• <60	0.66	0.39, 1.13 (0.13)		
Proteinuria at diagnosis (g/day)				
• >1.5	Reference Group			
• <1.5	1.77	1.10, 2.84 (0.01)		
LN class				
• III	Reference Group			
• IV	0.87	0.5, 1.47 (0.62)		
• III/IV + V	0.69	0.37, 1.31 (0.26)		
Number of Crescents	0.97	0.93, 1.01 (0.24)		
Activity Index	1	0.96, 1.05 (0.75)		
Chronicity Index	0.92	0.82, 1.04 (0.19)		
Interstitial fibrosis/Tubular atrophy				
• <25% *	Reference Group			
• >25% *	0.82	0.39, 1.72 (0.61)		
Induction treatment **				
• CYC	Reference Group			
• MPA	0.92	0.55, 1.56 (0.78)		

eGFR: estimated glomerular filtration rate using the CKD-EPI formula, SLEDAI: systemic lupus erythematosus disease activity index, anti-ds DNA: antibodies against double-stranded DNA, CYC: cyclophosphamide, MPA: mycophenolic acid. * refers to the percentage of the renal cortex involved by interstitial fibrosis and tubular atrophy, ** the two treatment groups were compared with and without the concomitant use of rituximab.

We further compared patients who achieved CR at 12-18-24 months versus those with PR or no response at the respective time points. We found that the only significant predictor of CR was baseline proteinuria <1.5 g/day (OR 16.9, $p = 0.008$ for month 12, OR 5.24, $p = 0.01$ for month 18 and OR 4, $p = 0.03$ for month 24) (Supplemental Table S2). Although achievement of CR in earlier time points was less frequent, baseline proteinuria <1.5 g/day was also found to be the only significant predictor of CR at 3 months (OR 9.4, $p < 0.001$) and 6 months (OR 5.3, $p = 0.004$), and, along with baseline eGFR > 60 mL/min (OR 4.04, $p = 0.02$), predicted CR at 9 months (OR 3.7, $p = 0.02$) (Supplemental Table S2).

3.4. Renal Flares and Determinants of Flares

Thirty-three percent (33/100) of patients had ≥ 1 renal flares in a median time of 38 months (IQR = 43); 30% (10/33) of flares were nephritic, and 70% (23/33) nephrotic. Repeat biopsy was performed in 91% (30/33) of cases, and a class switch was observed in 67% (20/30) of them. In all 30 repeat biopsies, active LN lesions were confirmed. In two of them, a pattern of focal segmental glomerulosclerosis was also described, which may have contributed to the nephrotic clinical presentation of these patients.

In univariate logistic regression analysis, longer time to response was identified as a significant risk factor of flare (OR 1.14, $p = 0.01$ for PR, OR 1.05, $p = 0.01$ for CR) (Table 3). Response (CR or PR) at 3 months (OR 1.05, $p = 0.9$), 6 months (OR 1.25, $p = 0.66$) and 9 months (OR 2.2, $p = 0.19$) after treatment did not significantly affect the risk of flare. Statistical significance was found for lack of response (CR or PR) at 12 (OR 3.8, $p = 0.04$), 18 (OR 4.9 $p = 0.01$) and 24 (OR 6.6, $p = 0.02$) months (Supplemental Table S3).

Table 3. Predictors of flares.

Variables	Univariate Models		Multivariate Model	
	OR	95% CIs (*p*-Value)	OR	95% CIs (*p*-Value)
Age (years)	0.95	0.92, 0.98 (0.02)	0.98	0.94, 1.03 (0.58)
Sex				
• Male	Reference Group			
• Female	0.5	0.19, 1.42 (0.2)		
Time from SLE diagnosis to LN (years)	0.93	0.84, 1.04 (0.23)		
Hypertension				
• No	Reference Group			
• Yes	0.96	0.37, 2.47 (0.94)		
Low C3				
• Yes	Reference Group			
• No	0.9	0.29, 2.96 (0.9)		
Low C4				
• Yes	Reference Group			
• No	0.3	0.09, 0.99 (0.05)		
Anti-dsDNA antibodies				
• Negative	Reference Group			
• Positive	0.96	0.29, 3.1 (0.94)		

Table 3. Cont.

Variables	Univariate Models		Multivariate Model	
	OR	95% CIs (p-Value)	OR	95% CIs (p-Value)
eGFR at diagnosis (mL/min/1.73 m^2)				
• >60	Reference Group			
• <60	0.7	0.27, 1.98 (0.5)		
Proteinuria at diagnosis (g/day)				
• <2	Reference Group			
• >2	3	1.14, 7.89 (0.02)		
LN class				
• III	Reference Group			
• IV	0.59	0.22, 1.55 (0.28)	0.38	0.09, 1.6 (0.19)
• III/IV + V	0.21	0.05, 0.8 (0.02)	0.13	0.01, 0.8 (0.02)
Number of Crescents	0.96	0.88, 1.05 (0.44)		
Activity Index	1.01	0.91, 1.11 (0.8)		
Chronicity Index	0.77	0.59, 1.01 (0.06)		
Interstitial fibrosis/Tubular atrophy				
• <25% *	Reference Group			
• >25% *	0.6	0.15, 2.4 (0.48)		
Induction treatment **				
• CYC	Reference Group			
• MPA	0.25	0.08, 0.8 (0.02)	0.14	0.03, 0.7 (0.01)
Time to PR (months)	1.14	1.02, 1.26 (0.01)		
Time to CR (months)	1.05	1.01, 1.1 (0.01)		
Time to CR/PR (months)	1.11	1.02, 1.21 (0.01)		
Proteinuria at 12 m (g/day)				
• <0.8	Reference Group			
• >0.8	3.38	1.14, 10 (0.02)	4.12	1.15, 14 (0.02)

eGFR: estimated glomerular filtration rate using the CKD-EPI formula, SLEDAI: systemic lupus erythematosus disease activity index, anti-ds DNA: antibodies against double-stranded DNA, CYC: cyclophosphamide, MPA: mycophenolic acid, CR: complete response, PR: partial response. * refers to the percentage of the renal cortex involved by interstitial fibrosis and tubular atrophy, ** the two treatment groups were compared with and without the concomitant use of rituximab.

Proteinuria >2 g/day at diagnosis (OR 3, $p = 0.02$), and proteinuria >0.8 g/day at 12 months (OR 3.38, $p = 0.02$) were significantly associated with a higher risk of flare. Conversely, parameters associated with a lower risk of flares were older age (OR 0.95, $p = 0.02$) and treatment with MPA (OR 0.25, $p = 0.02$) compared to treatment with CYC (whether these agents were used alone or in combination with RTX). Mixed classes were also found to reduce the risk of flare (OR 0.21, $p = 0.02$), but this association was significant only when mixed classes were compared to class III and not to class IV (Table 3).

Since proteinuria at diagnosis, as a variable, was found to be strongly associated with induction therapy, histological class, and proteinuria at 12 months, it was not included in the multivariate model for the risk of flare. Accordingly, time to remission was strongly correlated with proteinuria at 12 months and LN class and was not included in the multivariate model (Supplemental Table S4).

In the multivariate analysis, proteinuria >0.8 g/day at 12 months was a significant predictor of flare (OR 4.12, $p = 0.02$), while treatment with MPA (OR 0.14, $p = 0.01$) and mixed classes were associated with lower flare risk (OR 0.13, $p = 0.02$) (the latter only when compared to class III) (Table 3).

Baseline proteinuria >2 g/day (HR 2.56, $p = 0.02$) and proteinuria >0.8 g/day at 12 months (HR 2.57, $p = 0.01$) were also found to correlate with shorter time to flare (Figure 2).

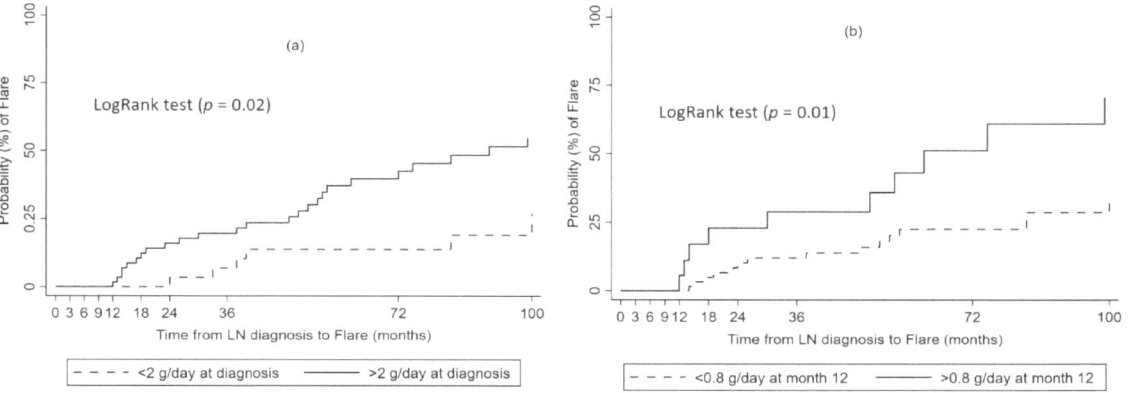

Figure 2. Kaplan–Meier survival estimates of probability for flare according to (**a**) Proteinuria at the time of LN diagnosis, (**b**) Proteinuria at 12 months.

3.5. Patient Survival

At a median follow-up time of 100 months, four deaths were reported. A 59-year-old and heavy smoker patient died due to lung cancer 8 years after LN diagnosis, during which he was on immunosuppressive treatment (he received CYC as induction treatment followed by MPA for 3 years and AZA, due mainly to extrarenal manifestations, for 5 years). One patient, aged 65, died due to bladder cancer 8 years after LN diagnosis. Interestingly, this patient had never received CYC. Two other patients, aged 30 and 38, died from sepsis (7 and 6 months after LN diagnosis, respectively). Both patients had presented with rapid deterioration of renal function and progressed to ESRD very soon after LN diagnosis.

3.6. Renal Survival

At the end of the follow-up period, 10% (10/100) of patients developed stage 3–4 CKD, and 12% (12/100) progressed to ESRD.

Six of 12 (50%) patients who reached ESRD were nonresponders, and in 5 of them, ESRD was developed in the first 9 months. Seven (58%) patients progressed to ESRD after 55–183 months from LN diagnosis. eGFR at the time of diagnosis, renal response, and time until ESRD are shown in Supplemental Table S5.

We defined the composite endpoint of stage 3–4 CKD and ESRD as adverse long-term renal outcomes. Of note, all patients who had a decrease of eGFR >25% of baseline values at the last follow-up had reached stage 3–4 CKD or ESRD.

In the univariate logistic regression analysis, adverse long-term renal outcome was significantly associated with baseline eGFR < 60 mL/min/1.73 m^2 (OR 6, $p = 0.001$), interstitial fibrosis/tubular atrophy >25% (OR 5.44, $p = 0.007$), proteinuria >0.8 g/day at 12 months (OR 9.5, $p = 0.003$) and longer time to response (OR 1.1, $p = 0.01$) (Table 4). The risk for stage 3–4 CKD or ESRD was greater for those not achieving any response after 6 months of treatment (OR 6.4, $p = 0.001$), while response at 3 months did not seem to affect long-term renal outcome significantly (OR 2.2, $p = 0.11$) (Supplemental Table S6).

Table 4. Predictors of long-term adverse renal outcome (stage 3–4 CKD, ESRD).

Variables	Univariate Models		Multivariate Model	
	OR	95% CIs (p-Value)	OR	95% CIs (p-Value)
Age (years)	1	0.96, 1.03 (0.9)		
Sex				
• Male	Reference Group			
• Female	0.8	0.2, 2.5 (0.7)		
Time from SLE diagnosis to LN (years)	1	0.9, 1.1 (0.9)		
Hypertension				
• No	Reference Group			
• Yes	2.28	0.83, 6.2 (0.1)		
Low C3				
• Yes	Reference Group			
• No	0.75	0.2, 3 (0.68)		
Low C4				
• Yes	Reference Group			
• No	1.6	0.53, 4.9 (0.4)		
Anti-dsDNA antibodies				
• Negative	Reference Group			
• Positive	0.45	0.1, 1.5 (0.2)		
eGFR at diagnosis (mL/min/1.73 m^2)				
• >60	Reference Group			
• <60	6	2, 16 (0.001)		
Proteinuria at diagnosis (g/day)				
• <1.5	Reference Group			
• >1.5	1.7	0.56, 5.12 (0.34)		
LN class				
• III	Reference Group			
• IV	0.59	0.19, 1.77 (0.34)		
• III/IV + V	0.62	0.17, 2.24 (0.47)		
Number of Crescents	1	0.93, 1.07 (0.91)		
Activity Index	1.03	0.92, 1.16 (0.5)		
Chronicity Index	1.13	0.87, 1.47 (0.34)		
Interstitial fibrosis/Tubular atrophy				
• <25% *	Reference Group			
• >25% *	5.44	1.59, 18 (0.007)	7.7	1.48, 40 (0.01)
Induction treatment **				
• CYC	Reference Group			
• MPA	1.02	0.35, 3 (0.95)		

Table 4. Cont.

Variables	Univariate Models		Multivariate Model	
	OR	95% CIs (p-Value)	OR	95% CIs (p-Value)
Time to PR (months)	1.14	1.04, 1.26 (0.006)		
Time to CR (months)	1.04	0.99, 1.1 (0.1)		
Time to CR/PR (months)	1.1	1.02, 1.2 (0.01)		
Proteinuria at 12 m (g/day)				
• <0.8	Reference Group			
• >0.8	9.5	1.84, 20 (0.003)	10.8	2.7, 42 (0.001)

eGFR: estimated glomerular filtration rate using the CKD-EPI formula, SLEDAI: systemic lupus erythematosus disease activity index, anti-ds DNA: antibodies against double-stranded DNA, CYC: cyclophosphamide, MPA: mycophenolic acid, CR: complete response, PR: partial response. * refers to the percentage of the renal cortex involved by interstitial fibrosis and tubular atrophy, ** the two treatment groups were compared with and without the concomitant use of rituximab.

eGFR at diagnosis was strongly correlated with baseline proteinuria, proteinuria at 12 months, and interstitial fibrosis/tubular atrophy. Therefore, it was excluded from the multivariate model. Time to remission was strongly correlated with baseline proteinuria, proteinuria at 12 months, and eGFR at diagnosis and was not included in the multivariate model either (Supplemental Table S7).

In multivariate analysis, proteinuria >0.8 g/day at 12 months (OR 10.8, $p = 0.001$) and interstitial fibrosis/tubular atrophy >25% at LN diagnosis (OR 7.7, $p = 0.01$) remained significant predictors of adverse renal outcome (Table 4).

4. Discussion

A major therapeutic goal in patients with LN is the long-term preservation of renal function by minimizing chronic active or relapsing disease and, at the same time, avoiding excessive drug toxicity. In this context, we need to identify predictors of renal response, relapse, and long-term adverse renal outcomes to optimize our therapeutic strategies. Short-term predictors can also serve as endpoints in large clinical trials investigating new therapeutic agents [14–17]. In our study, baseline proteinuria <1.5 g/day was the only significant predictor of time to complete response, while proteinuria >0.8 g/day at 12 months and treatment with CYC (compared to MPA) emerged as strong predictors of renal flare. We also showed that adverse long-term renal outcomes (stage 3–4 CKD, ESRD) could only be predicted by interstitial fibrosis/tubular atrophy >25% in baseline biopsy and proteinuria >0.8 g/day at 12 months.

In our study, response to treatment was achieved early after induction treatment; 59% of patients had a renal response at 3 months (26% CR, 33% PR), 67% at 6 months (43% CR, 24% PR), 88% at 12 months (69%CR, 19% PR) and 88% (71% CR, 17% PR) at 2 years. These results are encouraging compared to previous studies reporting 33–50% CR at 6 months, 49–68% CR at 12 months, and 63% CR at 2 years [9,14,18–24], although our population was predominantly Caucasian. Response to treatment has been associated with better long-term renal outcomes [25–28], with some studies reporting better renal survival in patients with CR than those with PR only [19,27]. In contrast, others did not find any significant differences [9]. Baseline renal function, proteinuria, hypertension, histological activity and chronicity indexes have been previously suggested as predictors of renal response [9,18,19,24,29–31]. In our study, baseline proteinuria >1.5 g/day emerged as the most significant predictor of early (i.e., at 3, 6, 9 months) and late complete response (i.e., at 12, 18 and 24 months). Time to response has not been fully addressed in previous studies, with some reporting a correlation with improved renal survival [28] and others a predictive role of baseline proteinuria [18,32]. Our study predicted time to CR only by baseline proteinuria >1.5 g/day.

Renal flare is a recognized predictor of progressive CKD and morbidity in LN patients [10,33]. Different studies report flare rates of 25–66% [14,34–36], largely depending on follow-up time and definitions of flare. In our study, 33% of patients experienced a relapse in a median time of 38 months. Few data are available regarding factors predictive of flare. Attainment of CR, rather than PR, shorter time to CR and maintenance treatment with MPA (compared to AZA) have been the main determinants of flare occurrence across studies [14,35–37]. In our study, although a longer time to either CR or PR correlated with a higher risk of flare, this correlation was significant only for responses at 12, 18 and 24 months. Induction treatment with MPA (compared to CYC) and proteinuria <0.8 g/day at 12 months were significantly associated with a lower risk of flare, with the latter finding adding to the value of 12-month proteinuria as a predictor of renal outcome. Proteinuria at the time of LN diagnosis, apart from affecting time to response, was also found to be a risk factor for flare. The cut-off level that was strongly associated with a higher flare risk was determined at 2 g/day. Baseline proteinuria >2 g/day and 12-month proteinuria >0.8 g/day were also found to correlate with a shorter time to flare. Interestingly, pure proliferative classes conferred a greater risk of flare when compared to mixed classes, but the difference was significant only between class III and mixed classes. Other baseline histological characteristics did not affect the risk of flare. However, studies have shown that the activity index of repeat, instead of initial, biopsy may predict flare occurrence and the time of flare [38,39].

Recent studies report cumulative renal survival rates in proliferative LN of 91, 81, 75 and 66% at 5, 10, 15 and 20 years, respectively, and 5-, 10- and 15-year cumulative incidence of ESRD of 3–11%, 6–19% and 19–25% respectively [40–43]. In our study, 22% of patients reached the composite renal outcome (stage 3–4 CKD or ESRD) in a median follow-up time of 100 months. Several studies have identified baseline parameters as predictors of long-term renal prognosis, such as creatinine, proteinuria, hypertension, activity and chronicity index [43,44], while others [15,16,18,28,40,44,45] highlight the importance of renal parameters at 12 months as single variables (i.e., proteinuria <0.7 g/day or <0.8 g/day) or as composite endpoint (i.e., renal response). Renal response definition, however, is not uniform across studies. The current study demonstrated that the only variables strongly associated with long-term adverse renal outcomes were proteinuria >0.8 g/day at 12 months and interstitial fibrosis/tubular atrophy >25% at the initial biopsy. Baseline proteinuria did not seem to affect renal survival significantly. Some studies have reported that activity and chronicity index, as well as interstitial fibrosis/tubular atrophy, correlate with a worse renal outcome when evaluated in repeat and not in initial biopsies [38,46]. In our study, interstitial fibrosis/tubular atrophy emerged as the only histologic parameter of the initial biopsy that could predict a worse renal outcome. Interstitial fibrosis at initial biopsy has already been associated with adverse renal outcomes [45,47]. These results imply that evaluating distinct components of the activity and chronicity indexes in initial and repeat biopsies may be of greater value in predicting renal response and long-term outcome than relying solely on activity and chronicity indexes. While some studies report that a very early response (i.e., at 3 months) can predict long-term renal outcomes [48,49], we did not find that such an early response significantly affected renal survival. In our study, a response at 6, 12, 18 and 24 months predicted a better renal outcome.

The use of an inception cohort of biopsy-proven proliferative (only) LN patients, the long follow-up time of 100 months, and the uniform approach in the setting of a specialized academic center constitute the main strengths of our study. The study's limitations are its retrospective design and the inclusion of almost exclusively Caucasian patients.

5. Conclusions

The current study highlights the value of baseline proteinuria <1.5 g/day as the only early predictor of time to complete response in patients with proliferative LN. It also demonstrates that induction treatment with mycophenolic acid significantly lowers the risk of renal flare. At the same time, 12-month proteinuria >0.8 g/day correlates significantly with flare occurrence and, along with interstitial fibrosis/tubular atrophy >25% at the initial biopsy, strongly predicts long-term renal outcome.

Supplementary Materials: The following supporting information can be downloaded at: https://www.mdpi.com/article/10.3390/jcm11175017/s1, Table S1: Differences in baseline characteristics between the two major induction treatment groups (mycophenolic acid versus cyclophosphamide); Table S2: Predictors of complete response at 3-6-9-12-18-24 months; Table S3: Response (CR or PR) at different time points as predictors of flare; Table S4: Statistical tests examining correlation between independent predictors of risk of flare; Table S5: Renal function at presentation, response to treatment and time to renal failure in patients with ESRD; Table S6: Responses at different time points as predictors of adverse renal outcome; Table S7: Statistical tests examining correlation between independent predictors of risk of adverse renal outcome; Figure S1: Kaplan-Meier survival estimates of probability for response according to [a] proliferative lupus nephritis class [b] treatment with cyclophosphamide versus MPA/MMF.

Author Contributions: Conceptualization, M.G.T.,J.B. and P.P.S.; Methodology, E.K., M.G.T. and I.M.; Software, I.M.; Validation, E.K., I.M.. S.M., P.P.S., J.B. and M.G.T.; Formal Analysis, I.M.; Investigation, E.K., S.M. and M.G.T.; Resources, E.K., S.M., G.L., P.P.S., J.B. and M.G.T.; Data Curation, E.K. and I.M.; Writing—Original Draft Preparation, E.K. and M.G.T.; Writing—Review & Editing, S.M., G.L., I.M., P.P.S. and J.B.; Visualization, E.K.; Supervision, M.G.T. and S.M.; Project Administration, M.G.T. and J.B.; Funding Acquisition, none.All authors have read and agreed to the published version of the manuscript.

Funding: No funding was received for this study.

Institutional Review Board Statement: The study was approved by the Institutional Review Board (protocol number 1725/14-12-2017) of Laiko General Hospital of Athens. The analysis included anonymized study data, and no patient consent was required.

Informed Consent Statement: Patients and/or the public were not involved in the design, conduct, reporting or dissemination plans of this research.

Data Availability Statement: The data supporting this study's findings are available from the corresponding author upon reasonable request.

Conflicts of Interest: The authors declare no conflict of interest.

References

1. Anders, H.-J.; Saxena, R.; Zhao, M.-H.; Parodis, I.; Salmon, J.E.; Mohan, C. Lupus nephritis. *Nat. Rev. Dis. Primers* **2020**, *6*, 7. [CrossRef] [PubMed]
2. Doria, A.; Iaccarino, L.; Ghirardello, A.; Zampieri, S.; Arienti, S.; Sarzi-Puttini, P.; Atzeni, F.; Piccoli, A.; Todesco, S. Long-term prognosis and causes of death in systemic lupus erythematosus. *Am. J. Med.* **2006**, *119*, 700–706. [CrossRef] [PubMed]
3. Yap, D.Y.; Tang, C.S.; Ma, M.K.; Lam, M.F.; Chan, T.M. Survival analysis and causes of mortality in patients with lupus nephritis. *Nephrol. Dial. Transplant.* **2012**, *27*, 3248–3254. [CrossRef] [PubMed]
4. Lerang, K.; Gilboe, I.M.; Steinar Thelle, D.; Gran, J.T. Mortality and years of potential life loss in systemic lupus erythematosus: A population-based cohort study. *Lupus* **2014**, *23*, 1546–1552. [CrossRef] [PubMed]
5. Costenbader, K.H.; Desai, A.; Alarcón, G.S.; Hiraki, L.T.; Shaykevich, T.; Brookhart, M.A.; Massarotti, E.; Lu, B.; Solomon, D.H.; Winkelmayer, W.C. Trends in the incidence, demographics, and outcomes of end-stage renal disease due to lupus nephritis in the US from 1995 to 2006. *Arthritis Rheum.* **2011**, *63*, 1681–1688. [CrossRef]
6. Tektonidou, M.; Dasgupta, A.; Ward, M.M. Risk of end-stage renal disease in patients with lupus nephritis, 1971-2015: A systematic review and Bayesian meta-analysis. *Arthritis Rheumatol.* **2016**, *68*, 1432–1441. [CrossRef]
7. Bastian, H.M.; Roseman, J.M.; McGwin, G.; Alarcón, G.S.; Friedman, A.W.; Fessler, B.J.; A Baethge, B.; Reveille, J.D.; LUMINA Study Group. Systemic lupus erythematosus in three ethnic groups. XII. Risk factors for lupus nephritis after diagnosis. *Lupus* **2002**, *11*, 152–160. [CrossRef]
8. Bertsias, G.K.; Tektonidou, M.; Amoura, Z.; Aringer, M.; Bajema, I.; Berden, J.H.; Boletis, J.; Cervera, R.; Dörner, T.; Doria, A.; et al. Joint European League Against Rheumatism and European Renal Association–European Dialysis and Transplant Association (EULAR/ERA-EDTA) recommendations for the management of adult and paediatric lupus nephritis. *Ann. Rheum. Dis.* **2012**, *71*, 1771–1782. [CrossRef]
9. Almalki, A.H.; Alrowaie, F.A.; Alhozali, H.M.; Almalki, N.K.; Alsubei, A.I.; Alturki, M.S.; Sadagah, L.F. Remission and long-term outcomes of proliferative lupus nephritis: Retrospective study of 96 patients from Saudi Arabia. *Lupus* **2019**, *28*, 1082–1090. [CrossRef]

10. Parikh, S.V.; Nagaraja, H.N.; Hebert, L.; Rovin, B.H. Renal flare as a predictor of incident and progressive CKD in patients with lupus nephritis. *Clin. J. Am. Soc. Nephrol.* **2014**, *9*, 279–284. [CrossRef]
11. Gladman, D.D.; Ibañez, D.; Urowitz, M.B. Systemic Lupus Erythematosus Disease Activity Index 2000. *J. Rheumatol.* **2002**, *29*, 288–291. [PubMed]
12. Kidney Disease: Improving Global Outcomes (KDIGO) Glomerulonephritis Work Group. KDIGO Clinical Practice Guideline for Glomerulonephritis. *Kidney Int. Suppl.* **2012**, *2*, 139–274.
13. Kidney Disease: Improving Global Outcomes (KDIGO) CKD Work Group. KDIGO clinical practice guideline for the evaluation and management of chronic kidney disease. *Kidney Int. Suppl.* **2013**, *3*, 1–150.
14. Ichinose, K.; Kitamura, M.; Sato, S.; Eguchi, M.; Okamoto, M.; Endo, Y.; Tsuji, S.; Takatani, A.; Shimizu, T.; Umeda, M.; et al. Complete renal response at 12 months after induction therapy is associated with renal relapse-free rate in lupus nephritis: Asinglecenter, retrospective cohort study. *Lupus* **2019**, *28*, 501–509. [CrossRef]
15. Dall'Era, M.; Cisternas, M.G.; Smilek, D.E.; Straub, L.; Houssiau, F.A.; Cervera, R.; Rovin, B.H.; Mackay, M. Predictors of long-term renal outcome in lupus nephritis trials: Lessons learned from the Euro-Lupus nephritis cohort. *Arthritis Rheumatol.* **2015**, *67*, 1305–1313. [CrossRef] [PubMed]
16. Tamirou, F.; Lauwerys, B.R.; Dall'Era, M.; Mackay, M.; Rovin, B.; Cervera, R.; AHoussiau, F. A proteinuria cut-off level of 0.7 g/day after 12 months of treatment best predicts long-term renal outcome in lupus nephritis: Data from the MAINTAIN Nephritis Trial. *Lupus Sci. Med.* **2015**, *2*, e000123. [CrossRef]
17. Ugolini-Lopes, M.R.; Seguro, L.P.C.; Castro, M.X.F.; Daffre, D.; Lopes, A.C.; Borba, E.F.; Bonfá, E. Early proteinuria response: A valid real-life situation predictor of long-term lupus renal outcome in an ethnically diverse group with severe biopsy-proven nephritis? *Lupus Sci. Med.* **2017**, *4*, e000213. [CrossRef]
18. Moroni, G.; Gatto, M.; Tamborini, F.; Quaglini, S.; Radice, F.; Saccon, F.; Frontini, G.; Alberici, F.; Sacchi, L.; Binda, V.; et al. Lack of EULAR/ERA-EDTA response at 1 year predicts poor long-term renal outcome in patients with lupus nephritis. *Ann. Rheum. Dis.* **2020**, *79*, 1077–1083. [CrossRef]
19. Chen, Y.E.; Korbet, S.M.; Katz, R.S.; Schwartz, M.M.; Lewis, E.J. Value of a complete or partial remission in severe lupus nephritis. *Clin. J. Am. Soc. Nephrol.* **2008**, *3*, 46–53. [CrossRef]
20. Ginzler, E.M.; Wofsy, D.; Isenberg, D.; Gordon, C.; Lisk, L.; Dooley, M.A. Mycophenolate mofetil or intravenous cyclophosphamide for induction treatment for lupus nephritis. *N. Engl. J. Med.* **2005**, *353*, 2219–2228. [CrossRef]
21. Appel, G.B.; Contreras, G.; Dooley, M.A.; Ginzler, E.M.; Isenberg, D.; Jayne, D.; Li, L.-S.; Mysler, E.; Sánchez-Guerrero, J.; Solomons, N.; et al. Mycophenolate mofetil versus cyclophosphamide for induction treatment of lupus nephritis. *J. Am. Soc. Nephrol.* **2009**, *20*, 1103–1112. [CrossRef] [PubMed]
22. Korbet, S.M.; Lewis, E.J.; Collaborative Study Group. Complete remission in severe lupus nephritis: Assessing the rate of loss in proteinuria. *Nephrol. Dial. Transplant.* **2012**, *27*, 2813–2819. [CrossRef]
23. Liu, G.; Wang, H.; Le, J.; Lan, L.; Xu, Y.; Yang, Y.; Chen, J.; Han, F. Early-stage predictors for treatment responses in patients with active lupus nephritis. *Lupus* **2019**, *28*, 283–289. [CrossRef] [PubMed]
24. Luís, M.S.; Bultink, I.E.; da Silva, J.A.; Voskuyl, A.E.; Inês, L.S. Early predictors of renal outcome in patients with proliferative lupus nephritis:a 36-month cohort study. *Rheumatology* **2021**, *60*, 5134–5141. [CrossRef] [PubMed]
25. Fernandes das Neves, M.; Irlapati RV, P.; Isenberg, D. Assessment of long-term remission in lupus nephritis patients: A retrospective analysis over 30 years. *Rheumatology* **2015**, *54*, 1403–1407. [CrossRef]
26. Pakchotanon, R.; Gladman, D.D.; Su, J.; Urowitz, M.B. Sustained complete renal remission is a predictor of reduced mortality, chronic kidney disease and endstage renal disease in lupus nephritis. *Lupus* **2018**, *27*, 468–474. [CrossRef]
27. Koo, H.S.; Kim, S.; Chin, H.J. Remission of proteinuria indicates good prognosis in patients with diffuse proliferative lupus nephritis. *Lupus* **2016**, *25*, 3–11. [CrossRef]
28. Pirson, V.; Enfrein, A.; Houssiau, F.A.; Tamirou, F. Absence of renal remission portends poor long-term kidney outcome in lupus nephritis. *Lupus Sci. Med.* **2021**, *8*, e000533. [CrossRef]
29. Moroni, G.; Quaglini, S.; Radice, A.; Trezzi, B.; Raffiotta, F.; Messa, P.; Sinico, R.A. The value of a panel of autoantibodies for predicting the activity of lupus nephritis at time of renal biopsy. *J. Immunol. Res.* **2015**, *2015*, 106904. [CrossRef]
30. Ichinose, K.; Kitamura, M.; Sato, S.; Fujikawa, K.; Horai, Y.; Matsuoka, N.; Tsuboi, M.; Nonaka, F.; Shimizu, T.; Fukui, S.; et al. Factors predictive of long-term mortality in lupus nephritis: A multicenter retrospective study of a Japanese cohort. *Lupus* **2019**, *28*, 295–303. [CrossRef]
31. McDonald, S.; Yiu, S.; Su, L.; Gordon, C.; Truman, M.; Lisk, L.; Solomons, N.; Bruce, I.N. Predictors of treatment response in a lupus nephritis population: Lessons from the Aspreva Lupus Management Study (ALMS) trial. *Lupus Sci. Med.* **2022**, *9*, e000584. [CrossRef] [PubMed]
32. Touma, Z.; Urowitz, M.B.; Ibañez, M.; Gladman, D.D. Time to recovery from proteinuria in patients with lupus nephritis receiving standard treatment. *J. Rheumatol.* **2014**, *41*, 688–697. [CrossRef]
33. Mosca, M.; Bencivelli, W.; Neri, R.; Pasquariello, A.; Batini, V.; Puccini, R.; Tavoni, A.; Bombardieri, S. Renal flares in 91 SLE patients with diffuse proliferative glomerulonephritis. *Kidney Int.* **2002**, *61*, 1502–1509. [CrossRef] [PubMed]
34. Sprangers, B.; Monahan, M.; Appel, G.B. Diagnosis and treatment of lupus nephritis flares—an update. *Nat. Rev. Nephrol.* **2012**, *8*, 709–717. [CrossRef] [PubMed]

35. Illei, G.G.; Takada, K.; Parkin, D.; Austin, H.A.; Crane, M.; Yarboro, C.H.; Vaughan, E.M.; Kuroiwa, T.; Danning, C.L.; Pando, J.; et al. Renal flares are common in patients with severe proliferative lupus nephritis treated with pulse immunosuppressive therapy: Long-term followup of a cohort of 145 patients participating in randomized controlled studies. *Arthritis Rheum.* **2002**, *46*, 995–1002. [CrossRef]
36. Yap, D.Y.; Tang, C.; Ma, M.K.; Mok, M.M.; Chan, G.C.; Kwan, L.P.; Chan, T.M. Longterm data on disease flares in patients with proliferative lupus nephritis in recent years. *J. Rheumatol.* **2017**, *44*, 1375–1383. [CrossRef] [PubMed]
37. So, M.W.; Koo, B.S.; Kim, Y.G.; Lee, C.-K.; Yoo, B. Predictive value of remission status after 6 months induction therapy in patients with proliferative lupus nephritis: A retrospective analysis. *Clin. Rheumatol.* **2011**, *30*, 1399–1405. [CrossRef] [PubMed]
38. Parodis, I.; Adamichou, C.; Aydin, S.; Gomez, A.; Demoulin, N.; Weinmann-Menke, J.; A Houssiau, F.; Tamirou, F. Per-protocol repeat kidney biopsy portends relapse and long-term outcome in incident cases of proliferative lupus nephritis. *Rheumatology* **2020**, *59*, 3424–3434. [CrossRef] [PubMed]
39. De Rosa, M.; Azzato, F.; Toblli, J.E.; De Rosa, G.; Fuentes, F.; Nagaraja, H.N.; Nash, R.; Rovin, B.H. A prospective observational cohort study highlights kidney biopsy findings of lupus nephritis patients in remission who flare following withdrawal of maintenance therapy. *Kidney Int.* **2018**, *94*, 788–794. [CrossRef]
40. Farinha, F.; Pepper, R.J.; Oliveira, D.G.; McDonnell, T.; Isenberg, D.A.; Rahman, A. Outcomes of membranous and proliferative lupus nephritis–analysis of a single-centre cohort with more than 30 years of follow-up. *Rheumatology* **2020**, *59*, 3314–3323. [CrossRef]
41. Mahajan, A.; Amelio, J.; Gairy, K.; Kaur, G.; A Levy, R.; Roth, D.; Bass, D. Systemic lupus erythematosus, lupus nephritis and end-stage renal disease: A pragmatic review mapping disease severity and progression. *Lupus* **2020**, *29*, 1011–1020. [CrossRef] [PubMed]
42. Hanly, J.G.; O'Keeffe, A.G.; Su, L.; Urowitz, M.B.; Romero-Diaz, J.; Gordon, C.; Bae, S.-C.; Bernatsky, S.; Clarke, A.E.; Wallace, D.J.; et al. The frequency and outcome of lupus nephritis: Results from an international inception cohort study. *Rheumatology* **2016**, *55*, 252–262. [CrossRef] [PubMed]
43. Moroni, G.; Vercelloni, P.G.; Quaglini, S.; Gatto, M.; Gianfreda, D.; Sacchi, L.; Raffiotta, F.; Zen, M.; Costantini, G.; Urban, M.L.; et al. Changing patterns in clinical–histological presentation and renal outcome over the last five decades in a cohort of 499 patients with lupusnephritis. *Ann. Rheum. Dis.* **2018**, *77*, 1318–1325. [CrossRef] [PubMed]
44. Yang, J.; Liang, D.; Zhang, H.; Liu, Z.; Le, W.; Zhou, M.; Hu, W.; Zeng, C. Long-term renal outcomes in a cohort of 1814 Chinese patients with biopsy-proven lupus nephritis. *Lupus* **2015**, *24*, 1468–1478. [CrossRef]
45. Vajgel, G.; Oliveira, C.B.L.; Costa, D.M.N.; Cavalcante, M.A.G.M.; Valente, L.M.; Sesso, R.; Crovella, S.; Kirsztajn, G.M.; Sandrin-Garcia, P. Initial renal histology and early response predict outcomes of Brazilian lupus nephritis patients. *Lupus* **2020**, *29*, 83–91. [CrossRef]
46. Gatto, M.; Radice, F.; Saccon, F.; Calatroni, M.; Frontini, G.; Trezzi, B.; Zen, M.; Ghirardello, A.; Tamborini, F.; Binda, V.; et al. Clinical and histological findings at second but not at first kidney biopsy predict end-stage kidney disease in a large multicentric cohort of patients with active lupus nephritis. *Lupus Sci. Med.* **2022**, *9*, 000689. [CrossRef]
47. Wilson, P.C.; Kashgarian, M.; Moeckel, G. Interstitial inflammation and tubular atrophy predict renal survival in lupus nephritis. *Clin. Kidney J.* **2018**, *11*, 207–218. [CrossRef]
48. Tamirou, F.; D'Cruz, D.; Sangle, S.; Remy, P.; Vasconcelos, C.; Fiehn, C.; Guttierez, M.D.M.A.; Gilboe, I.-M.; Tektonidou, M.; Blockmans, D.; et al. Long-term follow-up of the MAINTAIN Nephritis Trial, comparing azathioprine and mycophenolate mofetil as maintenance therapy of lupus nephritis. *Ann. Rheum. Dis.* **2016**, *75*, 526–531. [CrossRef]
49. Hanaoka, H.; Yamada, H.; Kiyokawa, T.; Iida, H.; Suzuki, T.; Yamasaki, Y.; Ooka, S.; Nagafuchi, H.; Okazaki, T.; Ichikawa, D.; et al. Lack of partial renal response by 12 weeks after induction therapy predicts poor renal response and systemic damage accrual in lupus nephritis class III or IV. *Arthritis Res. Ther.* **2017**, *19*, 4. [CrossRef]

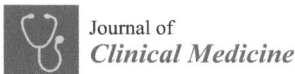

Article

Renal Tissue Expression of BAFF and BAFF Receptors Is Associated with Proliferative Lupus Nephritis

Miguel Marín-Rosales [1,2], Claudia Azucena Palafox-Sánchez [2,3,*], Ramón Antonio Franco-Topete [4], Francisco Josué Carrillo-Ballesteros [5], Alvaro Cruz [3], Diana Celeste Salazar-Camarena [2], José Francisco Muñoz-Valle [3] and Francisco Ramos-Solano [4]

[1] Departamento de Reumatología, Hospital General de Occidente, Secretaría de Salud Jalisco, Guadalajara 45170, Mexico
[2] Grupo de Inmunología Molecular, Centro Universitario de Ciencias de la Salud, Universidad de Guadalajara, Guadalajara 44340, Mexico
[3] Instituto de Investigación en Ciencias Biomédicas (IICB), Centro Universitario de Ciencias de la Salud, Universidad de Guadalajara, Guadalajara 44340, Mexico
[4] Departamento de Microbiología y Patología, Centro Universitario de Ciencias de la Salud, Universidad de Guadalajara, Guadalajara 44340, Mexico
[5] Departamento de Farmacobiología, Centro Universitario de Ciencias Exactas e Ingenierías, Universidad de Guadalajara, Guadalajara 44430, Mexico
* Correspondence: kklaumx@yahoo.com; Tel.: +52-333-815-0611

Abstract: Background: The B-cell activating factor (BAFF) controls the maturation and survival of B cells. An imbalance in this cytokine has been associated with systemic autoimmunity in SLE and lupus nephritis (LN). However, few investigations have evaluated the tissular expression of BAFF in LN. This study aimed to associate BAFF system expression at the tissular level with the proliferative LN classes. Methods: The analysis included eighteen kidney tissues, with sixteen LN (class III = 5, class IV = 6, class III/IV+V = 4, and class V = 1), and two controls. The tissular expression was evaluated with an immunochemistry assay. A Cytation5 imaging reader and ImageJ software were used to analyze the quantitative expression. A p-value < 0.05 was considered significant. Results: The expressions of BAFF, A proliferation-inducing ligand (APRIL), and their receptors were observed in glomerular, tubular, and interstitial zones, with BAFF being the most strongly expressed in the overall analysis. BAFF-Receptor (BR3), transmembrane activator and CALM interactor (TACI), and B-Cell maturation antigen (BCMA) displayed higher expressions in LN class IV in all zones analyzed ($p < 0.05$). Additionally, a positive correlation was found between APRIL, TACI, and BCMA at the glomerular level; BCMA and APRIL in the interstitial zone; and BR3, TACI, and BCMA in the tubule ($p < 0.05$). Conclusions: The expression of BAFF and BAFF receptors is mainly associated with LN class IV, emphasizing the participation of these receptors as an essential pathogenic factor in kidney involvement in SLE patients.

Keywords: systemic lupus erythematosus; proliferative lupus nephritis; BAFF system expression

1. Introduction

Lupus nephritis (LN) is the most frequent life-threatening clinical domain of systemic lupus erythematosus (SLE); renal involvement affects 30–70% of patients and shows high frequency and severity in Black and Latin-American Hispanic populations [1,2]. LN diagnosis is sustained based on clinical features and an evaluation of conventional biomarkers such as low complement serum concentration, high anti-dsDNA antibodies, and urinary findings [3,4]. However, kidney biopsy is the diagnostic gold standard and guides LN treatment, according to the 2003 International Society of Nephrology (ISN)/Renal Pathology Society (RPS) classification [5,6].

B-cell ontogeny is controlled through the BAFF system; this system is integrated by B-cell activating factor (BAFF), a proliferation-inducing ligand (APRIL), and their receptors, namely BAFF-Receptor (BR3), transmembrane activator and CALM interactor (TACI), and B-Cell maturation antigen (BCMA). BAFF and APRIL belong to the tumor necrosis factor (TNF) family and promote B-cell activation, proliferation, maturation, and survival through BR3, TACI, and BCMA receptors [7–11].

An imbalance in BAFF, APRIL, or their receptors in both murine models and humans has been associated with the development of autoimmune diseases, including SLE, Sjögren's Syndrome, and rheumatoid arthritis [11–18]. Regarding SLE, the serum concentration of BAFF and APRIL has been reported to be higher in SLE patients; these ligands were previously associated with the disease activity index and autoantibody levels and can predict a flare [13,14,19–25]. On the other hand, the soluble BCMA serum concentration was found to have a higher concentration and was correlated with the activity index in SLE patients [25]. Regarding the BAFF receptors, BR3, TACI, and BCMA were identified in CD3 T cells in SLE patients, and their expression varies according to SLE disease activity [21,23,25].

Given the growing need for diagnostic tools for LN, multiple new biomarkers have been associated with this domain [26], and BAFF and APRIL have been linked with renal activity in Mexican SLE patients [22,23]. Additionally, BAFF and their receptors were analyzed in situ in kidney tissues of LN patients, showing differential pattern expression according to LN classes [27]. However, the analysis did not include APRIL. Based on the association of the BAFF system with renal involvement, the poor renal prognosis for proliferative LN in Latin American SLE patients, and the small number of validated renal biomarkers, this study evaluated the renal tissue expression of BAFF, APRIL, BR3, TACI, and BCMA in patients with proliferative LN.

2. Materials and Methods

2.1. Study Tissues

A retrospective and descriptive study were conducted. This study included sixteen kidney tissues of LN patients classified as class III, IV, V, or V/III-IV according to the 2003 ISN/RPS classification [5]. All LN patients met the 2012 Systemic Lupus International Collaborating Clinics classification criteria for SLE [28] and were recruited at the rheumatology department of Hospital General de Occidente. Additionally, two kidney incisional biopsies without autoimmunity histopathological features were used as controls. All patients provided written informed consent according to the 2013 Declaration of Helsinki and actual national guidelines of the Health Ministry. The ethics and research committees of the Hospital General de Occidente, Jalisco, Mexico, approved the study under the number CI-561/18.

2.2. Immunohistochemical Staining

Kidney biopsies were fixed in 4% paraformaldehyde and embedded in paraffin using a tissue processor (TP1020; Leica Biosystems, Wetzlar, Germany). Tissues were sectioned at 5 µm, mounted on electrocharged slides, and deparaffinized at 60 °C for 30 min in a Dako Hybridizer (Dako Colorado Inc. Collins, CO, USA). Posteriorly, the tissues were rehydrated by immersion in xylene using graded ethanol dilutions followed by distilled water. According to Carrillo-Ballesteros et al., the immunohistochemical assay was standardized in amygdaline tissue [29]. Briefly, after rehydration of the tissue, epitope retrieval was performed with the Dako PT Link system (Dako Colorado Inc. Collins, CO, USA) at 90 degrees for 30 min, and the slides were submerged into the Dako PT Link cameras with a 1 mM EDTA buffer (pH = 9) for BAFF, APRIL, and BR3, as well as a 10 mM sodium citrate buffer (pH = 6) for TACI and BCMA. Later, all slides were cooled, and a 3% hydrogen peroxide—10% methanol solution was added to achieve an endogenous peroxidase blockade. Posteriorly, slides were incubated for 30 min with the following primary antibodies: rat monoclonal antibody to BAFF (Abcam, cat. no. ab16081, dilution 1:100), rabbit polyclonal antibody to APRIL (Abcam, cat. no. ab189263, dilution 1:50), mouse monoclonal antibody to BR3 (Abcam, cat. no. ab16232, dilution 1:250), rabbit polyclonal antibody to

TACI (Abcam, cat. no. ab79023, dilution 1:100), and rabbit polyclonal antibody to BCMA (Abcam, cat. no. ab5972, dilution 1:100). Following incubation with primary antibodies and buffer washing, the slides were incubated for 10 min with the universal post-primary antibody included in the BOND polymer refine detection system (Leica Biosystems, cat. no. DS9800), and diaminobenzidine (DAB) was employed for detection until the development of a red-brown color. Finally, slides were counterstained with Harris hematoxylin and reviewed under a microscope by two experienced pathologists.

2.3. Immunohistochemical Image Processing and Statistical Analysis

After slide tissue staining, three renal structures (glomerulus, tubule, and interstitial) were photographed in triplicate using a BioTek Citation|5 Cell Imaging Multimode Reader (Santa Clara, CA, USA) with 10× and 20× magnification. Later, the ImageJ v1.51j8 and DAB deconvolution plugin software (National Institute of Health, Bethesda, MD, USA. https://imagej.nih.gov/ij/, accessed on 15 January 2021) was used to analyze the photos and obtain the immunoreaction score. In the DAB layer, the pixel intensity value was represented in a range of 0–255 (the darkest shade and lightest shade represent 0 and 255, respectively), according to Chatterjee et al. [30]. The mean intensity default threshold was set in the ImageJ software under the "Image" menu using the "measure" tool from the "Analyze" menu. Later, the percentage of positive pixels was determined in the selected areas. Descriptive analysis included the median, interquartile range (IQR), and frequencies. Additionally, Fisher, Chi-square, Mann–Whitney U, Kruskal–Wallis and Dunn's post hoc, and Spearman correlation tests were used as appropriate. A p-value < 0.05 was considered significant.

3. Results

3.1. Histopathological Features of LN

Eighteen kidney tissues were included, including sixteen percutaneous biopsies of patients with LN, and two incisional biopsies were obtained by necropsy without histopathological features of autoimmunity. Thirteen (81%) LN cases were women, class IV represented 38% (6/16) of the cases, class III and class V+III/IV were 31% (5/16) and 25% (4/16) of the cases, respectively, and only 6% (1/16) were classified as class V. The wire-loop lesions and total renal activity index were associated with proliferative diffuse LN ($p < 0.05$). Table 1 shows all histopathological findings.

Table 1. Histopathological features of proliferative LN tissues.

	Class III ($n = 5$)	Class IV ($n = 6$)	Class V and V+III/IV ($n = 5$)	Total ($n = 16$)	p-Value
Glomerulus, (IQR)	23 (14-36)	27 (15-33)	30 (19-42)	25 (18-34)	0.837
Histopathological activity index, (IQR)	5 (5-6)	15 (12-16)	5 (4-6)	6 (5-14)	0.001
Histopathological chronicity index, (IQR)	4 (3-4)	3 (3-3)	3 (2-3)	3 (2-3)	0.239
Full-house phenomenon, (%)	4 (80)	6 (100)	5 (100)	15 (94)	0.279
Crescents, (%)	2 (40)	6 (100)	2 (40)	10 (62.5)	0.056
Glomerular sclerosis, (%)	4 (80)	4 (67)	4 (80)	12 (75)	0.356
Wire-loop lesions, (%)	0	5 (83)	0	5 (31)	0.002
Karyorrhexis, (%)	3 (60)	6 (100)	3 (60)	12 (75)	0.202
Neutrophilic infiltrated, (%)	3 (60)	6 (100)	3 (60)	12 (75)	0.202
Hyaline thrombus, (%)	1 (20)	3 (50)	0	4 (25)	0.155
Tubular atrophy, (%)	4 (80)	6 (100)	5 (100)	14 (88)	0.504
Tubular tumefaction, (%)	4 (80)	6 (100)	5 (100)	15 (94)	0.309
Tubular-interstitial infiltrated, (%)	5 (100)	4 (67)	3 (60)	12 (75)	0.288
Tubulointerstitial fibrosis, (%)	4 (80)	5 (83)	4 (80)	13 (81)	0.986

Data are shown as the median, IQR, frequencies, and percentages, as appropriate. The p-value was obtained using Fisher's test or Kruskal–Wallis and Dunn's post hoc test, as appropriate. LN: lupus nephritis; IQR: interquartile range.

3.2. Renal BAFF System Expression and Association with LN Classes

The LN tissues showed BAFF system expression at the glomerular, tubule, and interstitial levels. BAFF and BCMA were expressed in the glomerular epithelium membrane of the glomerulus, and TACI presented expression in glomerular resident cells. BAFF, APRIL, TACI, and BCMA were expressed at the tubular level, mainly in the cytoplasm of the tubular epithelium. Additionally, BR3, TACI, and BCMA demonstrated expression in inflammatory cells at an interstitial level. The control kidney tissues showed low BAFF expression in the tubular system, and APRIL, BR3, TACI, and BCMA were not expressed. Figure 1 shows BAFF system expression in tissues with LN and renal controls.

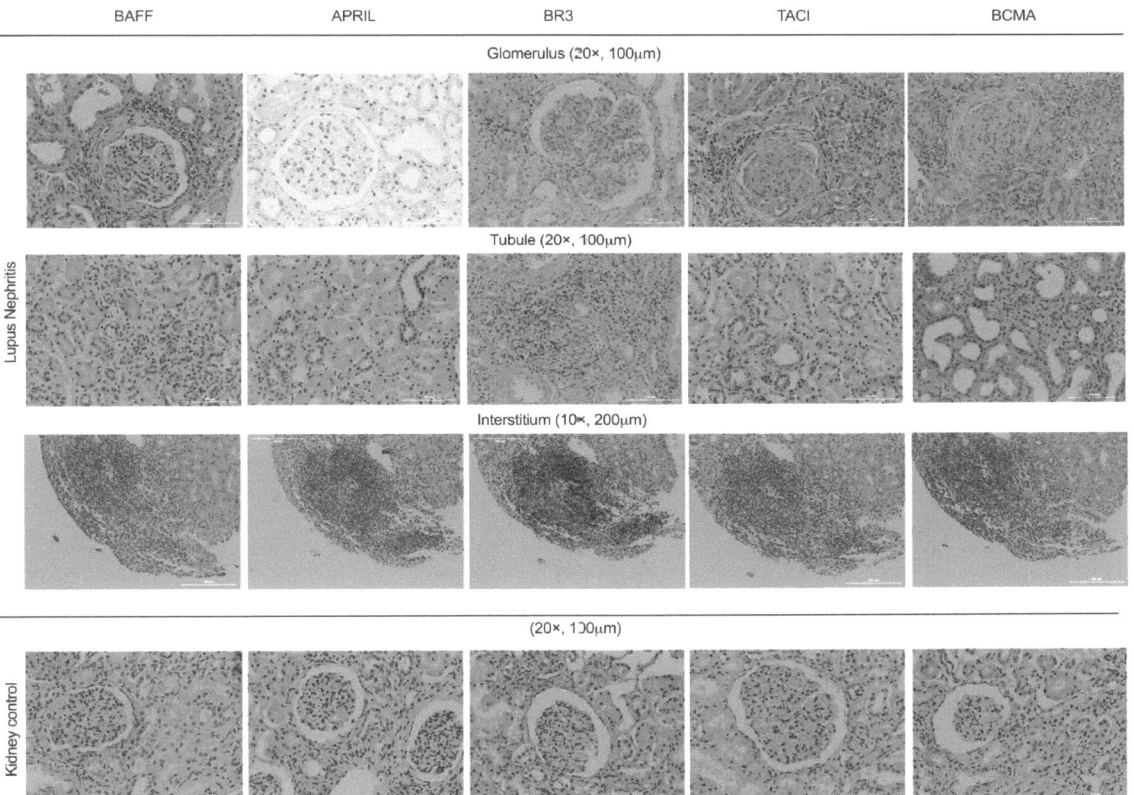

Figure 1. BAFF system expression in lupus nephritis tissues and kidney controls. Glomerular, tubular, and interstitial zones have a positive stain directed to BAFF system members. BR3 and TACI show more stains in the interstitial infiltration. Thus, APRIL was the lowest. The inflammatory cells in the interstitium could simulate an ectopic germinal center. Kidney control tissues did not show expression of BAFF, APRIL, or their receptors. BAFF: B-cells activating factor, APRIL: A proliferation-inducing ligand, BR3: BAFF receptor, TACI: Transmembrane activator and CALM interactor, BCMA: B-cell maturation antigen.

Based on the previous findings, ImageJ software was used to perform a quantitative expression analysis. For the LN tissues, the overall analysis indicated a higher percentage of BAFF expression [13.07% (IQR 9.62–19.91%)] than APRIL [8.86% (IQR 3.28–12.95%)], BR3 [6.93% (IQR 3.40–15.07%)], and BCMA [9.80% (IQR 5.32–12.95%)], with statistical significance ($p < 0.05$). Additionally, TACI [10.66% (IQR 7.74%–14.11%)] had higher expression than APRIL ($p < 0.05$) (see Figure 2d).

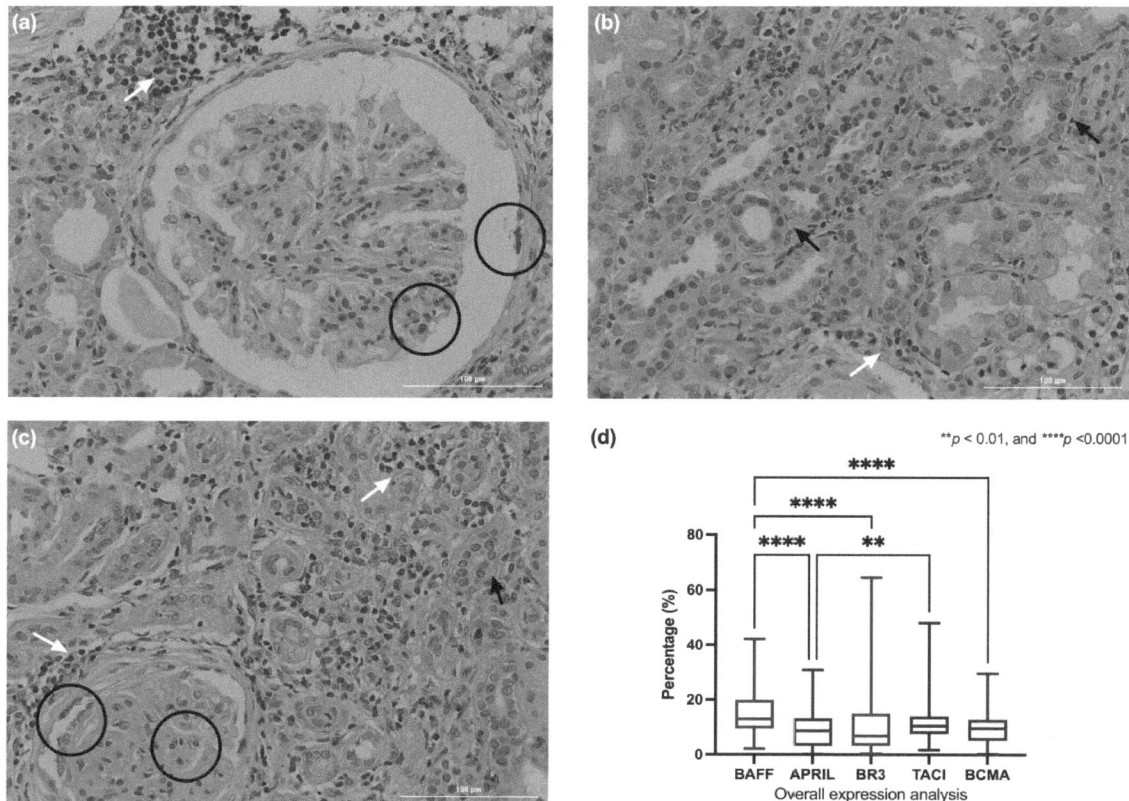

Figure 2. Overall analysis of BAFF system expression in LN. BAFF system expression according to glomerular, tubular, and interstitial zones is illustrated in (**a–c**). Black circles, black arrows, and white arrows indicate glomerular, tubular, and interstitial BAFF system expression, respectively. The overall expression analysis indicated a higher expression of BAFF and TACI than APRIL. Additionally, BAFF displays a higher expression of BR3 and BCMA (**d**). The p-value was obtained through Kruskal–Wallis and post hoc tests. Data are shown as the median with IQR. BAFF: B-cells activating factor, APRIL: A proliferation-inducing ligand, BR3: BAFF receptor, TACI: Transmembrane activator and CALM interactor, BCMA: B-cell maturation antigen, I IQR: Interquartile range.

After the overall analysis, the LN tissues were stratified according to the ISN/RPS 2003 classification, and BAFF system expression was evaluated in three zones: glomerulus, tubule, and interstitium. At the glomerular level, both ligands and the three BAFF receptors exhibited similar expression between the renal control and LN classes (Figure 3a–e). However, the classes of LN demonstrated different receptor pattern expressions, showing higher expressions of BR3, TACI, and BCMA in classes IV (Figure 3c–e).

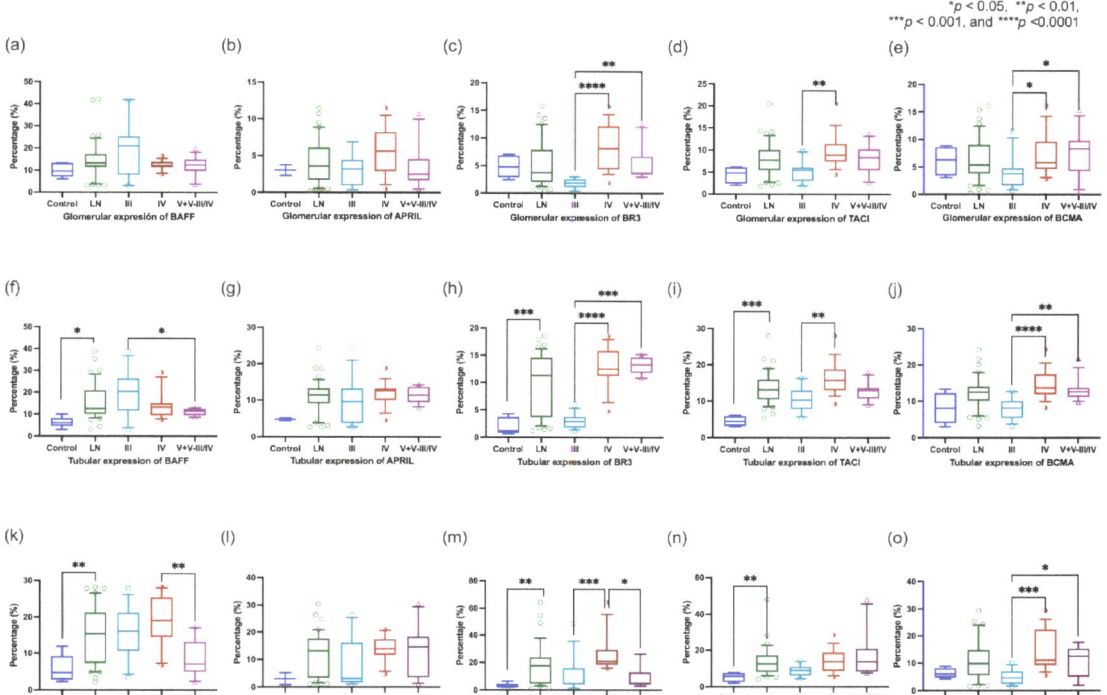

Figure 3. Association of BAFF system expression and proliferative LN classes according to glomerular, tubular, and interstitial zones. Glomerular expression of BR3 and BCMA was higher in class IV and V+V-III/IV groups than in class III. TACI showed a higher expression in class IV compared to class III (**c–e**). The tubular expression of BAFF was higher in the LN group, mainly in class III (**f**). The proliferative lesions (class IV) showed a higher expression of BR3, TACI, and BCMA (**h–j**). Compared to the interstitial BAFF system expression, BAFF, BR3, and TACI displayed higher expressions than the kidney controls (**k**). The Class IV group had higher expressions of BAFF, BR3, and BCMA (**k,m,o**). (**a,b,g,l,n**) did not show a statistical difference ($p > 0.05$). The p-value was obtained through Kruskal–Wallis and post hoc tests. Data are shown as median with IQR. BAFF: B-cells activating factor, APRIL: A proliferation-inducing ligand, BR3: BAFF receptor, TACI: Transmembrane activator and CALM interactor, BCMA: B-cell maturation antigen. IQR: Interquartile range, LN: lupus nephritis.

Similarly, the tubular zone was analyzed. BAFF, BR3, and TACI showed a higher percentage of expression than the renal controls, with statistical significance (Figure 3f,h,i). On the other hand, the tubular zone commonly expressed more APRIL and BCMA; however, no statistical significance was found (Figure 3g,j). When comparing BAFF system expression according to LN classes, classes IV and V+III/IV nephritis exhibited greater BR3, TACI, and BCMA expressions than the focal proliferative class (Figure 3h–j). In contrast, class III presented a higher expression of BAFF for another kind of nephritis (Figure 3a).

Additionally, expression analysis was performed in the interstitial zone. BAFF, BR3, and TACI exhibited higher expressions in LN compared to the control with statistical significance (Figure 3k,m,n). Otherwise, APRIL and BCMA showed a trend toward higher expression than the kidney controls; however, no statistical significance was found (Figure 3l,o). In the LN classes sub-analysis, BAFF, BR3, and BCMA expressions were higher in diffuse proliferative nephritis than in focal and membranous lesions (Figure 3k,m,o). On the other hand, TACI and APRIL did not show statistical significance (Figure 3l,n).

3.3. Correlation of Renal BAFF System Expression

Subsequently, a correlation analysis of BAFF system expression was performed. At the glomerular level (Figure 4a), APRIL displayed positive correlations with BR3 ($r^2 = 0.64$), TACI ($r^2 = 0.40$), and BCMA ($r^2 = 0.66$), with statistical significance ($p < 0.05$). Additionally, TACI and BCMA correlated positively ($r^2 = 0.40$, $p < 0.05$, Figure 4b). On the other hand, the tubular expression (Figure 4b) of BR3, TACI, and BCMA showed a positive correlation [BR3/TACI ($r^2 = 0.44$), BR3/BCMA ($r^2 = 0.51$), and TACI/BCMA ($r^2 = 0.47$), $p < 0.05$]. Additionally, analysis at the interstitial level (Figure 4c) demonstrated a positive correlation between APRIL and BCMA ($r^2 = 0.50$), as well as between BCMA and TACI ($r^2 = 0.43$), with statistical significance ($p < 0.05$).

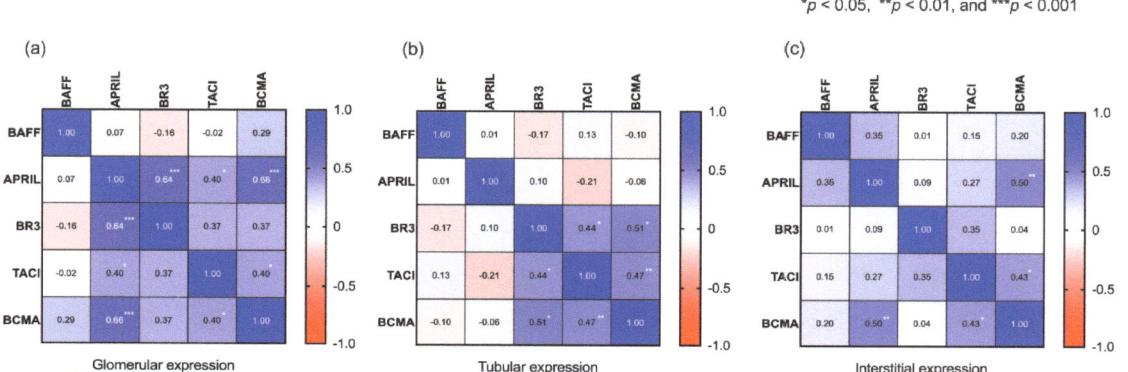

*$p < 0.05$, **$p < 0.01$, and ***$p < 0.001$

Figure 4. Matrix correlations of BAFF system expression according to zones. At the glomerular level, APRIL showed a positive correlation between all BAFF system receptors, and TACI correlated with BCMA (**a**). On the other hand, BR3, TACI, and BCMA showed a positive correlation at the tubular level (**b**). BCMA expression in the interstitium had a positive correlation with APRIL and TACI (**c**). The *p*-value was obtained through a Spearman rank correlation test. BAFF: B-cells activating factor, APRIL: A proliferation-inducing ligand, BR3: BAFF receptor, TACI: Transmembrane activator and CALM interactor, BCMA: B-cell maturation antigen.

4. Discussion

LN is the most frequent life-threatening complication among African and Latin American SLE patients. LN is considered a predictor of flare disease [31] and causes end-stage renal disease (ESRD) in 10–30% of cases [32]. Multiple conventional and new renal biomarkers have been associated with LN [26]. However, a kidney biopsy remains the diagnostic gold standard and guides treatment according to the histological findings.

This study associated the histopathological activity index and wire-loop lesions with LN-IV. The most frequent histopathological features were a full-house phenomenon, tubular tumefaction, tubular atrophy, and tubulointerstitial fibrosis. However, these typical pathological features for the diagnosis of LN had a sensitivity ranging from 68 to 80%, with a specificity of 80–96% [33]. On the other hand, fibrinoid necrosis, fibrous crescents, interstitial fibrosis, and tubular atrophy were associated with poor renal prognosis and ERSD [34]. Thus, searching for potential biomarkers for the diagnosis and treatment of LN is imperative.

BAFF system imbalance has been associated with LN and SLE flare [22,24]. BAFF, APRIL, and mRNA expression of these ligands have been identified at the urinary level in LN patients [35,36]. However, the serum and urinary concentrations did not show a correlation [35], and their links have not been elucidated. Thus, what is/are the sources of BAFF/APRIL at the urinary level?

Possible answers for the detection of both ligands at the urinary level include proteinuria associated with the loss of glomerular membrane integrity secondary to immune complex deposition. Additionally, the source of BAFF system ligands could be related to infiltrating immune cells and/or the local production of resident renal cells. This study identified the in situ expression of BAFF, APRIL, and their receptors in glomerular and tubular zones, as well as in inflammatory cells at the interstitial level in proliferative LN tissues, presenting similar findings to those reported by Suso et al. [27].

In murine models with LN, immune complex deposition induces the recruitment of immune cells, favoring BAFF secretion and altering the position of renal T cells. These events promote the formation of tertiary lymphoid structures [37]. Despite local BAFF overproduction, maintaining lymphoid structures requires chemokine CXCL13. In murine models, CXCL13 is secreted by podocytes in LN [38]; this chemokine has been associated with kidney graft rejection [39] and postulated as an allograft rejection biomarker [40]. However, this chemokine was not evaluated in the present study.

In addition to the role of podocytes related to murine nephritis, tubular epithelial cells could be involved in the BAFF system. All members of this system were expressed in the tubular epithelium in our study, showing a positive correlation between BR3, TACI, and BCMA receptors. Schwarting et al. associated tubular epithelial cells with ectopic BAFF overproduction and the histopathological activity index in LN. Additionally, an autocrine loop phenomenon was documented through in vitro assays [41]. For BAFF receptors, adipocytes, keratinocytes, and microglia, there are no immune cells with ectopic expression [42–44]. In LN murine models, the tubular cells showed mRNA and tissular expression of BAFF receptors [41]. Hence, resident cells could show an ectopic expression of these receptors and amplify local inflammation in patients with LN.

Belimumab, a monoclonal antibody with BAFF targeting, is the only biological treatment approved to treat non-renal clinical domains in SLE [45]. In addition to conventional treatment in LN, Belimumab increases the probability of completing renal remission with a similar rate of adverse events [46,47]. Even in refractory LN, adding Belimumab to the cyclophosphamide and rituximab scheme could improve the renal response with an adequate security profile [48]. The BAFF system expression in resident renal cells and inflammatory infiltrating cells described in this study could support the use of anti-BAFF treatment. Additionally, TACI deletion in murine models is associated with the protection of LN [16].

The main limitations of this study are a reduced number of patients, only the inclusion of proliferative nephritis, the study design, a lack of clinical data, and the absence of labeling of B cells and CXCL13. The information obtained could help generate new therapeutic and diagnostic targets in LN.

5. Conclusions

The expression of BAFF and its receptors is mainly associated with LN class IV, and both inflammatory cells and resident kidney cells are involved in the expression of this system. Together, our results emphasize BAFF system participation as an important pathogenic factor for kidney involvement in SLE patients. However, these results should be taken with caution.

Author Contributions: Conceptualization, M.M.-R. and C.A.P.-S.; methodology, R.A.F.-T., F.J.C.-B. and F.R.-S.; software, F.J.C.-B.; validation, R.A.F.-T.; formal analysis, M.M.-R. and D.C.S.-C.; investigation, M.M.-R. and A.C; resources, A.C. and C.A.P.-S.; data curation, A.C. and D.C.S.-C.; writing—original draft preparation, M.M.-R.; writing—review and editing, J.F.M.-V. and C.A.P.-S.; visualization, R.A.F.-T.; supervision, D.C.S.-C.; project administration, C.A.P.-S.; and funding acquisition, A.C. and C.A.P.-S. All authors have read and agreed to the published version of the manuscript.

Funding: This research was funded by Universidad de Guadalajara, grant number PRO-SNI 2018 to A.C. and PRO-SNI 2019 to C.A.P.S.

Institutional Review Board Statement: The study was conducted in accordance with the Declaration of Helsinki and was approved by the Ethics Committees of Hospital General de Occidente under the code CI-561/18 on 14 August 2018.

Informed Consent Statement: Informed consent was obtained from all subjects involved in the study.

Data Availability Statement: Not applicable.

Conflicts of Interest: The authors declare no conflict of interest.

References

1. Ortega, L.M.; Schultz, D.R.; Lenz, O.; Pardo, V.; Contreras, G.N. Lupus Nephritis: Pathologic Features, Epidemiology and a Guide to Therapeutic Decisions. *Lupus* **2010**, *19*, 557–574. [CrossRef] [PubMed]
2. Hernández Cruz, B.; Alonso, F.; Calvo Alén, J.; Pego-Reigosa, J.M.; López-Longo, F.J.; Galindo-Izquierdo, M.; Olivé, A.; Tomero, E.; Horcada, L.; Uriarte, E.; et al. Differences in Clinical Manifestations and Increased Severity of Systemic Lupus Erythematosus between Two Groups of Hispanics: European Caucasians versus Latin American Mestizos (Data from the RELESSER Registry). *Lupus* **2020**, *29*, 27–36. [CrossRef] [PubMed]
3. Soliman, S.; Mohan, C. Lupus Nephritis Biomarkers. *Clin. Immunol.* **2017**, *185*, 10–20. [CrossRef] [PubMed]
4. Hahn, B.H.; McMahon, M.A.; Wilkinson, A.; Wallace, W.D.; Daikh, D.I.; Fitzgerald, J.D.; Karpouzas, G.A.; Merrill, J.T.; Wallace, D.J.; Yazdany, J.; et al. American College of Rheumatology Guidelines for Screening, Case Definition, Treatment and Management of Lupus Nephritis. *Arthritis Care Res.* **2012**, *64*, 797. [CrossRef]
5. Weening, J.J.; D'Agati, V.D.; Schwartz, M.M.; Seshan, S.V.; Alpers, C.E.; Appel, G.B.; Balow, J.E.; Bruijn, J.A.; Cook, T.; Ferrario, F.; et al. The Classification of Glomerulonephritis in Systemic Lupus Erythematosus Revisited. *Kidney Int.* **2004**, *65*, 521–530. [CrossRef]
6. Kostopoulou, M.; Fanouriakis, A.; Cheema, K.; Boletis, J.; Bertsias, G.; Jayne, D.; Boumpas, D.T. Management of Lupus Nephritis: A Systematic Literature Review Informing the 2019 Update of the Joint EULAR and European Renal Association-European Dialysis and Transplant Association (EULAR/ERA-EDTA) Recommendations. *RMD Open* **2020**, *6*, 1–14. [CrossRef]
7. Schneider, P.; Mackay, F.; Steiner, V.; Hofmann, K.; Bodmer, J.-L.; Holler, N.; Ambrose, C.; Lawton, P.; Bixler, S.; Acha-Orbea, H.; et al. BAFF, a Novel Ligand of the Tumor Necrosis Factor Family, Stimulates B Cell Growth. *J. Exp. Med.* **1999**, *189*, 1747–1756. [CrossRef]
8. Hahne, M.; Kataoka, T.; Schröter, M.; Hofmann, K.; Irmler, M.; Bodmer, J.-L.; Schneider, P.; Bornand, T.; Holler, N.; French, L.; et al. APRIL, a New Ligand of the Tumor Necrosis Factor Family, Stimulates Tumor Cell Growth. *J. Exp. Med.* **1998**, *188*, 1185–1190. [CrossRef]
9. Ng, L.G.; Sutherland, A.; Newton, R.; Qian, F.; Cachero, T.G.; Scott, M.L.; Thompson, J.S.; Wheway, J.; Chtanova, T.; Groom, J.; et al. B Cell-Activating Factor Belonging to the TNF Family (BAFF)-R Is the Principal BAFF Receptor Facilitating BAFF Costimulation of Circulating T and B Cells. *J. Immunol.* **2004**, *173*, 807–817. [CrossRef]
10. Belnoue, E.; Pihlgren, M.; McGaha, T.; Tougne, C.; Rochat, A.-F.; Bossen, C.; Schneider, P.; Huard, B.; Lambert, P.-H.; Siegrist, C.-A. APRIL is critical for plasmablast survival in the bone marrow and poorly expressed by early-life bone marrow stromal cells. *Blood* **2008**, *111*, 2755–2764. [CrossRef]
11. Zhang, Y.; Li, J.; Zhang, Y.-M.; Zhang, X.-M.; Tao, J. Effect of TACI Signaling on Humoral Immunity and Autoimmune Diseases. *J. Immunol. Res.* **2015**, *2015*, 1–12. [CrossRef] [PubMed]
12. Mackay, F.; Woodcock, S.A.; Lawton, P.; Ambrose, C.; Baetscher, M.; Schneider, P.; Tschopp, J.; Browning, J. Mice Transgenic for Baff Develop Lymphocytic Disorders along with Autoimmune Manifestations. *J. Exp. Med.* **1999**, *190*, 1697–1710. [CrossRef] [PubMed]
13. Vincent, F.; Northcott, M.; Hoi, A.; Mackay, F.; Morand, E. Association of serum B cell activating factor from the tumour necrosis factor family (BAFF) and a proliferation-inducing ligand (APRIL) with central nervous system and renal disease in systemic lupus erythematosus. *Lupus* **2013**, *22*, 873–884. [CrossRef] [PubMed]
14. Vincent, F.B.; Kandane-Rathnayake, R.; Koelmeyer, R.; Hoi, A.; Harris, J.; Mackay, F.; Morand, E.F. Analysis of serum B cell-activating factor from the tumor necrosis factor family (BAFF) and its soluble receptors in systemic lupus erythematosus. *Clin. Transl. Immunol.* **2019**, *8*, e1047. [CrossRef]
15. Gross, J.A.; Johnston, J.; Mudri, S.; Enselman, R.; Dillon, S.R.; Madden, K.; Xu, W.; Parrish-Novak, J.; Foster, D.; Lofton-Day, C.; et al. TACI and BCMA are receptors for a TNF homologue implicated in B-cell autoimmune disease. *Nature* **2000**, *404*, 995–999. [CrossRef]
16. Arkatkar, T.; Jacobs, H.M.; Du, S.W.; Li, Q.-Z.; Hudkins, K.L.; Alpers, C.E.; Rawlings, D.J.; Jackson, S.W. TACI deletion protects against progressive murine lupus nephritis induced by BAFF overexpression. *Kidney Int.* **2018**, *94*, 728–740. [CrossRef]
17. Santillán-López, E.; Muñoz-Valle, J.F.; Oregon-Romero, E.; Espinoza-García, N.; Treviño-Talavera, B.A.; Salazar-Camarena, D.C.; Marín-Rosales, M.; Cruz, A.; Alvarez-Gómez, J.A.; Sagrero-Fabela, N.; et al. Analysis of *TNFSF13B* polymorphisms and BAFF expression in rheumatoid arthritis and primary Sjögren's syndrome patients. *Mol. Genet. Genom. Med.* **2022**, *10*, e1950. [CrossRef]

18. Groom, J.; Kalled, S.L.; Cutler, A.H.; Olson, C.; Woodcock, S.A.; Schneider, P.; Tschopp, J.; Cachero, T.G.; Batten, M.; Wheway, J.; et al. Association of BAFF/BLyS overexpression and altered B cell differentiation with Sjögren's syndrome. *J. Clin. Investig.* **2002**, *109*, 59–68. [CrossRef]
19. Becker-Merok, A.; Nikolaisen, C.; Nossent, H.C. B-lymphocyte activating factor in systemic lupus erythematosus and rheumatoid arthritis in relation to autoantibody levels, disease measures and time. *Lupus* **2006**, *15*, 570–576. [CrossRef]
20. Morel, J.; Roubille, C.; Planelles, L.; Rocha, C.; Fern, L.; Lukas, C.; Hahne, M.; Combe, B. Serum levels of tumour necrosis factor family members a proliferation-inducing ligand (APRIL) and B lymphocyte stimulator (BLyS) are inversely correlated in systemic lupus erythematosus. *Ann. Rheum. Dis.* **2009**, *68*, 997–1002. [CrossRef]
21. Salazar-Camarena, D.C.; Ortíz-Lazareno, P.; Marín-Rosales, M.; Cruz, A.; Muñoz-Valle, F.; Tapia-Llanos, R.; Orozco-Barocio, G.; Machado-Contreras, R.; Palafox-Sánchez, C.A. BAFF-R and TACI expression on CD3+ T cells: Interplay among BAFF, APRIL and T helper cytokines profile in systemic lupus erythematosus. *Cytokine* **2019**, *114*, 115–127. [CrossRef] [PubMed]
22. Marín-Rosales, M.; Cruz, A.; Salazar-Camarena, D.C.; Santillán-López, E.; Espinoza-García, N.; Muñoz-Valle, J.F.; Ramírez-Dueñas, M.G.; Oregón-Romero, E.; Orozco-Barocio, G.; Palafox-Sánchez, C.A. High BAFF expression associated with active disease in systemic lupus erythematosus and relationship with rs9514828C>T polymorphism in TNFSF13B gene. *Clin. Exp. Med.* **2019**, *19*, 183–190. [CrossRef] [PubMed]
23. Salazar-Camarena, D.C.; Ortiz-Lazareno, P.C.; Cruz, A.; Oregon-Romero, E.; Machado-Contreras, J.R.; Muñoz-Valle, J.F.; Orozco-López, M.; Marín-Rosales, M.; Palafox-Sánchez, C.A. Association of BAFF, APRIL serum levels, BAFF-R, TACI and BCMA expression on peripheral B-cell subsets with clinical manifestations in systemic lupus erythematosus. *Lupus* **2015**, *25*, 582–592. [CrossRef] [PubMed]
24. Petri, M.A.; van Vollenhoven, R.F.; Buyon, J.; Levy, R.A.; Navarra, S.V.; Cervera, R.; Zhong, Z.J.; Freimuth, W.W. Baseline Predictors of Systemic Lupus Erythematosus Flares: Data From the Combined Placebo Groups in the Phase III Belimumab Trials. *Arthritis Rheum.* **2013**, *65*, 2143–2153. [CrossRef] [PubMed]
25. Salazar-Camarena, D.C.; Palafox-Sánchez, C.A.; Cruz, A.; Marín-Rosales, M.; Muñoz-Valle, J.F. Analysis of the receptor BCMA as a biomarker in systemic lupus erythematosus patients. *Sci. Rep.* **2020**, *10*, 6236. [CrossRef] [PubMed]
26. Radin, M.; Miraglia, P.; Barinotti, A.; Fenoglio, R.; Roccatello, D.; Sciascia, S. Prognostic and Diagnostic Values of Novel Serum and Urine Biomarkers in Lupus Nephritis: A Systematic Review. *Am. J. Nephrol.* **2021**, *52*, 559–571. [CrossRef]
27. Suso, J.P.; Posso-Osorio, I.; Jiménez, C.A.; Naranjo-Escobar, J.; Ospina, F.E.; Sánchez, A.; Cañas, C.A.; Tobón, G.J. Profile of BAFF and its receptors' expression in lupus nephritis is associated with pathological classes. *Lupus* **2018**, *27*, 708–715. [CrossRef]
28. Petri, M.; Orbai, A.-M.; Alarcón, G.S.; Gordon, C.; Merrill, J.T.; Fortin, P.; Bruce, I.N.; Isenberg, D.; Wallace, D.J.; Nived, O.; et al. Derivation and validation of the Systemic Lupus International Collaborating Clinics classification criteria for systemic lupus erythematosus. *Arthritis Rheum.* **2012**, *64*, 2677–2686. [CrossRef]
29. Carrillo-Ballesteros, F.J.; Oregon-Romero, E.; Franco-Topete, R.A.; Govea-Camacho, L.H.; Cruz, A.; Muñoz-Valle, J.F.; Bustos-Rodríguez, F.J.; Pereira-Suárez, A.L.; Palafox-Sánchez, C.A. B-cell activating factor receptor expression is associated with germinal center B-cell maintenance. *Exp. Ther. Med.* **2019**, *17*, 2053–2060. [CrossRef]
30. Chatterjee, S.; Malhotra, R.; Varghese, F.; Bukhari, A.B.; Patil, A.; Budrukkar, A.; Parmar, V.; Gupta, S.; De, A. Quantitative Immunohistochemical Analysis Reveals Association between Sodium Iodide Symporter and Estrogen Receptor Expression in Breast Cancer. *PLoS ONE* **2013**, *8*, e54055. [CrossRef]
31. Inês, L.; Duarte, C.; Silva, R.S.; Teixeira, A.S.; Fonseca, F.P.; da Silva, J.A.P. Identification of clinical predictors of flare in systemic lupus erythematosus patients: A 24-month prospective cohort study. *Rheumatology* **2014**, *53*, 85–89. [CrossRef] [PubMed]
32. Tektonidou, M.G.; Dasgupta, A.; Ward, M.M. Risk of End-Stage Renal Disease in Patients With Lupus Nephritis, 1971-2015: A Systematic Review and Bayesian Meta-Analysis. *Arthritis Rheumatol.* **2016**, *68*, 1432–1441. [CrossRef] [PubMed]
33. Kudose, S.; Santoriello, D.; Bomback, A.S.; Stokes, M.B.; D'Agati, V.D.; Markowitz, G.S. Sensitivity and Specificity of Pathologic Findings to Diagnose Lupus Nephritis. *Clin. J. Am. Soc. Nephrol.* **2019**, *14*, 1605–1615. [CrossRef] [PubMed]
34. Rijnink, E.C.; Teng, Y.O.; Wilhelmus, S.; Almekinders, M.; Wolterbeek, R.; Cransberg, K.; Bruijn, J.A.; Bajema, I.M. Clinical and Histopathologic Characteristics Associated with Renal Outcomes in Lupus Nephritis. *Clin. J. Am. Soc. Nephrol.* **2017**, *12*, 734–737. [CrossRef]
35. Phatak, S.; Chaurasia, S.; Mishra, S.K.; Gupta, R.; Agrawal, V.; Aggarwal, A.; Misra, R. Urinary B cell activating factor (BAFF) and a proliferation-inducing ligand (APRIL): Potential biomarkers of active lupus nephritis. *Clin. Exp. Immunol.* **2017**, *187*, 376–382. [CrossRef]
36. Aguirre-Valencia, D.; Ríos-Serna, L.J.; Posso-Osorio, I.; Naranjo-Escobar, J.; López, D.; Bedoya-Joaqui, V.; Nieto-Aristizábal, I.; Castro, A.M.; Diaz-Ordoñez, L.; Navarro, E.P.; et al. Expression of BAFF, APRIL, and cognate receptor genes in lupus nephritis and potential use as urinary biomarkers. *J. Transl. Autoimmun.* **2020**, *3*, 100027. [CrossRef]
37. Kang, S.; Fedoriw, Y.; Brenneman, E.K.; Truong, Y.K.; Kikly, K.; Vilen, B.J. BAFF Induces Tertiary Lymphoid Structures and Positions T Cells within the Glomeruli during Lupus Nephritis. *J. Immunol.* **2017**, *198*, 1600281. [CrossRef]
38. Worthmann, K.; Gueler, F.; von Vietinghoff, S.; Davalos-Mißlitz, A.; Wiehler, F.; Davidson, A.; Witte, T.; Haller, H.; Schiffer, M.; Falk, C.S.; et al. Pathogenetic role of glomerular CXCL13 expression in lupus nephritis. *Clin. Exp. Immunol.* **2014**, *178*, 20–27. [CrossRef]

39. Kreimann, K.; Jang, M.-S.; Rong, S.; Greite, R.; Von Vietinghoff, S.; Schmitt, R.; Bräsen, J.H.; Schiffer, L.; Gerstenberg, J.; Vijayan, V.; et al. Ischemia Reperfusion Injury Triggers CXCL13 Release and B-Cell Recruitment After Allogenic Kidney Transplantation. *Front. Immunol.* **2020**, *11*, 1204. [CrossRef]
40. Schiffer, L.; Wiehler, F.; Bräsen, J.H.; Gwinner, W.; Greite, R.; Kreimann, K.; Thorenz, A.; Derlin, K.; Teng, B.; Rong, S.; et al. Chemokine CXCL13 as a New Systemic Biomarker for B-Cell Involvement in Acute T Cell-Mediated Kidney Allograft Rejection. *Int. J. Mol. Sci.* **2019**, *20*, 2552. [CrossRef]
41. Schwarting, A.; Relle, M.; Meineck, M.; Föhr, B.; Triantafyllias, K.; Weinmann, A.; Roth, W.; Weinmann-Menke, J. Renal tubular epithelial cell-derived BAFF expression mediates kidney damage and correlates with activity of proliferative lupus nephritis in mouse and men. *Lupus* **2018**, *27*, 243–256. [CrossRef] [PubMed]
42. Alexaki, V.-I.; Notas, G.; Pelekanou, V.; Kampa, M.; Valkanou, M.; Theodoropoulos, P.; Stathopoulos, E.N.; Tsapis, A.; Castanas, E. Adipocytes as Immune Cells: Differential Expression of TWEAK, BAFF, and APRIL and Their Receptors (Fn14, BAFF-R, TACI, and BCMA) at Different Stages of Normal and Pathological Adipose Tissue Development. *J. Immunol.* **2009**, *183*, 5948–5956. [CrossRef] [PubMed]
43. Alexaki, V.-I.; Pelekanou, V.; Notas, G.; Venihaki, M.; Kampa, M.; Dessirier, V.; Sabour-Alaoui, S.; Stathopoulos, E.N.; Tsapis, A.; Castanas, E. B-Cell Maturation Antigen (BCMA) Activation Exerts Specific Proinflammatory Effects in Normal Human Keratinocytes and Is Preferentially Expressed in Inflammatory Skin Pathologies. *Endocrinology* **2012**, *153*, 739–749. [CrossRef] [PubMed]
44. Kim, K.S.; Park, J.-Y.; Jou, I.; Park, S.M. Functional implication of BAFF synthesis and release in gangliosides-stimulated microglia. *J. Leukoc. Biol.* **2009**, *86*, 349–359. [CrossRef] [PubMed]
45. Blair, H.A.; Duggan, S.T. Belimumab: A Review in Systemic Lupus Erythematosus. *Drugs* **2018**, *78*, 355–366. [CrossRef]
46. Furie, R.; Rovin, B.H.; Houssiau, F.; Malvar, A.; Teng, Y.O.; Contreras, G.; Amoura, Z.; Yu, X.; Mok, C.-C.; Santiago, M.B.; et al. Two-Year, Randomized, Controlled Trial of Belimumab in Lupus Nephritis. *N. Engl. J. Med.* **2020**, *383*, 1117–1128. [CrossRef]
47. Shrestha, S.; Budhathoki, P.; Adhikari, Y.; Marasini, A.; Bhandari, S.; Mir, W.A.Y.; Shrestha, D.B. Belimumab in Lupus Nephritis: A Systematic Review and Meta-Analysis. *Cureus* **2021**, *13*, e20440. [CrossRef]
48. Atisha-Fregoso, Y.; Malkiel, S.; Harris, K.M.; Byron, M.; Ding, L.; Kanaparthi, S.; Barry, W.T.; Gao, W.; Ryker, K.; Tosta, P.; et al. Phase II Randomized Trial of Rituximab Plus Cyclophosphamide Followed by Belimumab for the Treatment of Lupus Nephritis. *Arthritis Rheumatol.* **2021**, *73*, 121–131. [CrossRef]

Disclaimer/Publisher's Note: The statements, opinions and data contained in all publications are solely those of the individual author(s) and contributor(s) and not of MDPI and/or the editor(s). MDPI and/or the editor(s) disclaim responsibility for any injury to people or property resulting from any ideas, methods, instructions or products referred to in the content.

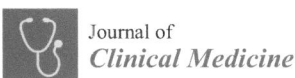

Journal of
Clinical Medicine

Review

Biomarkers in Systemic Lupus Erythematosus along with Metabolic Syndrome

Fernanda Isadora Corona-Meraz [1,2,*,†], Mónica Vázquez-Del Mercado [2,3,4], Flavio Sandoval-García [2,4], Jesus-Aureliano Robles-De Anda [2], Alvaro-Jovanny Tovar-Cuevas [1], Roberto-Carlos Rosales-Gómez [1], Milton-Omar Guzmán-Ornelas [1], Daniel González-Inostroz [2], Miguel Peña-Nava [2] and Beatriz-Teresita Martín-Márquez [2,4,*,†]

1. Multidisciplinary Health Research Center, Department of Biomedical Sciences, University Center of Tonala, University of Guadalajara, Guadalajara 45425, Jalisco, Mexico; alvaro.tovar@academicos.udg.mx (A.-J.T.-C.); roberto.rosales@academicos.udg.mx (R.-C.R.-G.); milton.guzman@academicos.udg.mx (M.-O.G.-O.)
2. Department of Molecular Biology and Genomics, Institute of Rheumatology and Musculoskeletal System Research, University Center of Health Sciences, University of Guadalajara, Guadalajara 44340, Jalisco, Mexico; dravme@hotmail.com (M.V.-D.M.); flavio.sandoval@academicos.udg.mx (F.S.-G.); jesus.robles@academicos.udg.mx (J.-A.R.-D.A.); dgi-17@hotmail.com (D.G.-I.); miguel.pena4206@alumnos.udg.mx (M.P.-N.)
3. Rheumatology Service, Internal Medicine Division, Civil Hospital of Guadalajara "Dr. Juan I. Menchaca", Guadalajara 44340, Jalisco, Mexico
4. Academic Group UDG-CA-703, "Immunology and Rheumatology", University Center of Health Sciences, University of Guadalajara, Guadalajara 44340, Jalisco, Mexico
* Correspondence: mariaf.corona@academicos.udg.mx (F.I.C.-M.); beatriz.martin@academicos.udg.mx (B.-T.M.-M.)
† These authors contributed equally to this work.

Abstract: Metabolic syndrome (MetS) is a group of physiological abnormalities characterized by obesity, insulin resistance (IR), and hypertriglyceridemia, which carry the risk of developing cardiovascular disease (CVD) and type 2 diabetes (T2D). Immune and metabolic alterations have been observed in MetS and are associated with autoimmune development. Systemic lupus erythematosus (SLE) is an autoimmune disease caused by a complex interaction of environmental, hormonal, and genetic factors and hyperactivation of immune cells. Patients with SLE have a high prevalence of MetS, in which elevated CVD is observed. Among the efforts of multidisciplinary healthcare teams to make an early diagnosis, a wide variety of factors have been considered and associated with the generation of biomarkers. This review aimed to elucidate some primary biomarkers and propose a set of assessments to improve the projection of the diagnosis and evolution of patients. These biomarkers include metabolic profiles, cytokines, cardiovascular tests, and microRNAs (miRs), which have been observed to be dysregulated in these patients and associated with outcomes.

Keywords: MetS; SLE; adipokines; CVD; microRNA

1. Introduction

Metabolic syndrome (MetS) is considered a noncommunicable disease in which the individual presents with three or more risk factors, including elevated blood pressure, large waist circumference, hyperglycemia, hypertriglyceridemia, low levels of high-density cholesterol (HDL-c), insulin resistance (IR), and increased blood pressure [1]. MetS is strongly associated with obesity and adiposity, determinants that resemble the phenotype of obesity-related IR, vascular stiffness, and endothelial dysfunction [2]. MetS is associated with cardiovascular disease (CVD), and one of the most critical etiological backgrounds of this pathology lies in the persistent metabolic alterations produced by adipose tissue dysfunction, which releases inflammatory cytokines, bioactive products such as adipokines, gaseous messengers, and microvesicles that alter the attached tissue phenotype and create reactions and molecules that are detectable at the systemic level [3,4].

The worldwide prevalence of MetS differs between populations due to different lifestyles. One of the most important modifiable factors is consuming a Western-pattern diet, characterized by processed and refined foods, red and processed meats, foods with added sugar and saturated and trans fats, and a low consumption of vegetables, fruits, nuts, and whole grains [5,6]. The prevalence of MetS differs between sexes, with females being the most affected [2,7–9].

On the other hand, immune–metabolic interactions observed in MetS have been associated with the development of autoimmune diseases, such as rheumatoid arthritis, ankylosing spondylitis, and systemic lupus erythematosus (SLE), among others [10].

SLE is the archetypical pathology of autoimmune diseases characterized by a wide range of clinical manifestations caused mainly by a complex interplay of environmental, hormonal, and genetic factors and the hyperactivation of immune cells [11].

In SLE, the breakdown of immune tolerance is essential for activating autoreactive B cells, consequently producing self-reactive antibodies. Autoantibodies such as anti-Smith (anti-Sm), anti-double-stranded DNA (anti-dsDNA), and anti-ribonucleoprotein (anti-RNP) are considered as hallmarks in SLE; nevertheless, these autoimmune diseases show a broad spectrum of more than 200 autoantibodies [12,13].

The mechanisms by which the autoantibodies cause tissue damage are mainly related to the accumulation of immune complexes, cytotoxicity, reactivity with autoantigens on the apoptotic cell surface, cell surface binding, and penetration into living cells [14].

During the clinical course of the disease, a wide range of organs may be affected, including skin, joints, lungs, heart, kidneys, hematological cells, and vascular and brain systems [12].

Regarding the vascular system, it has been documented that approximately 50% of SLE patients present with lupus vasculitis (LV), which mainly involves small- and medium-sized vessels. LV has many clinical forms that depend on the affected vessels and the site involved. The proposed pathogenic mechanism of LV is related to a complex interaction among vascular endothelium, immune cells, and their products, such as cytokines and autoantibodies, among which are antiphospholipid antibody (aPL) positivity, anti-endothelial cell antibodies, antineutrophil cytoplasmic antibodies (ANCA), and anti-dsDNA [15].

SLE patients are prone to suffer from cardiovascular diseases (CVDs) due to significant metabolic alterations in several pathways (i.e., lipoprotein metabolism) that might contribute to CVD pathology [16]. Indeed, a high prevalence of MetS has been reported in cohorts of SLE patients and is associated with increased disease activity, inflammation, and organ damage. MetS is recognized as a common comorbidity component of autoimmune diseases, where obesity has been associated with a low health-related quality of life in SLE patients [17].

Dietary intake and systemic metabolism are associated with the differentiation of the immune system. In this sense, it has been observed that the rates of autoimmunity are increasing in parallel with MetS, supporting the hypothesis that diet-induced obesity exacerbates autoimmune manifestations [18]. The activation of the immune system is necessary to initiate the production of interferon type I (IFN-I) and self-antigen-specific autoantibodies [19].

In experimental studies, obesity is related to the production of IFN-I by expanding plasmacytoid dendritic cells (pDCs) in visceral adipose tissue (VAT). Consequently, IFN-I impaired the number and function of T regulatory (Treg) cells, which could promote an autoimmune inflammatory microenvironment [17].

Since proinflammatory cytokines are a common underlying mechanism involving SLE and obesity, MetS probably triggers and contributes to overall inflammation, oxidative stress, and endothelial dysfunction [20].

Due to similarities in specific molecules' expression in SLE and MetS, it is relevant to identify predictive biomarkers that contribute to an early and timely diagnosis in conjunction with the clinical assessment.

2. Metabolic Dysregulation in SLE and Its Biomarkers

Reports have revealed that the prevalence of MetS in SLE patients in individual studies ranges between 3.3 and 45.2% [20]. In this regard, it has been reported that SLE patients exhibit a profound alteration in lipoprotein metabolism pathways characterized by an increase in serum levels of total cholesterol, triglycerides (TG), apolipoprotein B (ApoB), and LDL-c and reduced HDL-c and apolipoprotein A1 (ApoA1) [16,21].

Moreover, it has been shown that, in SLE, the values of oxidized and dysfunctional HDL-c increase, contributing to the development of atherosclerosis and promoting an inflammatory response of macrophages through the activation of nuclear factor kappa-light-chain-enhancer of activated B cells (NF-κB) and the formation of neutrophil extracellular traps (NETs) and lipoprotein oxidation [22].

Although lipid profile is a crucial standard for assessing CVD risk in SLE patients, glucose and insulin levels are essential for assessing IR, a clinical state characterized by reduced insulin efficacy associated with increased insulin release and elevated blood concentration in an attempt to obtain an effective response to circulating glucose levels [23].

MetS patients are prone to develop IR, and the increment of fat mass could result in adipose tissue inflammation, a source of proinflammatory cytokines that can potentiate systemic inflammation [24]. For instance, tumor necrosis factor-alpha (TNF-α) is considered a central proinflammatory cytokine studied in IR that modulates the activity and expression of enzymes blocking insulin function [25]. High levels of TNF-α have been found in SLE patients with active lupus, demonstrating the enhanced risk of IR in these patients [26].

On the other hand, insulin levels and the homeostasis model assessment-estimated insulin resistance (HOMA-IR) index are increased in patients with SLE and SLE with MetS compared to healthy controls [27]. Studies in the literature have shown that SLE patients manifest deficient insulin secretion and a greater risk of IR. For instance, Petri et al. found that 7% of SLE patients present with type 2 diabetes mellitus (T2D), and 10% had glucose intolerance, showing that T2D may be more frequent in these patients than is estimated [28]. El Magadmi and colleagues found hyperinsulinemia and reduced insulin sensitivity in a cohort of SLE patients, where 18% had MetS [29]. For their part, Contreras et al. noticed that the increased waist circumference, higher acid uric levels, and longer duration of hypertension are factors associated with IR in SLE patients [30].

Regarding the metabolic disturbance that can be detected in SLE, Tang et al. recently found that, by analyzing metabolite profiles using mass spectrometry techniques with multiple reaction monitoring, SLE patients show alterations in fatty acid and phospholipid catabolism and elevated levels of pyroglutamic acid and L-phenylalanine [31].

Considering that, in SLE, the production of autoantibodies is a hallmark of this autoimmune disease, it has been noticed that specific autoantibodies contribute to atherosclerosis in pathology, such as anti-HDL-IgG related to induce LDL to enter the endothelial cells (EC) and anti-apolipoprotein A1 (ApoA1)-IgG, which induces the activation of NF-kB and favors the expression of inflammatory factors, among which are TNF-α, interleukin-6 (IL-6), interleukin-8 (IL-8), C-C motif chemokine ligand 2 (CCL2), and metalloproteinase 9 [32].

Furthermore, it has been observed that antibodies against lipoprotein lipase (anti-LPL) have been associated with increased levels of TG, Apo-E, and Apo-B in patients with SLE [33]. In addition, the production of autoantibodies such as aPL that are anticardiolipin antibodies (aCL) and anti-β2-glycoprotein I antibodies (anti-β2GPI) could increase endothelial injury and promote the induction of the proinflammatory endothelial phenotype interacting with endothelial cells (EC) [32].

At this point, we consider it essential to illustrate that the differences in affinity of antibody and antigen interactions are discriminated by the fragment crystallizable region receptor (FcR) that induces different signals at the molecule level, resulting in various immunological reactions [14]. For instance, IgG isotype antiphospholipid antibodies display a more predictive value of the vascular manifestation than IgM, while IgA aPL can be more predictive for vascular events than IgM [34].

3. Cytokines and Adipokines in SLE along with MetS

Cytokine production is closely related to the immune system response. Elevated levels of proinflammatory cytokines have been observed in SLE and MetS. Whereas one principal goal in SLE cytokine profile analysis is to identify cytokines as biomarkers that can be used to identify disease status and predict flares, in MetS, the analysis of molecules related to metabolism regulation, such as adipokines, is essential.

In obesity, the adipose tissue expansion is a primary source of proinflammatory cytokines. During homeostatic conditions, the adipose tissue-resident immune cells produce anti-inflammatory cytokines such as interleukin 4 (IL-4), IL-5, IL-10, IL-13, and transforming growth factor beta (TGF-β). The adipose tissue macrophages (ATM) are polarized to an M2 phenotype and enrich the adipose immune system together with other immune cells such as regulatory invariant natural killer T cells (iNKT), type 2 innate lymphoid cells (ILC2), regulatory T cells (Treg), and eosinophils, among others [35]. Meanwhile, in obesity, saturated fatty acids induce the ATM to polarize to an M1 phenotype, producing IL-6, TNF-α, IL-12, and IL-1β, among other inflammatory factors contributing to the impairment of insulin signaling and promoting IR [36].

Since obesity and overweight are identified risk factors for the development of metabolic disturbances in SLE, quantifying proinflammatory cytokines results in utility for its diagnosis and management. Different studies on SLE have determined increased IL-6 levels and their association with disease activity. Ding et al. performed a meta-analysis of 24 studies that showed serum IL-6 levels in SLE patients are higher than those in healthy controls and correlate with SLE activity [37]. Furthermore, IL-6 has also been associated with metabolic disorders such as MetS and T2D, in which elevated levels of IL-6 have been observed in adipose tissue [38].

On the other hand, TNF-α is a proinflammatory cytokine detected in high concentrations in SLE and correlates with disease activity and lupus nephritis. However, TNF-α has been found as a mediator of inflammation and regulator of autoimmunity, exerting in SLE a dual role [39]. Regarding the role of TNF-α in MetS, some reports indicate that it acts as an essential inducer of atherosclerotic plaques by driving the expression of adhesion molecules and favoring the activation of immune cells within the arterial wall [40]. Moreover, it is well documented that TNF-α promotes lipolysis, increases free fatty acid (FFA), and influences metabolic dysregulations such as IR. Furthermore, TNF-α can inhibit insulin-stimulated tyrosine kinase activity of the insulin receptor and substrate by inducing serine phosphorylation and producing IR [41].

On the other hand, it is known that adipocytes are not considered energy storage cells only; they are active producers of a specific type of cytokines called adipokines, which exert endocrine, paracrine, and autocrine effects [19]. Adipocytes play a crucial role in energy homeostasis regulation. The mechanism by which they accomplish this is through the secretion of adiponectin, leptin, resistin, IFN-I, TNF-α, interleukin 1 (IL-1), IL-6, and plasmin activator inhibitor type 1 (PAI-1), which are cytokines that take part in cellular intercommunication and act as master regulators of inflammation and metabolism that could influence the metabolic dysregulation in SLE and MetS [5,42].

In an obese state, an imbalance of adipokines promotes a low-grade proinflammatory state, resulting in IR and vascular dysregulation [43]. In addition to the above, it is known that in an autoimmune context, adipokines are involved in inflammatory pathways that affect a wide range of cell types, influencing systemic inflammation, chronically damaging tissues and organs, and impacting quality of life. In order to consider adipokines as biomarker candidates for SLE and MetS, we will describe those mainly associated with both pathologies.

Leptin is the main adipokine produced by adipocytes, whose concentrations positively correlate with adipose tissue mass. Leptin is involved in low-grade inflammation due to overweight and obesity and is considered a proinflammatory adipokine [44]. In SLE patients, leptin is highly produced; however, it does not correlate with disease activity [45].

Hyperleptinemia and leptin resistance are closely associated with obesity and T2D, and lower leptin concentrations in circulation are correlated positively with improved insulin sensitivity, lipid metabolism, lower adiposity, and inflammation [23].

Adiponectin is an adipokine that exerts anti-inflammatory effects. It is a complex molecule produced by adipocytes of the white adipose tissue (WAT), and its concentrations are inversely correlated with body mass index (BMI). Some of adiponectin's functions are fatty acid biosynthesis and the inhibition of gluconeogenesis in the liver. It has been shown that, under systemic inflammation, adiponectin levels are modified, so an increase or decrease in its concentrations may be associated with pathophysiological conditions [44].

In SLE, higher adiponectin levels correlate positively with SLE severity and negatively with IR; however, when studies evaluate causal effects between circulating adiponectin levels and SLE, there are no relationship between circulating adiponectin levels and SLE risk [46].

Resistin is a cysteine-rich peptide hormone discovered in adipose tissue of rodents and detected in human peripheral blood mononuclear cells. Its functions are related to promoting immune response to inflammatory processes and enhancing heart, liver, and kidney diseases. In rodents, it has been found that WAT resistin secretion is associated with BMI and IR; in humans, the role of resistin in IR and T2D is controversial [47].

Adipsin is an adipokine mainly synthesized and secreted from WAT and exerts its functions by modulating glucose and lipid metabolism. Clinical data associate adipsin levels with BMI and visceral adipose tissue, whereas molecular assays reported that adipsin increases lipid accumulation and adipocyte differentiation through peroxisome proliferator-activated receptor (PPAR-γ) induction and complement component 3a (C3a) release [48]. Adipsin levels were found in higher concentrations in autoimmune diseases. However, further studies are needed to assess the association of adipsin with SLE [18].

Chemerin is an adipokine and chemoattractive protein that promotes inflammation, contributes to adipogenesis and glucose metabolism, and correlates with MetS [49]. In SLE, chemerin may serve as a marker of lupus nephritis (LN), where its circulating levels correlate with renal function [50].

Visfatin, also known as nicotinamide phosphoribosyl transferase (Nampt) was discovered as an insulin-mimetic adipokine produced mainly by visceral and subcutaneous adipose tissue, liver, immune cells, skeletal muscle, brain cells, cardiomyocytes, and renal glomeruli, among others. Its main functions are increasing glucose uptake by peripheral tissues, decreasing gluconeogenesis and glucose release, and stimulating the insulin cascade. In obesity, increased visfatin levels are related to a regulatory response to maintain glucose in stable levels; however, if the threshold is exceeded, visfatin is associated with inflammation and T2D, IR, CVD, and renal damage [51,52].

The role of visfatin in SLE is strongly associated with LN in humans and with pulmonary vasculitis and alveolar hemorrhage in experimental lupus models [53,54].

Omentin-1 is an adipokine expressed in higher levels in visceral adipose tissue; its concentrations decrease in overweight and obesity and increase after weight loss. Its biological activity is related to the enhancement of insulin-stimulated glucose uptake in human adipocytes [55]. Plasmatic omentin-1 levels were detected in differential expression between SLE patients with and without LN, suggesting that this adipokine could be employed as an auxiliary index [56].

Table 1 summarizes the results of different analyses in which adipokine serum or plasma levels were quantified in SLE and MetS studies.

Table 1. SLE and MetS adipokine levels.

Adipokines [1]	SLE	MetS	SLE and MetS	Ref.
Leptin	Increase	Increase	Increase with MetS	[45,57–59]
Adiponectin	Increase	Decrease	Decrease with MetS	[42,58,59]
Resistin	Increase	Increase	Increase with MetS	[42,58]
Chemerin	Increase (LN)	Increase	No data found	[50,60]
Visfatin	Increase (LN)	Increase	No data found	[51,54,61]
Omentin-1	Decrease	Decrease	No data found	[55,62]
Adipsin	Increase	Increase	No data found	[48,62]

[1] Serum or plasma levels. Abbreviatures: LN: lupus nephritis.

4. Cardiovascular Clinical Assessments in SLE

Systemic inflammation is associated with the disease progression, and metabolic dysregulation in SLE can accelerate cardiovascular complications. The proinflammatory response is caused not only by the autoimmune underlying condition but also by the adipose tissue, which, if sustained, will magnify the risk of developing other metabolic and cardiovascular diseases.

Metabolic dysregulation is part of the deteriorating clinical status of a patient with SLE due to the increased risk of CVD, which, according to several studies, is higher than in the general population [10]. Esdaile and colleagues noticed that SLE patients present with a >7-fold higher risk of coronary heart disease (CHD) or stroke and 17-fold risk of having severe CHD death. Nevertheless, traditional Framingham risk factors cannot fully explain the significant CHD risk increase and, therefore, could be multifactorial due to a proatherogenic lipid profile, immune dysregulation and inflammation, side effects of treatment, and microvascular dysfunction [63,64]. Subsequently, in the Hopkins Lupus cohort, Magder and Petri et al. described that patients with SLE have a risk of cardiovascular events 2.66 times higher than expected in the general population with similar levels of traditional risk factors [65].

Oliviera et al. suggested that SLE patients should be assessed with classical CVD-related risks and disease activity parameters, such as aberrant adaptive immune response, proinflammatory cytokine signaling, elevated IFN-I, dysregulated NET formation, dysfunctional HDL-c, and oxidative stress [66]. Likewise, to observe any increased CVD risk, the European Alliance of Associations for Rheumatology (EULAR) recommendations state the measurement of traditional and disease-associated cardiovascular risk factors as necessary. For example, blood pressure (<130/80 mm/Hg), urine protein/creatinine ratio (>500 mg/g), QRISK3 assessment, and the American College of Cardiology/American Heart Association risk equation, although it is recognized that further studies are needed to validate cut-off points in this population. In addition, risk scores for the systemic lupus erythematosus disease activity index (SLEDAI), lupus anticoagulant, and C3a measurements are recommended [66].

Regarding the evaluation of atheroma plaque formation and atherosclerosis, it is considered essential to measure coronary artery calcifications and carotid intima-media thickness by techniques such as pulse wave velocity (PWV) or endothelium-dependent flow-mediated vasodilatation (ED-FMD), which are considered biophysical markers of endothelial dysfunction [67].

In a meta-analysis performed for SLE, the patients presented significantly higher PWV than controls; these results were associated with BMI and disease duration [68]. On the other hand, in studies performed in brachial artery ED-FMD (baED-FMD), SLE patients had lower baED-FMD than controls, reflecting impaired endothelial function [67].

Analyses carried out in this regard performed on SLE patients showed that those patients formed 2.0 times more atherosclerotic plaques in the carotid and femoral arteries than patients with rheumatoid arthritis and T2D and presented with 32% more atherosclerosis in the carotid compared to healthy controls [69]. In relation to the data previously shown, it has been determined that the risk of myocardial infarction in SLE is 2 to 3 times higher than in the general population [70].

To obtain an accurate diagnosis, other diagnostic tools, such as magnetic resonance imaging (MRI), must be considered. For instance, Mavrogeni et al. detected by MRI 27.5% silent cardiac abnormalities/past abnormalities such as myocarditis, myocardial infarctions, or vasculitis [71]. It is necessary to consider that antiphospholipid syndrome (APS) adds significant inflammatory thrombotic and atherosclerotic risks since there is an increased endothelial risk due to decreased endothelial nitric oxide synthase. As a result of APS, the increased production of nitric oxide, proinflammatory cytokines, adhesion molecules, and reactive oxygen species (ROS) and the activation of monocytes and the classical complement pathway are generated, further contributing to vascular inflammation [72].

Likewise, the use of glucocorticoids has been associated with atherosclerosis, hypertension, T2D, hypercholesterolemia, and CVD, even with the use of doses lower than those recommended. Although their use produces potent anti-inflammatory effects by reducing B and T lymphocyte activity, prostaglandin synthesis, and cyclooxygenases, it was observed that one-third of SLE patients are resistant to this treatment, probably due to modifications in the glucocorticoid receptor [65,73].

On the other hand, hydroxychloroquine (HQC) has been used to treat inflammatory diseases such as SLE, other autoimmune and neoplastic disorders, and metabolic and infectious diseases. When HQC is used in patients with SLE, some signs and symptoms, such as fatigue, skin rashes, joint pain, mouth ulcers, and arthralgia, improve and inhibit the production of inflammatory cytokines [74,75]. In addition, a decrease in aortic stiffness, systemic vascular resistance, and increased elasticity of the large arteries has been noticed; therefore, HQC therapy in SLE exerts a protective effect on coronary artery disease [76,77].

One of the proposed HQC action mechanisms is the reduction in ROS production, which decreases oxidative stress and improves the endothelial function. On the other hand, it has been observed that HQC increases LDL-c receptor expression and decreases serum cholesterol and TG concentration. At the same time, HQC inhibits cytokine production, apoptosis, and autophagy. According to the EULAR recommendations, HQC is classified as one of the disease-modifying antirheumatic drugs (DMARDs), and its use is widely recommended [74,76].

5. MicroRNAs in SLE with MetS Background

About the etiopathogenesis of SLE, it is currently known that both genetic and epigenetic factors may contribute to the development of autoimmunity. Nevertheless, it is also accepted that microRNAs (miRs) could be considered valuable biomarkers in diagnosis, treatment response, and general disease monitoring. The miRs have been evaluated from different perspectives, and, at a certain point, the large number of miRs that have been reported becomes overwhelming; however, between SLE and MetS, the associations made punctually between both pathologies are rare.

The miRs, typically known as non-coding regulatory RNA, are a class of small RNAs (about 22–25 nucleotides) that exert a crucial role in regulating the expression of its target genes at the post-transcriptional level [61]. It has been observed that miRs control the immune system as epigenetic regulatory elements regulating cellular development and differentiation [78]. As for miR biogenesis, the process is known to be as follows: miR genes are transcribed to generate an extended primary transcript (pri-miRNA) and processed to generate pre-miRNA in the nuclei. After being exported to the cytoplasm, the pre-miRNAs are processed to mature miRs by RNase III Dicer and then loaded into Argonaute (Ago) to form the RNA-induced silencing complex (RISC) effector, which represses translation [79]. Thus, miRs are considered an essential contributor to regulating the genes involved in the immune response because the RISC can silence messenger RNA at the pre-translational, co-translational, and post-translational levels, regulating 40% of the genes that control the differentiation of immune cells. their functions, and autoantibodies' production [80].

The miR action is produced not only in the cells where they are synthesized but also can be transported to other target cells and found in the peripheral circulation. It also acts as a soluble marker sensitive to general health conditions. Furthermore, the most studied miRs in SLE are regulated by the expression of immune stimuli, like the presence of antigens, toll-like receptor (TLR) ligands, and inflammatory cytokines [81].

In SLE, NF-kB and IFN-I are deregulated pathways that interfere with inflammation. This pathway could be regulated by miR-146a and miR-155, which show potential for inhibition in the translation of IFN pathway signaling proteins such as TNF receptor-associated factor 6 (TRAF6), IL-1 receptor-associated kinase 1 (IRAK1), IFN regulatory factor 5 (IFN-5), and signal transducer and activator of transcription (STAT1) [82]. In a study by El-Akhras and colleagues in patients with SLE, they found that miR-146a was significantly increased in peripheral blood mononuclear cells (PBMC) and correlated positively with IL-6; based on these findings, they considered it a marketable marker for this autoimmune disease [83]. Additionally, Li et al. found in SLE patients that exosomal miR-155 is upregulated, whereas exosomal miR-146a was downregulated in SLE patients [84].

Regarding metabolic disturbances, it was observed that miR-146a is downregulated in obesity and correlates negatively with IL-6, TNF-α, and CD36 [85].

Another miR implicated in SLE pathology is miR-124, which modulates TLR-4-induced cytokine production by targeting signal transducers and STAT3 to decrease IL-6 production and TNF-α release. Zhang and colleagues found that miR-124 is downregulated in LN and could be considered as a significant diagnostic marker [86]. In addition, Yan et al. noticed that circulating miR-124-3p and miR-377-3p were significantly upregulated in SLE, where miR-124-3p is associated with antiC1q and C3, and miR-377-3p was determined as an independent predictor [87]. Concerning the influence of miR-124 in metabolic disorders, studies have revealed that miR-124 was highly expressed in T2D patients and related to lipid and glucose metabolism [88].

MiR-143/145 are intronic miRs expressed in endothelial cells that act in the differentiation and proliferation of vascular smooth muscle cells (VSMC) in the kidney; miR-145 is expressed in epithelial cells of proximal convoluted tubules and VSMC of renal vessels of children with LN, where its lower expression levels are related with the increase in vascular damage [81]. Moreover, increased levels of miR-143/145 in serum have been proposed as a potential diagnostic marker of SLE [89]. In T2D patients, miR-143 was detected in higher expression and associated with hypertension, increased body weight, glucose homeostasis, and impaired insulin activation [90].

Studies have observed that the miR-145 previously described acts as a positive regulator of the adipogenesis process and is related to the increase in adipose tissue/adipocytes in humans and rodents. Moreover, miR-145 promotes TNF-α secretion and lipolysis via NF-kB in vitro, showing their role in inflammation and cellular differentiation [91].

On the other hand, miR-125a negatively regulates the CCL5 upon activation of normal T cell expressed and secreted (RANTES); this proinflammatory cytokine is elevated in SLE and MetS [80].

Notably, the various treatment regimens for SLE can be considered a factor that may influence the expression of miRs and may be considered a biomarker of monitoring treatment response. For instance, Cecchi and colleagues observed that in SLE patients, rituximab affects the expression of circulating miRs, identifying a panel of five miRs, including miR-149-3p, miR-125b-5p, miR-199a-5p, miR-106b-3p, and miR-124-3p, as a potential target associated with proinflammatory cytokines and immune receptors [92]. These remarkable findings in the expression changes in miRs before and after treatment provide valuable information for future immunomodulation and diagnostic therapies of SLE.

6. MetS and SLE: A Harmful Relationship

MetS is a group of different physiological abnormalities with a metabolic background; in SLE, there is a high prevalence of MetS with a higher probability of developing heart disease [93,94]. Among the efforts of multidisciplinary health teams, proposals for early markers for detection, markers to assess the severity of the disease, and even markers to observe the response to treatment stand out. However, the more markers are studied, the more knowledge needs to appear; mainly, it has been observed how inflammation has a leading role in mediating both pathologies and, to a large extent, the release of cytokines mediates this inflammation [95]. In Figure 1, we propose a set of assessments to better project the diagnosis and evolution of patients with SLE and MetS. Biomarkers include metabolic, immunometabolic, clinical, and miR parameters, which are dysregulated in these patients and are associated with disease severity.

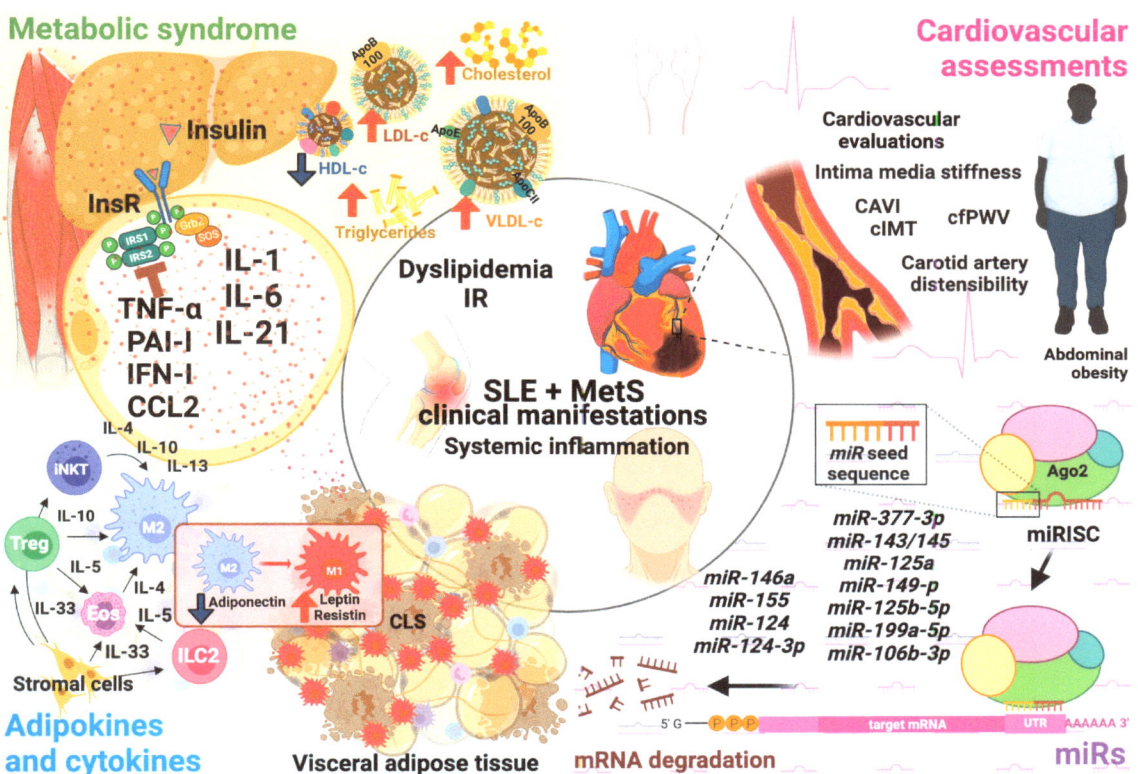

Figure 1. Systemic inflammation is the cornerstone where both pathologies converge and participate in the origin of clinical manifestations, development, and deterioration. Adipose tissue homeostasis becomes dysregulated as abnormal accumulation, and redistribution of body fat occurs during overweight and obesity due to chronic positive energy balance. This process modifies the immune cell population along with the T_H2 cytokine microenvironment. It overcomes angiogenic and tissue remodeling capabilities to overcome adipocyte hypoxia and oxidative and concomitant endoplasmic reticulum stress, leading to proinflammatory adipokine and cytokine turnover. The resulting decrease in adiponectin and increase in proinflammatory adipocytokines and immune cells locally interfere with insulin signaling and adipocyte fatty acid metabolism. As this T_H1 profile spreads through the bloodstream, other actively metabolic organs, such as the liver, muscle, and blood vessels, are affected by this deleterious condition and establish systemic inflammation, insulin resistance, and lipid dysregulation. Consequently, cardiovascular comorbidities develop, which, together with metabolic alterations, are already pathogenic features of SLE, exponentially increasing the severity,

activity, and clinical deterioration of the disease. MiRs are involved in all substantial parts of the etiology, pathophysiology, and progression of both SLE and MetS, as they are critical regulators of gene expression of cytokines, adipokines, cell growth factors, and metabolic switches. Moreover, their expression and regulatory activity can be modified by conditions such as hypoxia and interleukins, impacting their tissue and circulating levels, making them potential specific and sensitive biomarkers for diagnosis, disease development prediction, and disease severity progression. Abbreviatures: SLE: systemic lupus erythematosus; MetS: metabolic syndrome; IR: insulin resistance; InsR: insulin receptor; IRS-1: insulin receptor substrate-1; IRS-2: insulin receptor substrate-1; Grb2: growth factor receptor-bound protein 2; SOS: son of sevenless protein; ApoB: apolipoprotein B; LDL-c: low-density lipoprotein cholesterol; HDL-c: high-density lipoprotein cholesterol; VLDL-c: very-low-density lipoprotein cholesterol; TNF-α: tumor necrosis factor-alpha; PAI-1: plasminogen activator inhibitor-1; IFN-I: interferon type I; CCL2: C-C motif chemokine ligand 2; IL-1: interleukin-1; IL-6: interleukin-6; IL-21: interleukin-21; IL-4: interleukin-4; IL-10: interleukin-10; IL-13: interleukin-13; IL-5: interleukin-5; IL-33: interleukin-33; iNKT: invariant natural killer T cells; Treg: regulatory T cells; Eos: eosinophils; ILC2: type 2 innate lymphoid cells; M2: macrophages type 2; M1: macrophages type 1; CLS: crown-like structures; CAVI: cardio-ankle vascular index; cIMT: carotid intima-media thickness; cfPWV: carotid–femoral pulse wave; miR: microRNA; mRNA: messenger RNA; Ago2: argonaute-2; miRISC: miRNA-induced silencing complex; UTR: untranslated region; T_H1: T cell helper 1; T_H2: T cell helper 2. Created with BioRender.com. Agreement number VW26L47W1D.

In the clinical history of the disease, essential studies must be carried out on the patients, firstly, to define if the condition exists and, consequently, to determine the activity of the disease [96]. The constant stimulation of the immune system in SLE leads to the production of autoantibodies, the deposition of immune complexes, and the expression and secretion of cytokines. These cytokines are part of the activation of the cells of the immune system, which secrete more cytokines, creating a positive feedback cycle; this can cause the disease to become more severe at certain times [97]. Many of these cytokines also modulate their expression profile in MetS, and there is an exact association between these profiles and both diseases [98].

Few studies detail the presence or absence of MetS when evaluating cytokines or adipokines in SLE despite the relationship between both pathologies. Indeed, although the origin of inflammation is different, the mechanisms of execution of the immune system are similar.

Certainly, obesity has been considered a promoter of autoimmune diseases; in particular, the increase in fat mass has been associated with MetS and the inflammatory response, and it is located as an etiological factor of many diseases, including atherosclerosis, vascular events' mortality, and TD2 [99,100]. However, the precise mechanisms by which it favors the progression of said pathologies still need to be established.

Obesity is the leading cause of developing CVD, which has produced a significant number of causes of death in patients with SLE [100]. That is why continuous surveillance of CVD risk is so important. In a certain way, it is not so common for patients with autoimmune diseases to carry out close surveillance with a cardiologist. However, now it has become a clinical necessity due to the various studies that associate the increased risk in these patients.

Finally, among the newest markers are miRs, which have been studied in various pathologies, such as detection, in response to treatment, and even as future therapies. The miRs have been evaluated from different perspectives, and, at a certain point, the large number of miRs that have been reported becomes overwhelming; however, between SLE and MetS, the associations made punctually between both pathologies are rare.

7. Conclusions

SLE is a complex pathology with different clinical moments throughout its course, during which various factors intervene in the disease's severity and the appropriate immune response. On the other hand, MetS comprises metabolic alterations that, when present in a patient with SLE, potentiate the abnormal cellular imbalance and amplify the chances of exacerbation of the disease. SLE and MetS are closely connected so that factors in common such as diet, sex hormones, systemic and subclinical low-grade inflammation, treatment, T2D, IR, hyperlipidemia, cardiovascular abnormalities, and aberrant immune response are involved in the generation of markers that may be useful in daily clinical practice for the monitoring and selection of appropriate treatment. Metabolic profiles, proinflammatory molecules, adipokines, biophysical cardiovascular assessments, and miRs' quantification can be considered as a set of assessments that, in association with clinical findings, could elucidate a biologic–clinical causality to improve diagnosis, follow-up, and treatment in patients with SLE and MetS.

8. Perspectives

We consider it essential to perform a set of evaluations that include immunometabolic, biophysical, and epigenetic biomarkers; however, it should be considered that most human studies have limitations such as sample size, genetic variability, sex, age, dietary habits, and treatment, among others. Although experimental studies have been essential to elucidate the pathophysiological processes in MetS and SLE by controlling the intervening variables, the extrapolation of the results has been limited on some occasions. Therefore, we consider the relevance of the identification and quantification of biomarkers that present clinical correlation, predictive value, and sensitivity and that are non-invasive. About miRs, which are specific biomarkers to be detected in early diagnoses of various diseases (i.e., carcinomas), an advantage to consider is the quantification of expression levels in biological samples of easy access (serum, ductal lavage, urine, fecal matter) compared to invasive procedures (biopsy, cerebrospinal fluid, tissue by surgical procedure). In addition, it is possible to associate its expression with diverse clinical findings, which is essential to highlight the biological–clinical causality that will help with the other clinical tools that will allow premature diagnoses and the establishment of more accurate prognoses.

Author Contributions: Conceptualization, B.-T.M.-M., M.V.-D.M. and F.I.C.-M.; visualization, J.-A.R.-D.A., A.-J.T.-C. and R.-C.R.-G.; supervision, M.-O.G.-O., D.G.-I. and M.P.-N.; writing—original draft preparation, B.-T.M.-M., M.V.-D.M., F.I.C.-M., F.S.-G., M.-O.G.-O. and D.G.-I.; writing—review and editing, B.-T.M.-M., F.I.C.-M., J.-A.R-D.A., A.-J.T.-C., R.-C.R.-G. and F.S.-G. All authors have read and agreed to the published version of the manuscript.

Funding: This research received no external funding.

Conflicts of Interest: The authors declare no conflicts of interest.

References

1. Alkhulaifi, F.; Darkoh, C. Meal Timing, Meal Frequency and Metabolic Syndrome. *Nutrients* **2022**, *14*, 1719. [CrossRef] [PubMed]
2. Tsaban, G. Metabolic syndrome, LDL-hypercholesterolaemia, and cerebrocardiovascular risk: Sex matters. *Eur. J. Prev. Cardiol.* **2022**, *28*, 2018–2020. [CrossRef] [PubMed]
3. Perricone, C.; Ceccarelli, F. High Fat Diet, Metabolic Syndrome and Systemic Lupus Erythematosus: A Causal Loop. *Mediterr. J. Rheumatol.* **2020**, *31*, 172–173. [CrossRef] [PubMed]
4. Oikonomou, E.K.; Antoniades, C. The role of adipose tissue in cardiovascular health and disease. *Nat. Rev. Cardiol.* **2019**, *16*, 83–99. [CrossRef] [PubMed]
5. Clemente-Suarez, V.J.; Beltran-Velasco, A.I.; Redondo-Florez, L.; Martin-Rodriguez, A.; Tornero-Aguilera, J.F. Global Impacts of Western Diet and Its Effects on Metabolism and Health: A Narrative Review. *Nutrients* **2023**, *15*, 2749. [CrossRef] [PubMed]
6. Vrdoljak, J.; Kumric, M.; Vilovic, M.; Martinovic, D.; Rogosic, V.; Borovac, J.A.; Ticinovic Kurir, T.; Bozic, J. Can Fasting Curb the Metabolic Syndrome Epidemic? *Nutrients* **2022**, *14*, 456. [CrossRef] [PubMed]
7. Li, F.E.; Zhang, F.L.; Zhang, P.; Liu, D.; Liu, H.Y.; Guo, Z.N.; Yang, Y. Sex-based differences in and risk factors for metabolic syndrome in adults aged 40 years and above in Northeast China: Results from the cross-sectional China national stroke screening survey. *BMJ Open* **2021**, *11*, e038671. [CrossRef] [PubMed]
8. Azimi-Nezhad, M.; Aminisani, N.; Ghasemi, A.; Farimani, A.R.; Khorashadizadeh, F.; Mirhafez, S.R.; Hyde, M.; Shamshirgaran, S.M. Sex-specific prevalence of metabolic syndrome in older adults: Results from the Neyshabur longitudinal study on aging, Iran. *J. Diabetes Metab. Disord.* **2022**, *21*, 263–273. [CrossRef] [PubMed]
9. Ngwasiri, C.; Kinore, M.; Samadoulougou, S.; Kirakoya-Samadoulougou, F. Sex-specific-evaluation of metabolic syndrome prevalence in Algeria: Insights from the 2016-2017 non-communicable diseases risk factors survey. *Sci. Rep.* **2023**, *13*, 18908. [CrossRef]

10. Medina, G.; Vera-Lastra, O.; Peralta-Amaro, A.L.; Jimenez-Arellano, M.P.; Saavedra, M.A.; Cruz-Dominguez, M.P.; Jara, L.J. Metabolic syndrome, autoimmunity and rheumatic diseases. *Pharmacol. Res.* **2018**, *133*, 277–288. [CrossRef]
11. Nandakumar, K.S.; Nundel, K. Editorial: Systemic lupus erythematosus—Predisposition factors, pathogenesis, diagnosis, treatment and disease models. *Front. Immunol.* **2022**, *13*, 1118180. [CrossRef] [PubMed]
12. Irure-Ventura, J.; Lopez-Hoyos, M. Disease criteria of systemic lupus erythematosus (SLE); the potential role of non-criteria autoantibodies. *J. Transl. Autoimmun.* **2022**, *5*, 100143. [CrossRef] [PubMed]
13. Lou, H.; Ling, G.S.; Cao, X. Autoantibodies in systemic lupus erythematosus: From immunopathology to therapeutic target. *J. Autoimmun.* **2022**, *132*, 102861. [CrossRef] [PubMed]
14. Dema, B.; Charles, N. Autoantibodies in SLE: Specificities, Isotypes and Receptors. *Antibodies* **2016**, *5*, 2. [CrossRef] [PubMed]
15. Leone, P.; Prete, M.; Malerba, E.; Bray, A.; Susca, N.; Ingravallo, G.; Racanelli, V. Lupus Vasculitis: An Overview. *Biomedicines* **2021**, *9*, 1626. [CrossRef] [PubMed]
16. Urbain, F.; Ponnaiah, M.; Ichou, F.; Lhomme, M.; Materne, C.; Galier, S.; Haroche, J.; Frisdal, E.; Mathian, A.; Durand, H.; et al. Impaired metabolism predicts coronary artery calcification in women with systemic lupus erythematosus. *EBioMedicine* **2023**, *96*, 104802. [CrossRef] [PubMed]
17. Terrell, M.; Morel, L. The Intersection of Cellular and Systemic Metabolism: Metabolic Syndrome in Systemic Lupus Erythematosus. *Endocrinology* **2022**, *163*, bqac067. [CrossRef] [PubMed]
18. Taylor, E.B. The complex role of adipokines in obesity, inflammation, and autoimmunity. *Clin. Sci.* **2021**, *135*, 731–752. [CrossRef]
19. Crow, M.K. Pathogenesis of systemic lupus erythematosus: Risks, mechanisms and therapeutic targets. *Ann. Rheum. Dis.* **2023**, *82*, 999–1014. [CrossRef]
20. Apostolopoulos, D.; Vincent, F.; Hoi, A.; Morand, E. Associations of metabolic syndrome in SLE. *Lupus Sci. Med.* **2020**, *7*, e000436. [CrossRef]
21. Huang, S.; Zhang, Z.; Cui, Y.; Yao, G.; Ma, X.; Zhang, H. Dyslipidemia is associated with inflammation and organ involvement in systemic lupus erythematosus. *Clin. Rheumatol.* **2023**, *42*, 1565–1572. [CrossRef] [PubMed]
22. Kim, S.Y.; Yu, M.; Morin, E.E.; Kang, J.; Kaplan, M.J.; Schwendeman, A. High-Density Lipoprotein in Lupus: Disease Biomarkers and Potential Therapeutic Strategy. *Arthritis Rheumatol.* **2020**, *72*, 20–30. [CrossRef] [PubMed]
23. Hernandez-Negrin, H.; Ricci, M.; Mancebo-Sevilla, J.J.; Sanz-Canovas, J.; Lopez-Sampalo, A.; Cobos-Palacios, L.; Romero-Gomez, C.; Perez de Pedro, I.; Ayala-Gutierrez, M.D.M.; Gomez-Huelgas, R.; et al. Obesity, Diabetes, and Cardiovascular Risk Burden in Systemic Lupus Erythematosus: Current Approaches and Knowledge Gaps-A Rapid Scoping Review. *Int. J. Environ. Res. Public. Health* **2022**, *19*, 14768. [CrossRef]
24. Aruwa, C.E.; Sabiu, S. Adipose tissue inflammation linked to obesity: A review of current understanding, therapies and relevance of phyto-therapeutics. *Heliyon* **2024**, *10*, e23114. [CrossRef] [PubMed]
25. Li, M.; Chi, X.; Wang, Y.; Setrerrahmane, S.; Xie, W.; Xu, H. Trends in insulin resistance: Insights into mechanisms and therapeutic strategy. *Signal Transduct. Target. Ther.* **2022**, *7*, 216. [CrossRef]
26. Richter, P.; Macovei, L.A.; Mihai, I.R.; Cardoneanu, A.; Burlui, M.A.; Rezus, E. Cytokines in Systemic Lupus Erythematosus-Focus on TNF-alpha and IL-17. *Int. J. Mol. Sci.* **2023**, *24*, 14413. [CrossRef]
27. Garcia-Carrasco, M.; Mendoza-Pinto, C.; Munguia-Realpozo, P.; Etchegaray-Morales, I.; Velez-Pelcastre, S.K.; Mendez-Martinez, S.; Zamora-Ginez, I.; de Lara, L.G.V.; Galvez-Romero, J.L.; Escamilla-Marquez, M. Insulin Resistance and Diabetes Mellitus in Patients with Systemic Lupus Erythematosus. *Endocr. Metab. Immune Disord. Drug Targets* **2023**, *23*, 503–514. [CrossRef]
28. Petri, M.; Spence, D.; Bone, L.R.; Hochberg, M.C. Coronary artery disease risk factors in the Johns Hopkins Lupus Cohort: Prevalence, recognition by patients, and preventive practices. *Medicine* **1992**, *71*, 291–302. [CrossRef]
29. El Magadmi, M.; Ahmad, Y.; Turkie, W.; Yates, A.P.; Sheikh, N.; Bernstein, R.M.; Durrington, P.N.; Laing, I.; Bruce, I.N. Hyperinsulinemia, insulin resistance, and circulating oxidized low density lipoprotein in women with systemic lupus erythematosus. *J. Rheumatol.* **2006**, *33*, 50–56.
30. Contreras-Haro, B.; Hernandez-Gonzalez, S.O.; Gonzalez-Lopez, L.; Espinel-Bermudez, M.C.; Garcia-Benavides, L.; Perez-Guerrero, E.; Vazquez-Villegas, M.L.; Robles-Cervantes, J.A.; Salazar-Paramo, M.; Hernandez-Corona, D.M.; et al. Fasting triglycerides and glucose index: A useful screening test for assessing insulin resistance in patients diagnosed with rheumatoid arthritis and systemic lupus erythematosus. *Diabetol. Metab. Syndr.* **2019**, *11*, 95. [CrossRef]
31. Tang, K.T.; Chien, H.J.; Chang, Y.H.; Liao, T.L.; Chen, D.Y.; Lai, C.C. Metabolic disturbances in systemic lupus erythematosus evaluated with UPLC-MS/MS. *Clin. Exp. Rheumatol.* **2024**, *42*, 15–23. [CrossRef]
32. Moschetti, L.; Piantoni, S.; Vizzardi, E.; Sciatti, E.; Riccardi, M.; Franceschini, F.; Cavazzana, I. Endothelial Dysfunction in Systemic Lupus Erythematosus and Systemic Sclerosis: A Common Trigger for Different Microvascular Diseases. *Front. Med.* **2022**, *9*, 849086. [CrossRef] [PubMed]
33. Szabo, M.Z.; Szodoray, P.; Kiss, E. Dyslipidemia in systemic lupus erythematosus. *Immunol. Res.* **2017**, *65*, 543–550. [CrossRef]
34. Meroni, P.L.; Borghi, M.O. Antiphospholipid Antibody Assays in 2021: Looking for a Predictive Value in Addition to a Diagnostic One. *Front. Immunol.* **2021**, *12*, 726820. [CrossRef] [PubMed]
35. Huang, L.Y.; Chiu, C.J.; Hsing, C.H.; Hsu, Y.H. Interferon Family Cytokines in Obesity and Insulin Sensitivity. *Cells* **2022**, *11*, 4041. [CrossRef] [PubMed]
36. Liang, W.; Qi, Y.; Yi, H.; Mao, C.; Meng, Q.; Wang, H.; Zheng, C. The Roles of Adipose Tissue Macrophages in Human Disease. *Front. Immunol.* **2022**, *13*, 908749. [CrossRef]

37. Ding, J.; Su, S.; You, T.; Xia, T.; Lin, X.; Chen, Z.; Zhang, L. Serum interleukin-6 level is correlated with the disease activity of systemic lupus erythematosus: A meta-analysis. *Clinics* 2020, *75*, e1801. [CrossRef]
38. Banik, S.D.; Avila-Nava, A.; Lugo, R.; Chim Ake, R.; Gutierrez Solis, A.L. Association Between Low-Grade Inflammation and Hyperuricemia in Adults With Metabolic Syndrome in Yucatan, Mexico. *Can. J. Diabetes* 2022, *46*, 369–374. [CrossRef]
39. Ghorbaninezhad, F.; Leone, P.; Alemohammad, H.; Najafzadeh, B.; Nourbakhsh, N.S.; Prete, M.; Malerba, E.; Saeedi, H.; Tabrizi, N.J.; Racanelli, V.; et al. Tumor necrosis factor-alpha in systemic lupus erythematosus: Structure, function and therapeutic implications (Review). *Int. J. Mol. Med.* 2022, *49*, 43. [CrossRef]
40. Kim, C.W.; Oh, E.T.; Park, H.J. A strategy to prevent atherosclerosis via TNF receptor regulation. *FASEB J.* 2021, *35*, e21391. [CrossRef]
41. Sethi, J.K.; Hotamisligil, G.S. Metabolic Messengers: Tumour necrosis factor. *Nat. Metab.* 2021, *3*, 1302–1312. [CrossRef] [PubMed]
42. Gigante, A.; Iannazzo, F.; Navarini, L.; Sgariglia, M.C.; Margiotta, D.P.E.; Vaiarello, V.; Foti, F.; Afeltra, A.; Cianci, R.; Rosato, E. Metabolic syndrome and adipokine levels in systemic lupus erythematosus and systemic sclerosis. *Clin. Rheumatol.* 2021, *40*, 4253–4258. [CrossRef]
43. Turpin, T.; Thouvenot, K.; Gonthier, M.P. Adipokines and Bacterial Metabolites: A Pivotal Molecular Bridge Linking Obesity and Gut Microbiota Dysbiosis to Target. *Biomolecules* 2023, *13*, 1692. [CrossRef]
44. Neumann, E.; Hasseli, R.; Ohl, S.; Lange, U.; Frommer, K.W.; Muller-Ladner, U. Adipokines and Autoimmunity in Inflammatory Arthritis. *Cells* 2021, *10*, 216. [CrossRef]
45. Villa, N.; Badla, O.; Goit, R.; Saddik, S.E.; Dawood, S.N.; Rabih, A.M.; Mohammed, A.; Raman, A.; Uprety, M.; Calero, M.J.; et al. The Role of Leptin in Systemic Lupus Erythematosus: Is It Still a Mystery? *Cureus* 2022, *14*, e26751. [CrossRef] [PubMed]
46. Dan, Y.L.; Wang, P.; Cheng, Z.; Wu, Q.; Wang, X.R.; Wang, D.G.; Pan, H.F. Circulating adiponectin levels and systemic lupus erythematosus: A two-sample Mendelian randomization study. *Rheumatology* 2021, *60*, 940–946. [CrossRef]
47. Peng, X.; Huang, J.; Zou, H.; Peng, B.; Xia, S.; Dong, K.; Sun, N.; Tao, J.; Yang, Y. Roles of plasma leptin and resistin in novel subgroups of type 2 diabetes driven by cluster analysis. *Lipids Health Dis.* 2022, *21*, 7. [CrossRef]
48. Guo, D.; Liu, J.; Zhang, P.; Yang, X.; Liu, D.; Lin, J.; Wei, X.; Xu, B.; Huang, C.; Zhou, X.; et al. Adiposity Measurements and Metabolic Syndrome Are Linked Through Circulating Neuregulin 4 and Adipsin Levels in Obese Adults. *Front. Physiol.* 2021, *12*, 667330. [CrossRef] [PubMed]
49. Sun, J.X.; Zhang, C.; Cheng, Z.B.; Tang, M.Y.; Liu, Y.Z.; Jiang, J.F.; Xiao, X.; Huang, L. Chemerin in atherosclerosis. *Clin. Chim. Acta* 2021, *520*, 8–15. [CrossRef]
50. Jialal, I. Chemerin levels in metabolic syndrome: A promising biomarker. *Arch. Physiol. Biochem.* 2021, *129*, 1009–1011. [CrossRef]
51. Abdalla, M.M.I. Role of visfatin in obesity-induced insulin resistance. *World J. Clin. Cases* 2022, *10*, 10840–10851. [CrossRef] [PubMed]
52. Erten, M. Visfatin as a Promising Marker of Cardiometabolic Risk. *Acta Cardiol. Sin.* 2021, *37*, 464–472. [CrossRef]
53. Tumurkhuu, G.; Casanova, N.G.; Kempf, C.L.; Ercan Laguna, D.; Camp, S.M.; Dagvadorj, J.; Song, J.H.; Reyes Hernon, V.; Travelli, C.; Montano, E.N.; et al. eNAMPT/TLR4 inflammatory cascade activation is a key contributor to SLE Lung vasculitis and alveolar hemorrhage. *J. Transl. Autoimmun.* 2023, *6*, 100181. [CrossRef]
54. Ali, A.Y.; Abdullah, H.; Abdallah, M.F.H.; Fayed, A. Impact of Adipokines in Brachial Artery Flow-mediated Dilatation in Lupus Nephritis. *Saudi J. Kidney Dis. Transpl.* 2022, *33*, 272–279. [CrossRef] [PubMed]
55. Salvoza, N.; Giraudi, P.; Gazzin, S.; Bonazza, D.; Palmisano, S.; de Manzini, N.; Zanconati, F.; Raseni, A.; Sirianni, F.; Tiribelli, C.; et al. The potential role of omentin-1 in obesity-related metabolic dysfunction-associated steatotic liver disease: Evidence from translational studies. *J. Transl. Med.* 2023, *21*, 906. [CrossRef] [PubMed]
56. Zhang, T.P.; Li, H.M.; Leng, R.X.; Li, X.P.; Li, X.M.; Pan, H.F.; Ye, D.Q. Plasma levels of adipokines in systemic lupus erythematosus patients. *Cytokine* 2016, *86*, 15–20. [CrossRef] [PubMed]
57. Kim, J.E.; Kim, J.S.; Jo, M.J.; Cho, E.; Ahn, S.Y.; Kwon, Y.J.; Ko, G.J. The Roles and Associated Mechanisms of Adipokines in Development of Metabolic Syndrome. *Molecules* 2022, *27*, 334. [CrossRef] [PubMed]
58. Kuo, C.Y.; Tsai, T.Y.; Huang, Y.C. Insulin resistance and serum levels of adipokines in patients with systemic lupus erythematosus: A systematic review and meta-analysis. *Lupus* 2020, *29*, 1078–1084. [CrossRef] [PubMed]
59. Kamel, S.M.; Abdel Azeem Abd Elazeem, M.; Mohamed, R.A.; Kamel, M.M.; Abdel Aleem Abdelaleem, E.A. High serum leptin and adiponectin levels as biomarkers of disease progression in Egyptian patients with active systemic lupus erythematosus. *Int. J. Immunopathol. Pharmacol.* 2023, *37*, 3946320231154988. [CrossRef]
60. Su, X.; Cheng, Y.; Zhang, G.; Wang, B. Chemerin in inflammatory diseases. *Clin. Chim. Acta* 2021, *517*, 41–47. [CrossRef]
61. Jiang, Y.; Zhou, L. The Value of Visfatin in the Prediction of Metabolic Syndrome: A Systematic Review and Meta-Analysis. *Horm. Metab. Res.* 2023, *55*, 610–616. [CrossRef] [PubMed]
62. Chougule, D.; Nadkar, M.; Venkataraman, K.; Rajadhyaksha, A.; Hase, N.; Jamale, T.; Kini, S.; Khadilkar, P.; Anand, V.; Madkaikar, M.; et al. Adipokine interactions promote the pathogenesis of systemic lupus erythematosus. *Cytokine* 2018, *111*, 20–27. [CrossRef] [PubMed]
63. Esdaile, J.M.; Abrahamowicz, M.; Grodzicky, T.; Li, Y.; Panaritis, C.; du Berger, R.; Cote, R.; Grover, S.A.; Fortin, P.R.; Clarke, A.E.; et al. Traditional Framingham risk factors fail to fully account for accelerated atherosclerosis in systemic lupus erythematosus. *Arthritis Rheum.* 2001, *44*, 2331–2337. [CrossRef] [PubMed]

64. Tobin, R.; Patel, N.; Tobb, K.; Weber, B.; Mehta, P.K.; Isiadinso, I. Atherosclerosis in Systemic Lupus Erythematosus. *Curr. Atheroscler. Rep.* **2023**, *25*, 819–827. [CrossRef] [PubMed]
65. Magder, L.S.; Petri, M. Incidence of and risk factors for adverse cardiovascular events among patients with systemic lupus erythematosus. *Am. J. Epidemiol.* **2012**, *176*, 708–719. [CrossRef] [PubMed]
66. Drosos, G.C.; Vedder, D.; Houben, E.; Boekel, L.; Atzeni, F.; Badreh, S.; Boumpas, D.T.; Brodin, N.; Bruce, I.N.; Gonzalez-Gay, M.A.; et al. EULAR recommendations for cardiovascular risk management in rheumatic and musculoskeletal diseases, including systemic lupus erythematosus and antiphospholipid syndrome. *Ann. Rheum. Dis.* **2022**, *81*, 768–779. [CrossRef]
67. Mak, A.; Kow, N.Y.; Schwarz, H.; Gong, L.; Tay, S.H.; Ling, L.H. Endothelial dysfunction in systemic lupus erythematosus—A case-control study and an updated meta-analysis and meta-regression. *Sci. Rep.* **2017**, *7*, 7320. [CrossRef]
68. Wang, P.; Mao, Y.M.; Zhao, C.N.; Liu, L.N.; Li, X.M.; Li, X.P.; Pan, H.F. Increased Pulse Wave Velocity in Systemic Lupus Erythematosus: A Meta-Analysis. *Angiology* **2018**, *69*, 228–235. [CrossRef] [PubMed]
69. Liu, Y.; Kaplan, M.J. Cardiovascular disease in systemic lupus erythematosus: An update. *Curr. Opin. Rheumatol.* **2018**, *30*, 441–448. [CrossRef]
70. Samuelsson, I.; Parodis, I.; Gunnarsson, I.; Zickert, A.; Hofman-Bang, C.; Wallen, H.; Svenungsson, E. Myocardial infarctions, subtypes and coronary atherosclerosis in SLE: A case-control study. *Lupus Sci. Med.* **2021**, *8*, e000515. [CrossRef]
71. Mavrogeni, S.; Koutsogeorgopoulou, L.; Markousis-Mavrogenis, G.; Bounas, A.; Tektonidou, M.; Lliossis, S.C.; Daoussis, D.; Plastiras, S.; Karabela, G.; Stavropoulos, E.; et al. Cardiovascular magnetic resonance detects silent heart disease missed by echocardiography in systemic lupus erythematosus. *Lupus* **2018**, *27*, 564–571. [CrossRef] [PubMed]
72. Tektonidou, M.G. Cardiovascular disease risk in antiphospholipid syndrome: Thrombo-inflammation and atherothrombosis. *J. Autoimmun.* **2022**, *128*, 102813. [CrossRef] [PubMed]
73. Stojan, G.; Petri, M. The risk benefit ratio of glucocorticoids in SLE: Have things changed over the past 40 years? *Curr. Treatm Opt. Rheumatol.* **2017**, *3*, 164–172. [CrossRef]
74. Dima, A.; Jurcut, C.; Chasset, F.; Felten, R.; Arnaud, L. Hydroxychloroquine in systemic lupus erythematosus: Overview of current knowledge. *Ther. Adv. Musculoskelet. Dis.* **2022**, *14*, 1759720X211073001. [CrossRef] [PubMed]
75. Wakiya, R.; Ueeda, K.; Nakashima, S.; Shimada, H.; Kameda, T.; Mansour, M.M.F.; Kato, M.; Miyagi, T.; Sugihara, K.; Mizusaki, M.; et al. Effect of add-on hydroxychloroquine therapy on serum proinflammatory cytokine levels in patients with systemic lupus erythematosus. *Sci. Rep.* **2022**, *12*, 10175. [CrossRef] [PubMed]
76. Floris, A.; Piga, M.; Mangoni, A.A.; Bortoluzzi, A.; Erre, G.L.; Cauli, A. Protective Effects of Hydroxychloroquine against Accelerated Atherosclerosis in Systemic Lupus Erythematosus. *Mediat. Inflamm.* **2018**, *2018*, 3424136. [CrossRef]
77. Yang, D.H.; Leong, P.Y.; Sia, S.K.; Wang, Y.H.; Wei, J.C. Long-Term Hydroxychloroquine Therapy and Risk of Coronary Artery Disease in Patients with Systemic Lupus Erythematosus. *J. Clin. Med.* **2019**, *8*, 796. [CrossRef]
78. Hiramatsu-Asano, S.; Wada, J. Therapeutic Approaches Targeting miRNA in Systemic Lupus Erythematosus. *Acta Med. Okayama* **2022**, *76*, 359–371. [CrossRef]
79. Luo, B.; Zhou, K.; Liufu, Y.; Huang, X.; Zeng, H.; Zhang, Z. Novel insight into miRNA biology and its role in the pathogenesis of systemic lupus erythematosus. *Front. Immunol.* **2022**, *13*, 1059887. [CrossRef]
80. Chi, M.; Ma, K.; Li, Y.; Quan, M.; Han, Z.; Ding, Z.; Liang, X.; Zhang, Q.; Song, L.; Liu, C. Immunological Involvement of MicroRNAs in the Key Events of Systemic Lupus Erythematosus. *Front. Immunol.* **2021**, *12*, 699684. [CrossRef]
81. So, B.Y.F.; Yap, D.Y.H.; Chan, T.M. MicroRNAs in Lupus Nephritis-Role in Disease Pathogenesis and Clinical Applications. *Int. J. Mol. Sci.* **2021**, *22*, 10737. [CrossRef] [PubMed]
82. Testa, U.; Pelosi, E.; Castelli, G.; Labbaye, C. miR-146 and miR-155: Two Key Modulators of Immune Response and Tumor Development. *Noncoding RNA* **2017**, *3*, 22. [CrossRef] [PubMed]
83. El-Akhras, B.A.; Talaat, R.M.; El-Masry, S.A.; Bassyouni, I.H.; El-Sayed, I.H.; Ali, Y.B. Crosstalk between miR-146a and pro-inflammatory cytokines in patients with systemic lupus erythematosus. *Int. J. Immunopathol. Pharmacol.* **2023**, *37*, 3946320231154998. [CrossRef] [PubMed]
84. Li, W.; Liu, S.; Chen, Y.; Weng, R.; Zhang, K.; He, X.; He, C. Circulating Exosomal microRNAs as Biomarkers of Systemic Lupus Erythematosus. *Clinics* **2020**, *75*, e1528. [CrossRef] [PubMed]
85. Benbaibeche, H.; Hichami, A.; Oudjit, B.; Haffaf, E.M.; Kacimi, G.; Koceir, E.A.; Khan, N.A. Circulating mir-21 and mir-146a are associated with increased cytokines and CD36 in Algerian obese male participants. *Arch. Physiol. Biochem.* **2022**, *128*, 1461–1466. [CrossRef]
86. Zhang, L.; Zhang, X.; Si, F. MicroRNA-124 represents a novel diagnostic marker in human lupus nephritis and plays an inhibitory effect on the growth and inflammation of renal mesangial cells by targeting TRAF6. *Int. J. Clin. Exp. Pathol.* **2019**, *12*, 1578–1588. [PubMed]
87. Yan, L.; Jiang, L.; Wang, B.; Hu, Q.; Deng, S.; Huang, J.; Sun, X.; Zhang, Y.; Feng, L.; Chen, W. Novel microRNA biomarkers of systemic lupus erythematosus in plasma: miR-124-3p and miR-377-3p. *Clin. Biochem.* **2022**, *107*, 55–61. [CrossRef] [PubMed]
88. Duan, X.K.; Sun, Y.X.; Wang, H.Y.; Xu, Y.Y.; Fan, S.Z.; Tian, J.Y.; Yu, Y.; Zhao, Y.Y.; Jiang, Y.L. miR-124 is upregulated in diabetic mice and inhibits proliferation and promotes apoptosis of high-glucose-induced beta-cells by targeting EZH2. *World J. Diabetes* **2023**, *14*, 209–221. [CrossRef] [PubMed]
89. Stypinska, B.; Wajda, A.; Walczuk, E.; Olesinska, M.; Lewandowska, A.; Walczyk, M.; Paradowska-Gorycka, A. The Serum Cell-Free microRNA Expression Profile in MCTD, SLE, SSc, and RA Patients. *J. Clin. Med.* **2020**, *9*, 161. [CrossRef]

90. Aladel, A.; Khatoon, F.; Khan, M.I.; Alsheweir, A.; Almutairi. M.G.; Almutairi, S.O.; Almutairi, F.K.; Osmonaliev, K.; Beg, M.M.A. Evaluation of miRNA-143 and miRNA-145 Expression and Their Association with Vitamin-D Status Among Obese and Non-Obese Type-2 Diabetic Patients. *J. Multidiscip. Healthc.* **2022**, *15*, 2979–2990. [CrossRef]
91. Deiuliis, J.A. MicroRNAs as regulators of metabolic disease: Pathophysiologic significance and emerging role as biomarkers and therapeutics. *Int. J. Obes.* **2016**, *40*, 88–101. [CrossRef] [PubMed]
92. Cecchi, I.; Perez-Sanchez, C.; Sciascia, S.; Radin, M.; Arias de la Rosa, I.; Barbarroja Puerto, N.; Scudeler, L.; Perez-Sanchez, L.; Patino Trives, A.M.; Aguirre Zamorano, M.A.; et al. Circulating microRNAs as potential biomarkers for monitoring the response to in vivo treatment with Rituximab in systemic lupus erythematosus patients. *Autoimmun. Rev.* **2020**, *19*, 102488. [CrossRef]
93. Rochlani, Y.; Pothineni, N.V.; Kovelamudi, S.; Mehta, J.L. Metabolic syndrome: Pathophysiology, management, and modulation by natural compounds. *Ther. Adv. Cardiovasc. Dis.* **2017**, *11*, 215–225. [CrossRef] [PubMed]
94. DelOlmo-Romero, S.; Medina-Martinez, I.; Gil-Gutierrez, R.; Pocovi-Gerardino, G.; Correa-Rodriguez, M.; Ortego-Centeno, N.; Rueda-Medina, B. Metabolic syndrome in systemic lupus erythematosus patients under Mediterranean diet. *Med. Clin.* **2023**, *162*, 259–264. [CrossRef] [PubMed]
95. Akhil, A.; Bansal, R.; Anupam, K.; Tandon, A.; Bhatnagar, A. Systemic lupus erythematosus: Latest insight into etiopathogenesis. *Rheumatol. Int.* **2023**, *43*, 1381–1393. [CrossRef] [PubMed]
96. White, F. Application of Disease Etiology and Natural History to Prevention in Primary Health Care: A Discourse. *Med. Princ. Pract.* **2020**, *29*, 501–513. [CrossRef]
97. Ameer, M.A.; Chaudhry, H.; Mushtaq, J.; Khan, O.S.; Babar, M.; Hashim, T.; Zeb, S.; Tariq, M.A.; Patlolla, S.R.; Ali, J.; et al. An Overview of Systemic Lupus Erythematosus (SLE) Pathogenesis, Classification, and Management. *Cureus* **2022**, *14*, e30330. [CrossRef]
98. Wang, Y.; Huang, Z.; Xiao, Y.; Wan, W.; Yang, X. The shared biomarkers and pathways of systemic lupus erythematosus and metabolic syndrome analyzed by bioinformatics combining machine learning algorithm and single-cell sequencing analysis. *Front. Immunol.* **2022**, *13*, 1015882. [CrossRef] [PubMed]
99. Tsigalou, C.; Vallianou, N.; Dalamaga, M. Autoantibody Production in Obesity: Is There Evidence for a Link Between Obesity and Autoimmunity? *Curr. Obes. Rep.* **2020**, *9*, 245–254. [CrossRef]
100. Li, X.; Zhu, J.; Zhao, W.; Zhu, Y.; Zhu, L.; Shi, R.; Wang, Z.; Pan, H.; Wang, D. The Causal Effect of Obesity on the Risk of 15 Autoimmune Diseases: A Mendelian Randomization Study. *Obes. Facts* **2023**, *16*, 598–605. [CrossRef]

Disclaimer/Publisher's Note: The statements, opinions and data contained in all publications are solely those of the individual author(s) and contributor(s) and not of MDPI and/or the editor(s). MDPI and/or the editor(s) disclaim responsibility for any injury to people or property resulting from any ideas, methods, instructions or products referred to in the content.

Review

Urinary Biomarkers for Lupus Nephritis: A Systems Biology Approach

Mohamed H. Omer [1,†], Areez Shafqat [2,*,†], Omar Ahmad [2], Juzer Nadri [2], Khaled AlKattan [2] and Ahmed Yaqinuddin [2]

1. School of Medicine, Cardiff University, Cardiff CF14 4YS, UK; omermh2@cardiff.ac.uk
2. College of Medicine, Alfaisal University, Riyadh 11533, Saudi Arabia; oahmad@alfaisal.edu (O.A.); juzernadri@gmail.com (J.N.); kkattan@alfaisal.edu (K.A.); ayaqinuddin@alfaisal.edu (A.Y.)
* Correspondence: ashafqat@alfaisal.edu
† These authors have contributed equally to the work.

Abstract: Systemic lupus erythematosus (SLE) is the prototypical systemic autoimmune disorder. Kidney involvement, termed lupus nephritis (LN), is seen in 40–60% of patients with systemic lupus erythematosus (SLE). After the diagnosis, serial measurement of proteinuria is the most common method of monitoring treatment response and progression. However, present treatments for LN—corticosteroids and immunosuppressants—target inflammation, not proteinuria. Furthermore, subclinical renal inflammation can persist despite improving proteinuria. Serial kidney biopsies—the gold standard for disease monitoring—are also not feasible due to their inherent risk of complications. Biomarkers that reflect the underlying renal inflammatory process and better predict LN progression and treatment response are urgently needed. Urinary biomarkers are particularly relevant as they can be measured non-invasively and may better reflect the compartmentalized renal response in LN, unlike serum studies that are non-specific to the kidney. The past decade has overseen a boom in applying cutting-edge technologies to dissect the pathogenesis of diseases at the molecular and cellular levels. Using these technologies in LN is beginning to reveal novel disease biomarkers and therapeutic targets for LN, potentially improving patient outcomes if successfully translated to clinical practice.

Keywords: lupus nephritis; proteomics; transcriptomics; metabolomics; microRNAs; biomarkers

1. Introduction

Systemic lupus erythematosus (SLE) is a multisystem autoimmune disorder with heterogeneous clinical manifestations [1]. It most commonly affects women of childbearing age. Lupus nephritis (LN) describes renal involvement in SLE, affecting approximately 40–60% of patients, with African Americans being at higher risk both of LN development and severe forms of LN [2,3]. Patients with LN usually present with findings of nephritic (e.g., hematuria, generalized edema, hypertension) and/or nephrotic (generalized edema, frothy urine) glomerular disease. Urinalysis often reveals proteinuria and hematuria with red blood cell (RBC) casts. Other routinely performed investigations for LN include renal function tests, 24 h urinary proteinuria or spot urine protein-to-creatinine ratio, complement levels, and serologies to assess for anti-double stranded DNA (dsDNA) and anti-nuclear antibodies (ANAs).

The presence of LN portends a poor prognosis in patients with SLE, associated with a significant morbidity and mortality burden [4]. Despite advancements in immunomodulatory therapies, approximately 30% of patients with LN develop end-stage kidney disease, requiring renal replacement therapy [5,6].

The gold standard technique for diagnosing and monitoring LN remains a kidney biopsy [7,8]. The pattern of glomerular disease on renal biopsy is also used to classify LN into six distinct subtypes. However, a kidney biopsy is an invasive technique with an array of potential complications [9]. Moreover, patients with LN often require repeated kidney biopsies to assess disease activity, which is associated with a compounding risk of adverse events [7,8]. On the other hand, traditional serum and urinary biomarkers such as complement levels, glomerular filtration rate, and urine protein-to-creatinine ratios offer limited specificity. They also cannot distinguish LN from other etiologies of nephritis [10–12]. Furthermore, the treatment for LN—corticosteroids and immunosuppressants—targets the immune response, not proteinuria [13]. It is possible for inflammation to subsist despite improving proteinuria.

Hence, a need emerges to identify novel markers that meet the following requirements: they reflect the biology of LN; they can be measured easily, preferably through a non-invasive, routinely collectible sample such as urine; and their temporal changes reflect disease activity in a manner that can reflect a change in clinical state, such as disease progression and treatment response. Thoroughly assessing lupus nephritis requires a protocol that combines novel biomarkers with clinical disease activity scores, renal biopsy findings, conventional laboratory markers such as proteinuria and renal function tests, and imaging tools.

In the era of precision medicine and novel immuno-technologies, multi-omic techniques represent a novel strategy to identify potential biomarkers for LN [14,15]. Omics describes a comprehensive assessment of a particular set of molecules. The most utilized example of a genomics approach is genome-wide association studies (GWASs), for instance, in which the genotype of several thousands of individuals is analyzed for genetic markers, and statistically significant differences in the frequency of a genetic variant between cases and controls are taken as evidence of an association between that genetic variant and disease [16]. The techniques used for transcriptomic, proteomic, and metabolomic analyses—the main aspects of multi-omics discussed in this review—are detailed in their corresponding sections.

This review discusses the application of multi-omics technologies on urine to identify biomarkers for LN that reflect its disease burden/severity and can also be used to monitor treatment responses, thereby providing an alternative to the current gold standard of renal biopsies that are invasive and consequently carry inherent risks and contraindications and can be unfeasible to conduct serially in individual patients.

2. Urinary Transcriptomics

Transcriptomics involves the quantitative and/or qualitative analysis of different types of RNA molecules (e.g., mRNA and non-coding RNAs, such as microRNAs) expressed in a given sample. Microarray-based analysis was historically the primary method for global transcriptional profiling. RNA sequencing (RNAseq), either in bulk (i.e., bulk-RNAseq) or at the single-cell level (i.e., scRNA-seq), subsequently emerged and is now increasingly used. ScRNA-seq reveals the gene expression patterns of individual cells in tissues and has revealed a previously underappreciated complexity of cellular transcripts that change in health and disease and are contingent upon the organ of context and tissue microenvironment.

The application of transcriptomics approaches to urine is an emerging approach to identifying predictive biomarkers that better reflect disease severity and treatment response than proteinuria [17,18]. Most studies compare scRNA-seq findings of renal biopsy specimens between patients with LN and controls to identify disease-associated phenotypes in renal parenchymal cells and immune cells that may be candidates for being considered therapeutic targets [19,20].

ScRNA-seq findings of non-lesional, non-sun-exposed skin biopsies of patients with LN and healthy controls showed that upregulated keratinocyte IFN responses could distinguish patients with LN from controls [21,22]. These findings indicate that transcriptomic analyses of a readily accessible site such as the skin could represent a novel biomarker for LN monitoring. In the kidneys, an interferon and pro-fibrotic signature elaborated by renal tubular epithelial cells has been associated with a failure to respond to treatment [22]. Similarly, the expression of several transcripts in serial kidney biopsy pre- and post-treatment related to innate and adaptive immune cell activation, including interferon responses, can distinguish treatment responders from non-responders [23].

MicroRNAs

MicroRNAs are non-coding RNA molecules that regulate the stability of mRNA, thereby controlling its translation into protein and regulating an array of physiological and pathological processes [24,25]. In the context of LN, several microRNAs contributing mechanistically to various pathophysiological processes in LN—from the modulation of inflammatory responses to pathways related to renal fibrosis—have been identified as potential diagnostic biomarkers and indicators of disease activity (Figure 1) [26].

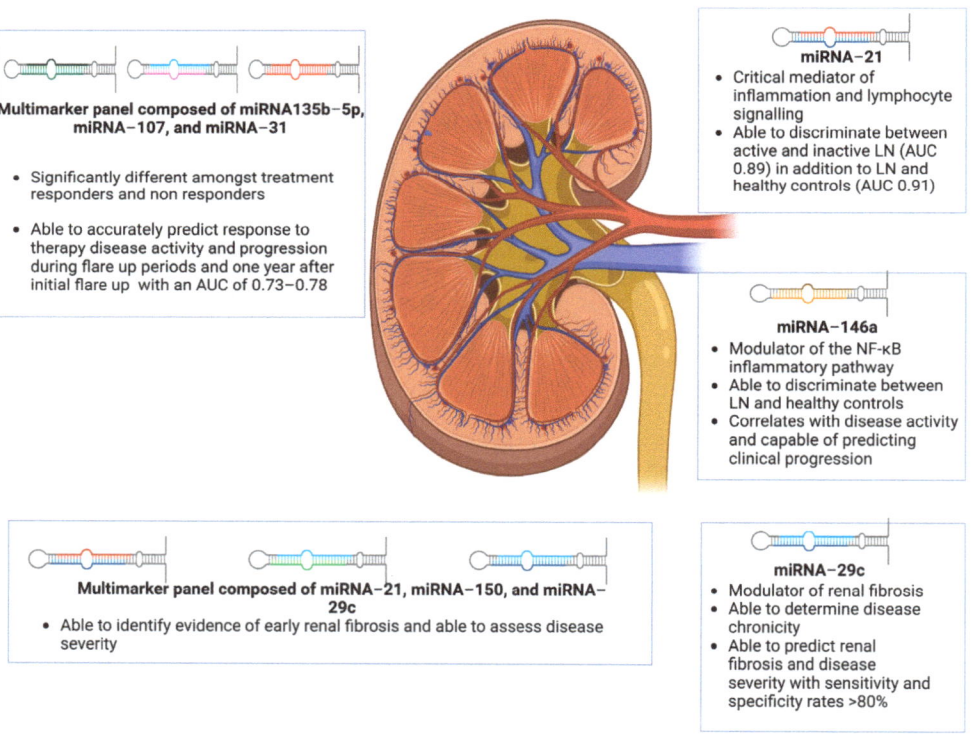

Figure 1. An overview of urinary microRNAs associated with lupus nephritis. This figure was created using BioRender.com.

Both urinary and plasma microRNAs are often quantified non-invasively using a real-time quantitative polymerase chain reaction (RT-qPCR), owing to this method's high sensitivity, cost, and time efficiency [25,27]. MiRNA-21, a critical mediator of inflammation that upregulates interleukin-6- and NF-κB-associated pathways and modulates lymphocyte signaling, was one of the first identified microRNAs associated with LN [28–31]. Urinary miRNA-21 could distinguish between inactive and active LN in a cohort study of 55 patients with SLE and 30 healthy controls with an area under the curve (AUC) of 0.89 [32].

Furthermore, in 52 patients with LN, miRNA-21 could distinguish between healthy controls and patients with LN with a sensitivity of 86% and an AUC of 0.91 [33]. Urinary miRNA-146a, also a modulator of the NF-κB inflammatory pathway, could similarly accurately discriminate patients with LN from healthy controls [34,35]. Interestingly, miRNA-146a also correlated directly with disease activity and histological features, indicating its potential to predict disease severity and response to therapy [36]. Finally, miRNA-29c, a key modulator of renal fibrosis, has recently been shown to accurately determine renal chronicity and disease severity in LN with a sensitivity and specificity of over 80% [37–39].

Recently, a paradigm shift has emerged in urinary transcriptomics with the development of novel biomarker panels utilizing several microRNAs with differing utilities to accurately aid in diagnosing and assessing disease activity [39–42]. For instance, a recent panel using three microRNAs (miRNA-21, miRNA-150, and miRNA-29c) was evaluated in a cohort study of 45 patients with LN and 20 controls [39]. This microRNA panel showed that changes in these individual microRNA levels correlated significantly with the LN chronicity index (CI), which was a significant predictor of renal fibrosis recorded by immunohistochemistry. Additionally, evaluating a separate panel consisting of three microRNAs (miRNA-135b-5p, miRNA-107, and miRNA-31) in a cohort of 42 patients with LN, comprising 21 responders and 21 non-responders, revealed significant differences amongst responders and non-responders [43]. They could accurately predict disease activity and progression during flare-up periods and one year following the initial flare-up (AUC of 0.73–0.78).

3. Urinary Proteomics

Proteomics approaches broadly characterize peptide abundance or interactions in a specific sample. The primary technique applied to proteomic study is spectrometry (MS). Mass cytometry adds more resolution to proteomics, which allows us to identify the proteins expressed by different cell types. The advent of mass spectroscopy also led to large-scale metabolomic analyses aimed at characterizing the abundance of molecules like fatty acids, amino acids, and carbohydrates. Mass spectroscopy imaging has been devised to provide spatial context about the proteins and metabolites present within a sample lost in bulk-level mass spectroscopy.

The application of urinary proteomic techniques to identify biomarker proteins has demonstrated excellent potential across several systemic and renal disorders [44]. Identifying urinary biomarker proteins can facilitate the non-invasive diagnosis of LN while aiding in the characterization of disease activity and severity. Additionally, urinary proteomics can pave the way for identifying biomarkers that predict responsiveness to therapy and propensity toward relapse [45].

Two primary approaches underpin the utilization of urinary proteomics in the context of LN biomarker discovery [46]. Targeted proteomics offers a unique perspective as it involves the study of proteins with an established pathophysiological role in the context of LN. Although limited in scope, this approach allows the identification of biomarkers that have biological credibility as they are directly involved in the immunopathogenesis of LN. On the other hand, untargeted proteomics in the form of unbiased discovery proteomics allows for discovering a wide array of potential urinary protein biomarkers that are upregulated or downregulated in patients with LN.

3.1. Pro-Inflammatory Biomarkers

Urine proteomics has revealed that numerous cytokines, including IL-17, TWEAK, and MCP-1, can be elevated in patients with LN and positively correlate with disease activity [12]. Screening 1000 urinary protein biomarkers in 30 patients with LN and correlating the urinary protein signature with a single-cell transcriptomic analysis of renal biopsy specimens, Fava et al. demonstrated a robust link between urinary chemokine signals and renal immune cell infiltration, indicating that this approach may be more reflective of the immune status of the kidney than urinary proteinuria—currently widely utilized [47]. This approach also allowed for the stratification of patients with LN over a gradient of IFNγ-inducible chemokines, thereby adding biologically relevant information beyond traditional histological classifications [47]. Furthermore, these findings indicate the possibility of dynamically tracking LN status non-invasively through urine samples over time in a manner that could guide treatment decisions [47].

Recent urinary proteomic studies have revealed a consistent elevation in IL-16 in the urine of patients with active LN [48]. IL-16, a potent T-cell chemoattractant, significantly correlates with renal activity and the NIH indices—histopathology-based scoring systems designed to quantify the severity and progression of LN [49]. Moreover, an early decline in urinary IL-16 at 3 months correlated with treatment response to immunosuppression—a response determined based on UPCR, serum creatinine, and the dose of prednisone—outperforming traditional measures like UPCR [48]. In addition to its predictive value for treatment response, IL-16 can distinguish between proliferative LN and pure membranous LN with an AUC of 0.89 [49]. Additionally, urinary IL-16 abundance correlated with single-cell RNA sequencing analyses of renal biopsies, indicating that IL-16 is produced by infiltrating immune cells in LN kidneys, supporting its utility as a biomarker for monitoring intrarenal immune activity [49]. In 225 patients with LN, urine proteomic signatures showed that fibrous crescents were similar to activity-related lesions despite being considered inactive lesions [48]. Despite their classification under the NIH chronicity index, an inflammatory signature including CD73, MMP9, MIP1b, and IL-8 was identified in fibrous crescents, highlighting the potential for tailored interventions [50].

Beyond IL-16, CD163—a macrophage-specific hemoglobin scavenger receptor upregulated during inflammation—has been consistently identified as a urinary biomarker through ELISA and single-cell transcriptomics techniques in patients with LN [51–53]. Urinary CD163, closely following IL-16, significantly correlates with LN severity indicated by the NIH activity index and histological activity [48,54]. Urinary CD163 concentration improved considerably by week 12 in complete treatment responders, with a decline at three months predicting a one-year response more accurately than proteinuria [48]. Elevated CD163 levels across all LN classes, especially in proliferative forms, were closely linked to disease activity and treatment response, highlighting its utility as a non-invasive marker for tracking LN progression and therapeutic efficacy [48].

In addition to cytokines, a urine proteomic analysis has unveiled numerous signaling molecules as biomarkers of LN pathogenesis [14]. The application of extensive proteomics revealed a panel of six biomarkers (ICAM2, FABP4, FASLG, IGFBP-2, SELE, and TNFSF13B/BAFF) that effectively distinguished (AUC ROC > 0.8) patients with LN and active renal disease (AR) from those with inactive disease (iSLE), with the majority also showing a strong correlation with clinical disease activity [55]. Other promising urine biomarkers—such as Angptl4, L-selectin, TPP1, and TGFβ1—also had high ROC AUC values for distinguishing patients with lupus and AR from those with iSLE, with the combination of Angptl4, L-selectin, and TPP1 yielding the highest discrimination with an AUC of 0.97 [56]. Urinary L-selectin and Angptl4 preceded or coincided with worsening renal disease activity as measured by the renal domains of the Systemic Lupus Erythematosus Disease Activity Index (rSLEDAI), supporting a causal relationship between their elevation and LN severity [56]. However, not all these urinary proteins are suitable for diagnosing LN, as their levels may rise in other conditions causing chronic kidney disease [56]. For instance, Angptl4, L-selectin, and TPP1 were elevated in CKD secondary to numerous cases, TGFβ1 was only increased in FSGS, and urinary Angptl4 correlated with the CKD stage (correlation coefficient: 0.56; $p < 0.0001$) [56]. Additional urinary biomarkers such as ORM1 hold potential for the early detection of LN, even before the onset of significant proteinuria [57]. Another study on 92 patients investigated the use of high-throughput proteomics to identify urine-based markers for tracking kidney disease activity and damage in patients with LN monitored by the NIH activity index (NIH-AI) and chronicity index (NIH-CI) scores [58]. The study identified eight urinary markers (ApoA-II, vWF, IL-1α, IGFBP2, IL-6Rβ, KIM-1, DBH, and fetuin-A) and developed two predictive algorithms with over 88% specificity and 93% accuracy [58]. As longitudinal kidney biopsies are not typically performed for disease monitoring, these urinary markers hold promise for non-invasively tracking changes in LN status over time.

The role of a complement in LN is gaining attention due to the emergence of complement-targeting therapeutics [59]. In a study of 30 patients with LN, the kidney deposition of Membrane Attack Complex (MAC)—the terminal product of complement activation—was positively associated with tubulointerstitial fibrosis and atrophy (IFTA) and proteinuria, which are predictors of progression to ESKD [60]. Urinary proteomic assays in 46 patients with LN demonstrated that patients with more severe IFTA had a higher ratio of C9 to CD59 than those with no/mild IFTA [60]. Urinary complement activation markers also correlated with the increased expression of genes involved in TGFβ and PDGFRβ signaling, indicating a potential link between terminal complement pathway activation in kidney tubules and critical growth factors in developing kidney fibrosis in LN [61,62]. These findings align with transcriptomic data demonstrating that TGFβ1 can stimulate the expression of C3 in the kidneys and with studies showing that PDGFRβ-positive pericytes can secrete complement factor C1q in murine models of renal fibrosis [63,64]. TGFβ has been recognized for its crucial role in activating pro-apoptotic pathways, leading to renal fibrosis in patients with lupus, which can contribute to persistent immune stimulation and epitope spreading, consequently worsening autoimmunity [65].

3.2. Rail Score

A combination approach that utilizes both targeted and untargeted proteomics techniques to generate a novel biomarker panel represents an excellent strategy for biomarker development in the context of LN. This strategy has led to the recent development of the Renal Activity Index for Lupus Nephritis (RAIL) [45]. The RAIL score was developed by selecting urinary biomarkers from targeted and untargeted proteomics studies and applying multivariate regression analyses to identify the six most discriminative urinary biomarkers for LN—NGAL, MCP-1, KIM-1, ceruloplasmin, adiponectin, and hemopexin.

The RAIL score represents a novel biomarker panel comprising six urinary protein biomarkers, two from targeted proteomics and four from untargeted proteomic techniques. The two proteins utilized in the RAIL identified via targeted proteomics are neutrophil gelatinase-associated lipocalin (NGAL) and monocyte chemoattractant protein-1 (MCP-1). Mechanistically, NGAL represents a nephroprotective protein consistently upregulated in patients with various forms of renal injury in renal epithelial cells [66]. In contrast, MCP-1 is a chemokine that regulates immune cells' diffuse infiltration into renal tissue, facilitating the ongoing inflammatory cascade in LN [67]. Targeted proteomic techniques include enzyme-linked immunosorbent assays (ELISAs) to accurately quantify NGAL and MCP-1 in urinary samples amongst patients with LN [68]. Numerous cross-sectional and prospective cohort studies have shown that NGAL and MCP-1 significantly increase in patients with LN [69–73]. Moreover, higher levels of NGAL and MCP-1 were correlated with heightened disease activity, and these biomarkers could predict subsequent relapses and disease flares accurately [74–77]. The findings of these cohort studies, which jointly included approximately three hundred patients, led to the incorporation of MCP-1 and NGAL into the RAIL score.

In contrast, the other four biomarkers incorporated in the RAIL score were identified using unbiased discovery proteomics techniques, such as mass spectrometry. Four primary proteomic discovery studies pioneered the identification of novel urinary biomarkers in the context of LN [77–81]. These studies compared urine proteomic signatures across approximately 300 patients with LN and controls. They identified ~30 target proteins through the utilization of techniques such as surface-enhanced laser desorption–ionization time-of-flight mass spectrometry (SELDI-TOF) and matrix-assisted laser desorption–ionization time-of-flight mass spectrometry (MALDI-TOF-MS/MS). Identified proteins were then validated in further targeted proteomics studies utilizing ELISA techniques [81–84]. Subsequently, four of these proteins were selected in the RAIL score, including ceruloplasmin, adiponectin, hemopexin, and kidney injury molecule-1 (KIM-1). Mechanistically, hemopexin and ceruloplasmin represent antioxidant proteins that are increased in subjects with LN, potentially as an indicator of ongoing inflammation [85,86]. Furthermore, KIM-1 is in the nephron and is upregulated during kidney damage to facilitate the clearance of damaged cells [87,88]. Finally, adiponectin suppresses inflammation that can be upregulated in patients with LN [89]. Figure 2 provides an illustrative demonstration of the RAIL biomarkers and their function in the kidney. Importantly, proteins such as NGAL and KIM-1 are not specific for LN and reflect kidney injury secondary to a variety of causes (reviewed here: [90]).

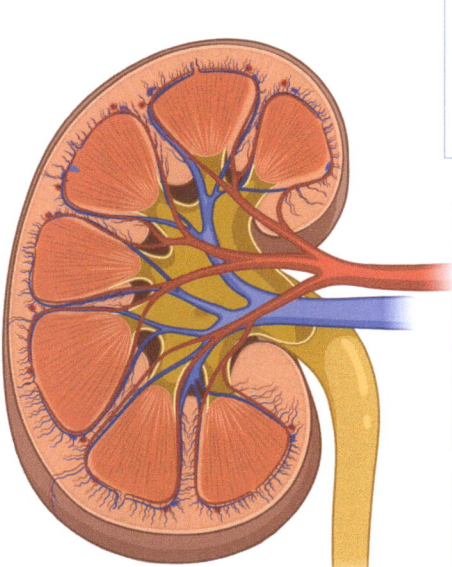

Figure 2. An overview of the components of the RAIL score. This figure was created using BioRender.com.

The first study to validate the RAIL score was conducted in a cohort of 46 children and adolescents and demonstrated outstanding efficacy with the capability to identify over 90% of LN cases [91]. Furthermore, the RAIL score outperformed conventional diagnostic scores that utilized traditional serum and laboratory biomarkers. Following this, the RAIL score was validated in a further study using 79 adult patients with LN, and it demonstrated excellent efficacy with an AUC of 0.88, indicating excellent diagnostic capacity [92]. Additionally, a third study set out to validate the predictive accuracy of the RAIL score in predicting response to therapy and disease flares amongst a cohort of 87 patients with LN [93]. In the study, the RAIL biomarkers could accurately predict response to therapy and propensity towards relapse, highlighting that these biomarkers not only hold diagnostic potential but are also capable of predicting the prognosis. RAIL scores could also distinguish clinically active LN from inactive LN or healthy controls in pediatric patients with SLE and decreased by ≥1 point in patients with complete remission [94]. Importantly, the RAIL score outperformed the rSLEDAI in capturing high LN activity (AUC of 0.79 vs. 0.62, respectively). Furthermore, the RAIL score could reveal subclinical/low–moderate LN activity in patients with an rSLEDAI of 0 who had a kidney biopsy more than 3 months ago [95], underscoring its potential as a method to routinely monitor subclinical kidney disease [94].

4. Urinary Metabolomics

Metabolomics approaches involve comprehensively profiling low-molecular-weight metabolites in a given biological sample. Nuclear magnetic resonance (NMR) spectroscopy and mass spectrometry are the main methods for conducting metabolomic analyses. Numerous studies have leveraged these techniques to identify novel biomarkers associated with various healthy and disease states, including cardiovascular disease [96], neurodegenerative disease [97], aging [98], pregnancy complications [99], and autoimmune diseases [100].

In this regard, NMR spectroscopy of serum of patients with LN, patients with SLE and without LN, and healthy controls has demonstrated that patients with LN have higher levels of lipoproteins (VLDL and LDL), but lower levels of acetate, than patients with SLE [101,102]. NMR spectroscopy of serum was used to describe that a combination of three metabolites (neuritic acid, C1q, and cystatin-C) could distinguish patients with SLE and LN from those without LN with an AUC of 0.9 [103]. Interestingly, these metabolomic changes are reversed upon treatment with cyclophosphamide-based therapy for 6 months, with LDL/VLDL levels decreasing and acetate levels increasing, with these changes also correlated with SLEDAI, renal SLEDAI, and serum C3 and C4 levels [102]. These findings indicate that serum-based metabolomics can distinguish patients with LN from SLE without LN and from healthy controls, as well as identify differential responses to treatment, which can thereby be used for monitoring therapy response.

Urinary metabolomics approaches in LN have been used to identify metabolites differentially affected in distinct histological classes of LN and monitor treatment responses. Compared to healthy controls, urinary pyruvate, citrate, fumarate, malate, and α-ketoglutarate are significantly decreased in patients with LN [104,105]. Comparing NMR-based metabolomic profiling in seven patients with class III/IV LN vs. class V LN, Romick-Rosendale et al. showed that urinary citrate was significantly lower in class V LN. In contrast, urinary taurine and Hippurate were markedly lower in class III/IV LN than type V LN [106]. In another study of six patients with pure class III/IV LN, seven patients with pure class V LN, and seven with mixed type III/IV + V LN, the ratio of picolinic acid to tryptophan (Pic/Trp) in urine was significantly lower in patients with type V LN than those with class III/IV. Combining the Pic/Trp ratio with eGFR and the urinary protein-to-creatinine ratio (UPCR) could distinguish the LN classification of pure type III/IV vs. pure type V LN with an AUC of 0.91, outperforming eGFR alone (0.499) and UCPR alone (0.444), which are current laboratory measures for monitoring LN [104].

In the context of treatment response, urinary citrate, which was significantly lower in patients with LN than healthy controls and distinguished between them with an AUC of 0.91, increased 6 months after induction therapy with cyclophosphamide for LN [105]. Urinary citrate levels also correlated moderately but significantly with C3 ($r = 0.362$; $p = 0.03$) and UPCR ($r = -0.346$; $p = 0.039$). Although urinary acetate levels—higher in patients with LN than healthy controls at the disease diagnosis—did not decrease significantly post-treatment, they did correlate significantly with SLEDAI ($r = 0.337$; $p = 0.048$). Considering this evidence and serum-based metabolomics studies that identified LN biomarkers, these findings pave the way for monitoring LN treatment response through routine blood samples or non-invasively through urine instead of renal biopsies. However, it remains to be investigated to what degree these treatment-related changes are brought about by clinically beneficial treatment responses or as an independent effect of these medications on the serum and urine metabolome [107].

5. Conclusions and Perspectives

Table 1 provides an overview of the transcriptomic, proteomic, and metabolomic biomarkers discussed within this review. Utilizing urinary transcriptomics, proteomics, and metabolomics in LN holds tremendous potential to aid in establishing accurate diagnoses and predicting the therapeutic response and prognosis. It is unlikely that urinary microRNAs and the RAIL biomarkers will replace conventional diagnostic modalities such as kidney biopsies and other traditional biomarkers. However, an approach utilizing urinary microRNAs, the RAIL and other pro-inflammatory biomarkers, and urinary metabolites in combination with conventional diagnostic methods offers a unique perspective toward enhancing diagnostic and prognostic accuracy. Moreover, urinary multi-omic protocols can eliminate the need for multiple kidney biopsies amongst patients with LN, as urinary microRNA, metabolites, and protein biomarkers can predict disease activity, reducing the repeated utilization of invasive procedures. Developing a multi-parameter urinary panel incorporating different types of multi-omic biomarkers could facilitate the generation of a novel, non-invasive modality that integrates emerging immuno-technologies to accurately aid in the disease diagnosis, predict the prognosis and therapeutic response, and assess the presence of chronic disease and renal architectural damage. Finally, such biomarkers can provide novel insights into the pathophysiology of the disease and its mechanisms, leading to advances in the understanding and targeted treatment of the disease.

Table 1. Summary of biomarkers for lupus nephritis.

Biomarker	Association	References
Urinary Transcriptomics		
miRNA-21	Distinguished inactive and active LN (AUC = 0.89) and differentiated healthy controls from patients with LN (sens.: 86%; AUC = 0.91).	[28–33]
miRNA-146a	Accurately discriminates patients with LN from healthy controls, directly correlates with disease activity and histological features.	[34–36]
miRNA-29c	Key modulator of renal fibrosis, accurately determines renal chronicity and disease severity in LN (sens.: >80%; spec.: >80%).	[37–39]
MicroRNA Panel (miRNA-21, miRNA-150, miRNA-29c)	Correlated significantly with the LN chronicity index.	[39]
MicroRNA Panel (miRNA-135b-5p, miRNA-107, miRNA-31)	Predicting disease activity and progression, showing significant differences between responders and non-responders during flare-ups and one year after (AUC = 0.73–0.78).	[43]
Urinary Proteomics		
IL-16	Correlates with renal activity and NIH indices, predictive of treatment response, distinguishes LN types with high accuracy (AUC of 0.89).	[48,49]
CD73, MMP9, MIP1b, IL-8	Identifies fibrous crescents.	[50]
CD163	Correlates with LN severity and treatment response, predicts one-year response more accurately than traditional measures.	[48,51–54]
Proteomic Panel (ICAM2, FABP4, FASLG, IGFBP-2, SELE, TNFSF13B/BAFF)	Distinguishes active renal disease from inactive disease in patients with LN with high accuracy (AUC > 0.8), correlates with clinical disease activity.	[55]

Table 1. Cont.

Biomarker	Association	References
Angptl4, L-selectin, TPP1, TGFβ1	High discrimination power for active vs. inactive disease (highest AUC of 0.97 with a combination), indicates causal relationship with LN severity.	[56]
ORM1	Early detection of LN.	[57]
Urinary apoA-II, vWF, IL-1α, IGFBP2, IL-6Rβ, KIM-1, DBH, Fetuin-A	Identified for tracking kidney disease activity and damage in LN, with high specificity and accuracy.	[58]
Complement Activation Markers (C9-to-CD59 Ratio)	Associated with tubulointerstitial fibrosis and proteinuria, indicators of ESRD progression; linked with TGFβ and PDGFRβ signaling in kidney fibrosis development.	[60–64]
NGAL	Upregulated in renal epithelial cells during renal injury. Significantly increases in patients with LN, correlates with disease activity, and predicts relapses and disease flares.	[66,69–77]
MCP-1	Elevated levels associated with increased disease activity and predictive of disease progression.	[67,69–77]
Ceruloplasmin	Antioxidant protein increased in LN, potentially indicating ongoing inflammation.	[86]
Adiponectin	Anti-inflammatory protein upregulated in patients with LN.	[89]
Hemopexin	Antioxidant protein increased in subjects with LN, indicating ongoing inflammation.	[85]
KIM-1	Upregulated during kidney damage for the clearance of damaged cells.	[87]
RAIL Score (NGAL, MCP-1, Ceruloplasmin, Adiponectin, Hemopexin, KIM-1)	Diagnostic capability (over 90% identification rate of LN cases in children and adolescents; AUC of 0.88 in adults). Excellent predictive accuracy for response to therapy and disease flares.	[90–95]
Urinary Metabolomics		
Serum Lipoproteins (VLDL, LDL), Acetate Levels	Higher VLDL and LDL but lower acetate levels in patients with LN compared to healthy controls. Changes upon treatment correlate with disease activity and treatment response.	[101,102]
Serum Neuritic Acid, C1q, Cystatin-C	Can distinguish patients with SLE and LN from those without LN (AUC = 0.9). Levels reverse upon treatment.	[103]
Urinary Pyruvate, Citrate, Fumarate, Malate, α-Ketoglutarate	Significantly decreased in patients with LN compared to healthy controls.	[104,105]
Urinary Citrate	Significantly lower in class V LN compared to class III/IV. Increases after treatment, correlating with treatment response.	[105,106]
Urinary Taurine and Hippurate	Markedly lower in class III/IV LN than class V.	[106]
Urinary-Picolinic-Acid-to-Tryptophan Ratio (Pic/Trp)	Lower in type V LN than in class III/IV; combined with eGFR and UPCR, distinguishes LN classes with high accuracy (AUC of 0.91).	[104]
Urinary Acetate	Higher in patients with LN at diagnosis; correlates with disease activity (SLEDAI), but does not significantly decrease post-treatment.	[106]

Angptl4: Angiopoietin-like 4; C1q: Complement component 1q; DBH: Dopamine beta-hydroxylase; FABP4: Fatty acid binding protein 4; FASLG: Fas ligand; ICAM2: Intercellular adhesion molecule 2; IGFBP-2: Insulin-like growth factor binding protein 2; IL: Interleukin; IL-1α: Interleukin 1 alpha; IL-6Rβ: Interleukin 6 receptor beta; KIM-1: Kidney injury molecule-1; L-selectin: L-selectin; LDL: Low-density lipoprotein; MCP-1: Monocyte chemoattractant protein-1; MIP1b: Macrophage inflammatory protein 1 beta; miRNA: microRNA; MMP9: Matrix metallopeptidase 9; NGAL: Neutrophil gelatinase-associated lipocalin; ORM1: Orosomucoid 1; SELE: Selectin E; TGFβ1: Transforming growth factor beta 1; TNFSF13B/BAFF: Tumor necrosis factor superfamily member 13B/B-cell activating factor; TPP1: Tripeptidyl peptidase 1; VLDL: Very-low-density lipoprotein; vWF: von Willebrand factor.

Nonetheless, several challenges and limitations remain in utilizing urinary transcriptomics and proteomics in the clinical setting. More extensive prospective studies across diverse patient cohorts remain a need to validate the findings of urinary biomarkers, including the RAIL biomarkers and urinary microRNAs. In 368 adolescents and young adults, RAIL biomarkers amongst the healthy controls demonstrated substantial variations in biomarker levels due to age and gender [108]. Moreover, several studies have found conflicting evidence regarding quantifying specific urinary microRNAs in the context of lupus nephritis [109]. Hence, validation studies establishing reference ranges for these urinary biomarkers to distinguish healthy controls from patients with LN accurately are needed.

Additionally, cutting-edge quantitative transcriptomic, proteomic, and metabolomic techniques are required to quantify these biomarkers accurately in the clinical setting. The majority of the studies validating the RAIL biomarkers utilized ELISA techniques for protein quantification; however, given the emergence of novel approaches such as mass spectrometry to quantify proteins, the incorporation of these techniques in the clinical setting is required owing to their accuracy and potential cost-effectiveness when utilized at a grander scale [110]. On the other hand, the majority of studies quantifying urinary microRNAs used RT-qPCR to quantify microRNAs; however, the emergence of next-generation sequencing technology offers unique perspectives toward the quantification of microRNAs due to its greater sensitivity and capacity to quantify total microRNA signatures [111]. Additionally, mechanistic research efforts are required to further elucidate the contribution of identified biomarkers towards the pathophysiology of LN. The confounding effect of treatment (including corticosteroids and immunosuppressants), patient comorbidities, and lifestyle factors on urinary transcriptomic, proteomic, and metabolomic findings must also be better understood, as this could majorly affect the interpretation of findings in individual patients. Finally, collaborative efforts are needed between scientists and clinicians to bridge the gap and raise awareness regarding the tremendous utility of these biomarkers in the clinical setting. Metabolomics approaches are increasingly utilized in the field of cardiovascular disease prevention and management in the form of composite metabolomic risk scores or lipidomic scores, which signals increasing clinician awareness of these novel approaches. Nevertheless, more must be done to increase knowledge of these technologies if they are to be introduced widely into clinical care, including the possibility of integrating their basics into the medical education curriculum.

Author Contributions: Conceptualization, M.H.O.; writing—original draft preparation, M.H.O., A.S., O.A. and J.N.; writing—review and editing, K.A. and A.Y. All authors have read and agreed to the published version of the manuscript.

Funding: This research received no external funding.

Institutional Review Board Statement: Not applicable.

Informed Consent Statement: Not applicable.

Data Availability Statement: Not applicable.

Acknowledgments: Figures were created using Biorender.com.

Conflicts of Interest: The authors declare no conflicts of interest.

References

1. Tsokos, G.C. Systemic Lupus Erythematosus. *N. Engl. J. Med.* **2011**, *365*, 2110–2121. [CrossRef]
2. Almaani, S.; Meara, A.; Rovin, B.H. Update on Lupus Nephritis. *Clin. J. Am. Soc. Nephrol.* **2017**, *12*, 825–835. [CrossRef] [PubMed]
3. Anders, H.-J.; Saxena, R.; Zhao, M.-H.; Parodis, I.; Salmon, J.E.; Mohan, C. Lupus nephritis. *Nat. Rev. Dis. Primers* **2020**, *6*, 7. [CrossRef] [PubMed]
4. Luo, W.; Farinha, F.; Isenberg, D.A.; Rahman, A. Survival analysis of mortality and development of lupus nephritis in patients with systemic lupus erythematosus up to 40 years of follow-up. *Rheumatology* **2022**, *62*, 200–208. [CrossRef] [PubMed]
5. Fasano, S.; Milone, A.; Nicoletti, G.F.; Isenberg, D.A.; Ciccia, F. Precision medicine in systemic lupus erythematosus. *Nat. Rev. Rheumatol.* **2023**, *19*, 331–342. [CrossRef] [PubMed]

6. Kernder, A.; Richter, J.G.; Fischer-Betz, R.; Winkler-Rohlfing, B.; Brinks, R.; Aringer, M.; Schneider, M.; Chehab, G. Delayed diagnosis adversely affects outcome in systemic lupus erythematosus: Cross sectional analysis of the LuLa cohort. *Lupus* **2021**, *30*, 431–438. [CrossRef] [PubMed]
7. Fanouriakis, A.; Kostopoulou, M.; Cheema, K.; Anders, H.J.; Aringer, M.; Bajema, I.; Boletis, J.; Frangou, E.; Houssiau, F.A.; Hollis, J.; et al. 2019 Update of the Joint European League against Rheumatism and European Renal Association-European Dialysis and Transplant Association (EULAR/ERA-EDTA) recommendations for the management of lupus nephritis. *Ann. Rheum. Dis.* **2020**, *79*, 713–723. [CrossRef] [PubMed]
8. Hahn, B.H.; McMahon, M.A.; Wilkinson, A.; Wallace, W.D.; Daikh, D.I.; Fitzgerald, J.D.; Karpouzas, G.A.; Merrill, J.T.; Wallace, D.J.; Yazdany, J.; et al. American College of Rheumatology guidelines for screening, treatment, and management of lupus nephritis. *Arthritis Care Res.* **2012**, *64*, 797–808. [CrossRef]
9. Antonis, F.; Myrto, K.; Jeanette, A.; Martin, A.; Laurent, A.; Sang-Cheol, B.; John, B.; Ian, N.B.; Ricard, C.; Andrea, D.; et al. EULAR recommendations for the management of systemic lupus erythematosus: 2023 update. *Ann. Rheum. Dis.* **2024**, *83*, 15. [CrossRef]
10. Soliman, S.; Mohan, C. Lupus nephritis biomarkers. *Clin. Immunol.* **2017**, *185*, 10–20. [CrossRef]
11. Mok, C.C. Biomarkers for lupus nephritis: A critical appraisal. *J. Biomed. Biotechnol.* **2010**, *2010*, 638413. [CrossRef] [PubMed]
12. Palazzo, L.; Lindblom, J.; Mohan, C.; Parodis, I. Current Insights on Biomarkers in Lupus Nephritis: A Systematic Review of the Literature. *J. Clin. Med.* **2022**, *11*, 5759. [CrossRef] [PubMed]
13. Rovin, B.H.; Ayoub, I.M.; Chan, T.M.; Liu, Z.-H.; Mejía-Vilet, J.M.; Floege, J. KDIGO 2024 Clinical Practice Guideline for the management of LUPUS NEPHRITIS. *Kidney Int.* **2024**, *105*, S1–S69. [CrossRef]
14. Zhang, T.; Duran, V.; Vanarsa, K.; Mohan, C. Targeted urine proteomics in lupus nephritis—A meta-analysis. *Expert Rev. Proteom.* **2020**, *17*, 767–776. [CrossRef] [PubMed]
15. Dias, R.; Hasparyk, U.G.; Lopes, M.P.; de Barros, J.L.V.M.; Simões e Silva, A.C. Novel Biomarkers for Lupus Nephritis in the "OMICS" Era. *Curr. Med. Chem.* **2021**, *28*, 6011–6044. [CrossRef] [PubMed]
16. Hasin, Y.; Seldin, M.; Lusis, A. Multi-omics approaches to disease. *Genome Biol.* **2017**, *18*, 83. [CrossRef] [PubMed]
17. Solé, C.; Goicoechea, I.; Goñi, A.; Schramm, M.; Armesto, M.; Arestin, M.; Manterola, L.; Tellaetxe, M.; Alberdi, A.; Nogueira, L.; et al. The Urinary Transcriptome as a Source of Biomarkers for Prostate Cancer. *Cancers* **2020**, *12*, 513. [CrossRef] [PubMed]
18. Dubois, J.; Rueger, J.; Haubold, B.; Far, R.K.-K.; Sczakiel, G. Transcriptome analyses of urine RNA reveal tumor markers for human bladder cancer: Validated amplicons for RT-qPCR-based detection. *Oncotarget* **2021**, *12*, 1011–1023. [CrossRef] [PubMed]
19. Arazi, A.; Rao, D.A.; Berthier, C.C.; Davidson, A.; Liu, Y.; Hoover, P.J.; Chicoine, A.; Eisenhaure, T.M.; Jonsson, A.H.; Li, S.; et al. The immune cell landscape in kidneys of patients with lupus nephritis. *Nat. Immunol.* **2019**, *20*, 902–914. [CrossRef] [PubMed]
20. Deng, Y.; Zheng, Y.; Li, D.; Hong, Q.; Zhang, M.; Li, Q.; Fu, B.; Wu, L.; Wang, X.; Shen, W.; et al. Expression characteristics of interferon-stimulated genes and possible regulatory mechanisms in lupus patients using transcriptomics analyses. *EBioMedicine* **2021**, *70*, 103477. [CrossRef]
21. Der, E.; Ranabothu, S.; Suryawanshi, H.; Akat, K.M.; Clancy, R.; Morozov, P.; Kustagi, M.; Czuppa, M.; Izmirly, P.; Belmont, H.M.; et al. Single cell RNA sequencing to dissect the molecular heterogeneity in lupus nephritis. *JCI Insight* **2017**, *2*, e93009. [CrossRef] [PubMed]
22. Der, E.; Suryawanshi, H.; Morozov, P.; Kustagi, M.; Goilav, B.; Ranabothu, S.; Izmirly, P.; Clancy, R.; Belmont, H.M.; Koenigsberg, M.; et al. Tubular cell and keratinocyte single-cell transcriptomics applied to lupus nephritis reveal type I IFN and fibrosis relevant pathways. *Nat. Immunol.* **2019**, *20*, 915–927. [CrossRef]
23. Parikh, S.V.; Malvar, A.; Song, H.; Shapiro, J.; Mejia-Vilet, J.M.; Ayoub, I.; Almaani, S.; Madhavan, S.; Alberton, V.; Besso, C.; et al. Molecular profiling of kidney compartments from serial biopsies differentiate treatment responders from non-responders in lupus nephritis. *Kidney Int.* **2022**, *102*, 845–865. [CrossRef] [PubMed]
24. Bartel, D.P. MicroRNAs. *Cell* **2004**, *116*, 281–297. [CrossRef] [PubMed]
25. Condrat, C.E.; Thompson, D.C.; Barbu, M.G.; Bugnar, O.L.; Boboc, A.; Cretoiu, D.; Suciu, N.; Cretoiu, S.M.; Voinea, S.C. miRNAs as Biomarkers in Disease: Latest Findings Regarding Their Role in Diagnosis and Prognosis. *Cells* **2020**, *9*, 276. [CrossRef] [PubMed]
26. Tsokos, G.C.; Lo, M.S.; Reis, P.C.; Sullivan, K.E. New insights into the immunopathogenesis of systemic lupus erythematosus. *Nat. Rev. Rheumatol.* **2016**, *12*, 716–730. [CrossRef] [PubMed]
27. Schmittgen, T.D.; Lee, E.J.; Jiang, J.; Sarkar, A.; Yang, L.; Elton, T.S.; Chen, C. Real-time PCR quantification of precursor and mature microRNA. *Methods* **2008**, *44*, 31–38. [CrossRef]
28. Dai, Y.; Huang, Y.S.; Tang, M.; Lv, T.Y.; Hu, C.X.; Tan, Y.H.; Xu, Z.M.; Yin, Y.B. Microarray analysis of microRNA expression in peripheral blood cells of systemic lupus erythematosus patients. *Lupus* **2007**, *16*, 939–946. [CrossRef] [PubMed]
29. Jenike, A.E.; Halushka, M.K. miR-21: A non-specific biomarker of all maladies. *Biomark. Res.* **2021**, *9*, 18. [CrossRef]
30. Stagakis, E.; Bertsias, G.; Verginis, P.; Nakou, M.; Hatziapostolou, M.; Kritikos, H.; Iliopoulos, D.; Boumpas, D.T. Identification of novel microRNA signatures linked to human lupus disease activity and pathogenesis: miR-21 regulates aberrant T cell responses through regulation of PDCD4 expression. *Ann. Rheum. Dis.* **2011**, *70*, 1496–1506. [CrossRef]
31. Kumarswamy, R.; Volkmann, I.; Thum, T. Regulation and function of miRNA-21 in health and disease. *RNA Biol.* **2011**, *8*, 706–713. [CrossRef] [PubMed]

32. Khoshmirsafa, M.; Kianmehr, N.; Falak, R.; Mowla, S.J.; Seif, F.; Mirzaei, B.; Valizadeh, M.; Shekarabi, M. Elevated expression of miR-21 and miR-155 in peripheral blood mononuclear cells as potential biomarkers for lupus nephritis. *Int. J. Rheum. Dis.* **2018**, *22*, 458–467. [CrossRef] [PubMed]
33. Nakhjavani, M.; Etemadi, J.; Pourlak, T.; Mirhosaini, Z.; Zununi Vahed, S.; Abediazar, S. Plasma levels of miR-21, miR-150, miR-423 in patients with lupus nephritis. *Iran. J. Kidney Dis.* **2019**, *13*, 198–206.
34. Labbaye, C.; Testa, U. The emerging role of MIR-146A in the control of hematopoiesis, immune function and cancer. *J. Hematol. Oncol.* **2012**, *5*, 13. [CrossRef] [PubMed]
35. Perez-Hernandez, J.; Forner, M.J.; Pinto, C.; Chaves, F.J.; Cortes, R.; Redon, J. Increased Urinary Exosomal MicroRNAs in Patients with Systemic Lupus Erythematosus. *PLoS ONE* **2015**, *10*, e0138618. [CrossRef] [PubMed]
36. Perez-Hernandez, J.; Martinez-Arroyo, O.; Ortega, A.; Galera, M.; Solis-Salguero, M.A.; Chaves, F.J.; Redon, J.; Forner, M.J.; Cortes, R. Urinary exosomal miR-146a as a marker of albuminuria, activity changes and disease flares in lupus nephritis. *J. Nephrol.* **2020**, *34*, 1157–1167. [CrossRef] [PubMed]
37. Huang, H.; Huang, X.; Luo, S.; Zhang, H.; Hu, F.; Chen, R.; Huang, C.; Su, Z. The MicroRNA MiR-29c Alleviates Renal Fibrosis via TPM1-Mediated Suppression of the Wnt/β-Catenin Pathway. *Front. Physiol.* **2020**, *11*, 331. [CrossRef] [PubMed]
38. Solé, C.; Cortés-Hernández, J.; Felip, M.L.; Vidal, M.; Ordi-Ros, J. miR-29c in urinary exosomes as predictor of early renal fibrosis in lupus nephritis. *Nephrol. Dial. Transplant.* **2015**, *30*, 1488–1496. [CrossRef] [PubMed]
39. Solé, C.; Moliné, T.; Vidal, M.; Ordi-Ros, J.; Cortés-Hernández, J. An Exosomal Urinary miRNA Signature for Early Diagnosis of Renal Fibrosis in Lupus Nephritis. *Cells* **2019**, *8*, 773. [CrossRef]
40. Lu, S.; Kong, H.; Hou, Y.; Ge, D.; Huang, W.; Ou, J.; Yang, D.; Zhang, L.; Wu, G.; Song, Y.; et al. Two plasma microRNA panels for diagnosis and subtype discrimination of lung cancer. *Lung Cancer* **2018**, *123*, 44–51. [CrossRef]
41. Ying, L.; Du, L.; Zou, R.; Shi, L.; Zhang, N.; Jin, J.; Xu, C.; Zhang, F.; Zhu, C.; Wu, J.; et al. Development of a serum miRNA panel for detection of early stage non-small cell lung cancer. *Proc. Natl. Acad. Sci. USA* **2020**, *117*, 25036–25042. [CrossRef] [PubMed]
42. Nagaraj, S.; Zoltowska, K.M.; Laskowska-Kaszub, K.; Wojda, U. microRNA diagnostic panel for Alzheimer's disease and epigenetic trade-off between neurodegeneration and cancer. *Ageing Res. Rev.* **2019**, *49*, 125–143. [CrossRef] [PubMed]
43. Garcia-Vives, E.; Solé, C.; Moliné, T.; Vidal, M.; Agraz, I.; Ordi-Ros, J.; Cortés-Hernández, J. The Urinary Exosomal miRNA Expression Profile is Predictive of Clinical Response in Lupus Nephritis. *Int. J. Mol. Sci.* **2020**, *21*, 1372. [CrossRef] [PubMed]
44. Hudler, P.; Kocevar, N.; Komel, R. Proteomic approaches in biomarker discovery: New perspectives in cancer diagnostics. *Sci. World J.* **2014**, *2014*, 260348. [CrossRef] [PubMed]
45. Aljaberi, N.; Bennett, M.; Brunner, H.I.; Devarajan, P. Proteomic profiling of urine: Implications for lupus nephritis. *Expert Rev. Proteom.* **2019**, *16*, 303–313. [CrossRef] [PubMed]
46. Sobsey, C.A.; Ibrahim, S.; Richard, V.R.; Gaspar, V.; Mitsa, G.; Lacasse, V.; Zahedi, R.P.; Batist, G.; Borchers, C.H. Targeted and Untargeted Proteomics Approaches in Biomarker Development. *Proteomics* **2020**, *20*, 1900029. [CrossRef] [PubMed]
47. Fava, A.; Buyon, J.; Mohan, C.; Zhang, T.; Belmont, H.M.; Izmirly, P.; Clancy, R.; Trujillo, J.M.; Fine, D.; Zhang, Y.; et al. Integrated urine proteomics and renal single-cell genomics identify an IFN-γ response gradient in lupus nephritis. *JCI Insight* **2020**, *5*, e138345. [CrossRef] [PubMed]
48. Fava, A.; Buyon, J.; Magder, L.; Hodgin, J.; Rosenberg, A.; Demeke, D.S.; Rao, D.A.; Arazi, A.; Celia, A.I.; Putterman, C.; et al. Urine proteomic signatures of histological class, activity, chronicity, and treatment response in lupus nephritis. *JCI Insight* **2024**, *9*, e172569. [CrossRef]
49. Fava, A.; Rao, D.A.; Mohan, C.; Zhang, T.; Rosenberg, A.; Fenaroli, P.; Belmont, H.M.; Izmirly, P.; Clancy, R.; Trujillo, J.M.; et al. Urine Proteomics and Renal Single-Cell Transcriptomics Implicate Interleukin-16 in Lupus Nephritis. *Arthritis Rheumatol.* **2022**, *74*, 829–839. [CrossRef]
50. Celia, A.I.; Hodgin, J.; Demeke, D.; Rosenberg, A.; Magder, L.; Buyon, J.; Diamond, B.; James, J.A.; Apruzzese, W.; Fenaroli, P.; et al. POS0297 PROTEOMIC ANALYSIS OF HISTOLOGICAL LESIONS LUPUS NEPHRITIS IDENTIFIES AN INFLAMMATORY SIGNATURE OF FIBROUS CRESCENTS. *Ann. Rheum. Dis.* **2023**, *82*, 390–391. [CrossRef]
51. Mejia-Vilet, J.M.; Zhang, X.L.; Cruz, C.; Cano-Verduzco, M.L.; Shapiro, J.P.; Nagaraja, H.N.; Morales-Buenrostro, L.E.; Rovin, B.H. Urinary Soluble CD163: A Novel Noninvasive Biomarker of Activity for Lupus Nephritis. *J. Am. Soc. Nephrol.* **2020**, *31*, 1335–1347. [CrossRef] [PubMed]
52. Peterson, K.S.; Huang, J.-F.; Zhu, J.; D'Agati, V.; Liu, X.; Miller, N.; Erlander, M.G.; Jackson, M.R.; Winchester, R.J. Characterization of heterogeneity in the molecular pathogenesis of lupus nephritis from transcriptional profiles of laser-captured glomeruli. *J. Clin. Investig.* **2004**, *113*, 1722–1733. [CrossRef] [PubMed]
53. Huang, Y.-J.; Lin, C.-H.; Yang, H.-Y.; Luo, S.-F.; Kuo, C.-F. Urine Soluble CD163 Is a Promising Biomarker for the Diagnosis and Evaluation of Lupus Nephritis. *Front. Immunol.* **2022**, *13*, 935700. [CrossRef]
54. Zhang, T.; Li, H.; Vanarsa, K.; Gidley, G.; Mok, C.C.; Petri, M.; Saxena, R.; Mohan, C. Association of Urine sCD163 With Proliferative Lupus Nephritis, Fibrinoid Necrosis, Cellular Crescents and Intrarenal M2 Macrophages. *Front. Immunol.* **2020**, *11*, 671. [CrossRef] [PubMed]
55. Li, Y.; Tang, C.; Vanarsa, K.; Thai, N.; Castillo, J.; Lea, G.A.B.; Lee, K.H.; Kim, S.; Pedroza, C.; Wu, T.; et al. Proximity extension assay proteomics and renal single cell transcriptomics uncover novel urinary biomarkers for active lupus nephritis. *J. Autoimmun.* **2024**, *143*, 103165. [CrossRef] [PubMed]

56. Vanarsa, K.; Soomro, S.; Zhang, T.; Strachan, B.; Pedroza, C.; Nidhi, M.; Cicalese, P.; Gidley, C.; Dasari, S.; Mohan, S.; et al. Quantitative planar array screen of 1000 proteins uncovers novel urinary protein biomarkers of lupus nephritis. *Ann. Rheum. Dis.* **2020**, *79*, 1349–1361. [CrossRef] [PubMed]
57. Kwon, O.C.; Lee, E.J.; Yeom, J.; Hong, S.; Lee, C.K.; Yoo, B.; Park, M.C.; Kim, K.; Kim, Y.G. Discovery of urine biomarkers for lupus nephritis via quantitative and comparative proteome analysis. *Clin. Transl. Med.* **2021**, *11*, e638. [CrossRef] [PubMed]
58. Akhgar, A.; Sinibaldi, D.; Zeng, L.; Farris, A.B., 3rd; Cobb, J.; Battle, M.; Chain, D.; Cann, J.A.; Illei, G.G.; Lim, S.S.; et al. Urinary markers differentially associate with kidney inflammatory activity and chronicity measures in patients with lupus nephritis. *Lupus Sci. Med.* **2023**, *10*, e000747. [CrossRef] [PubMed]
59. Mastellos, D.C.; Hajishengallis, G.; Lambris, J.D. A guide to complement biology, pathology and therapeutic opportunity. *Nat. Rev. Immunol.* **2024**, *24*, 118–141. [CrossRef]
60. Wang, S.; Wu, M.; Chiriboga, L.; Zeck, B.; Goilav, B.; Wang, S.; Jimenez, A.L.; Putterman, C.; Schwarz, D.; Pullman, J.; et al. Membrane attack complex (MAC) deposition in renal tubules is associated with interstitial fibrosis and tubular atrophy: A pilot study. *Lupus Sci. Med.* **2022**, *9*, e000576. [CrossRef]
61. Meng, X.-m.; Nikolic-Paterson, D.J.; Lan, H.Y. TGF-β: The master regulator of fibrosis. *Nat. Rev. Nephrol.* **2016**, *12*, 325–338. [CrossRef]
62. Wang, S.; Broder, A.; Shao, D.; Kesarwani, V.; Boderman, B.; Aguilan, J.; Sidoli, S.; Suzuki, M.; Greally, J.M.; Saenger, Y.M.; et al. Urine Proteomics Link Complement Activation with Interstitial Fibrosis/Tubular Atrophy in Lupus Nephritis Patients. *Semin. Arthritis Rheum.* **2023**, *63*, 152263. [CrossRef]
63. Liu, T.; Yang, M.; Xia, Y.; Jiang, C.; Li, C.; Jiang, Z.; Wang, X. Microarray-based analysis of renal complement components reveals a therapeutic target for lupus nephritis. *Arthritis Res. Ther.* **2021**, *23*, 223. [CrossRef]
64. Xavier, S.; Sahu, R.K.; Landes, S.G.; Yu, J.; Taylor, R.P.; Ayyadevara, S.; Megyesi, J.; Stallcup, W.B.; Duffield, J.S.; Reis, E.S.; et al. Pericytes and immune cells contribute to complement activation in tubulointerstitial fibrosis. *Am. J. Physiol.-Ren. Physiol.* **2017**, *312*, F516–F532. [CrossRef]
65. Sciascia, S.; Cozzi, M.; Barinotti, A.; Radin, M.; Cecchi, I.; Fenoglio, R.; Mancardi, D.; Wilson Jones, G.; Rossi, D.; Roccatello, D. Renal Fibrosis in Lupus Nephritis. *Int. J. Mol. Sci.* **2022**, *23*, 14317. [CrossRef] [PubMed]
66. Bolignano, D.; Donato, V.; Coppolino, G.; Campo, S.; Buemi, A.; Lacquaniti, A.; Buemi, M. Neutrophil Gelatinase–Associated Lipocalin (NGAL) as a Marker of Kidney Damage. *Am. J. Kidney Dis.* **2008**, *52*, 595–605. [CrossRef] [PubMed]
67. Haller, H.; Bertram, A.; Nadrowitz, F.; Menne, J. Monocyte chemoattractant protein-1 and the kidney. *Curr. Opin. Nephrol. Hypertens.* **2016**, *25*, 42–49. [CrossRef]
68. Harlan, R.; Zhang, H. Targeted proteomics: A bridge between discovery and validation. *Expert Rev. Proteom.* **2014**, *11*, 657–661. [CrossRef] [PubMed]
69. Noris, M.; Bernasconi, S.; Casiraghi, F.; Sozzani, S.; Gotti, E.; Remuzzi, G.; Mantovani, A. Monocyte chemoattractant protein-1 is excreted in excessive amounts in the urine of patients with lupus nephritis. *Lab. Investig.* **1995**, *73*, 804–809.
70. Marks, S.D.; Shah, V.; Pilkington, C.; Tullus, K. Urinary monocyte chemoattractant protein-1 correlates with disease activity in lupus nephritis. *Pediatr. Nephrol.* **2010**, *25*, 2283–2288. [CrossRef]
71. Brunner, H.I.; Mueller, M.; Rutherford, C.; Passo, M.H.; Witte, D.; Grom, A.; Mishra, J.; Devarajan, P. Urinary neutrophil gelatinase–associated lipocalin as a biomarker of nephritis in childhood-onset systemic lupus erythematosus. *Arthritis Rheum.* **2006**, *54*, 2577–2584. [CrossRef] [PubMed]
72. El Shahawy, M.S.; Hemida, M.H.; Abdel-Hafez, H.A.; El-Baz, T.Z.; Lotfy, A.-W.M.; Emran, T.M. Urinary neutrophil gelatinase-associated lipocalin as a marker for disease activity in lupus nephritis. *Scand. J. Clin. Lab. Investig.* **2018**, *78*, 264–268. [CrossRef]
73. Gómez-Puerta, J.A.; Ortiz-Reyes, B.; Urrego, T.; Vanegas-García, A.L.; Muñoz, C.H.; González, L.A.; Cervera, R.; Vásquez, G. Urinary neutrophil gelatinase-associated lipocalin and monocyte chemoattractant protein 1 as biomarkers for lupus nephritis in Colombian SLE patients. *Lupus* **2017**, *27*, 637–646. [CrossRef]
74. Rovin, B.H.; Song, H.; Birmingham, D.J.; Hebert, L.A.; Yu, C.Y.; Nagaraja, H.N. Urine Chemokines as Biomarkers of Human Systemic Lupus Erythematosus Activity. *J. Am. Soc. Nephrol.* **2005**, *16*, 467–473. [CrossRef]
75. Suzuki, M.; Wiers, K.M.; Klein-Gitelman, M.S.; Haines, K.A.; Olson, J.; Onel, K.B.; O'Neil, K.; Passo, M.H.; Singer, N.G.; Tucker, L.; et al. Neutrophil gelatinase-associated lipocalin as a biomarker of disease activity in pediatric lupus nephritis. *Pediatr. Nephrol.* **2008**, *23*, 403–412. [CrossRef] [PubMed]
76. Hinze, C.H.; Suzuki, M.; Klein-Gitelman, M.; Passo, M.H.; Olson, J.; Singer, N.G.; Haines, K.A.; Onel, K.; O'Neil, K.; Silverman, E.D.; et al. Neutrophil gelatinase-associated lipocalin is a predictor of the course of global and renal childhood-onset systemic lupus erythematosus disease activity. *Arthritis Rheum.* **2009**, *60*, 2772–2781. [CrossRef]
77. Singh, R.G.; Usha; Rathore, S.S.; Behura, S.K.; Singh, N.K. Urinary MCP-1 as diagnostic and prognostic marker in patients with lupus nephritis flare. *Lupus* **2012**, *21*, 1214–1218. [CrossRef] [PubMed]
78. Suzuki, M.; Ross, G.F.; Wiers, K.; Nelson, S.; Bennett, M.; Passo, M.H.; Devarajan, P.; Brunner, H.I. Identification of a urinary proteomic signature for lupus nephritis in children. *Pediatr. Nephrol.* **2007**, *22*, 2047–2057. [CrossRef] [PubMed]
79. Aggarwal, A.; Gupta, R.; Negi, V.S.; Rajasekhar, L.; Misra, R.; Singh, P.; Chaturvedi, V.; Sinha, S. Urinary haptoglobin, alpha-1 anti-chymotrypsin and retinol binding protein identified by proteomics as potential biomarkers for lupus nephritis. *Clin. Exp. Immunol.* **2017**, *188*, 254–262. [CrossRef]

80. Zhang, X.; Jin, M.; Wu, H.; Nadasdy, T.; Nadasdy, G.; Harris, N.; Green-Church, K.; Nagaraja, H.; Birmingham, D.J.; Yu, C.-Y.; et al. Biomarkers of lupus nephritis determined by serial urine proteomics. *Kidney Int.* **2008**, *74*, 799–807. [CrossRef]
81. Brunner, H.I.; Bennett, M.R.; Mina, R.; Suzuki, M.; Petri, M.; Kiani, A.N.; Pendl, J.; Witte, D.; Ying, J.; Rovin, B.H.; et al. Association of noninvasively measured renal protein biomarkers with histologic features of lupus nephritis. *Arthritis Rheum.* **2012**, *64*, 2687–2697. [CrossRef]
82. Suzuki, M.; Wiers, K.; Brooks, E.B.; Greis, K.D.; Haines, K.; Klein-Gitelman, M.S.; Olson, J.; Onel, K.; O'Neil, K.M.; Silverman, E.D.; et al. Initial validation of a novel protein biomarker panel for active pediatric lupus nephritis. *Pediatr. Res.* **2009**, *65*, 530–536. [CrossRef] [PubMed]
83. Go, D.J.; Lee, J.Y.; Kang, M.J.; Lee, E.Y.; Lee, E.B.; Yi, E.C.; Song, Y.W. Urinary vitamin D-binding protein, a novel biomarker for lupus nephritis, predicts the development of proteinuric flare. *Lupus* **2018**, *27*, 1600–1615. [CrossRef] [PubMed]
84. Wu, T.; Du, Y.; Han, J.; Singh, S.; Xie, C.; Guo, Y.; Zhou, X.J.; Ahn, C.; Saxena, R.; Mohan, C. Urinary angiostatin—A novel putative marker of renal pathology chronicity in lupus nephritis. *Mol. Cell. Proteom.* **2013**, *12*, 1170–1179. [CrossRef]
85. Tolosano, E.; Altruda, F. Hemopexin: Structure, Function, and Regulation. *DNA Cell Biol.* **2002**, *21*, 297–306. [CrossRef] [PubMed]
86. Hellman, N.E.; Gitlin, J.D. Ceruloplasmin metabolism and function. *Annu. Rev. Nutr.* **2002**, *22*, 439–458. [CrossRef]
87. Han, W.K.; Bailly, V.; Abichandani, R.; Thadhani, R.; Bonventre, J.V. Kidney Injury Molecule-1 (KIM-1): A novel biomarker for human renal proximal tubule injury. *Kidney Int.* **2002**, *62*, 237–244. [CrossRef]
88. Bonventre, J.V. Kidney Injury Molecule-1 (KIM-1): A specific and sensitive biomarker of kidney injury. *Scand. J. Clin. Lab. Investig.* **2008**, *68*, 78–83. [CrossRef]
89. Achari, A.E.; Jain, S.K. Adiponectin, a Therapeutic Target for Obesity, Diabetes, and Endothelial Dysfunction. *Int. J. Mol. Sci.* **2017**, *18*, 1321. [CrossRef]
90. Desanti De Oliveira, B.; Xu, K.; Shen, T.H.; Callahan, M.; Kiryluk, K.; D'Agati, V.D.; Tatonetti, N.P.; Barasch, J.; Devarajan, P. Molecular nephrology: Types of acute tubular injury. *Nat. Rev. Nephrol.* **2019**, *15*, 599–612. [CrossRef]
91. Brunner, H.I.; Bennett, M.R.; Abulaban, K.; Klein-Gitelman, M.S.; O'Neil, K.M.; Tucker, L.; Ardoin, S.P.; Rouster-Stevens, K.A.; Onel, K.B.; Singer, N.G.; et al. Development of a Novel Renal Activity Index of Lupus Nephritis in Children and Young Adults. *Arthritis Care Res.* **2016**, *68*, 1003–1011. [CrossRef] [PubMed]
92. Gulati, G.; Bennett, M.R.; Abulaban, K.; Song, H.; Zhang, X.; Ma, Q.; Brodsky, S.V.; Nadasdy, T.; Haffner, C.; Wiley, K.; et al. Prospective validation of a novel renal activity index of lupus nephritis. *Lupus* **2017**, *26*, 927–936. [CrossRef] [PubMed]
93. Brunner, H.I.; Bennett, M.R.; Gulati, G.; Abulaban, K.; Klein-Gitelman, M.S.; Ardoin, S.P.; Tucker, L.B.; Rouster-Stevens, K.A.; Witte, D.; Ying, J.; et al. Urine Biomarkers to Predict Response to Lupus Nephritis Therapy in Children and Young Adults. *J. Rheumatol.* **2017**, *44*, 1239–1248. [CrossRef]
94. Cody, E.M.; Wenderfer, S.E.; Sullivan, K.E.; Kim, A.H.J.; Figg, W.; Ghumman, H.; Qiu, T.; Huang, B.; Devarajan, P.; Brunner, H.I. Urine biomarker score captures response to induction therapy with lupus nephritis. *Pediatr. Nephrol.* **2023**, *38*, 2679–2688. [CrossRef] [PubMed]
95. Aljaberi, N.; Wenderfer, S.E.; Mathur, A.; Qiu, T.; Jose, S.; Merritt, A.; Rose, J.; Devarajan, P.; Huang, B.; Brunner, H. Clinical measurement of lupus nephritis activity is inferior to biomarker-based activity assessment using the renal activity index for lupus nephritis in childhood-onset systemic lupus erythematosus. *Lupus Sci. Med.* **2022**, *9*, e000631. [CrossRef] [PubMed]
96. Nurmohamed, N.S.; Kraaijenhof, J.M.; Mayr, M.; Nicholls, S.J.; Koenig, W.; Catapano, A.L.; Stroes, E.S. Proteomics and lipidomics in atherosclerotic cardiovascular disease risk prediction. *Eur. Heart J.* **2023**, *44*, 1594–1607. [CrossRef]
97. Jové, M.; Portero-Otín, M.; Naudí, A.; Ferrer, I.; Pamplona, R. Metabolomics of human brain aging and age-related neurodegenerative diseases. *J. Neuropathol. Exp. Neurol.* **2014**, *73*, 640–657. [CrossRef] [PubMed]
98. Panyard, D.J.; Yu, B.; Snyder, M.P. The metabolomics of human aging: Advances, challenges, and opportunities. *Sci. Adv.* **2022**, *8*, eadd6155. [CrossRef]
99. Yu, J.; Ren, J.; Ren, Y.; Wu, Y.; Zeng, Y.; Zhang, Q.; Xiao, X. Using metabolomics and proteomics to identify the potential urine biomarkers for prediction and diagnosis of gestational diabetes. *Ebiomedicine* **2024**, *101*, 105008. [CrossRef] [PubMed] [PubMed Central]
100. Alonso, A.; Julià, A.; Vinaixa, M.; Domènech, E.; Fernández-Nebro, A.; Cañete, J.D.; Ferrándiz, C.; Tornero, J.; Gisbert, J.P.; Nos, P.; et al. Urine metabolome profiling of immune-mediated inflammatory diseases. *BMC Med.* **2016**, *14*, 133. [CrossRef]
101. Guleria, A.; Pratap, A.; Dubey, D.; Rawat, A.; Chaurasia, S.; Sukesh, E.; Phatak, S.; Ajmani, S.; Kumar, U.; Khetrapal, C.L.; et al. NMR based serum metabolomics reveals a distinctive signature in patients with Lupus Nephritis. *Sci. Rep.* **2016**, *6*, 35309. [CrossRef] [PubMed]
102. Guleria, A.; Phatak, S.; Dubey, D.; Kumar, S.; Zanwar, A.; Chaurasia, S.; Kumar, U.; Gupta, R.; Aggarwal, A.; Kumar, D.; et al. NMR-Based Serum Metabolomics Reveals Reprogramming of Lipid Dysregulation Following Cyclophosphamide-Based Induction Therapy in Lupus Nephritis. *J. Proteome Res.* **2018**, *17*, 2440–2448. [CrossRef] [PubMed]
103. Zhang, Y.; Gan, L.; Tang, J.; Liu, D.; Chen, G.; Xu, B. Metabolic profiling reveals new serum signatures to discriminate lupus nephritis from systemic lupus erythematosus. *Front. Immunol.* **2022**, *13*, 967371. [CrossRef] [PubMed]
104. Anekthanakul, K.; Manocheewa, S.; Chienwichai, K.; Poungsombat, P.; Limjiasahapong, S.; Wanichthanarak, K.; Jariyasopit, N.; Mathema, V.B.; Kuhakarn, C.; Reutrakul, V.; et al. Predicting lupus membranous nephritis using reduced picolinic acid to tryptophan ratio as a urinary biomarker. *iScience* **2021**, *24*, 103355. [CrossRef]

105. Ganguly, S.; Kumar, U.; Gupta, N.; Guleria, A.; Majumdar, S.; Phatak, S.; Chaurasia, S.; Kumar, S.; Aggarwal, A.; Kumar, D.; et al. Nuclear magnetic resonance-based targeted profiling of urinary acetate and citrate following cyclophosphamide therapy in patients with lupus nephritis. *Lupus* **2020**, *29*, 782–786. [CrossRef] [PubMed]
106. Romick-Rosendale, L.E.; Brunner, H.I.; Bennett, M.R.; Mina, R.; Nelson, S.; Petri, M.; Kiani, A.; Devarajan, P.; Kennedy, M.A. Identification of urinary metabolites that distinguish membranous lupus nephritis from proliferative lupus nephritis and focal segmental glomerulosclerosis. *Arthritis Res. Ther.* **2011**, *13*, R199. [CrossRef] [PubMed]
107. Zhang, T.; Mohan, C. Caution in studying and interpreting the lupus metabolome. *Arthritis Res. Ther.* **2020**, *22*, 172. [CrossRef] [PubMed]
108. Bennett, M.R.; Ma, Q.; Ying, J.; Devarajan, P.; Brunner, H. Effects of age and gender on reference levels of biomarkers comprising the pediatric Renal Activity Index for Lupus Nephritis (p-RAIL). *Pediatr. Rheumatol. Online J.* **2017**, *15*, 74. [CrossRef]
109. Roointan, A.; Gholaminejad, A.; Shojaie, B.; Hudkins, K.L.; Gheisari, Y. Candidate MicroRNA Biomarkers in Lupus Nephritis: A Meta-analysis of Profiling Studies in Kidney, Blood and Urine Samples. *Mol. Diagn. Ther.* **2022**, *27*, 141–158. [CrossRef]
110. Rozanova, S.; Barkovits, K.; Nikolov, M.; Schmidt, C.; Urlaub, H.; Marcus, K. Quantitative Mass Spectrometry-Based Proteomics: An Overview. *Methods Mol. Biol.* **2021**, *2228*, 85–116. [CrossRef]
111. Siddika, T.; Heinemann, I.U. Bringing MicroRNAs to Light: Methods for MicroRNA Quantification and Visualization in Live Cells. *Front. Bioeng. Biotechnol.* **2021**, *8*, 619583. [CrossRef] [PubMed]

Disclaimer/Publisher's Note: The statements, opinions and data contained in all publications are solely those of the individual author(s) and contributor(s) and not of MDPI and/or the editor(s). MDPI and/or the editor(s) disclaim responsibility for any injury to people or property resulting from any ideas, methods, instructions or products referred to in the content.

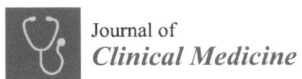

Article

Comparison of Clinical and Laboratory Characteristics in Lupus Nephritis vs. Non-Lupus Nephritis Patients—A Comprehensive Retrospective Analysis Based on 921 Patients

Joanna Kosałka-Węgiel [1,2,*], Radosław Dziedzic [3], Andżelika Siwiec-Koźlik [2], Magdalena Spałkowska [4], Mamert Milewski [2], Anita Wach [2], Lech Zaręba [5], Stanisława Bazan-Socha [2,6] and Mariusz Korkosz [1,2]

[1] Jagiellonian University Medical College, Department of Rheumatology and Immunology, Jakubowskiego 2, 30-688 Kraków, Poland; mariusz.korkosz@uj.edu.pl

[2] University Hospital, Department of Rheumatology, Immunology and Internal Medicine, Jakubowskiego 2, 30-688 Kraków, Poland; lek.andzelika.siwiec@gmail.com (A.S.-K.); mamert.mmm@gmail.com (M.M.); anita.wach@gmail.com (A.W.); stanislawa.bazan-socha@uj.edu.pl (S.B.-S.)

[3] Jagiellonian University Medical College, Doctoral School of Medical and Health Sciences, Św. Łazarza 16, 31-530 Kraków, Poland; radoslawjozefdziedzic@gmail.com

[4] Jagiellonian University Medical College, Department of Dermatology, Botaniczna 3, 31-501 Kraków, Poland; magdalena.spalkowska@uj.edu.pl

[5] University of Rzeszów, College of Natural Sciences, Institute of Computer Science, Pigonia 1, 35-310 Rzeszów, Poland; lzareba@ur.edu.pl

[6] Jagiellonian University Medical College, Department of Internal Medicine, Faculty of Medicine, Jakubowskiego 2, 30-688 Kraków, Poland

* Correspondence: joanna.kosalka@uj.edu.pl; Tel.: +48-12-400-31-10

Abstract: Background: Lupus nephritis (LN) is an inflammation of the kidneys that is related to systemic lupus erythematosus (SLE). This study aimed to evaluate the differences in clinical and laboratory characteristics between LN and non-LN SLE patients. **Methods**: We conducted a retrospective analysis of medical records collected from SLE patients treated at the University Hospital in Kraków, Poland, from 2012 to 2022. All patients met the 2019 European League Against Rheumatism and the American College of Rheumatology (EULAR/ACR) criteria for SLE. **Results**: Among 921 SLE patients, LN was documented in 331 (35.94%). LN patients were younger at SLE diagnosis (29 vs. 37 years; $p < 0.001$) and had a male proportion that was 2.09 times higher than the non-LN group (16.62% vs. 7.97%; $p < 0.001$). They were more often diagnosed with serositis and hematological or neurological involvement ($p < 0.001$ for all). Hypertension and hypercholesterolemia occurred more frequently in these patients ($p < 0.001$ for both). LN patients exhibited a higher frequency of anti-dsDNA, anti-histone, and anti-nucleosome antibodies ($p < 0.001$ for all). Conversely, the non-LN group had a 1.24-fold (95% CI: 1.03–1.50; $p = 0.021$) increase in the odds ratio of having positive anti-cardiolipin IgM antibody results. LN patients were more frequently treated with immunosuppressants. The risk factors for experiencing at least three LN flares included female sex, younger age at the onset of LN or SLE, LN occurring later than SLE onset, the presence of anti-nucleosome or anti-dsDNA antibodies, and certain SLE manifestations such as myalgia, arthritis, proteinuria > 3.5 g/day, and pathological urinary casts in the urine sediment. **Conclusions**: LN patients differ from non-LN patients in the age of SLE diagnosis, treatment modalities, and autoantibody profile and have more frequent, severe manifestations of SLE. However, we still need more prospective studies to understand the diversity of LN and its progression in SLE patients.

Keywords: systemic lupus erythematosus; lupus nephritis; prognostic factors; EULAR/ACR; ISN/RPS

1. Introduction

Systemic lupus erythematosus (SLE) is an autoimmune disease characterized by the abnormal activation of autoreactive T and B cells, subsequent production of autoantibodies, activation of complement, and immune-complex deposition, which results in tissue and also organ damage [1–3]. SLE is diagnosed predominantly in women of young age, interestingly, with a female-to-male ratio of about 15:1 [4]. Other risk factors for SLE development include race other than Caucasian, genetic determinants (i.e., gene variants located on the X chromosome, such as *IRAK1*, *MECP2*, and *TLR7*), hormonal factors (i.e., estrogens, progesterone, and prolactin), immune abnormalities, and environmental factors (i.e., ultraviolet light exposure, urban areas, cigarette smoking, and viral and bacterial infections) [5–8].

Kidney involvement is one of the most common and severe manifestations of SLE, affecting up to 75% of patients during the course of the disease [9–11]. It typically develops in the early stages of SLE, especially within the first 3–5 years, but it can also present at initial diagnosis [12]. The manifestation of lupus nephritis (LN) varies from subclinical laboratory abnormalities to overt nephritis, nephrotic syndrome, and rapidly progressive renal failure [13,14]. Additionally, up to 30% of patients with LN will develop ESKD within 5 years of onset [12]. Risk factors for progressive kidney disease are not fully recognized but include neuropsychiatric lupus, pediatric onset, male sex, race other than Caucasian, poor socioeconomic status, hypertension, impaired renal function at the time of renal biopsy, anemia, presence of anti-dsDNA antibodies, persistent hypocomplementemia, frequent relapses or incomplete remission, and proteinuria > 4 g per day at diagnosis [10,15,16].

Histologically, there are six distinct classes of nephropathy classified by the International Society of Nephrology/Renal Pathology Society (ISN/RPS) that represent different manifestations and severities of renal involvement in SLE [9]. Patients with proliferative forms of LN are at the highest risk for kidney replacement therapy [12]. Additionally, crescentic glomerulonephritis, thrombotic microangiopathy, or extensive tubulointerstitial damage increase the risk for a worse renal prognosis in LN patients [15,16]. Patients with LN have a higher mortality ratio and die earlier than SLE patients without LN [12]; therefore, early LN diagnosis and prompt treatment initiation are vital to prevent disease progression. Many studies have been carried out on LN cases to determine the predictors of a more unfavorable prognosis; however, their results are inconsistent [11,17,18]. Furthermore, data on the Polish LN population remains scarce [19–22]. Thus, we aimed to retrospectively evaluate the clinical and laboratory data, including histology, disease follow-up, and treatment modalities, in a large cohort of 921 Polish SLE patients, including 331 subjects with LN. We also examined which factors impact LN development and further prognosis, which could be useful for clinicians.

2. Patients and Methods

2.1. Study Population

We retrospectively reviewed the medical records of all SLE cases diagnosed and treated in the University Hospital, Kraków, Poland, from January 2012 to June 2022. At the time of data collection, all patients met the European League Against Rheumatism and the American College of Rheumatology (EULAR/ACR) criteria from 2019 for SLE [23].

This paper is a continuation of our previous manuscript on LN, in which detailed information on our methods has been provided [24]. Briefly, we recorded data on sex, current age, age at first SLE symptoms and diagnosis, the time between the onset of SLE symptoms and diagnosis, duration of the disease, family history of SLE and other autoimmune diseases, clinical and laboratory SLE manifestations, internist comorbidities, miscarriages in women, different treatment modalities, and cause of and age at death (if applicable). The evaluated clinical manifestations included general symptoms, lymphadenopathy, skin lesions, oral or nasopharyngeal ulcerations, photosensitivity, joint involvement, serositis, hematologic domain (leukopenia, lymphopenia, anemia, hemolytic anemia, thrombocytopenia, macrophage activation syndrome, and thrombotic thrombocytopenic purpura), kidney, nervous system and respiratory tract involvement, Raynaud's phenomenon, and lupoid hepatitis. All of them were defined in detail in our previous paper [24]. We also collected data on family history concerning SLE and other autoimmune diseases in the first- and second-line degrees of the ascending and descending relatives.

Next, we divided patients into two subgroups: the first comprised those with LN diagnosis (LN patients), and the second consisted of patients without LN diagnosis (non-LN patients). LN was confirmed either by a renal biopsy and classified according to the ISN/RPS criteria or based on overt renal symptoms (proteinuria, active urinary sediment) during a lupus flare [2]. The evaluation of LN was extended to age at LN diagnosis, histologic type of nephropathy according to the ISN/RPS criteria (if kidney biopsy was performed), numbers of LN exacerbations, and diagnosis of ESKD, if applicable [25]. We also analyzed internal disease comorbidities such as arterial hypertension, diabetes mellitus, hypercholesterolemia, atrial fibrillation, lower extremity peripheral artery disease, heart failure, malignant tumor, or any thromboembolic events. The recorded treatment modalities included corticosteroids, hydroxychloroquine or chloroquine, azathioprine, methotrexate, cyclosporine A, mycophenolate mofetil, cyclophosphamide, sulfasalazine, immunoglobulins intravenously in suppressive doses, and biological agents (belimumab, rituximab, and anifrolumab) used currently or in the past. We also reported if a patient had a splenectomy or plasmapheresis in their medical records.

We received approval for the research from the Bioethics Committee of the Jagiellonian University Medical College (No: 118.6120.41.2023, on 15 June 2023). Furthermore, all procedures adhered to the ethical principles outlined in the Declaration of Helsinki.

2.2. Laboratory Analysis

We used routine laboratory techniques to measure complete blood cell count (CBC), lipid profile, haptoglobin, creatinine with estimated glomerular filtration rate (eGFR, using Modification of Diet in Renal Disease formula), 24 h urine protein excretion, urinary sediment analysis, direct antiglobulin test, and blood group designation [26]. Anti-nuclear antibodies (ANAs) were evaluated by an indirect immunofluorescence (IIF) technique using Hep-2 cells. Extractable Nuclear Antigen (ENA) testing was conducted when ANA (IIF) results were positive. Anti-Sjögren's-syndrome-related antigen A (SSA), anti-Sjögren's-syndrome-related antigen B (SSB), anti-histone, anti-nucleosome, anti-Smith (Sm), and anti-ribonucleoprotein (RNP) antibodies and autoantibodies were identified by an enzyme-linked immunosorbent assay (ELISA) or a line-blot immunoassay. Anti-double-stranded DNA (anti-dsDNA) antibodies were assayed by IIF using *Crithidia luciliae* as a substrate. Anti-myeloperoxidase (MPO) and anti-proteinase three (PR3) antibodies were assessed using a standardized ELISA technique. Serum complement levels (C3c and C4) and rheumatoid factor (RF) were assessed by nephelometry. Laboratory tests for hypercoagulability were also included, such as lupus anticoagulant (LA), anti-cardiolipin (aCL), anti-beta-2-glycoprotein I (anti-β2GPI) antibodies (both in IgM and IgG classes), antithrombin activity, protein C activity, free protein S level, activity of factor VIII, and presence of factor V Leiden and prothrombin G20210A gene variants. All of them were measured using routine laboratory techniques.

2.3. Statistical Elaboration

The results were analyzed using STATISTICA Tibco 13.3 software (StatSoft Inc., Tulsa, OK, USA). Categorical variables are presented as frequencies (number of cases) with relative frequencies (percentages) and compared using the Chi^2 test or the exact Fisher test. The normality of data distribution was evaluated using the Shapiro-Wilk test. All continuous variables were non-normally distributed and thus were presented as median with Q1–Q3 ranges and compared using the Mann-Whitney test. To calculate the odds ratio (OR) with a 95% confidence interval (CI), the cut-off points were calculated based on receiver operating characteristic (ROC) curves. Cluster analysis was performed using the k-means method. A significance threshold of two-sided p-values below 0.05 was employed for all analyses.

3. Results

3.1. Demographic Characteristics

The summary of demographic parameters is provided in Table 1. The study included 921 SLE patients. Among them, 331 (35.94%) represented the LN cases, with the most common being class IV (diffuse proliferative glomerulonephritis), identified in 91 (50.56%) out of 180 performed renal biopsies. Detailed characteristics of the kidney specimen histology are provided in our previous publication [24].

Table 1. Demographic characteristics of 921 patients with systemic lupus erythematosus.

Characteristics	LN Patients $n = 331$	Non-LN Patients $n = 590$	p-Value
Age of onset			
Adult onset (age of onset $\geq$ 18 years), n (%)	286 (86.9%)	544 (93.8%)	<0.001 *
Juvenile onset (age of onset < 18 years), n (%)	43 (13.1%)	36 (6.2%)	
Sex of patients			
Female, n (%)	276 (83.38%)	543 (92.04%)	<0.001 *
Male, n (%)	55 (16.62%)	47 (7.96%)	
Disease characteristics			
Age at first symptoms, years	28 (20.75–39)	34 (24–46)	<0.001 *
Age at onset, years	29 (22–41)	37 (27–49)	<0.001 *
Time delay between onset of symptoms and diagnosis, years	0 (0–1)	0.5 (0–3)	<0.001 *
Age at last visit, years	44 (35–57)	52 (41–63)	<0.001 *
Disease duration, years	13 (6–20)	14 (8–22)	0.76

Categorical variables are presented as numbers with percentages, continuous variables are presented as median with Q1–Q3 ranges, and an asterisk marks the statistically significant differences. Abbreviations: LN—lupus nephritis, n—number.

The treatment modalities based on the kidney biopsy classes are summarized in Table 2. As presented, LN patients regarding the class of nephropathy differ in the frequency of usage of specific immunosuppressive medications such as cyclophosphamide and plasmapheresis.

In 207 (62.53%) LN patients, kidney manifestations were present at SLE diagnosis, while in 122 (36.86%) patients, it was diagnosed at a median of 5.5 years later ($p < 0.001$). Patients with confirmed LN were diagnosed with SLE at a median of 8 years earlier (29 vs. 37 years, respectively; $p < 0.001$) and two-fold more frequently in childhood or teenage years ($p < 0.001$), with the first symptoms appearing at a median of 6 years earlier (28 vs. 34 years, respectively; $p < 0.001$) than in the remaining group. Consequently, the time delay between symptom onset and diagnosis was a median of 0.5 years shorter in the LN group (0 vs. 0.5 years, respectively; $p < 0.001$). On the other hand, the disease duration from diagnosis to analysis was similar in both groups (median: 13 vs. 14 years, respectively; $p = 0.76$). Women constituted the majority of cases in both SLE subgroups; however, SLE was diagnosed 2.09 times more frequently in men in the LN cases ($p < 0.001$).

In 157 individuals (17.05%), there were reported cases of systemic autoimmune disorders among close relatives, with no significant differences observed between the two studied subgroups ($p > 0.05$). Additionally, Hashimoto's disease was reported in 16 individuals (1.74% overall), type 1 diabetes mellitus in 4 individuals (0.43% overall), Graves–Basedov disease in 3 individuals (0.33% overall), Sjögren's syndrome in 2 individuals (0.22% overall), systemic sclerosis in 1 individual (0.11% overall), granulomatosis with polyangiitis in 1 individual (0.11% overall), dermatomyositis in 1 individual (0.11% overall), mixed connective tissue disease in 1 individual (0.11% overall), celiac disease in 1 individual (0.11% overall), ulcerative colitis in 1 individual (0.11% overall), myasthenia gravis in 1 individual (0.11%

overall), immune thrombocytopenia in 1 individual (0.11% overall), autoimmune hepatitis in 1 individual (0.11% overall), Addison–Biermer anemia in 1 individual (0.11% overall), and undifferentiated connective tissue disease in 1 individual (0.11% overall).

Table 2. Characteristics of treatment in 180 lupus nephritis patients who underwent kidney biopsy.

Treatment	I n = 3	II n = 33	III n = 26	IV n = 91	V n = 22	VI n = 5	p-Value
Glucocorticoids oral and/or intravenous, n (%)	3 (100.0%)	33 (100.0%)	25 (96.2%)	90 (98.9%)	22 (100.0%)	5 (100.0%)	0.31
Chloroquine or hydroxychloroquine, n (%)	2 (66.7%)	21 (63.6%)	18 (69.2%)	56 (61.5%)	12 (54.5%)	4 (80.0%)	0.79
Azathioprine, n (%)	2 (66.7%)	16 (48.5%)	14 (53.8%)	43 (47.3%)	12 (54.5%)	4 (80.0%)	0.71
Methotrexate, n (%)	1 (33.3%)	2 (6.1%)	5 (19.2%)	14 (15.4%)	6 (27.3%)	2 (40.0%)	0.24
Cyclosporine, n (%)	0 (0.0%)	2 (6.1%)	2 (7.7%)	16 (17.6%)	5 (22.7%)	1 (20.0%)	0.42
Belimumab, n (%)	1 (33.3%)	1 (3.0%)	1 (3.8%)	8 (8.8%)	0 (0.0%)	0 (0.0%)	0.21
Mycophenolate mofetil, n (%)	1 (33.3%)	20 (60.6%)	15 (57.7%)	72 (79.1%)	18 (81.8%)	5 (100.0%)	0.06
Cyclophosphamide, n (%)	1 (33.3%)	15 (45.5%)	18 (69.2%)	77 (84.6%)	18 (81.8%)	5 (100.0%)	<0.001 *
Rituximab, n (%)	0 (0.0%)	1 (3.0%)	0 (0.0%)	10 (11.0%)	3 (13.6%)	0 (0.0%)	0.30
Immunoglobulins, n (%)	0 (0.0%)	1 (3.0%)	1 (3.8%)	2 (2.2%)	2 (9.1%)	1 (20.0%)	0.34
Plasmapheresis, n (%)	0 (0.0%)	2 (6.1%)	1 (3.8%)	3 (3.3%)	2 (9.1%)	2 (40.0%)	0.027 *
Sulfasalazine, n (%)	1 (33.3%)	0 (0.0%)	0 (0.0%)	4 (4.4%)	2 (9.1%)	0 (0.0%)	0.053

Categorical variables are presented as numbers and an asterisk marks the statistically significant differences. Abbreviations: n—number.

3.2. Lupus Nephritis Is Related to More Severe Clinical Immunosuppressive Treatment

Table 3 presents the frequencies of systemic involvement other than kidney-related involvement in the SLE cohort. In the LN group, the most common were hematological (95.17%), joint (84.29%), and constitutional symptoms (80.97%). Non-LN patients exhibited similar predominant clinics, with joint (92.88%), hematological (89.66%), and mucocutaneous signs (87.3%) being the most frequent. Comparing LN to non-LN cases, the former group was characterized by more severe manifestations. For instance, diffuse alveolar hemorrhage (4.75 times; $p = 0.024$), central nervous system involvement (3.03 times; $p < 0.001$), pleural effusion (2.22 times; $p < 0.001$), and pericardial effusion (2.22 times; $p < 0.001$) were more common in LN. Additionally, we reported fever (1.33 times; $p < 0.001$), fatigue or weakness (1.11 times; $p = 0.037$), hematological signs (1.06 times; $p = 0.006$) such as lymphopenia (1.15 times; $p < 0.001$), hemolytic anemia (1.9 times; $p = 0.001$), or anemia of any cause (1.29 times; $p < 0.001$), and peripheral nervous system involvement (1.87 times; $p = 0.037$) more frequently in LN. On the other hand, we documented mucocutaneous signs (1.17 fold; $p < 0.001$) such as lupus malar rash (1.21 fold; $p = 0.016$) or other skin changes (1.14 fold; $p = 0.007$), photosensitivity (1.43 fold; $p < 0.001$), and Raynaud's phenomenon (1.56 times; $p < 0.001$) less frequently in LN patients.

Table 3. Cumulative frequencies of systemic involvement in all enrolled patients.

Clinical Manifestations	LN Patients n = 331	Non-LN Patients n = 590	p-Value
Constitutional manifestations, n (%)	268 (80.97%)	461 (78.14%)	0.35
Fever, n (%)	166 (52.87%)	233 (39.9%)	<0.001 *
Fatigue/weakness, n (%)	222 (70.03%)	366 (62.89%)	0.037 *
Myalgias, n (%)	122 (38.49%)	222 (38.21%)	0.99
Weight loss, n (%)	81 (25.80%)	121 (20.75%)	0.10
Lymphadenopathy, n (%)	64 (20.25%)	114 (19.52%)	0.86
Mucocutaneus manifestations, n (%)	248 (74.92%)	515 (87.30%)	<0.001 *
Lupus malar rash, n (%)	130 (39.88%)	285 (48.39%)	0.016 *
Discoid rash, n (%)	22 (6.77%)	52 (8.83%)	0.33
Urticaria, n (%)	26 (8.00%)	51 (8.66%)	0.83
Cutaneous vasculitis, n (%)	23 (7.08%)	36 (6.11%)	0.67
Alopecia, n (%)	85 (26.07%)	161 (27.33%)	0.74
Oral and/or nasal ulcers, n (%)	51 (15.69%)	92 (15.62%)	0.95
Photosensitivity, n (%)	89 (27.38%)	231 (39.22%)	<0.001 *
Other skin changes [1], n (%)	206 (62.61%)	421 (71.48%)	0.007 *
Joint manifestations, n (%)	279 (84.29%)	548 (92.88%)	<0.001 *
Arthritis, n (%)	194 (59.69%)	385 (65.59%)	0.09
Arthralgia, n (%)	279 (84.80%)	545 (92.37%)	<0.001 *
Serositis, n (%)	122 (37.08%)	112 (18.98%)	<0.001 *
Pleural effusion, n (%)	90 (27.44%)	73 (12.37%)	<0.001 *
Pericardial effusion, n (%)	75 (23.44%)	62 (10.56%)	<0.001 *
Pericarditis, n (%)	12 (3.65%)	25 (4.24%)	0.79
Hematological manifestations, n (%)	315 (95.17%)	529 (89.66%)	0.006 *
Leucopenia [2], n (%)	209 (65.11%)	362 (62.31%)	0.44
Lymphopenia [3], n (%)	261 (83.65%)	414 (72.89%)	<0.001 *
Anemia [4], n (%)	272 (84.47%)	381 (65.69%)	<0.001 *
Hemolytic anemia [5], n (%)	42 (30.43%)	42 (16.03%)	0.001 *
Thrombocytopenia [6], n (%)	110 (34.16%)	182 (31.33%)	0.42
Direct Coombs test, n (%)	29 (36.25%)	31 (41.33%)	0.63
Macrophage activation syndrome, n (%)	5 (1.53%)	3 (0.51%)	0.23
Thrombotic thrombocytopenic purpura [7], n (%)	1 (0.30%)	1 (0.17%)	0.75
Kidney involvement, n (%)	331 (100%)	0 (0%)	<0.001 *
24 h urinary protein excretion > 0.5 g/day, n (%)	300 (96.46%)	0 (0%)	<0.001 *
24 h urinary protein excretion > 3.5 g/day, n (%)	158 (58.74%)	0 (0%)	<0.001 *
Urinary casts, n (%)	138 (61.06%)	0 (0%)	<0.001 *
Erythrocyturia, n (%)	229 (84.81%)	0 (0%)	<0.001 *
Leukocyturia, n (%)	242 (84.62%)	0 (0%)	<0.001 *
Neurological abnormality, n (%)	59 (17.82%)	45 (7.63%)	<0.001 *
Central nervous system involvement, n (%)	44 (13.37%)	26 (4.41%)	<0.001 *
Peripheral nervous system involvement, n (%)	24 (7.29%)	23 (3.90%)	0.037

Table 3. *Cont.*

Clinical Manifestations	LN Patients n = 331	Non-LN Patients n = 590	p-Value
Raynaud's phenomenon, n (%)	61 (18.48%)	170 (28.81%)	<0.001 *
Lung involvement, n (%)	30 (9.06%)	49 (8.31%)	0.79
Interstitial lung disease, n (%)	19 (5.76%)	30 (5.08%)	0.78
Diffuse alveolar hemorrhage, n (%)	8 (2.42%)	3 (0.51%)	0.024 *
Pulmonary hypertension, n (%)	9 (2.80%)	22 (3.75%)	0.57
Lupoid hepatitis, n (%)	13 (3.94%)	31 (5.25%)	0.46

Categorical variables are presented as numbers with percentages, and an asterisk marks the statistically significant differences. Abbreviations: n—number; LN—lupus nephritis. [1]—erythema, livedo racemosa, livedo reticularis; [2]—<4000/mm^3 or diagnosis in a medical history; [3]—<1500/mm^3 or diagnosis based on a medical history; [4]—≤12 g/dL in women, ≤13.5 g/dL in men, or diagnosis based on medical history; [5]—anemia with a positive direct Coombs test or anemia with a decreased level of haptoglobin or diagnosis based on a medical history; [6]—<100,000/mm^3 or diagnosis based on a medical history; [7]—confirmed with ADAMTS-13 level.

3.3. Arterial Hypertension and Hypercholesterolemia Were the Only Internal Disease Comorbidities with a Higher Prevalence in the Lupus Nephritis Group

In general, the SLE subtype differed regarding the analyzed internal medicine comorbidities, except for arterial hypertension and hypercholesterolemia (Table 4), which were 1.75 times and 1.81 times more frequent in LN, respectively ($p < 0.001$ for both). Overall, ESKD was reported in 23 cases (6.95%) in the LN group and 3 cases (0.51%) in the non-LN group ($p < 0.001$), where it was related to concomitant internal diseases.

Table 4. Cumulative frequencies of comorbidities in all included patients.

Comorbidities [1]	LN Patients n = 331	Non-LN Patients n = 590	p-Value
Hypertension, n (%)	241 (72.81%)	246 (41.69%)	<0.001 *
Diabetes mellitus, n (%)	38 (11.48%)	58 (9.83%)	0.50
Heart failure [2], n (%)	23 (6.95%)	24 (4.07%)	0.08
Hypercholesterolemia [3], n (%)	223 (67.58%)	220 (37.29%)	<0.001 *
Atrial fibrillation, n (%)	14 (4.23%)	19 (3.22%)	0.54
Peripheral artery disease, n (%)	11 (3.33%)	39 (6.61%)	0.05
End-stage kidney disease, n (%)	23 (6.97%)	2 (0.34%)	<0.001 *
Monoclonal gammopathy of undetermined significance, n (%)	9 (2.72%)	10 (1.69%)	0.42
Malignant tumor, n (%)	31 (9.37%)	61 (10.37%)	0.71
Artery thrombotic episode, n (%)	100 (30.21%)	219 (37.12%)	0.041 *
Stroke, n (%)	21 (6.34%)	52 (8.81%)	0.23
Transient ischemic attack, n (%)	6 (1.81%)	10 (1.69%)	0.89
Myocardial infarct, n (%)	88 (26.59%)	184 (31.19%)	0.16
Thrombotic episode in another artery, n (%)	7 (2.11%)	15 (2.54%)	0.85
Venous thrombotic episode, n (%)	61 (18%)	108 (18%)	0.97
Deep venous thrombosis, n (%)	50 (15%)	91 (15%)	0.97
Pulmonary embolism, n (%)	14 (4%)	25 (4%)	0.88
Deep venous thrombosis and pulmonary embolism, n (%)	8 (2%)	11 (2%)	0.75
Thrombotic episode in another venous, n (%)	8 (2%)	11 (2%)	0.75
Miscarriage, n (%)	32 (13.06%) [4]	79 (18.16%) [4]	0.11

Categorical variables are presented as numbers with percentages, and an asterisk marks the statistically significant differences. [1]—comorbidities present or in the past; [2]—symptoms of heart failure or LVEF ≤ 40% or a diagnosis based on medical history; [3]—LDL > 3 mmol/L or pharmacotherapy with statin or a diagnosis based on medical history; [4]—% of women with miscarriage from number of women with systemic lupus erythematous. Abbreviations: LDL—low-density lipoprotein, LN—lupus nephritis, LVEF—left ventricular ejection fraction, n—number.

3.4. The Mortality Rates Were Similar in Lupus and Non-Lupus Nephritis Cases

Throughout the median follow-up period of 14 years, a total of 47 (5.57%) SLE patients died, with 16 (5.28%) in the LN group and 31 (5.73%) in the non-LN group ($p = 0.79$). Among the deceased, the predominant causes of death included infections (10 cases, 21.28% overall), followed by SLE exacerbation (4 cases, 8.51% overall) and malignancies (4 cases, 8.51% overall), with no significant differences observed between subgroups ($p > 0.05$ for all).

Statistically significant factors influencing mortality in all SLE patients include male sex, presence of aCL antibodies in IgG or IgM classes, presence of aβ2GPI in IgM class antibodies, internal comorbidities (arterial hypertension, diabetes mellitus, heart failure, hypercholesterolemia, atrial fibrillation, and peripheral artery disease), malignant tumor, monoclonal gammopathy of undetermined significance, thromboembolic episodes (myocardial infarction, deep vein thrombosis), rituximab administration, and certain SLE manifestations (fever, weight loss, fatigue/weakness, arthritis, pericardial or pleural effusion, hemolytic anemia, thrombocytopenia, macrophage activation syndrome, erythrocyturia or urinary casts in urine sediment, diffuse alveolar hemorrhage, and pulmonary hypertension).

3.5. Lupus Nephritis Was Associated with a Higher Frequency of Anti-dsDNA, Anti-Nucleosome, and Anti-Histone Antibodies

As expected, anti-dsDNA antibodies were more common in the LN group (84.44% vs. 62.48%; $p < 0.001$). Amongst the whole cohort, patients with an anti-dsDNA titer of 1:80 or more in indirect immunofluorescence had a 1.76 OR (95% CI: 1.52–2.04; $p < 0.001$) of suffering from LN. In LN, we also documented anti-nucleosome (45.89% vs. 28.62%; $p < 0.001$) and anti-histone antibodies (37.66% vs. 22.1%; $p < 0.001$) more frequently. Detailed information is shown in Table 5. Interestingly, in the presence of any of those three antibodies ($n = 553$, 72.1%), juvenile-onset SLE, recurrent fever, concomitant antiphospholipid antibodies, pleural effusion, lymphopenia, hemolytic anemia, proteinuria, leucocyturia, erythrocyturia, and granular casts in the urine sediment were reported more frequently ($p < 0.05$ for all).

Table 5. Laboratory findings in all included patients.

Laboratory Parameter (Number of Patients with Analyzed Parameter)	LN Patients $n = 331$	Non-LN Patients $n = 590$	p-Value
Rheumatoid factor, n (%)	33 (20.89%)	130 (38.01%)	<0.001 *
ANA—IIF assay, n (%)	331 (100%)	590 (100%)	
Anti-SSA antibodies [1], n (%)	156 (49.37%)	364 (65.94%)	<0.001 *
Anti-SSB antibodies [1], n (%)	72 (22.78%)	181 (32.79%)	0.002 *
Anti-histone antibodies [1], n (%)	119 (37.66%)	122 (22.1%)	<0.001 *
Anti-nucleosome antibodies [1], n (%)	145 (45.89%)	158 (28.62%)	<0.001 *
Anti-Smith antibodies [1], n (%)	41 (13.08%)	71 (12.39%)	0.97
Anti-RNP antibodies [1], n (%)	77 (24.44%)	114 (20.69%)	0.23
Anti-dsDNA antibodies [1], n (%)	163 (51.58%)	174 (31.75%)	<0.001 *
Anti-dsDNA antibodies [2], n (%)	266 (84.44%)	323 (62.48%)	<0.001 *
Anti-PR3 antibodies [3], n (%)	5 (6.49%)	2 (2.99%)	0.56
Anti-MPO antibodies [3], n (%)	9 (11.11%)	5 (7.14%)	0.58
Antiphospholipid antibodies			
Lupus anticoagulant, n (%)	64 (25.60%)	128 (30.62%)	0.19
Anti-cardiolipin antibodies IgG or IgM, n (%)	150 (55.56%)	270 (56.84%)	0.83

Table 5. Cont.

Laboratory Parameter (Number of Patients with Analyzed Parameter)	LN Patients $n = 331$	Non-LN Patients $n = 590$	p-Value
Anti-cardiolipin antibodies IgG, n (%)	120 (44.78%)	187 (40.30%)	0.27
Anti-cardiolipin antibodies IgM, n (%)	91 (34.08%)	195 (42.12%)	0.039 *
Anti-β2 glycoprotein I IgG or IgM, n (%)	46 (20.91%)	110 (29.1%)	0.035 *
Anti-β2 glycoprotein I IgG, n (%)	29 (13.62%)	66 (17.84%)	0.22
Anti-β2 glycoprotein I IgM, n (%)	27 (12.68%)	80 (21.68%)	0.009 *

Categorical variables are presented as numbers with percentages, and an asterisk marks the statistically significant differences. [1]—Immunoblotting assay; [2]—CLIFT (the *Crithidia luciliae* immunofluorescence test); [3]—ELISA (Enzyme-Linked Immunosorbent Assay). Abbreviations: ANA—anti-nuclear antibodies, dsDNA—double stranded DNA, IIF—indirect immunofluorescence, MPO—myeloperoxidase, PR3—proteinase 3, RNP—ribonucleoprotein, LN—lupus nephritis, n—number.

Furthermore, as expected, the presence of anti-dsDNA antibodies in the whole cohort was associated with a higher number of renal exacerbations, as well as with an increased mortality rate ($p = 0.043$), atrial fibrillation ($p = 0.011$), malignancy ($p = 0.039$), and other SLE manifestations (myalgia, vasculitis, photosensitivity, and Raynaud's phenomenon; $p < 0.05$ for all). On the other hand, anti-nucleosome antibodies in LN were associated with myocardial infarct ($p = 0.013$), as well as lymphadenopathy, arthritis, pericardial effusion, leucopenia, and central system nervous involvement ($p < 0.05$ for all). In turn, anti-histone antibodies were linked to oral and/or nasal ulcers and arthritis, arthralgia, pericardial effusion, leucopenia, and central system nervous involvement ($p < 0.05$ for all). Surprisingly, neither SLE subgroup differed in the frequency of anti-Sm antibody presence. On the other hand, anti-SSA and anti-SSB antibodies were observed more often in non-LN than in LN patients (65.94% vs. 49.37% for anti-SSA antibodies, $p < 0.001$; and 32.79% vs. 22.78% for anti-SSB antibodies, $p = 0.002$). No differences were observed in ABO blood groups and Rh blood types between both LN groups.

3.6. Antiphospholipid Antibodies and Arterial Thrombotic Episodes Were Reported More Frequently in the Non-Lupus Nephritis Group

Regarding antiphospholipid antibodies, there was a greater prevalence of anti-CL antibodies in the IgM class among non-LN individuals compared to those with LN (42.12% vs. 34.08%; $p = 0.039$). Furthermore, our findings indicate a 1.24-fold increase (95% CI: 1.03–1.50; $p = 0.021$) in the OR of positive aCL antibodies in the IgM class among non-LN patients as opposed to those with LN. Additionally, LN exhibited a lower incidence of arterial thrombotic episodes compared to non-LN cases (30.21% vs. 37.12%; $p = 0.041$). Notably, in LN patients, we observed a 0.85-fold decrease (95% CI: 0.74–0.98; $p = 0.026$) in the OR of arterial thrombotic episodes, with no significant difference in venous thrombotic episodes between the two groups. In contrast, individuals with the presence of aCL in the IgM class showed a higher OR for strokes (1.96-fold; 95% CI: 1.03–3.76; $p = 0.032$) and DVT (1.79-fold; 95% CI: 1.09–2.95; $p = 0.016$) within the non-LN group. For more details, see Tables 4 and 5. We found no differences in antithrombin and protein C activity, free protein S level, level and activity of factor VIII, frequency of factor V Leiden and G20210A prothrombin gene variants between LN and non-LN patients.

3.7. Lupus Nephritis Is Related to a More Aggressive Immunosuppressive Treatment

The administration of immunosuppressive therapy in SLE patients is detailed in Table 6. In both SLE subgroups, corticosteroids were the most commonly used (99.39% of LN patients and 94.06% of non-LN patients). Additionally, in LN patients, chloroquine or hydroxychloroquine (99.39%), mycophenolate mofetil (65.22%), and cyclophosphamide (64.51%) were more commonly used, whereas in non-LN chloroquine or hydroxychloroquine (82.88%), azathioprine (33.45%) and methotrexate (22.54%). Obviously, more aggressive treatment modes, including mycophenolate mofetil, cyclophosphamide, rituximab, immunoglobulins, or plasmapheresis, have been reported in LN than in non-LN individuals.

Table 6. Treatment received by all enrolled patients.

Treatment	LN Patients $n = 331$	Non-LN Patients $n = 590$	p-Value
Glucocorticoids oral and/or intravenous, n (%)	327 (99.39%)	554 (94.06%)	<0.001 *
Chloroquine or hydroxychloroquine, n (%)	328 (99.39%)	489 (82.88%)	0.06
Azathioprine, n (%)	166 (51.08%)	197 (33.45%)	<0.001 *
Methotrexate, n (%)	56 (17.39%)	133 (22.54%)	0.06
Cyclosporine, n (%)	38 (11.73%)	39 (6.62%)	0.036 *
Belimumab, n (%)	19 (5.92%)	21 (3.57%)	0.09
Mycophenolate mofetil, n (%)	210 (65.22%)	90 (15.28%)	<0.001 *
Cyclophosphamide, n (%)	209 (64.51%)	72 (12.22%)	<0.001 *
Rituximab, n (%)	21 (6.54%)	8 (1.36%)	<0.001 *
Immunoglobulins, n (%)	17 (5.28%)	11 (1.87%)	0.010 *
Plasmapheresis, n (%)	27 (8.41%)	4 (0.68%)	<0.001 *
Sulfasalazine, n (%)	12 (3.73%)	36 (6.11%)	0.13
Anifrolumab, n (%)	4 (1.24%)	6 (1.02%)	0.35
Splenectomy, n (%)	1 (0.31%)	4 (0.68%)	0.80

Categorical variables are presented as numbers with percentages, and an asterisk marks the statistically significant differences. Abbreviations: LN—lupus nephritis, n—number.

3.8. Cluster Analysis

Next, we performed cluster analysis in both studied SLE subgroups (Tables 7 and 8). In LN (Table 7), we revealed three different clusters: cluster 1 ($n = 23$) comprised patients with ESKD (LN patients with ESKD), cluster 2 ($n = 203$) consisted of patients without ESKD and with a time of less than one year from the first SLE symptoms to the SLE diagnosis (LN patients with early-onset SLE without ESKD), and cluster 3 ($n = 104$) consisted of patients without ESKD but with a time of at least one year from the first SLE symptoms to the SLE diagnosis (LN patients with late-onset SLE without ESKD). Compared with the remaining ones, cluster 1 was characterized by a higher frequency of pleural effusion, skin changes diagnosed as erythema, livedo racemosa, livedo reticularis, a higher frequency of class VI glomerulonephritis according to the ISN/RPS classification system in renal biopsy, and a higher rate of mortality. Patients in cluster 1 were also administered immunoglobulins and plasmapheresis more often. Moreover, cases in cluster 1 vs. cluster 2 more often had hemolytic anemia and thrombocytopenia, while women more frequently had miscarriages. Interestingly, patients in cluster 3 vs. clusters 1 and 2 were younger at the time of SLE diagnosis and suffered from arthritis more often. Clusters were comparable according to age and other internal comorbidities, autoantibody profile, and thrombotic episodes.

In the non-LN group (Table 8), we indicated two different clusters based on the time delay from the first SLE symptoms to the diagnosis. Cluster 4 had patients with less than one year from the first symptoms to diagnosis (non-LN patients with early-onset SLE) and cluster 5 had patients with one year or more (non-LN patients with late-onset SLE). The first one included 288 patients, whereas the second had 290 cases. Patients in cluster 4 were older at the time of SLE diagnosis and presented with a longer duration of the disease. Regarding clinics, both clusters were similar, except for a higher frequency of malar rash and a lower frequency of hemolytic anemia documented in those from cluster 5. They were also administered azathioprine more often.

Table 7. Three clusters among lupus nephritis patients based on the time from the first systemic lupus erythematosus symptoms to the disease diagnosis and the presence of end stage kidney disease.

Features	Cluster 1 LN Patients with ESKD $n = 23$	Cluster 2 LN Patients with Early-Onset SLE without ESKD $n = 203$	Cluster 3 LN Patients with Late-Onset SLE without ESKD $n = 104$	p-Value
Juvenile onset (age of onset < 18 years), n (%)	17 (73.91%)	172 (84.31%) #	97 (95.10%) *	0.003
Other skin changes [1], n (%)	8 (34.78%)	125 (61.88%) *	73 (70.19%) **	0.007
Pleural effusion, n (%)	12 (52.17%)	55 (27.23%) *	23 (22.33%) **	0.002
Arthritis, n (%)	10 (43.48%)	112 (56.57%) #	72 (69.23%) *	0.003
Hemolytic anemia [2], n (%)	7 (70.00%)	24 (29.27%) *	11 (23.91%)	0.020
Thrombocytopenia [3], n (%)	14 (60.87%)	55 (27.92%) **,#	41 (40.20%)	0.002
Miscarriages, n (%)	5 (26.32%)	13 (8.67%) *	14 (18.18%)	0.030
LN class VI [4], n (%)	3 (27.27%)	1 (0.88%) **	1 (1.72%) *	0.020
Death, n (%)	6 (37.5%)	8 (4.12%) **	2 (2.15%) **	<0.001
Plasmapheresis, n (%)	8 (34.78%)	14 (7.18%) **	5 (4.85%) **	0.004

Categorical variables are presented as numbers with percentages. *—$p < 0.05$ in comparison with cluster 1; **—$p < 0.01$ in comparison with cluster 1; #—$p < 0.05$ in comparison with cluster 3; [1]—erythema, livedo racemosa, livedo reticularis; [2]—anemia with a positive direct Coombs test, anemia with a decreased level of haptoglobin, or a diagnosis based on medical history; [3]—<100,000/mm^3 or diagnosis based on medical history; [4]—according to the International Society of Nephrology/Renal Pathology Society criteria. In two (0.6%) LN cases, the time of first kidney manifestation in the SLE course was unknown. Abbreviations: ESKD—end-stage kidney disease, LN—lupus nephritis, n—number, SLE—systemic lupus erythematosus.

Table 8. Two clusters among non-lupus nephritis patients based on the time from the first systemic lupus erythematosus symptoms to the SLE diagnosis.

Features	Cluster 4 Non-LN Patients with Early-Onset SLE $n = 288$	Cluster 5 Non-LN Patients with Late-Onset SLE $n = 290$	p-Value
Juvenile onset (age of onset < 18 years), n (%)	259 (89.93%)	283 (97.59%)	<0.001
Lupus malar rash, n (%)	155 (53.82%)	126 (43.60%)	0.016
Direct Coombs test, n (%)	12 (29.27%)	19 (55.88%)	<0.001
Diabetes mellitus, n (%)	36 (12.50%)	18 (6.21%)	<0.001
Azathioprine, n (%)	114 (39.58%)	82 (28.28%)	0.004

Categorical variables are presented as numbers with percentages. In two (0.6%) LN cases, the time of first kidney manifestation in the SLE course was unknown. Abbreviations: LN—lupus nephritis, n—number, SLE—systemic lupus erythematosus.

3.9. Multiple Lupus Nephritis Exacerbations Are Related to the Distinct Clinical Picture

In the entire LN group, we documented renal flares in 191 (57.7%) patients, with one renal exacerbation in 58 (17.52%) cases, two renal exacerbations in 44 (14.06%) patients, and at least three renal exacerbations in 19 (5.74%) cases. The exact number of renal flares was unknown in 19 LN patients (5.74%).

Notably, LN patients with at least three renal flares exhibited distinct clinical characteristics. They were more frequently women (92.06% vs. 80.32%; $p = 0.026$), 5 years younger at the onset of SLE (medians: 25 vs. 30 years; $p = 0.015$), and 12 years younger at LN diagnosis (medians: 27 vs. 39 years; $p < 0.001$). Surprisingly, however, in those with multiple kidney exacerbations, LN was diagnosed less frequently during SLE onset (49.21% vs. 65.46%; $p = 0.02$). Furthermore, these patients reported more frequent myalgia (53.23% vs. 34.44%; $p = 0.006$), arthritis (72.13% vs. 56.22%; $p = 0.021$), nephrotic proteinuria (85.25% vs. 52.24%; $p < 0.001$), pathological urinary casts in the urine sediment (78.43% vs. 56.55%; $p = 0.001$), and end-stage kidney disease (ESKD) (14.52% vs. 5.22%; $p = 0.006$) in their medical history. Conversely, lymphopenia was the only manifestation found less frequently in those LN patients (6.67% vs. 21.1%; $p = 0.01$).

Additionally, the LN groups were similar in other SLE manifestations ($p > 0.05$ for all). Treatment modalities more frequently used in LN patients with at least three renal flares included azathioprine (69.84% vs. 46.75%; $p = 0.001$), cyclosporine A (25.4% vs. 7.76%; $p < 0.001$), mycophenolate mofetil (82.54% vs. 62.04%; $p = 0.003$), cyclophosphamide (95.24% vs. 57.32%; $p < 0.001$), and rituximab (17.74% vs. 4.08%; $p < 0.001$); however, there were no differences between groups in treatment with corticosteroids, chloroquine or hydroxychloroquine, methotrexate, belimumab, immunoglobulins, sulfasalazine, anifrolumab, plasmapheresis, and splenectomy ($p > 0.05$ for all). Additionally, both groups differed in autoantibody profile and kidney biopsy results. Those with multiple renal flares exhibited a higher frequency of anti-nucleosome (58.06% vs. 42.02%; $p = 0.023$) and anti-dsDNA antibodies (93.33% vs. 81.59%; $p = 0.022$), were class VI more frequently (6.38% vs. 1.55%; $p = 0.012$), and were class II less frequently (21.71% vs. 6.38%; $p = 0.004$) in histological investigations. In other ANA types identified by an immunoblot assay test and a histological renal biopsy, patterns were similar ($p > 0.05$ for all).

4. Discussion

In this study, we provide significant insights into the demographic, clinical, and laboratory profiles within a cohort comprising both LN and non-LN patients. Our findings revealed significant differences between LN and non-LN patients in several clinically relevant features. These distinctions could serve as valuable prognostic indicators for predicting which SLE patients might be at an increased risk of developing LN in the future. LN patients were younger at the time of SLE diagnosis. Obviously, women constituted the majority of cases in both SLE groups, but the percentage of men in the LN group was slightly higher. In LN, we also documented concomitant mucocutaneous manifestations, joint involvement, serositis, hematological abnormalities, and neurological involvement more frequently, along with hypertension and hypercholesterolemia as concomitant internal diseases. Patients with LN had a higher prevalence of anti-dsDNA, anti-histone, and anti-nucleosome antibodies. Conversely, aCL and anti-β2GPI in both IgM classes and thrombotic episodes (strokes and deep venous thrombosis) were reported more frequently in the non-LN group, similarly to the presence of anti-SSA and anti-SSB antibodies. In both SLE subgroups, corticosteroids were the most common therapy regimen, although as expected, LN patients were more frequently treated with immunosuppressants such as azathioprine, mycophenolate mofetil, cyclophosphamide, and rituximab.

In general, renal involvement appeared in about one-third of our SLE cohort. This frequency is similar to another report in a prospective multi-ethnic/racial SLE inception cohort, where LN occurred in 38.3% of SLE patients [14]. Furthermore, Jourde-Chiche et al. [27] highlighted the risk factors for LN relapses, encompassing antiphospholipid syndrome, higher baseline proteinuria, low C3 complement, higher Systemic Lupus Erythematosus Diseases Activity Index (SLEDAI) at inclusion, lower eGFR, lower serum albumin, lower hemoglobin levels, and lower leucocyte, lymphocyte, and eosinophil counts. In addition, Rovin et al. [15] have suggested that a decrease in complement levels and an elevation in anti-dsDNA antibodies are associated with a high likelihood of subsequent clinical LN relapse. Our findings are only partially consistent with theirs, because in addition to proteinuria, urinary protein excretion of more than 3.5 g/day, and a presence of anti-dsDNA antibodies, other significant risk factors for LN flares included female sex, younger age at LN or SLE onset, LN occurring later than SLE onset, the presence of anti-nucleosome antibodies, and several SLE manifestations such as myalgia, arthritis, and pathological urinary casts in the urine sediment. On the contrary, in our cohort, we observed that lymphopenia was associated with a lower number of renal flares. Next, we noticed a higher presence of juvenile-onset SLE in the LN group, which also stays in line with the report by Font et al. [28]. Furthermore, the shortened delay between symptom onset and SLE diagnosis in LN further underscores the urgency of promptly identifying and addressing renal involvement. Another reported risk factor for the development of LN is male sex [29], which is consistent with our findings.

The LN group was characterized by more severe clinical manifestations in our study. These patients often had general symptoms, including fever and fatigue/weakness, but also had life-threatening complications more frequently, such as serositis with pleural and pericardial effusion. Furthermore, these patients also had diffuse alveolar hemorrhage and central nervous system involvement more frequently, which interestingly were associated with specific antibody types such as anti-nucleosome or anti-histone. Neuropsychiatric SLE is a serious SLE complication [30,31]; thus, potential factors are needed to predict its development. For example, a study by Su et al. [32] specified that positive anti-SSA antibodies were related to peripheral neuropathy among LN patients and suggested their usefulness as a biomarker of this disease. We did not find this association, which may have a genetic or racial relationship. Next, the LN group had hematological manifestations such as lymphopenia, anemia, and hemolytic anemia more often. That observation also did not mirror those published by Hanly et al. [14] in a study with a large SLE cohort. Regardless of some discretions, the conditions listed above in our patients led to a worse clinical prognosis [33].

On the contrary, non-LN patients were characterized by a higher presence of mucocutaneous manifestations, photosensitivity, and Raynaud's phenomenon with a higher prevalence of joint involvement. These observations are in line with the current literature [14]. Nevertheless, the symptoms listed above were also perceived as common disease flares in ESKD SLE patients [34], similar to Raynaud's phenomenon. These may be a strong predictor for a poor long-term outcome in LN patients, according to a report published by Yadav et al. [35], and may therefore be linked to a worse clinical prognosis of SLE.

In turn, we did not observe any differences regarding the occurrence of several autoimmune diseases in the family history of LN and non-LN patients, but psoriasis, rheumatoid arthritis, and SLE were diagnosed most frequently in LN patients. This observation is novel, since it has previously been shown that only SLE presence in family members was a risk factor for autoimmune disorders [36].

In our dataset, we observed a higher prevalence of arterial hypertension and hypercholesterolemia in LN, which were associated with an increased mortality rate and ESKD in LN [37]; however, we found no significant differences in diabetes mellitus, heart failure, atrial fibrillation, malignant tumors, peripheral artery disease, myocardial infarct, ischemic stroke, and venous thromboembolism between the analyzed LN and non-LN patients. Thus, one might speculate that the presence of SLE itself, regardless of renal involvement, is a risk factor for those comorbidities [38–41].

The standardized mortality ratios in SLE cohorts are up to 5.3 times higher than those in age-matched healthy controls [42]. The mortality rate in our study remains comparable between LN and non-LN groups. Infections, SLE exacerbations, and emerging malignancies were the primary cause of death, consistent with the findings presented by Kandane-Rathnayake et al. [43]. These comparable mortality rates underscore the persistent need for effective management of SLE flares but also the prevention of infections whenever possible (utilizing antibiotic therapy when necessary and vaccinations) and regular oncological screenings independent from kidney involvement. Next, based on the literature, some prognostic factors are associated with higher mortality rates in SLE. They include male sex, age of at least 50 at SLE diagnosis, renal and lung involvement, thrombocytopenia, SLEDAI of at least 20 points, hypertension, ischemic heart disease, antiphospholipid syndrome (APS), and thrombotic episodes [44–46]. Our results align with those presented by other authors; however, other comorbidities such as diabetes mellitus, heart failure, hypercholesterolemia, atrial fibrillation, and malignancy were also associated with a higher mortality rate. Additionally, thrombocytopenia as a hematological manifestation was linked to a poor prognosis in our study, as well as hemolytic anemia of any case, including macrophage activation syndrome. What is noteworthy is that, apart from renal and lung involvements, arthritis, serositis, and general symptoms were also associated with a higher risk of death. Our data suggest that patients with SLE should undergo regular monitoring and, if necessary, immunosuppressive treatment to prevent the occurrence of serious SLE manifestations. Furthermore, an interdisciplinary approach and oncological screenings are essential in managing this group of patients.

As anticipated, LN patients exhibited a distinct pattern of autoantibody types with anti-nucleosome, anti-histone, and anti-dsDNA antibodies as the most important. Based on the literature, their association with LN is still not fully elucidated, however [47,48]. Interestingly, a study by Choi et al. [49] revealed that patients with simultaneous positivity in all of the above antibodies had higher disease activity with more advanced histopathological changes in renal biopsies, as well as a more rapid decline in renal function. We did not observe that association; however, the IV class according to ISN/RPS was the most prevalent among the 83 patients who exhibited them all, which was identified in 29 (34.94%) cases. Furthermore, anti-dsDNA antibodies were not only a predictor of LN development [29] but also poor prognosis in LN [50]. This is consistent with our results, since the presence of anti-dsDNA antibodies was linked to an increased LN exacerbation rate, malignancy, and a higher death risk. Additionally, we noted an increased incidence of anti-nucleosome antibodies in patients who experienced a myocardial infarct, which is a new finding. Interestingly, in contrast to many studies, we did not observe a higher prevalence of anti-Sm antibodies in LN cases. This may be related to the race specification, since anti-Sm antibodies are more frequently documented in African Americans, at least in some reports [51,52]. On the other hand, we observed a higher presence of rheumatoid factor and anti-SSA with anti-SSB antibodies in the non-LN group, suggesting a decreased association with LN.

The subsequent important finding of our study is the association between aCL antibodies and thrombotic episodes in non-LN subjects. The existing literature indicates that the presence of any type of antiphospholipid antibodies (aPLAs) in LN is linked to an unfavorable long-term prognosis and reduced renal survival attributed to thrombotic events [53]; however, it is necessary to note that SLE itself also increases the risk of arterial thromboembolism [54]. Moreover, according to a recent meta-analysis conducted by Domingues et al. [55], the presence of antiphospholipid antibodies in SLE is associated with a three- to five-fold increased risk of specific microvascular renal lesions; however, data from the previous literature did not report an association between antiphospholipid antibodies and LN [56,57], similar to us. All thromboembolic events occurred with a comparable incidence in both SLE groups, except for those with non-LN and the presence of aCL in the IgM class, as compared to the remaining in the same subgroup. This observation is unexpected, since the presence of LN is a strong predictor of thrombotic events, especially venous ones [58].

The detailed data on immunosuppressive therapy showed distinct patterns in medication usage between LN and non-LN cases. More than 99% of LN patients were on corticosteroids orally/intravenously, which are a flagship example of drugs used in SLE patients with affected kidneys [59]. Next, more aggressive treatment modalities, including azathioprine, cyclosporine, mycophenolate mofetil, cyclophosphamide, rituximab, immunoglobulins, and plasmapheresis were more commonly used in LN. Nevertheless, the efficacy of immunosuppressive agent-induction therapy for lupus nephritis is still being investigated [60].

Importantly, given the complexity of SLE, it is worth pointing out the role of genetic and environmental factors in the development and progression of LN. Genetic predispositions, such as specific HLA alleles and polymorphisms in immune-related genes, can increase the susceptibility to LN [61]. For example, genetic variants in genes expressed in the kidney (including *TNFRSF1B*, *KLK1*, *KLK3*, *ACE*, *AGT*, and *APOL1*) may result in increased susceptibility to kidney injury and, as a result, in progression to lupus nephritis [62]. Environmental factors, including infections, medications, and exposure to UV light, can trigger disease onset and exacerbate flares in genetically predisposed SLE/LN individuals [63–65]. Understanding the interplay between these genetic and environmental factors can help identify at-risk patients and develop personalized treatment strategies.

The final issue that is worth discussing is the cluster analysis based on the presence of ESKD in LN patients and the time delay from the first symptoms to SLE diagnosis in non-LN patients, which showed intriguing subgroup analyses in both LN and non-LN patients, delineating variations in clinical presentation, outcomes, and treatment responses. The groups are heterogeneous, but there are specific patterns in their clinical characteristics. Therefore, it may be possible to anticipate the course of the disease based on given features, i.e., the occurrence of certain additional complications; thus, it may help in optimizing therapy accordingly.

Our study has some limitations. Firstly, the study's retrospective nature may introduce inherent biases in data collection and patient selection. Next, the study has a single-center design that may limit the generalizability of the results to a larger population. We did not collect patient-reported outcomes, such as quality-of-life questionnaires, which might best assess the patient's well-being, including the impact of disease and treatment mode. Also, we did not analyze other imaging and laboratory test results, such as echocardiography. Finally, some of the presented relationships may be incidental and not represent a cause-and-effect relationship. Therefore, while our study provides valuable insights, these limitations highlight the need for cautious interpretation of the results.

5. Conclusions

In conclusion, the present study significantly contributes to the understanding of SLE and LN by revealing distinct demographic, clinical and laboratory features in affected individuals. Indeed, LN patients were younger at first symptoms and at disease onset but were also more often characterized by the presence of mucocutaneous, joint, and hematological manifestations and suffered more often from internal comorbidities such as hypertension, hypercholesterolemia, and end-stage kidney disease. Next, this group presented a more frequent occurrence of autoantibodies with a higher usage of immunosuppressive treatment. Furthermore, ESKD patients were characterized by a less frequent juvenile onset and a higher prevalence of skin changes and hematologic disturbances such as hemolytic anemia and thrombocytopenia.

Early identification and tailored treatment of LN are crucial given their association with more severe SLE manifestations and specific autoantibody profiles. Clinicians should prioritize monitoring high-risk patients, particularly those in the abovementioned groups, in terms of clinical and laboratory state, including autoantibody profile. Implementing comprehensive patient monitoring practices also addressing internist comorbidities, such as hypertension and hypercholesterolemia, can improve outcomes. Nevertheless, more prospective studies with diverse cohorts would be beneficial in understanding the diversity of LN and its progression in SLE patients.

Author Contributions: Conceptualization, J.K.-W., M.M., S.B.-S. and M.K.; methods, J.K.-W., R.D., S.B.-S. and M.K.; software, J.K.-W. and R.D.; validation, J.K.-W., R.D., S.B.-S. and M.K.; formal analysis, J.K.-W., R.D. and L.Z.; investigation, J.K.-W., A.S.-K., M.S. and A.W.; resources, J.K.-W.; data curation, J.K.-W., R.D. and L.Z.; writing—original draft preparation, J.K.-W. and R.D.; writing—review and editing, A.S.-K., M.S., M.M., A.W., L.Z., S.B.-S. and M.K.; visualization, J.K.-W. and R.D.; supervision, S.B.-S. and M.K.; project administration, J.K.-W. All authors have read and agreed to the published version of the manuscript.

Funding: This work was supported by the Research Grant of Jagiellonian University Medical College No. N41/DBS/000936 (to J.K.-W.).

Institutional Review Board Statement: The study was conducted in accordance with the guidelines of the Declaration of Helsinki and was approved by the Bioethical Committee of Jagiellonian University (Kraków, Poland) (Approval No.: 118.6120.41.2023, on 15 June 2023).

Informed Consent Statement: Patient consent was waived due to a retrospective study design.

Data Availability Statement: The data presented in this study are available on reasonable request from the corresponding author.

Conflicts of Interest: The authors declare no conflicts of interest.

References

1. Durcan, L.; O'Dwyer, T.; Petri, M. Management Strategies and Future Directions for Systemic Lupus Erythematosus in Adults. *Lancet* **2019**, *393*, 2332–2343. [CrossRef]
2. Kosalka, J.; Jakiela, B.; Musial, J. Changes of Memory B- and T-Cell Subsets in Lupus Nephritis Patients. *Folia Histochem. Cytobiol.* **2016**, *54*, 32–41. [CrossRef]
3. Jakiela, B.; Kosałka, J.; Plutecka, H.; Bazan-Socha, S.; Sanak, M.; Musiał, J. Facilitated Expansion of Th17 Cells in Lupus Nephritis Patients. *Clin. Exp. Immunol.* **2018**, *194*, 283–294. [CrossRef]
4. Klein, A.; Polliack, A.; Gafter-Gvili, A. Systemic Lupus Erythematosus and Lymphoma: Incidence, Pathogenesis and Biology. *Leuk. Res.* **2018**, *75*, 45–49. [CrossRef]
5. Ruiz-Irastorza, G.; Khamashta, M.A.; Castellino, G.; Hughes, G.R. Systemic Lupus Erythematosus. *Lancet* **2001**, *357*, 1027–1032. [CrossRef]
6. Schur, P.H. Laboratory Testing for the Diagnosis, Evaluation, and Management of Systemic Lupus Erythematosus: Still More Questions for the next Generations. *Clin. Immunol.* **2016**, *172*, 117–121. [CrossRef]
7. Battaglia, M.; Garrett-Sinha, L.A. Bacterial Infections in Lupus: Roles in Promoting Immune Activation and in Pathogenesis of the Disease. *J. Transl. Autoimmun.* **2021**, *4*, 100078. [CrossRef]
8. Speyer, C.B.; Costenbader, K.H. Cigarette Smoking and the Pathogenesis of Systemic Lupus Erythematosus. *Expert Rev. Clin. Immunol.* **2018**, *14*, 481–487. [CrossRef]
9. Anders, H.-J.; Saxena, R.; Zhao, M.; Parodis, I.; Salmon, J.E.; Mohan, C. Lupus Nephritis. *Nat. Rev. Dis. Primers* **2020**, *6*, 7. [CrossRef] [PubMed]
10. Parodis, I.; Tamirou, F.; Houssiau, F.A. Prediction of Prognosis and Renal Outcome in Lupus Nephritis. *Lupus Sci. Med.* **2020**, *7*, e000389. [CrossRef]
11. Saleh, M.; Eltoraby, E.E.; Tharwat, S.; Nassar, M.K. Clinical and Histopathological Features and Short-Term Outcomes of Lupus Nephritis: A Prospective Study of 100 Egyptian Patients. *Lupus* **2020**, *29*, 993–1001. [CrossRef]
12. Parikh, S.V.; Almaani, S.; Brodsky, S.; Rovin, B.H. Update on Lupus Nephritis: Core Curriculum 2020. *Am. J. Kidney Dis.* **2020**, *76*, 265–281. [CrossRef]
13. Gasparotto, M.; Gatto, M.; Binda, V.; Doria, A.; Moroni, G. Lupus Nephritis: Clinical Presentations and Outcomes in the 21st Century. *Rheumatology* **2020**, *59*, v39–v51. [CrossRef] [PubMed]
14. Hanly, J.G.; O'Keeffe, A.G.; Su, L.; Urowitz, M.B.; Romero-Diaz, J.; Gordon, C.; Bae, S.-C.; Bernatsky, S.; Clarke, A.E.; Wallace, D.J.; et al. The Frequency and Outcome of Lupus Nephritis: Results from an International Inception Cohort Study. *Rheumatology* **2016**, *55*, 252–262. [CrossRef]
15. Rovin, B.H.; Caster, D.J.; Cattran, D.C.; Gibson, K.L.; Hogan, J.J.; Moeller, M.J.; Roccatello, D.; Cheung, M.; Wheeler, D.C.; Winkelmayer, W.C.; et al. Management and Treatment of Glomerular Diseases (Part 2): Conclusions from a Kidney Disease: Improving Global Outcomes (KDIGO) Controversies Conference. *Kidney Int.* **2019**, *95*, 281–295. [CrossRef]
16. Mahmoud, G.A.; Zayed, H.S.; Ghoniem, S.A. Renal Outcomes among Egyptian Lupus Nephritis Patients: A Retrospective Analysis of 135 Cases from a Single Centre. *Lupus* **2015**, *24*, 331–338. [CrossRef]
17. Davidson, A.; Aranow, C.; Mackay, M. Lupus Nephritis: Challenges and Progress. *Curr. Opin. Rheumatol.* **2019**, *31*, 682–688. [CrossRef] [PubMed]
18. Almaani, S.; Meara, A.; Rovin, B.H. Update on Lupus Nephritis. *Clin. J. Am. Soc. Nephrol.* **2017**, *12*, 825–835. [CrossRef]
19. Wermut, W.; Hebanowski, M.; Mlotowski, T.; Stolarczyk, J. Lupus nephritis in patients observed at the II Department of Internal Diseases of the Medical Academy in Gdańsk. *Pol. Tyg. Lek.* **1977**, *32*, 89–93. [PubMed]
20. Szymanik-Grzelak, H.; Barabasz, M.; Wikiera-Magott, I.; Banaszak, B.; Wieczorkiewicz-Płaza, A.; Bieniaś, B.; Drożynska-Duklas, M.; Tkaczyk, M.; Pańczyk-Tomaszewska, M. Retrospective Analysis of Clinical and Pathomorphological Features of Lupus Nephritis in Children. *Adv. Med. Sci.* **2021**, *66*, 128–137. [CrossRef]
21. Perkowska-Ptasinska, A.; Bartczak, A.; Wagrowska-Danilewicz, M.; Halon, A.; Okon, K.; Wozniak, A.; Danilewicz, M.; Karkoszka, H.; Marszałek, A.; Kowalewska, J.; et al. Clinicopathologic Correlations of Renal Pathology in the Adult Population of Poland. *Nephrol. Dial. Transplant.* **2017**, *32*, ii209–ii218. [CrossRef] [PubMed]
22. Zwolińska, D.; Kiliś-Pstrusińska, K.; Wikiera, I.; Medyńska, A. [Lupus nephritis in children]. *Pol. Merkur. Lek.* **2000**, *8*, 454–456.
23. Aringer, M. EULAR/ACR Classification Criteria for SLE. *Semin. Arthritis Rheum.* **2019**, *49*, S14–S17. [CrossRef] [PubMed]
24. Kosałka-Węgiel, J.; Dziedzic, R.; Siwiec-Koźlik, A.; Spałkowska, M.; Milewski, M.; Żuk-Kuwik, J.; Zaręba, L.; Bazan-Socha, S.; Korkosz, M. Clinical and Laboratory Characteristics of Early-Onset and Delayed-Onset Lupus Nephritis Patients: A Single-Center Retrospective Study. *Rheumatol. Int.* **2024**, *44*, 1283–1294. [CrossRef] [PubMed]
25. Kaczmarczyk, K.; Kosalka, J.; Soja, J.; Kuzniewski, M.; Musial, J.; Okon, K. Renal Interstitial Mast Cell Counts Differ across Classes of Proliferative Lupus Nephritis. *Folia Histochem. Cytobiol.* **2014**, *52*, 218–224. [CrossRef] [PubMed]

26. Levey, A.S.; Titan, S.M.; Powe, N.R.; Coresh, J.; Inker, L.A. Kidney Disease, Race, and GFR Estimation. *Clin. J. Am. Soc. Nephrol.* **2020**, *15*, 1203–1212. [CrossRef]
27. Jourde-Chiche, N.; Costedoat-Chalumeau, N.; Baumstarck, K.; Loundou, A.; Bouillet, L.; Burtey, S.; Caudwell, V.; Chiche, L.; Couzi, L.; Daniel, L.; et al. Weaning of Maintenance Immunosuppressive Therapy in Lupus Nephritis (WIN-Lupus): Results of a Multicentre Randomised Controlled Trial. *Ann. Rheum. Dis.* **2022**, *81*, 1420–1427. [CrossRef]
28. Font, J.; Cervera, R.; Espinosa, G.; Pallares, L.; Ramos-Casals, M.; Jimenez, S.; Garcia-Carrasco, M.; Seisdedos, L.; Ingelmo, M. Systemic Lupus Erythematosus (SLE) in Childhood: Analysis of Clinical and Immunological Findings in 34 Patients and Comparison with SLE Characteristics in Adults. *Ann. Rheum. Dis.* **1998**, *57*, 456–459. [CrossRef]
29. Chan, S.C.W.; Wang, Y.-F.; Yap, D.Y.H.; Chan, T.M.; Lau, Y.L.; Lee, P.P.W.; Lai, W.M.; Ying, S.K.Y.; Tse, N.K.C.; Leung, A.M.H.; et al. Risk and Factors Associated with Disease Manifestations in Systemic Lupus Erythematosus—Lupus Nephritis (RIFLE-LN): A Ten-Year Risk Prediction Strategy Derived from a Cohort of 1652 Patients. *Front. Immunol.* **2023**, *14*, 1200732. [CrossRef]
30. Williams, W.; Shah, D.; Sargeant, L.A. The Clinical and Epidemiologic Features in 140 Patients with Lupus Nephritis in a Predominantly Black Population from One Center in Kingston, Jamaica. *Am. J. Med. Sci.* **2004**, *327*, 324–329. [CrossRef]
31. Liu, Y.; Tu, Z.; Zhang, X.; Du, K.; Xie, Z.; Lin, Z. Pathogenesis and Treatment of Neuropsychiatric Systemic Lupus Erythematosus: A Review. *Front. Cell Dev. Biol.* **2022**, *10*, 998328. [CrossRef] [PubMed]
32. Su, Y.-J.; Huang, C.-R.; Chang, W.-N.; Tsai, N.-W.; Kung, C.-T.; Lin, W.-C.; Huang, C.-C.; Su, C.-M.; Cheng, B.-C.; Chang, Y.-T.; et al. The Association between Autoantibodies and Peripheral Neuropathy in Lupus Nephritis. *BioMed Res. Int.* **2014**, *2014*, 524940. [CrossRef] [PubMed]
33. Kammoun, K.; Jarraya, F.; Bouhamed, L.; Kharrat, M.; Makni, S.; Hmida, M.B.; Makni, H.; Kaddour, N.; Boudawara, T.; Bahloul, Z.; et al. Poor Prognostic Factors of Lupus Nephritis. *Saudi J. Kidney Dis. Transpl.* **2011**, *22*, 727–732.
34. Barrera-Vargas, A.; Quintanar-Martínez, M.; Merayo-Chalico, J.; Alcocer-Varela, J.; Gómez-Martín, D. Risk Factors for Systemic Lupus Erythematosus Flares in Patients with End-Stage Renal Disease: A Case–Control Study. *Rheumatology* **2016**, *55*, 429–435. [CrossRef]
35. Kang, E.-S.; Ahn, S.M.; Oh, J.S.; Kim, Y.-G.; Lee, C.-K.; Yoo, B.; Hong, S. Long-Term Renal Outcomes of Patients with Non-Proliferative Lupus Nephritis. *Korean J. Intern. Med.* **2023**, *38*, 769–776. [CrossRef]
36. Ulff-Møller, C.J.; Simonsen, J.; Kyvik, K.O.; Jacobsen, S.; Frisch, M. Family History of Systemic Lupus Erythematosus and Risk of Autoimmune Disease: Nationwide Cohort Study in Denmark 1977–2013. *Rheumatology* **2017**, *56*, 957–964. [CrossRef]
37. Drakoulogkona, O.; Barbulescu, A.L.; Rica, I.; Musetescu, A.E.; Ciurea, P.L. The Outcome of Patients with Lupus Nephritis and the Impact of Cardiovascular Risk Factors. *Curr. Health Sci. J.* **2011**, *37*, 70–74.
38. Fedorchenko, Y.; Mahmudov, K.; Abenov, Z.; Zimba, O.; Yessirkepov, M. Diabetes Mellitus in Rheumatic Diseases: Clinical Characteristics and Treatment Considerations. *Rheumatol. Int.* **2023**, *43*, 2167–2174. [CrossRef] [PubMed]
39. Kostopoulou, M.; Nikolopoulos, D.; Parodis, I.; Bertsias, G. Cardiovascular Disease in Systemic Lupus Erythematosus: Recent Data on Epidemiology, Risk Factors and Prevention. *Curr. Vasc. Pharmacol.* **2020**, *18*, 549–565. [CrossRef]
40. Choi, M.Y.; Flood, K.; Bernatsky, S.; Ramsey-Goldman, R.; Clarke, A.E. A Review on SLE and Malignancy. *Best Pract. Res. Clin. Rheumatol.* **2017**, *31*, 373–396. [CrossRef]
41. Chen, Y.; Fu, C.; Pu, S.; Xue, Y. Systemic Lupus Erythematosus Increases Risk of Incident Atrial Fibrillation: A Systematic Review and Meta-Analysis. *Int. J. Rheum. Dis.* **2022**, *25*, 1097–1106. [CrossRef] [PubMed]
42. Singh, R.R.; Yen, E.Y. SLE Mortality Remains Disproportionately High, despite Improvements over the Last Decade. *Lupus* **2018**, *27*, 1577–1581. [CrossRef] [PubMed]
43. Kandane-Rathnayake, R.; Golder, V.; Louthrenoo, W.; Chen, Y.-H.; Cho, J.; Lateef, A.; Hamijoyo, L.; Luo, S.-F.; Wu, Y.-J.J.; Navarra, S.V.; et al. Lupus Low Disease Activity State and Remission and Risk of Mortality in Patients with Systemic Lupus Erythematosus: A Prospective, Multinational, Longitudinal Cohort Study. *Lancet Rheumatol.* **2022**, *4*, e822–e830. [CrossRef] [PubMed]
44. Kasitanon, N.; Magder, L.S.; Petri, M. Predictors of Survival in Systemic Lupus Erythematosus. *Medicine* **2006**, *85*, 147–156. [CrossRef] [PubMed]
45. Abu-Shakra, M.; Urowitz, M.B.; Gladman, D.D.; Gough, J. Mortality Studies in Systemic Lupus Erythematosus. Results from a Single Center. II. Predictor Variables for Mortality. *J. Rheumatol.* **1995**, *22*, 1265–1270. [PubMed]
46. Ruiz-Irastorza, G.; Egurbide, M.-V.; Ugalde, J.; Aguirre, C. High Impact of Antiphospholipid Syndrome on Irreversible Organ Damage and Survival of Patients with Systemic Lupus Erythematosus. *Arch. Intern. Med.* **2004**, *164*, 77–82. [CrossRef] [PubMed]
47. Mortensen, E.S.; Fenton, K.A.; Rekvig, O.P. Lupus Nephritis. *Am. J. Pathol.* **2008**, *172*, 275–283. [CrossRef] [PubMed]
48. Bonanni, A.; Vaglio, A.; Bruschi, M.; Sinico, R.A.; Cavagna, L.; Moroni, G.; Franceschini, F.; Allegri, L.; Pratesi, F.; Migliorini, P.; et al. Multi-Antibody Composition in Lupus Nephritis: Isotype and Antigen Specificity Make the Difference. *Autoimmun. Rev.* **2015**, *14*, 692–702. [CrossRef] [PubMed]
49. Choi, S.-E.; Park, D.-J.; Kang, J.-H.; Lee, S.-S. Significance of Co-Positivity for Anti-dsDNA, -Nucleosome, and -Histone Antibodies in Patients with Lupus Nephritis. *Ann. Med.* **2023**, *55*, 1009–1017. [CrossRef]
50. Lin, S.; Zhang, J.; Chen, B.; Li, D.; Liang, Y.; Hu, Y.; Liu, X.; Bai, Y.; Chen, C. Role of Crescents for Lupus Nephritis in Clinical, Pathological and Prognosis: A Single-Center Retrospective Cohort Study. *Eur. J. Med. Res.* **2023**, *28*, 60. [CrossRef]
51. Ward, M.M.; Studenski, S. Clinical Manifestations of Systemic Lupus Erythematosus. Identification of Racial and Socioeconomic Influences. *Arch. Intern. Med.* **1990**, *150*, 849–853. [CrossRef]

52. Ishizaki, J.; Saito, K.; Nawata, M.; Mizuno, Y.; Tokunaga, M.; Sawamukai, N.; Tamura, M.; Hirata, S.; Yamaoka, K.; Hasegawa, H.; et al. Low Complements and High Titre of Anti-Sm Antibody as Predictors of Histopathologically Proven Silent Lupus Nephritis without Abnormal Urinalysis in Patients with Systemic Lupus Erythematosus. *Rheumatology* **2015**, *54*, 405–412. [CrossRef]
53. Yap, D.Y.H.; Thong, K.M.; Yung, S.; Tang, C.; Ma, B.M.Y.; Chan, T.M. Antiphospholipid Antibodies in Patients with Lupus Nephritis: Clinical Correlations and Associations with Long-Term Outcomes. *Lupus* **2019**, *28*, 1460–1467. [CrossRef] [PubMed]
54. Mok, C.C.; Tong, K.H.; To, C.H.; Siu, Y.P.; Ho, L.Y.; Au, T.C. Risk and Predictors of Arterial Thrombosis in Lupus and Non-Lupus Primary Glomerulonephritis: A Comparative Study. *Medicine* **2007**, *86*, 203–209. [CrossRef]
55. Domingues, V.; Chock, E.Y.; Dufrost, V.; Risse, J.; Seshan, S.V.; Barbhaiya, M.; Sartelet, H.; Erkan, D.; Wahl, D.; Zuily, S. Increased Risk of Acute and Chronic Microvascular Renal Lesions Associated with Antiphospholipid Antibodies in Patients with Systemic Lupus Erythematosus: A Systematic Review and Meta-Analysis. *Autoimmun. Rev.* **2022**, *21*, 103158. [CrossRef] [PubMed]
56. Mehrani, T.; Petri, M. IgM Anti-ß$_2$ Glycoprotein I Is Protective Against Lupus Nephritis and Renal Damage in Systemic Lupus Erythematosus. *J. Rheumatol.* **2011**, *38*, 450–453. [CrossRef]
57. Sachse, C.; Lüthke, K.; Hartung, K.; Fricke, M.; Liedvogel, B.; Kalden, J.R.; Peter, H.H.; Lakomek, H.J.; Henkel, E.; Deicher, H.; et al. Significance of Antibodies to Cardiolipin in Unselected Patients with Systemic Lupus Erythematosus: Clinical and Laboratory Associations. *Rheumatol. Int.* **1995**, *15*, 23–29. [CrossRef] [PubMed]
58. Choojitarom, K.; Verasertniyom, O.; Totemchokchyakarn, K.; Nantiruj, K.; Sumethkul, V.; Janwityanujit. S. Lupus Nephritis and Raynaud's Phenomenon Are Significant Risk Factors for Vascular Thrombosis in SLE Patients with Positive Antiphospholipid Antibodies. *Clin. Rheumatol.* **2008**, *27*, 345–351. [CrossRef]
59. Houssiau, F.A.; Lauwerys, B.R. Current Management of Lupus Nephritis. *Best Pract. Res. Clin. Rheumatol.* **2013**, *27*, 319–328. [CrossRef]
60. Kaneko, M.; Jackson, S.W. Recent Advances in Immunotherapies for Lupus Nephritis. *Pediatr. Nephrol.* **2023**, *38*, 1001–1012. [CrossRef]
61. Iwamoto, T.; Niewold, T.B. Genetics of Human Lupus Nephritis. *Clin. Immunol.* **2017**, *185*, 32–39. [CrossRef] [PubMed]
62. Munroe, M.E.; James, J.A. Genetics of Lupus Nephritis: Clinical Implications. *Semin. Nephrol.* **2015**, *35*, 396–409. [CrossRef] [PubMed]
63. Refai, R.H.; Hussein, M.F.; Abdou, M.H.; Abou-Raya, A.N. Environmental Risk Factors of Systemic Lupus Erythematosus: A Case–Control Study. *Sci. Rep.* **2023**, *13*, 10219. [CrossRef] [PubMed]
64. Bai, H.; Jiang, L.; Li, T.; Liu, C.; Zuo, X.; Liu, Y.; Hu, S.; Sun, L.; Zhang, M.; Lin, J.; et al. Acute Effects of Air Pollution on Lupus Nephritis in Patients with Systemic Lupus Erythematosus: A Multicenter Panel Study in China. *Environ. Res.* **2021**, *195*, 110875. [CrossRef]
65. Díaz-Coronado, J.C.; Rojas-Villarraga, A.; Hernandez-Parra, D.; Betancur-Vásquez, L.; Lacouture-Fierro, J.; Gonzalez-Hurtado, D.; González-Arango, J.; Uribe-Arango, L.; Gaviria-Aguilar, M.C.; Pineda-Tamayo, R.A. Clinical and Sociodemographic Factors Associated with Lupus Nephritis in Colombian Patients: A Cross-Sectional Study. *Reumatol. Clínica* **2021**, *17*, 351–356. [CrossRef]

Disclaimer/Publisher's Note: The statements, opinions and data contained in all publications are solely those of the individual author(s) and contributor(s) and not of MDPI and/or the editor(s). MDPI and/or the editor(s) disclaim responsibility for any injury to people or property resulting from any ideas, methods, instructions or products referred to in the content.

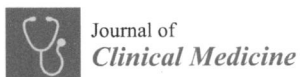

Article

High Interleukin 21 Levels in Patients with Systemic Lupus Erythematosus: Association with Clinical Variables and rs2221903 Polymorphism

Noemí Espinoza-García [1], Diana Celeste Salazar-Camarena [2], Miguel Marín-Rosales [2,3], María Paulina Reyes-Mata [2], María Guadalupe Ramírez-Dueñas [4], José Francisco Muñoz-Valle [4], Itzel María Borunda-Calderón [5], Aarón González-Palacios [2] and Claudia Azucena Palafox-Sánchez [2,4,*]

[1] Doctorado en Ciencias en Biología Molecular en Medicina (DCBMM), Centro Universitario de Ciencias de la Salud, Universidad de Guadalajara, Guadalajara 44340, Jalisco, Mexico; noemi.espinoza@academicos.udg.mx

[2] Grupo de Inmunología Molecular, Centro Universitario de Ciencias de la Salud, Universidad de Guadalajara, Guadalajara 44340, Jalisco, Mexico; celeste.salazar@academicos.udg.mx (D.C.S.-C.); miguel.marin@academicos.udg.mx (M.M.-R.); paulina.reyes@academicos.udg.mx (M.P.R.-M.); aaron.gonzalez@academicos.udg.mx (A.G.-P.)

[3] Hospital General de Occidente, Secretaría de Salud Jalisco, Guadalajara 45170, Jalisco, Mexico

[4] Instituto de Investigación en Ciencias Biomédicas (IICB), Centro Universitario de Ciencias de la Salud, Universidad de Guadalajara, Guadalajara 44340, Jalisco, Mexico; maria.rduenas@academicos.udg.mx (M.G.R.-D.); jose.mvalle@academicos.udg.mx (J.F.M.-V.)

[5] Doctorado en Ciencias Biomédicas (DCB), Centro Universitario de Ciencias de la Salud, Universidad de Guadalajara, Guadalajara 44340, Jalisco, Mexico; itzel.borunda2324@alumnos.udg.mx

* Correspondence: claudia.palafox@academicos.udg.mx; Tel.: +52-33-10585200 (ext. 342000)

Citation: Espinoza-García, N.; Salazar-Camarena, D.C.; Marín-Rosales, M.; Reyes-Mata, M.P.; Ramírez-Dueñas, M.G.; Muñoz-Valle, J.F.; Borunda-Calderón, I.M.; González-Palacios, A.; Palafox-Sánchez, C.A. High Interleukin 21 Levels in Patients with Systemic Lupus Erythematosus: Association with Clinical Variables and rs2221903 Polymorphism. *J. Clin. Med.* **2024**, *13*, 4512. https://doi.org/10.3390/jcm13154512

Academic Editor: Matteo Piga

Received: 15 July 2024
Revised: 30 July 2024
Accepted: 31 July 2024
Published: 2 August 2024

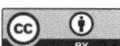

Copyright: © 2024 by the authors. Licensee MDPI, Basel, Switzerland. This article is an open access article distributed under the terms and conditions of the Creative Commons Attribution (CC BY) license (https://creativecommons.org/licenses/by/4.0/).

Abstract: Background: Systemic lupus erythematosus (SLE) is an autoimmune disease characterized by autoantibody production and diverse tissue and organ inflammatory affections. Interleukin 21 (IL-21) is implicated in B cell survival, proliferation, differentiation, class switching, and immunoglobulin production; therefore, it is considered a key cytokine in the pathogenesis of SLE. However, its association with disease activity and clinical phenotypes remains unclear. We aimed to evaluate the association of IL-21 levels with the disease activity and clinical phenotypes in patients with SLE. Also, we analyzed the *IL21* polymorphisms associated with increased IL-21 levels. **Methods:** The IL-21 serum levels were determined using the enzyme-linked immunosorbent assay (ELISA) method. The rs2221903 and rs2055979 polymorphisms were assessed in 300 healthy controls (HCs) and 300 patients with SLE by the polymerase chain reaction–restriction fragment length polymorphism (PCR-RFLP) technique. The levels of IL-21 were monitored during follow-up visits in 59 patients with SLE. **Results:** The patients with SLE showed higher IL-21 levels compared to the HCs. The IL-21 levels did not correlate with Mex-SLEDAI and were not different in patients with inactive, mild–moderate, and severe disease. The IL-21 levels were increased in patients with hematological affection. The ROC curve analysis revealed that the IL-21 levels had good predictive power in discriminating among patients with SLE and HCs. In a follow-up analysis, the levels of IL-21 remained higher in the patients with SLE even when the patients were in remission. Also, the rs2221903 polymorphism was associated with increased IL-21 levels. **Conclusions:** This study highlights the importance of IL-21 as a key cytokine in SLE. IL-21 levels are higher in patients with SLE and remain increased regardless of disease activity. According to the ROC analysis, IL-21 is a potential biomarker of SLE. Further longitudinal studies are needed to explore the relationship between IL-21 and the clinical phenotypes of SLE.

Keywords: Interleukin 21; systemic lupus erythematosus; *IL21* polymorphism

1. Introduction

Systemic lupus erythematosus (SLE) is a chronic autoimmune disease characterized by autoantibody production, immune complex formation, and inflammatory tissue damage [1]. In the SLE pathogenesis, diverse cytokines are involved in the onset, progression, and exacerbation of the disease, including interferon-alpha (IFNα), tumor necrosis factor-alpha (TNFα), interleukin (IL) 6, IL-10, IL-12, IL-17, IL-21, IL-27, and B cell-activating factor (BAFF), among others [2–6], highlighting SLE as a complex multi-cytokine disease.

IL-21 is a pleiotropic cytokine produced by T follicular helper (Tfh) cells, circulating Tfh (cTfh), T peripheral helper (Tph) cells, T helper 17 (Th17), T helper 9 (Th9) cells, and Natural Killer T cells [7–10]. These cells can help B cells through IL-21 [9], promoting B cell activation and differentiation, affinity maturation, class switching, and antibody production [11–13]. It has been reported that IL-21 levels are increased in patients with SLE compared to controls [4,14,15]. To our knowledge, lupus nephritis is the only clinical phenotype associated with IL-21 levels [15]. However, studies show heterogeneous results regarding the correlation between IL-21 levels and clinical variables in patients with SLE [16,17]. In a previous study, we found that patients with SLE have increased frequencies of IL-21+ cTfh and Tph cells, which are maintained independently of the disease activity [18]. The crucial role of IL-21 in SLE development is underscored by its elevated levels in affected patients compared to controls, and its persistence at high levels further highlights its significance.

Among the factors associated with the disease, genetic factors, including single-nucleotide polymorphisms (SNPs), have a special contribution. The SNPs rs2221903 (+3268 T>C) and rs2055979 (+1439 C>A), localized in the second intron of the *IL21* gene, have been associated with increased IL-21 levels [4,19]. Both polymorphisms have been associated with autoimmune diseases, such as rheumatoid arthritis [20] and multiple sclerosis [21,22]. In the context of SLE, the rs2221903 and rs2055979 SNPs have been studied by several research groups with discordant results [4,19,23].

This study aimed to evaluate the IL-21 levels in patients with SLE and compare them with healthy controls, as well as to analyze their association with disease activity, clinical phenotype, and *IL21* polymorphisms (rs2221903 and rs2055979).

2. Materials and Methods

2.1. Subjects

This study included 600 subjects: 300 HCs (273 females and 27 males) and 300 patients with SLE (283 females and 17 males). The patients with SLE were classified according to the American College of Rheumatology's 1997 revised criteria [24] and were recruited through consecutive non-randomized selection methods in the rheumatology department of the Hospital General de Occidente, Guadalajara, Mexico. The Mexican versions of the Systemic Lupus Disease Activity Index (Mex-SLEDAI) [25] and the Systemic Lupus International Collaborating Clinics (SLICC) damage index [26] scores were applied to all patients with SLE at the moment of inclusion. The exclusion criteria were patients with overlap syndromes, pregnancy, biological therapy, and current infection. Subjects included as HCs were recruited through clinical assessments under protocols of blood donation in a blood bank, excluding subjects with chronic diseases; also, all subjects included were similar to the patients with SLE in age and gender, and they were all unrelated individuals with no first-degree family suffering from some autoimmune disease. All participants were Mexican mestizos from western Mexico [27]. The clinical activity groups for the patients with SLE were stratified according to the Mex-SLEDAI score as follows: inactive (0–1), mild–moderate (2–6), and severe ($\geq$7) disease. Most patients were undergoing pharmacological treatment; however, none were undergoing biological therapy. In addition, a follow-up analysis was performed on 59 patients with SLE.

This study was approved by the Ethics and Research Committee from Hospital General de Occidente (no. CEI-146/21 and no. CI-146/21). Before inclusion, all participants were required to sign an informed consent form. The present study was carried out following the ethical standards and principles established in the Declaration of Helsinki and the research committees from the participant institutions [28].

2.2. Quantification of IL-21 Serum Levels and Anti-dsDNA Antibodies

Serum was obtained from peripheral blood samples from patients with SLE and HCs and stored at $-20\ °C$ until use. The IL-21 levels were determined in 278 patients with SLE and 170 HC using an ELISA assay (ELISA MAX™ Deluxe Set Human IL-21: cat. No 433804, BioLegend, CA, USA), performed following the manufacturer's instructions. The ELISA kit sensitivity is 16 pg/mL, and the detection limit range is 31.3–2000 pg/mL. Samples were analyzed undiluted in duplicate and read at 450 and 570 nm using the Multiskan™ Go Microplate Spectrophotometer (Thermo Fisher Scientific, Waltham, WA, USA). The results of anti-double-stranded DNA (anti-dsDNA) antibody test were taken from medical records. The anti-dsDNA antibody test was performed by Crithidia luciliae indirect immunofluorescence method.

2.3. Genotyping of IL21 rs2221903 and rs2055979 Polymorphisms

Genomic DNA (gDNA) was purified from peripheral blood samples of patients with SLE and HCs using the modified Miller's technique [29]. The rs2221903 and rs2055979 polymorphisms were genotyped using the polymerase chain reaction–restriction fragment length polymorphism (PCR-RFLP) technique. The amplification of the DNA fragment containing the rs2221903 (+3268 T>C) polymorphism was performed using the following primers: forward: 5′-TGGACACTGACGCCCATATTGA-3′ and reverse: 5′-AAG GCAGTTTAGTGGCGACAGC-3′. For the rs2055979 (+1439 C>A) SNP, the following primers were used: forward: 5′-CAG CCA GGA AAC TCT GGA AAG AA-3′ and reverse: 5′-GCTCTGAACCCAAACACTCTCATTT-3′ [4]. Both PCRs were carried out in a total volume of 25 µL containing the following: 1X PCR buffer, 4 mM $MgCl_2$, 2.5 mM dNTPs, 2 µM of each primer, 0.5 units of Taq DNA polymerase (Invitrogen Life Technologies, Carlsbad, CA, USA), and 100 ng of gDNA. The PCR cycling conditions used were as follows: initial denaturation cycle at 95 °C for 5 min, followed by 32 cycles of denaturation for 50 s at 95 °C, annealing for 30 s at 65 °C, extension for 30 s at 72 °C, and final extension for 5 min at 72 °C.

The amplified 230 bp PCR product of the rs2221903 (+3268 T>C) polymorphism was subjected to digestion with 3 IU of the *MboII* restriction enzyme (New England BioLabs®, Ipswich, MA, USA) for 1 h at 37 °C. The resulting restriction fragments based on the genotype were TT: 230 bp; TC: 230, 149, and 81 bp; and CC: 149 and 81 bp. As for the rs2055979 (+1439 C>A) polymorphism, the 212 bp PCR product was digested using 5 IU of *NlaIII* restriction enzyme (New England BioLabs®, Ipswich, MA, USA) for 1 h at 37 °C. In this case, the restriction fragments and genotypes were CC: 158 and 54 bp; CA: 212, 158, and 54 bp; and AA: 212 bp. The digested PCR products were resolved in 6% polyacrylamide gels and stained with $AgNO_3$.

2.4. Statistical Analysis

The data were analyzed using software packages from IBM SPSS statistics v25 (IBM Corporation; Armonk, NY, USA) and GraphPad Prism v10.2.3 (GraphPad Software Incorporation; La Jolla, CA, USA). The Kolmogorov–Smirnov test was used to assess variable distribution. Categorical variables are presented as absolute values and percentages, whereas continuous variables are presented as medians and 25th–75th percentiles. According to the case, the Kruskal–Wallis test, post hoc Dunn's test, Mann–Whitney U test, and Wilcoxon test were used to compare groups. The Receiver Operator Characteristic (ROC) curve analysis was used to evaluate the IL-21 sensitivity and specificity in discriminating between patients with SLE and controls. The Chi-square test was used to calculate the Hardy–Weinberg equilibrium. Genotypic and allelic frequencies of *IL21* polymorphisms were determined by direct counting, and comparison was performed using the Chi-square test or Fisher's exact test. The Odds Ratios (ORs) and 95% confidence intervals (95% CI) were calculated to determine the risk of SLE associated with the *IL21* SNPs. The haplotype inference was calculated by the EM algorithm and the SHEsis software platform [30,31]. The *p*-value was adjusted using Bonferroni correction when appropriate, and a *p*-value < 0.05 was considered with statistical significance.

3. Results

3.1. Subjects' Demographic and Clinical Characteristics

The demographic and clinical characteristics of patients with SLE are summarized in Table 1. The median ages were 35 [interquartile range (IQR) 25–48] years old for patients with SLE and 29 (IQR 25–38) years old for HCs. The median of disease evolution was 4 (IQR 1.4–11) years for patients with SLE. Eighty-one percent of patients with SLE had inactive or mild–moderate disease activity according to Mex-SLEDAI, with a median score value of 2 (IQR 1–6); additionally, most patients had no damage with a median score of 0 (IQR 0–1) according to the SLICC damage index. Concerning treatment, prednisone was prescribed in 68% with a median dosage of 10 (IQR 5–20) mg/day, followed by antimalarial drugs (58.3%) and azathioprine (48%).

Table 1. Demographic and clinical characteristics in patients with SLE.

Variables	SLE (*n* = 300)
Demographic features	
Age, years; median (p25–p75)	35 (25–48)
Gender (F/M)	283/17
Disease features	
Disease duration, years; median (p25–p75)	4 (1.4–11.0)
Mex-SLEDAI score; median (p25–p75)	2 (1–6)
Inactive, *n* (%)	123 (41.0)
Mild–moderate, *n* (%)	124 (41.3)
Severe, *n* (%)	53 (17.7)
SLICC score; median (p25–p75)	0 (0–1)
Non-damage, *n* (%)	201 (67.0)
Damage, *n* (%)	99 (33.0)
Clinical domain	
Hematologic [†], *n* (%)	134 (44.7)
Mucocutaneous [‡], *n* (%)	102 (34.0)
Constitutional [§], *n* (%)	76 (25.3)
Renal [¶], *n* (%)	66 (22.0)
Musculoskeletal [††], *n* (%)	51 (17.0)
Neuropsychiatric [‡‡], *n* (%)	19 (6.3)
Serosal [§§], *n* (%)	12 (4.0)
Treatment	
Prednisone, *n* (%)	204 (68.0)
rednisone dose; median (p25–p75)	10 (5.0–20.0)
Antimalarial, *n* (%)	175 (58.3)
Azathioprine, *n* (%)	144 (48.0)
Methotrexate, *n* (%)	55 (18.3)
Mycophenolate Mofetil, *n* (%)	28 (9.3)
Cyclophosphamide, *n* (%)	27 (9.0)
Autoantibodies	
Antinuclear antibodies, *n* (%)	277/287 (96.5)
Anti-dsDNA, *n* (%)	180/268 (67.2)
Anti-RNP, *n* (%)	45/122 (36.9)
Anti-Ro, *n* (%)	40/123 (32.5)
Anti-Sm, *n* (%)	32/141 (22.7)
Anti-La, *n* (%)	17/128 (13.3)

Table 1. Cont.

Variables	SLE (n = 300)
Biochemical analysis	
Glucose (mg/dL)	91 (39.0–383.0)
Serum creatinine (mg/dL)	0.9 (0.1–10.2)
Serum urea (mg/dL)	36.5 (1.5–2.7)
Blood cell count	
Hemoglobin	12.6 (4.1–19.8)
Hematocrit	38.6 (8.3–58.1)
Leukocytes	5.7 (4.3–7.45)
Lymphocytes	1.3 (0.8–1.9)
Neutrophils	3.8 (2.6–5.2)
Platelets	243 (188–294)
ESR (mm/h)	33.0 (1.0–135.0)

The data are shown as the median and p25–p75; Mex-SLEDAI: inactive (score of 0–1), mild–moderate (score 2–6), or severe ($\geq$7); SLICC: non-damage (SLICC score of 0) or damage (SLICC score > 1); [†] hematologic: leukopenia, lymphopenia, and thrombocytopenia; [‡] mucocutaneous: malar rash, alopecia, oral ulcers, and photosensitivity; [§] constitutional: fatigue; [¶] renal: persistent proteinuria (>0.5 g/day) and cellular casts; [††] musculoskeletal: articular involvement; [‡‡] neuropsychiatric: neurologic damage, psychosis, and convulsions; [§§] serosal: Raynaud's phenomenon and serositis. SLE, Systemic Lupus Erythematosus; Mex-SLEDAI, Mexican version of the Systemic Lupus Erythematosus Disease Activity Index; SLICC, Systemic Lupus International Collaborating Clinics; ESR, Erythrocyte Sedimentation Rate.

3.2. Association of IL-21 Levels with Clinical Phenotype of Patients with SLE

The IL-21 levels were higher in patients with SLE [110.5 (IQR 92.7–136.5) pg/mL] compared with the HCs [61.7 (IQR 37.4–91.6) pg/mL; $p < 0.0001$. Figure 1a]. The IL-21 levels were compared according to the clinical phenotype of patients with SLE. All patients with SLE with inactive disease, mild–moderate disease activity, and severe disease activity had higher IL-21 levels in comparison with the HCs [109.4 (IQR 92.7–91.6) pg/mL, 113.1 (IQR 91.6–137.0) pg/mL, and 105.7 (IQR 94.9–123.3) pg/mL vs. 61.7 (IQR 37.4–91.6) pg/mL, respectively; $p < 0.0001$; Figure 1b]. However, according to the disease activity, no significant differences were observed in the IL-21 levels between patients with SLE. When the patients with SLE were stratified according to clinical domains, the patients with SLE with hematological affection showed higher levels of IL-21 vs. no hematological affection [116.7 (101.5–143.8) pg/mL vs. 105.7 (87.4–131.0) pg/mL; $p = 0.0018$; Figure 1c], and other clinical domains did not show statistical difference ($p > 0.05$). Also, when the patients with SLE were classified according to chronicity [chronicity (−) 113.1 (IQR 90.5–143.0) pg/mL vs. chronicity (+) 108.9 (IQR 98.5–129.3) pg/mL; $p = 0.8213$; Figure 1d] and anti-dsDNA status [anti-dsDNA (−) 108.9 (IQR 95.5–130.3) pg/mL vs. anti-dsDNA (+) 114–1 (IQR 92.7–139.2) pg/mL; $p = 0.5209$; Figure 1e], no statistical difference was found. On the other hand, the IL-21 levels did not correlate with the Mex-SLEDAI score or anti-dsDNA concentration ($p > 0.05$).

An ROC curve analysis was conducted to evaluate the ability of the IL-21 levels to distinguish between patients with SLE and HCs. The AUC was 0.794, meaning this cytokine showed good predictive power in discriminating between patients with SLE and controls ($p < 0.0001$, Figure 1f).

Regarding treatment, the IL-21 cytokine levels in the patients with SLE showed no significant difference between those receiving treatment and the untreated patients. The concentration remained consistent at 121.3 (IQR 105.5–162.1) pg/mL for the untreated patients and 115.1 (IQR 104.7–139.6) pg/mL for the treated patients ($p = 0.4019$, Figure 2a). This finding was similar even in patients undergoing the induction treatment concerning those in the maintenance phase [117.1 (IQR 96.6–145.9) vs. 115.1 (IQR 101.5–139.2) pg/mL, respectively; $p = 0.9831$; Figure 2b].

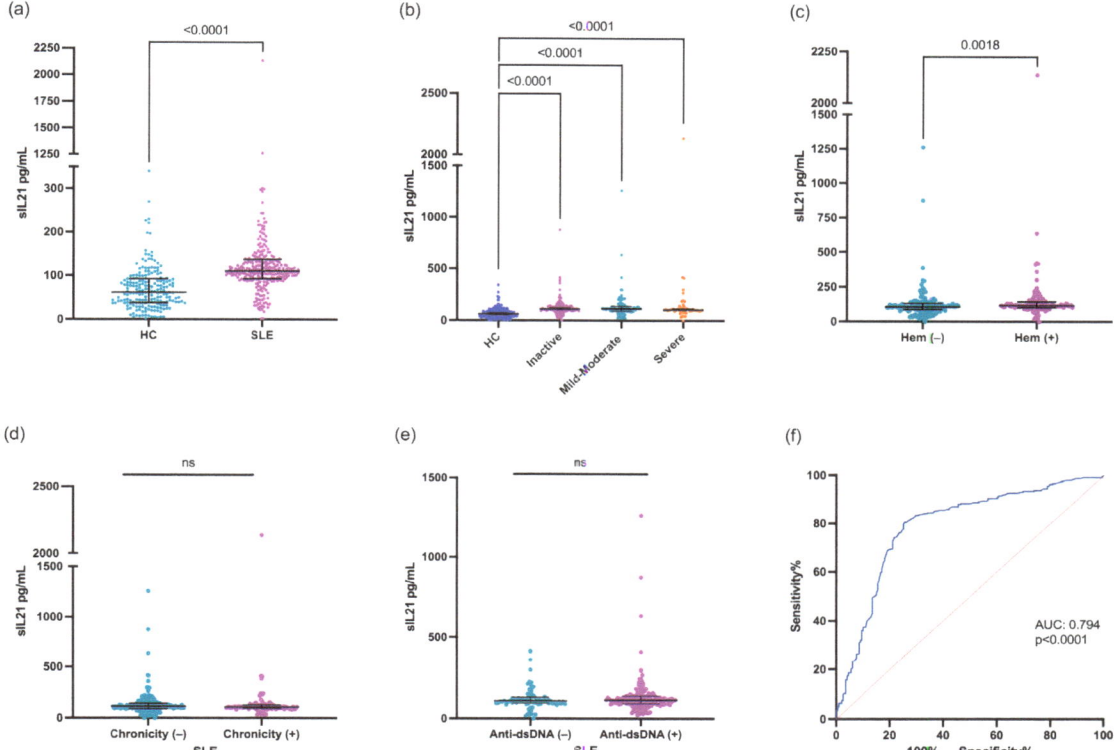

Figure 1. Evaluation of IL-21 levels according to clinical characteristics in patients with SLE. Comparison of IL-21 levels between HCs and patients with SLE (**a**), IL-21 levels according to disease activity (**b**), hematological domain (**c**) and chronicity (**d**), IL-21 levels according to anti-dsDNA status (**e**), and IL-21 performance as biomarker diagnosis in SLE (**f**). Patients with SLE were stratified according to Mex-SLEDAI score as follows: inactive (0–1), mild–moderate (2–6), and severe ($\geq$7) disease. Hematological domain (Hem) included lymphopenia (<1.2 × 10^3/μL), leukopenia (<4.0 × 10^3/μL), thrombocytopenia (<100 × 10^3/μL), and hemolytic anemia. Data are shown as median and IQR. p-value was obtained through Mann–Whitney U test, Kruskal–Wallis test with Dunn's post hoc test, and Spearman's correlation test, according to case. Area Under the Curve was calculated through ROC curves. ns, no significative.

Finally, we analyzed the IL-21 levels in 59 patients with SLE during recruitment and the follow-up visits. The patients were categorized according to whether they had remission or active disease. Interestingly, the concentration of this cytokine remained similar in both groups (as shown in Figure 2c; $p > 0.05$). Even when we compared the data between the paired analyses, the IL-21 levels remained consistent regardless of whether the patients were in remission or had active disease (Figure 2d,e; $p > 0.05$).

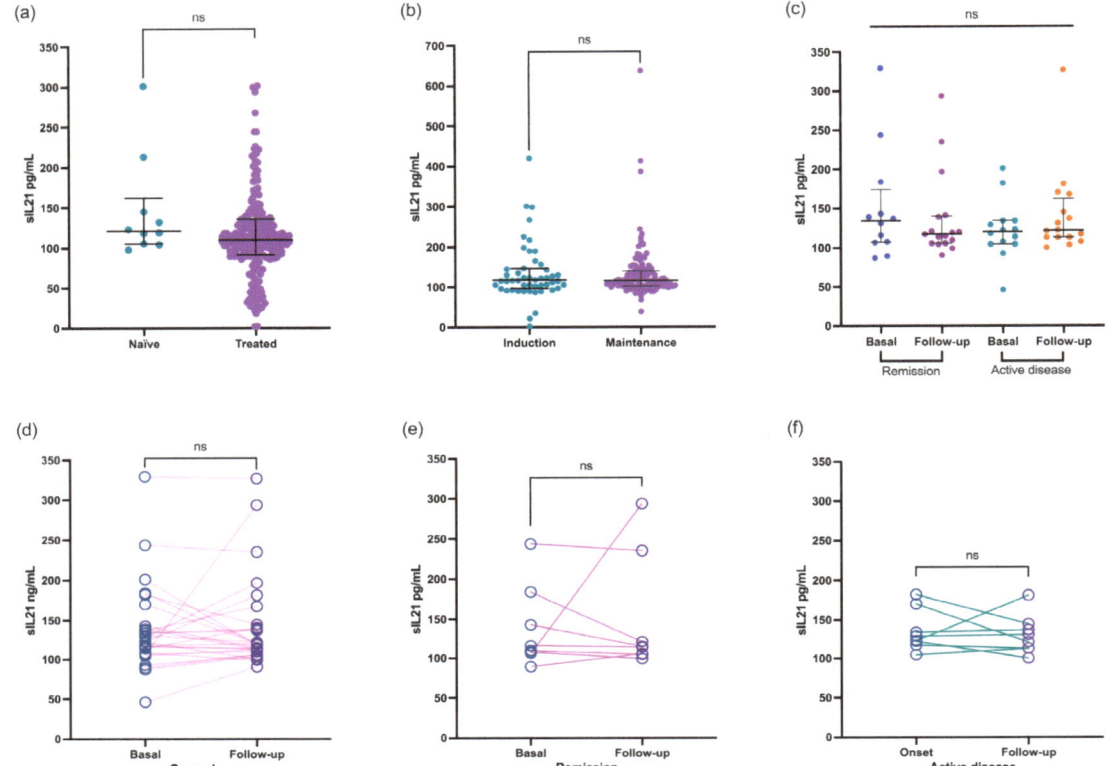

Figure 2. Comparison of IL-21 levels in patients with SLE based on type of treatment. Patients with SLE who were either treatment-naïve or treated showed similar concentrations of IL-21 (**a**) regardless of whether they were undergoing induction or maintenance treatment (**b**). IL-21 level comparison between patients with SLE at basal and follow-up recruitment stratified according to remission and active disease (**c**). Paired comparison of IL2-1 in patients with SLE at baseline and follow-up (**d**), as well as stratified by remission (**e**) and active (**f**) disease groups. Data are shown as median and IQR. *p*-value was obtained through Mann–Whitney U test and Wilcoxon test according to case. ns, no significative.

3.3. Genotype and Allele Frequencies of rs2221903 and rs2055979 Polymorphisms

The genotype and allele frequency distribution of the rs2221903 and rs2055979 polymorphisms in the patients with SLE and HCs are shown in Table 2. Both polymorphisms were in Hardy–Weinberg equilibrium, with similar observed and expected frequencies in the HCs ($p > 0.05$). There were significant differences in the genotype and allele frequencies of the rs2221903 polymorphism between the patients with SLE and HCs, with a higher proportion of the C allele observed in the SLE group. According to this, the C allele as well as the TC and CC genotypes from the rs2221903 polymorphism were associated with a higher risk of SLE (OR = 1.75, 95% CI, 1.17–2.61, and $p = 0.005$; OR = 1.58, 95% CI, 1.02–2.46, and $p = 0.039$; and OR = 6.56, 95% CI, 1.07–75.60, and $p = 0.046$, respectively). In addition, the dominant model from the rs2221903 polymorphism was associated with increased SLE susceptibility (TT vs. TC+CC, OR = 1.71, 95% CI 1.11–2.62, $p = 0.014$). On the other hand, the genotype and allele frequencies of the rs2055979 polymorphism observed in the patients with SLE were not significantly different from those of the HCs.

Table 2. Frequencies of genotypes, alleles, and haplotypes of *IL21* gene polymorphisms.

	HC n = 300 (%)	SLE n = 300 (%)	p-Value	OR (95% CI)	p_c-Value
rs2221903 (+3268 T>C)					
TT	258 (86.29)	236 (78.67)	1	-	-
TC	40 (13.38)	58 (19.33)	**0.039**	**1.58 (1.02–2.46)**	0.078
CC	1 (0.33)	6 (2.00)	**0.046** †	**6.56 (1.07–75.60)**	0.092
T	556 (92.98)	530 (88.33)	1	-	-
C	42 (7.02)	70 (11.67)	**0.005**	**1.75 (1.17–2.61)**	-
Dominant model					
TT	258 (86.29)	236 (78.67)	1	-	-
TC + CC	41 (13.71)	64 (21.33)	**0.014**	**1.71 (1.11–2.62)**	-
Recessive model					
TT + TC	298 (99.67)	294 (98.00)	1	-	-
CC	1 (0.33)	6 (2.00)	0.058 †	0.16 (0.02–1.37)	-
rs2055979 (+1439 C>A)					
CC	90 (30.00)	87 (29.00)	1	-	-
CA	153 (51.00)	154 (51.33)	0.830	1.04 (0.72–1.51)	1
AA	57 (19.00)	59 (19.67)	0.775	1.07 (0.67–1.71)	1
C	333 (55.50)	328 (54.67)	1	-	-
A	267 (44.50)	272 (45.33)	0.772	1.03 (0.82–1.30)	-
Dominant model					
CC	90 (30.00)	87 (29.00)	1	-	-
CA + AA	210 (70.00)	213 (71.00)	0.788	1.05 (0.74–1.49)	-
Recessive model					
CC + CA	243 (81.00)	241 (80.33)	1	-	-
AA	57 (19.00)	59 (19.67)	0.836	0.96 (0.64–1.44)	-
Haplotype ‡					
TC	292.13 (48.68)	261.14 (43.50)	1	0.81 (0.64–1.02)	-
TA	263.87 (43.98)	268.86 (44.81)	0.281	1.14 (0.90–1.44)	0.562
CC	39.87 (6.64)	66.86 (11.14)	**0.004**	**1.87 (1.21–2.85)**	**0.008**

‡ The haplotype analysis included the rs2221903 (+3268 T>C) and rs2055979 (+1439 C>A) polymorphisms of the IL21 gene. All haplotypes with a frequency <0.03 were excluded from the analysis. Bonferroni correction was applied to the p-values to control for multiple comparisons, and the results are shown as corrected p-values (p_c-value). The statistical tests used for the allelic and genotype frequencies included the Chi-square test and † Fisher's exact test according to the case. A p-value < 0.05 was considered statistically significant. The values in bold indicate statistically significant results. Abbreviations: CI, confidence interval; HC, healthy control; OR, odds ratio; SLE, systemic lupus erythematosus.

3.4. Haplotype Analysis

The rs2221903 and rs2055979 polymorphisms showed a strong linkage disequilibrium (D' = 0.88, r' = 0.047, p = 0.01). As shown in Table 2, the CC haplotype was associated with increased SLE susceptibility (OR = 1.87, 95% CI, 1.21–2.85, p = 0.004).

3.5. Association of rs2221903 and rs2055979 Polymorphisms with IL-21 Levels, SLICC Damage Index, and Anti-dsDNA Antibodies

According to the rs2221903 polymorphism, SLE carriers of the CT genotype showed higher IL-21 levels [120.7 pg/mL (IQR 99.8–166.9)] than carriers of the TT genotype [107.8 ng/mL (91.6–130.5)] with a statistical difference (p = 0.0236, Figure 3a). This finding was consistent when comparing the IL-21 levels through the dominant model [TT vs. TC+CC, 107.8 pg/mL (IQR 91.6–130.5) vs. 118.2 pg/mL (IQR 101.5–167.6), p = 0.0041, Figure 3b]. In contrast, the IL-21 levels were similar when analyzed according to the rs2055979 genotypes as well as for the rs2055979 and rs2221903 haplotypes (Figure S1).

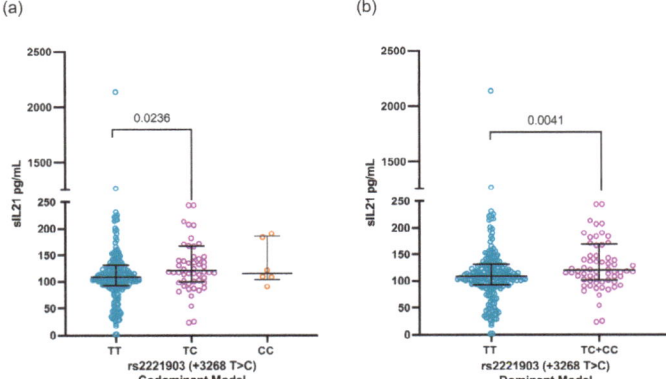

Figure 3. Comparison of IL-21 levels based on codominant and dominant models of rs2221903 polymorphism (+3268 T>C) in *IL21* gene. IL-21 levels according to codominant model (**a**) and dominant model (**b**) of rs2055979 polymorphism of *IL21* gene. Data are shown as median and IQR. *p*-value was obtained through Mann–Whitney U test and Kruskal–Wallis test with Dunn's post hoc test according to case. IQR, interquartile range; HCs, healthy controls; SLE, systemic lupus erythematosus.

4. Discussion

SLE is an autoimmune disorder characterized by autoantibody production and multiorgan affection [1]. The SLE pathogenesis involves different factors; nevertheless, the aberrant expression of different cytokines plays an important role in the disease's onset, establishment, and propagation [2–6]. IL-21 is an important cytokine produced by different T cell subpopulations such as Tfh, cTfh, Tph, and Th17 cells. Experimentally, it has been proven that IL-21 is necessary for B cell expansion, class switching, and plasma cell development during lupus-like onset in animal models [32,33]. IL-21 in vitro stimulation, along with costimulatory signaling, increases the proportion of memory and plasma B cells [34]. Also, increased Tph cells and IL-21 have been associated with extrafollicular B cell activation and auto-antibody production [35]. In patients with SLE, Tfh cells and activated B cells were positively correlated with the IL-21 levels [16]. The blockade of IL-21 reduces dsDNA autoantibodies and total IgG as well as immunoglobulin deposits in mice [36]. IL-21 has been linked to lupus nephritis due to its role in enhancing antibody production through T cell-dependent B cell stimulation [15,37]. The above highlights the importance of IL-21 and underscores the relevance of monitoring its levels in patients with SLE. This approach provides insights into how serum cytokines can be linked to the clinical aspects of the patient.

Patients with SLE in this study showed increased IL-21 levels compared with the HCs (110.5 pg/mL vs. 61.7 pg/mL, $p < 0.0001$). There were no significant correlations between the levels of IL-21 and disease activity evaluated by the Mex-SLEDAI index, and inactive patients showed similar IL-21 levels to those with mild–moderate and severe disease. The correlation between IL-21 and disease activity is highly heterogeneous in the literature. Some studies have identified a significant association between IL-21 and high disease activity [15,16,38], whereas others found no significant relationship between IL-21 levels and disease activity [14,17,39,40]. The inconsistent results regarding the IL-21 levels and their association with disease activity may be attributed to the heterogeneity in the clinical features of patients with SLE, including the disease evolution, level of disease activity, as well as different stratifications of disease activity indices.

While the IL-21 levels are not definitively linked to disease activity, they have been found to be higher in patients with SLE. This suggests that IL-21 may play a role in the initial development and onset of SLE, impacting clinical symptoms at diagnosis and during periods of high disease activity. However, its expression appears to be unrelated to clinical manifestations in long-term cases of established SLE.

It is important to evaluate the possible biomarkers in SLE according to clinical phenotype. Therefore, we analyzed IL-21 in the group of patients according to clinical phenotypes. We found that patients with SLE with hematological involvement had higher IL-21 levels than their counterparts. The main hematological affections in our patients were cytopenias. Regarding this, it is possible that IL-2 deficiency, induced by lymphopenia, reduces the expansion and maintenance of Tregs and therefore favors greater proliferation of effector T cells and increasing IL-21 levels IL-21, in turn, promotes the activity of effector T cells and counteracts the suppression of Tregs, creating a positive feedback loop that exacerbates immune dysregulation [41]. Previously, a single study associated IL-21 levels with lupus nephritis [15]. Our study did not find differences between IL-21 levels and other clinical domains, nor did it find differences in the damage index (chronicity). However, there were only 19 patients with lupus nephritis included in this study; therefore, our results might not be representative. The clinical phenotype is crucial for understanding biomarkers in patients with SLE. Unfortunately, our study included a heterogeneous mix of clinical phenotypes, making it difficult to compare subcategories due to the small number of patients in each group. Additionally, most reports in the literature do not specify the proportion of clinical phenotypes, further complicating comparisons.

As mentioned before, IL-21 plays a crucial role in IL-21R-expressing B cells by facilitating the activation, class switching, and differentiation of B cells for antibody production. In the context of SLE, it promotes the production of autoantibodies such as anti-dsDNA among others [32,33]. The IL-21 levels were not different among patients with positive anti-dsDNA antibodies versus those with negative anti-dsDNA antibodies. Similarly, other groups that studied patients with SLE reported a lack of association of IL-21 levels and anti-dsDNA antibodies [15,40]. In contrast, B cells from patients with SLE highly express the IL-21 receptor and respond to IL-21 in vitro to produce higher antibody levels; moreover, the IL-21 receptor correlates with anti-dsDNA antibodies [42]. Autoantibody production is a complex process that involves cytokines and costimulatory molecules through follicular and extrafollicular T cell and B cell interaction.

Another important cytokine for antibody production is BAFF, which is also correlated with IL-21 levels in patients with SLE [15]. Therefore, even when IL-21 levels are not correlated with antibody production, its function could be observed through the IL-21 receptor and other molecules involved in antibody production. It is possible that during the onset of the disease, IL-21 is positively correlated with antibody production. According to this hypothesis, in newly diagnosed Sjogren's syndrome, the IL-21 levels correlate with the total IgG levels [43]; this association could be due to different molecular pathogenesis among different autoimmune diseases or, again, due to recently diagnosed Sjogren's syndrome compared to patients with long-term SLE. A limitation in our study is that anti-dsDNA antibodies were qualitatively assessed; therefore, we cannot assure the lack of association between anti-dsDNA antibodies and IL-21 levels. It would be of great interest to quantitatively measure the anti-dsDNA antibodies and analyze other molecules and cytokines involved in autoantibody production, such as IL-21R and BAFF.

In 59 patients with SLE, the IL-21 levels were measured in a follow-up visit. The analysis showed that IL-21 is stable throughout time regardless of remission or active disease. In the study by Reynolds et al., in patients with long-evolution SLE disease, the IL-21 levels are stable in a follow-up quantification (around 5 months) [17]. The clinical characteristics of the patients are similar between our patients and those in their report. We previously found that IL-21-producing cTfh and Tph cells are higher in patients with SLE compared to the controls and that there were no differences according to disease activity [18]. Therefore, the expression of IL-21 seems to be constant in patients with long-term SLE disease. We further analyzed whether the IL-21 levels could be different according to the treatment of patients with SLE. The IL-21 levels did not show a statistical difference between the treated and untreated patients. In an experimental SLE treatment model, it was found that glucocorticoid reduces IL-21 expression and Tfh cells [44]. Tfh cells from patients with SLE reduce IL-21 production after glucocorticoid treatment in vitro [45]. Induction therapy in patients with untreated lupus nephritis reduced the IL-21 levels [37]. Also, in a cohort of patients with recently diagnosed myasthenia gravis, glucocorticoid treatment reduced the IL-21 levels and *IL21* mRNA in PBMC [46]. In patients with new-onset SLE, the treatment reduced Tfh cells and IL-21 levels [16]. The scenarios described above include new-onset cases of autoimmune diseases (both patients and experimental models) and in vitro stimulation. These results align with our findings and reinforce the hypothesis that there are differences in biomarkers according to disease evolution: new-onset or highly active patients versus long-term established SLE. Specifically, new-onset patients exhibited variable IL-21 levels based on treatment and disease activity, whereas patients with long-term evolution maintained higher IL-21 levels. Unfortunately, other reports of IL-21 levels do not compare treated and untreated patients, which would help support our findings. Additionally, the treatment is taken as a whole given the heterogenous prescription of patients. It would be of great interest to classify patients to compare types of treatments. Further longitudinal studies that include IL-21+ T cell populations with new patients and an extended follow-up are needed to understand IL-21's role in the SLE pathogenesis and determine its clinical utility as a biomarker.

Finally, we evaluated the association of the *IL21* gene SNPs (rs2221903 and rs2055979) and IL-21 levels in SLE. Our results show that the C allele of the rs2221903 polymorphism is associated with SLE susceptibility in the Mexican population (OR = 1.75). Also, the rs2221903 polymorphism was associated with higher IL-21 levels. To the best of our knowledge, this is the first report that shows an association between the *IL21* gene rs2221903 polymorphism with SLE susceptibility and increased IL-21 levels in the Mexican population. The role of intronic SNPs is not well defined, but it is reported to be associated with functional consequences as they may influence mRNA translation [47]. However, other reports have failed to find an association between IL-21 levels and the rs2221903 polymorphism in patients with SLE [4,38]. On the other hand, the rs2055979 polymorphism was not associated with IL-21 levels or disease clinical variables in SLE.

Previously, the rs2221903 polymorphism has been associated with an increased risk of SLE in the Chinese, European American, African American, and Caucasian populations [19,23,48] but not in other populations such as Hispanic, Gullah, and Egyptian, as well as in another Chinese study [4,23,38]. Also, we did not find any association between the rs2055979 polymorphism and SLE, which is congruent with the findings of Sawalha et al. for European American, African American, Hispanic American, and Gullah populations [23]. However, a study in the Chinese population found an association between polymorphisms and SLE [4]. These discrepancies could be explained in part by the genetic ancestry of the studied populations. The genetic ancestry of the Mexican population from western Mexico is a mixture of European (64.6%), Native American (30.8%), and African ($\approx$8%) ancestries [49]. Also, the Mexican mestizo population has a small proportion of Asian ancestry (1–1.4%) [49].

In addition, we found a strong linkage disequilibrium between the rs2221903 and rs2055979 polymorphisms, which was similar to that previously reported in the Chinese and Mexican populations [4,20]. The TC and TA haplotypes were the most frequent in both the HCs and patients with SLE, whereas the CC haplotype was more frequent in the SLE group. We found that the CC haplotype was associated with an increased risk for SLE (OR = 1.87, 95% CI, 1.21–2.85, p = 0.004), which was also similar to the finding reported by Ding et al. in a Chinese population [48]. A meta-analysis analyzed seven articles with heterogeneous results and finally pointed out that the rs2221903 CC genotype is associated with SLE risk [19]. Also, the A allele of rs2055979 was associated with SLE risk [4]; however, in another study, this polymorphism was not associated with SLE risk [23]. Therefore, more research is needed to conclude the association of these SNPs with SLE.

Our findings highlight the importance of IL-21 in the SLE pathogenesis; however, further longitudinal studies are needed to define the role of IL-21 in patients with SLE according to the remission and exacerbation of the disease activity, considering the different clinical phenotypes. Furthermore, it would be interesting to analyze the expression of intracellular IL-21 in T cell subpopulations, including IL-21 expression in the affected tissues, to elucidate IL-21's molecular mechanisms that are directly involved in SLE. A limitation of this study is that mRNA expression was not evaluated; therefore, we do not know the relationship between gene expression and cytokine levels. The polymorphisms rs2221903 and rs2055979 exhibit heterogeneous results across various reports regarding their association with the disease, potentially due to ethnicity-specific outcomes or the presence of other polymorphisms in proximity that are yet to be discovered. According to our study, in the Mexican mestizo population, the rs2221903 polymorphism is associated with increased IL-21 levels and SLE susceptibility, while rs2055979 is not associated with these.

Further studies are still necessary to obtain a better understanding of IL-21's role in SLE, the expression throughout the disease evolution, the association of IL-21 levels with clinical variables in SLE in longitudinal studies, and the action of its polymorphism to the risk of SLE.

5. Conclusions

This study highlights the importance of IL-21 as a key cytokine in SLE. The IL-21 levels are higher in patients with SLE and remain increased regardless of disease activity. The rs2221903 polymorphism of the *IL21* gene is associated with higher IL-21 levels and increased susceptibility to SLE in the Mexican population. According to the ROC analysis, IL-21 is a potential biomarker of SLE. Further longitudinal studies are needed to explore the relationship between IL-21 and the clinical phenotypes of SLE.

Supplementary Materials: The following supporting information can be downloaded at https://www.mdpi.com/article/10.3390/jcm13154512/s1, Figure S1. The IL-21 levels according to the rs2055979 (+1439 C>A) genotype and rs2055979 and rs2221903 haplotypes in the *IL21* gene. The IL-21 levels according to the rs2055979 (+1439 C>A) genotype (a) and rs2055979 and rs2221903 haplotypes (b) of the *IL21* gene. The data are shown as the median and IQR. The *p*-value was obtained through the Kruskal–Wallis test with Dunn's post hoc test. IQR: interquartile range.

Author Contributions: Conceptualization, N.E.-G. and C.A.P.-S.; methodology, D.C.S.-C. and M.M.-R.; software, A.G.-P. and M.G.R.-D.; formal analysis, N.E.-G., M.M.-R. and I.M.B.-C.; investigation, N.E.-G., D.C.S.-C. and M.M.-R.; writing—original draft preparation, N.E.-G.; writing—review and editing, M.P.R.-M. and C.A.P.-S.; supervision, J.F.M.-V.; funding acquisition, C.A.P.-S. All authors have read and agreed to the published version of the manuscript.

Funding: This research was supported by the Fondo de Desarrollo Científico de Jalisco para atender retos sociales "FODECIJAL 2023" grant 10586-2023 to CAPS from Consejo Estatal de Ciencia y Tecnología de Jalisco (COECYTJAL); and by Fondos para Proyectos de Impulso a la Investigación (PIN 2022-III) grant to CAPS from Centro Universitario de Ciencias de la Salud, Universidad de Guadalajara.

Institutional Review Board Statement: This study was conducted in accordance with the Declaration of Helsinki and the research committees from the participating institutions. This study was approved by the Ethics and Research Committee of Hospital General de Occidente (no. CEI-146/21 and no. CI-146/21).

Informed Consent Statement: Before inclusion, all participants were required to sign an informed consent form.

Data Availability Statement: The data used to support the findings of this study will be available upon request to the corresponding authors.

Acknowledgments: We thank all the subjects who participated in our study.

Conflicts of Interest: The authors declare no conflicts of interest.

References

1. Rahman, A.; Isenberg, D.A. Mechanisms of Disease: Systemic Lupus Erythematosus. *N. Engl. J. Med.* **2008**, *358*, 929–939. [CrossRef]
2. Bengtsson, A.A.; Sturfelt, G.; Truedsson, L.; Blomberg, J.; Alm, G.; Vallin, H.; Rönnblom, L. Activation of Type I Interferon System in Systemic Lupus Erythematosus Correlates with Disease Activity but Not with Antiretroviral Antibodies. *Lupus* **2016**, *9*, 664–671. [CrossRef] [PubMed]
3. Duarte, A.L.B.P.; Dantas, A.T.; De Ataíde Mariz, H.; Dos Santos, F.A.; Da Silva, J.C.; Da Rocha, L.F.; Galdino, S.L.; Galdino Da Rocha Pitta, M. Decreased Serum Interleukin 27 in Brazilian Systemic Lupus Erythematosus Patients. *Mol. Biol. Rep.* **2013**, *40*, 4889–4892. [CrossRef]
4. Lan, Y.; Luo, B.; Wang, J.L.; Jiang, Y.W.; Wei, Y.S. The Association of Interleukin-21 Polymorphisms with Interleukin-21 Serum Levels and Risk of Systemic Lupus Erythematosus. *Gene* **2014**, *538*, 94–98. [CrossRef] [PubMed]
5. Robak, E.; Kulczycka-Siennicka, L.; Gerlicz, Z.; Kierstan, M.; Korycka-Wolowiec, A.; Sysa-Jedrzejowska, A. Correlations between Concentrations of Interleukin (IL)-17A, IL-17B and IL-17F, and Endothelial Cells and Proangiogenic Cytokines in Systemic Lupus Erythematosus Patients. *Eur. Cytokine Netw.* **2013**, *24*, 60–68. [CrossRef]
6. Sun, Z.; Zhang, R.; Wang, H.; Jiang, P.; Zhang, J.; Zhang, M.; Gu, L.; Yang, X.; Zhang, M.; Ji, X. Serum IL-10 from Systemic Lupus Erythematosus Patients Suppresses the Differentiation and Function of Monocyte-Derived Dendritic Cells. *J. Biomed. Res.* **2012**, *26*, 456–466. [CrossRef] [PubMed]
7. Jin, X.; Chen, J.; Wu, J.; Lu, Y.; Li, B.; Fu, W.; Wang, W.; Cui, D. Aberrant Expansion of Follicular Helper T Cell Subsets in Patients with Systemic Lupus Erythematosus. *Front. Immunol.* **2022**, *13*, 928359. [CrossRef]
8. Pontarini, E.; Murray-Brown, W.J.; Croia, C.; Lucchesi, D.; Conway, J.; Rivellese, F.; Fossati-Jimack, L.; Astorri, E.; Prediletto, E.; Corsiero, E.; et al. Unique Expansion of IL-21+ Tfh and Tph Cells under Control of ICOS Identifies Sjögren's Syndrome with Ectopic Germinal Centres and MALT Lymphoma. *Ann. Rheum. Dis.* **2020**, *79*, 1588–1599. [CrossRef]
9. Tian, Y.; Zajac, A.J. IL-21 and T Cell Differentiation: Consider the Context. *Trends Immunol.* **2016**, *37*, 557. [CrossRef]
10. Yang, Y.; Zhang, M.; Ye, Y.; Ma, S.; Fan, L.; Li, Z. High Frequencies of Circulating Tfh-Th17 Cells in Myasthenia Gravis Patients. *Neurol. Sci.* **2017**, *38*, 1599–1608. [CrossRef]
11. Coquet, J.M.; Kyparissoudis, K.; Pellicci, D.G.; Besra, G.; Berzins, S.P.; Smyth, M.J.; Godfrey, D.I. IL-21 Is Produced by NKT Cells and Modulates NKT Cell Activation and Cytokine Production. *J. Immunol.* **2007**, *178*, 2827–2834. [CrossRef] [PubMed]
12. Kuchen, S.; Robbins, R.; Sims, G.P.; Sheng, C.; Phillips, T.M.; Lipsky, P.E.; Ettinger, R. Essential Role of IL-21 in B Cell Activation, Expansion, and Plasma Cell Generation during CD4 + T Cell-B Cell Collaboration. *J. Immunol.* **2007**, *179*, 5886–5896. [CrossRef] [PubMed]
13. Spolski, R.; Leonard, W.J. Interleukin-21: A Double-Edged Sword with Therapeutic Potential. *Nat. Rev. Drug Discov.* **2014**, *13*, 379–395. [CrossRef] [PubMed]
14. Lee, J.; Shin, E.K.; Lee, S.Y.; Her, Y.M.; Park, M.K.; Kwok, S.K.; Ju, J.H.; Park, K.S.; Kim, H.Y.; Cho, M.L.; et al. Oestrogen Up-Regulates Interleukin-21 Production by CD4+ T Lymphocytes in Patients with Systemic Lupus Erythematosus. *Immunology* **2014**, *142*, 573–580. [CrossRef] [PubMed]
15. Shater, H.; Fawzy, M.; Farid, A.; El-Amir, A.; Fouad, S.; Madbouly, N. The Potential Use of Serum Interleukin-21 as Biomarker for Lupus Nephritis Activity Compared to Cytokines of the Tumor Necrosis Factor (TNF) Family. *Lupus* **2022**, *31*, 55–64. [CrossRef] [PubMed]
16. Wang, L.; Zhao, P.; Ma, L.; Shan, Y.; Jiang, Z.; Wang, J.; Jiang, Y. Increased Interleukin 21 and Follicular Helper T-like Cells and Reduced Interleukin 10+ B Cells in Patients with New-Onset Systemic Lupus Erythematosus. *J. Rheumatol.* **2014**, *41*, 1781–1792. [CrossRef] [PubMed]
17. Reynolds, J.A.; McCarthy, E.M.; Haque, S.; Ngamjanyaporn, P.; Sergeant, J.C.; Lee, E.; Lee, E.; Kilfeather, S.A.; Parker, B.; Bruce, I.N. Cytokine Profiling in Active and Quiescent SLE Reveals Distinct Patient Subpopulations. *Arthritis Res. Ther.* **2018**, *20*, 173. [CrossRef] [PubMed]
18. Sagrero-Fabela, N.; Ortíz-Lazareno, P.C.; Salazar-Camarena, D.C.; Cruz, A.; Cerpa-Cruz, S.; Muñoz-Valle, J.F.; Marín-Rosales, M.; Alvarez-Gómez, J.A.; Palafox-Sánchez, C.A. BAFFR Expression in Circulating T Follicular Helper (CD4+CXCR5+PD-1+) and T Peripheral Helper (CD4+CXCR5−PD-1+) Cells in Systemic Lupus Erythematosus. *Lupus* **2023**, *32*, 1093–1104. [CrossRef]
19. Qi, J.H.; Qi, J.; Xiang, L.N.; Nie, G. Association between IL-21 Polymorphism and Systemic Lupus Erythematosus: A Meta-Analysis. *Genet. Mol. Res.* **2015**, *14*, 9595–9603. [CrossRef]
20. Carreño-Saavedra, N.M.; Reyes-Pérez, I.V.; Machado-Sulbaran, A.C.; Martínez-Bonilla, G.E.; Ramírez-Dueñas, M.G.; Muñoz-Valle, J.F.; Olaya-Valdiviezo, V.; García-Iglesias, T.; Martínez-García, E.A.; Sánchez-Hernández, P.E. IL-21 (Rs2055979 and Rs2221903)/IL-21R (Rs3093301) Polymorphism and High Levels of IL-21 Are Associated with Rheumatoid Arthritis in Mexican Patients. *Genes* **2023**, *14*, 878. [CrossRef]
21. Ali Abdulla, A.; Abdulaali Abed, T.; Razzaq Abdul-Ameer, W. Impact of IL-21 Gene Polymorphisms (Rs2055979) and the Levels of Serum IL-21 on the Risk of Multiple Sclerosis. *Arch. Razi Inst.* **2022**, *77*, 71–76. [CrossRef]
22. Gharibi, T.; Kazemi, T.; Aliparasti, M.R.; Farhoudi, M.; Almasi, S.; Dehghanzadeh, R.; Seyfizadeh, N.; Babaloo, Z. Investigation of IL-21 Gene Polymorphisms (Rs2221903, Rs2055979) in Cases with Multiple Sclerosis of Azerbaijan, Northwest Iran. *Am. J. Clin. Exp. Immunol.* **2015**, *4*, 7. Available online: https://www.ncbi.nlm.nih.gov/pmc/articles/PMC4494115/ (accessed on 6 May 2020).

23. Sawalha, A.H.; Kaufman, K.M.; Kelly, J.A.; Adler, A.J.; Aberle, T.; Kilpatrick, J.; Wakeland, E.K.; Li, Q.Z.; Wandstrat, A.E.; Karp, D.R.; et al. Genetic Association of Interleukin-21 Polymorphisms with Systemic Lupus Erythematosus. *Ann. Rheum. Dis.* **2008**, *67*, 458–461. [CrossRef]
24. Hochberg, M.C. Updating the American College of Rheumatology Revised Criteria for the Classification of Systemic Lupus Erythematosus. *Arthritis Rheum.* **1997**, *40*, 1725. [CrossRef]
25. Guzman, J.; Cardiel, M.H.; Arce-Salinas, A.; Sanchez-Guerrero, J.; Alarcon-Segovia, D. Measurement of Disease Activity in Systemic Lupus Erythematosus. Prospective Validation of 3 Clinical Indices. *J. Rheumatol.* **1992**, *19*, 1551–1558. Available online: https://pubmed.ncbi.nlm.nih.gov/1464867/ (accessed on 6 May 2020). [PubMed]
26. Gladman, D.D.; Ibañez, D.; Urowltz, M.B. Systemic Lupus Erythematosus Disease Activity Index 2000. *J. Rheumatol.* **2002**, *29*, 288–291. [CrossRef]
27. Gorodezky, C.; Alaez, C.; Vázquez-García, M.N.; De La Rosa, G.; Infante, E.; Balladares, S.; Toribio, R.; Pérez-Luque, E.; Muñoz, L. The Genetic Structure of Mexican Mestizos of Different Locations: Tracking Back Their Origins through MHC Genes, Blood Group Systems, and Microsatellites. *Hum. Immunol.* **2001**, *62*, 979–991. [CrossRef] [PubMed]
28. World Medical Asociation (AMM). *Declaración de Helsinki de la AMM—Principios Éticos para las Investigaciones Médicas en Seres Humanos*; World Medical Asociation Inc.: Ferney-Voltaire, France, 2013; pp. 1–8.
29. Miller, S.A.; Dykes, D.D.; Polesky, H.F. A Simple Salting out Procedure for Extracting DNA from Human Nucleated Cells. *Nucleic Acids Res.* **1988**, *16*, 1215. [CrossRef]
30. Li, Z.; Zhang, Z.; He, Z.; Tang, W.; Li, T.; Zeng, Z.; He, L.; Shi, Y. A Partition-Ligation-Combination-Subdivision Em Algorithm for Haplotype Inference with Multiallelic Markers: Update of the SHEsis (http://Analysis.Bio-x.cn). *Cell Res.* **2009**, *19*, 519–523. [CrossRef]
31. Shi, Y.Y.; He, L. SHEsis, a Powerful Software Platform for Analyses of Linkage Disequilibrium, Haplotype Construction, and Genetic Association at Polymorphism Loci. *Cell Res.* **2005**, *15*, 97–98. [CrossRef]
32. Long, D.; Chen, Y.; Wu, H.; Zhao, M.; Lu, Q. Clinical Significance and Immunobiology of IL-21 in Autoimmunity. *J. Autoimmun.* **2019**, *99*, 1–14. [CrossRef]
33. Ren, H.M.; Lukacher, A.E.; Rahman, Z.S.M.; Olsen, N.J. New Developments Implicating IL-21 in Autoimmune Disease. *J. Autoimmun.* **2021**, *122*, 102689. [CrossRef]
34. Nakou, M.; Papadimitraki, E.D.; Fanouriakis, A.; Bertsias, G.K.; Choulaki, C.; Goulidaki, N.; Sidiropoulos, P.; Boumpas, D.T. Interleukin-21 Is Increased in Active Systemic Lupus Erythematosus Patients and Contributes to the Generation of Plasma B Cells. *Clin. Exp. Rheumatol.* **2013**, *31*, 0172–0179. Available online: https://www.clinexprheumatol.org/abstract.asp?a=5562 (accessed on 5 March 2020).
35. Makiyama, A.; Chiba, A.; Noto, D.; Murayama, G.; Yamaji, K.; Tamura, N.; Miyake, S. Expanded Circulating Peripheral Helper T Cells in Systemic Lupus Erythematosus: Association with Disease Activity and B Cell Differentiation. *Rheumatology* **2019**, *58*, 1861–1869. [CrossRef]
36. Herber, D.; Brown, T.P.; Liang, S.; Young, D.A.; Collins, M.; Dunussi-Joannopoulos, K. IL-21 Has a Pathogenic Role in a Lupus-Prone Mouse Model and Its Blockade with IL-21R.Fc Reduces Disease Progression. *J. Immunol.* **2007**, *178*, 3822–3830. [CrossRef]
37. Wang, N.; Gao, C.; Cui, S.; Qin, Y.; Zhang, C.; Yi, P.; Di, X.; Liu, S.; Li, T.; Gao, G.; et al. Induction Therapy Downregulates the Expression of Th17/Tfh Cytokines in Patients with Active Lupus Nephritis. *Am. J. Clin. Exp. Immunol.* **2018**, *7*, 67. Available online: https://www.ncbi.nlm.nih.gov/pmc/articles/PMC6146154/ (accessed on 10 June 2024).
38. Ahmed, Y.M.; Erfan, D.M.; Hafez, S.F.; Shehata, I.H.; Morshedy, N.A. The Association of Single Nucleotide Polymorphism of Interleukin-21 Gene and Serum Interleukin-21 Levels with Systemic Lupus Erythematosus. *Egypt. J. Med. Human. Genet.* **2017**, *18*, 129–136. [CrossRef]
39. Hagn, M.; Ebel, V.; Sontheimer, K.; Schwesinger, E.; Lunov, O.; Beyer, T.; Fabricius, D.; Barth, T.F.E.; Viardot, A.; Stilgenbauer, S.; et al. CD5+ B Cells from Individuals with Systemic Lupus Erythematosus Express Granzyme B. *Eur. J. Immunol.* **2010**, *40*, 2060–2069. [CrossRef]
40. Hirahara, S.; Katsumata, Y.; Kawasumi, H.; Kawaguchi, Y.; Harigai, M. Serum Levels of Soluble Programmed Cell Death Protein 1 and Soluble Programmed Cell Death Protein Ligand 2 Are Increased in Systemic Lupus Erythematosus and Associated with the Disease Activity. *Lupus* **2020**, *29*, 686–696. [CrossRef] [PubMed]
41. Chevalier, N.; Thorburn, A.N.; Macia, L.; Tan, J.; Juglair, L.; Yagita, H.; Yu, D.; Hansbro, P.M.; Mackay, C.R. Inflammation and Lymphopenia Trigger Autoimmunity by Suppression of IL-2-Controlled Regulatory T Cell and Increase of IL-21-Mediated Effector T Cell Expansion. *J. Immunol.* **2014**, *193*, 4845–4858. [CrossRef] [PubMed]
42. Wang, S.; Wang, J.; Kumar, V.; Karnell, J.L.; Naiman, B.; Gross, P.S.; Rahman, S.; Zerrouki, K.; Hanna, R.; Morehouse, C.; et al. IL-21 Drives Expansion and Plasma Cell Differentiation of Autoreactive CD11chiT-Bet+ B Cells in SLE. *Nat. Commun.* **2018**, *9*, 1758. [CrossRef]
43. Kang, K.Y.; Kim, H.O.; Kwok, S.K.; Ju, J.H.; Park, K.S.; Sun, D.I.; Jhun, J.Y.; Oh, H.J.; Park, S.H.; Kim, H.Y. Impact of Interleukin-21 in the Pathogenesis of Primary Sjögren's Syndrome: Increased Serum Levels of Interleukin-21 and Its Expression in the Labial Salivary Glands. *Arthritis Res. Ther.* **2011**, *13*, R179. [CrossRef]
44. Shen, C.; Xue, X.; Zhang, X.; Wu, L.; Duan, X.; Su, C. Dexamethasone Reduces Autoantibody Levels in MRL/Lpr Mice by Inhibiting Tfh Cell Responses. *J. Cell Mol. Med.* **2021**, *25*, 8329–8337. [CrossRef]

45. Feng, X.; Wang, D.; Chen, J.; Lu, L.; Hua, B.; Li, X.; Tsao, B.P.; Sun, L. Inhibition of Aberrant Circulating Tfh Cell Proportions by Corticosteroids in Patients with Systemic Lupus Erythematosus. *PLoS ONE* **2012**, *7*, e51982. [CrossRef]
46. Li, Y.; Rauniyar, V.K.; Yin, W.F.; Hu, B.; Ouyang, S.; Xiao, B.; Yang, H. Serum IL-21 Levels Decrease with Glucocorticoid Treatment in Myasthenia Gravis. *Neurol. Sci.* **2014**, *35*, 29–34. [CrossRef]
47. Sauna, Z.E.; Kimchi-Sarfaty, C. Understanding the Contribution of Synonymous Mutations to Human Disease. *Nat. Rev. Genet.* **2011**, *12*, 683–691. [CrossRef]
48. Ding, L.; Wang, S.; Chen, G.M.; Leng, R.X.; Pan, H.F.; Ye, D.Q. A Single Nucleotide Polymorphism of IL-21 Gene Is Associated with Systemic Lupus Erythematosus in a Chinese Population. *Inflammation* **2012**, *35*, 1781–1785. [CrossRef]
49. Martínez-Cortés, G.; Salazar-Flores, J.; Gabriela Fernández-Rodríguez, L.; Rubi-Castellanos, R.; Rodríguez-Loya, C.; Velarde-Félix, J.S.; Franciso Mũoz-Valle, J.; Parra-Rojas, I.; Rangel-Villalobos, H. Admixture and Population Structure in Mexican-Mestizos Based on Paternal Lineages. *J. Hum. Genet.* **2012**, *57*, 568–574. [CrossRef] [PubMed]

Disclaimer/Publisher's Note: The statements, opinions and data contained in all publications are solely those of the individual author(s) and contributor(s) and not of MDPI and/or the editor(s). MDPI and/or the editor(s) disclaim responsibility for any injury to people or property resulting from any ideas, methods, instructions or products referred to in the content.

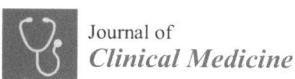 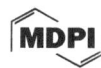

Article

Clinical Predictors of Mood Disorders and Prevalence of Neuropsychiatric Symptoms in Patients with Systemic Lupus Erythematosus

María Recio-Barbero [1,2], Janire Cabezas-Garduño [1,3], Jimena Varona [4], Guillermo Ruiz-Irastorza [1,2,4,*], Igor Horrillo [1,2,5], J. Javier Meana [1,2,5], Borja Santos-Zorrozúa [1] and Rafael Segarra [1,2,3,5]

1. BioBizkaia Health Research Institute, 48903 Barakaldo, Spain; maria.reciobarbero@bio-bizkaia.eus (M.R.-B.); janire.cabezasgarduno@osakidetza.eus (J.C.-G.); jimena.varonaperez@osakidetza.eus (J.V.); igor.horrillo@ehu.eus (I.H.); javier.meana@ehu.eus (J.J.M.); borja.santoszorrozua@bio-bizkaia.eus (B.S.-Z.); rafael.segarraechevarria@osakidetza.eus (R.S.)
2. University of the Basque Country, UPV/EHU, 48940 Leioa, Spain
3. Department of Psychiatry, Cruces University Hospital, 48903 Barakaldo, Spain
4. Autoimmune Disease Unit, Department of Internal Medicine, Cruces University Hospital, 48903 Barakaldo, Spain
5. Centro de Investigación Biomédica en Red de Salud Mental, CIBERSAM ISCIII, 48940 Leioa, Spain
* Correspondence: guillermo.ruiz@ehu.eus

Abstract: **Background/Objectives:** We aimed to determine the prevalence and clinical correlations of mood disorders in a sample of systemic lupus erythematosus (SLE) patients. Hence, we hypothesized that the prevalence of mood disorders would be lower than reported in the literature and that patients would remain clinically stable and show less damage accrual despite low-dose corticosteroid prescription. **Methods:** In total, 92 SLE outpatients gave informed consent to participate in this cross-sectional study. Psychiatric and autoimmune clinical data were obtained, and a structured psychiatric interview was performed. The main clinical scales for the assessment of clinical symptomatology were included. To examine the potential relationships of presenting a mood disorder in SLE, clinical correlations and multivariate analyses were performed. **Results:** Mood disorders were the most prevalent disorder reported by SLE patients (16%), followed by adjustment disorders (5%). A significant proportion of patients presented psychosocial disturbances that did not meet the ICD-10 criteria for psychiatric diagnosis. According to the cut-off criterion for the Montgomery–Åsberg Depression Rating Scale (MADRS), up to 27% of the sample met the clinical criteria for depression. The multivariate analysis revealed a relationship between the presence of a mood disorder with total scores of the MADRS and the Young Mania Rating Scale (YMRS). **Conclusions:** The prevalence of mood disorders in patients with SLE was lower than previously reported. Although self-report clinical scales are useful for assessing clinical symptomatology, they should not be used in place of a comprehensive standardized interview conducted by a trained mental health specialist. Multidisciplinary teamwork is required for the early identification and therapeutic management of autoimmune patients with neuropsychiatric disorders.

Keywords: mood disorders; depressive disorder; neuropsychiatric lupus; systemic lupus erythematosus; autoimmune disorders

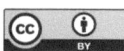

1. Introduction

Systemic lupus erythematosus (SLE) is a chronic autoimmune disease with the potential to affect multiple organ systems. The etiology of SLE includes the interaction between genetic and environmental components, resulting in immune dysregulation and the breakdown of self-tolerance [1]. Humoral immunity plays a major role in the pathogenesis of SLE, with the production of a wide range of autoantibodies, some of them with a well-defined pathogenic activity, such as anti-DNA in lupus nephritis, anti-Ro in neonatal lupus, and antiphospholipid in thrombotic events [1]. However, the disease is much more complex, with the participation of cellular compartments of both the adaptive and innate immune response, which results in a broad spectrum of clinical manifestations [1]. Female gender strongly influences the pathogenesis, with a resultant female/male ratio of 10/1 [2]. The course of lupus includes periods of remission and flares, leading to chronic inflammation [3,4], which, if not treated promptly and adequately, can cause irreversible organ damage, thus reducing survival and the health-related quality of life [4–6].

SLE symptoms may also present with related neuropsychological disturbances. Indeed, patients suffering from autoimmune diseases such as multiple sclerosis and rheumatoid arthritis, in addition to SLE, have reported a higher incidence of neuropsychiatric disturbances, with prevalence rates ranging from 15% to 75% [7–10]. Nervous system disturbances are frequently reported in SLE [1] and may affect both the central nervous system (CNS) and the peripheral nervous system (PNS), resulting in a wide range of diffuse neurologic and neuropsychiatric conditions (e.g., headache, acute confusional state, seizures, psychosis, mood disorders, and cognitive dysfunction) [3].

While nervous system involvement in SLE remains one of the major causes of morbidity and mortality [5], its etiology and pathogenesis remain unclear [11]. In other words, SLE encompasses a wide spectrum of clinical features, among which physical and neuropsychiatric symptoms, together with psychosocial disturbances, appear to stand out [12]. Aiming to identify the most prevalent neuropsychiatric disorders in SLE patients, in 1999, the American College of Rheumatology (ACR) proposed a classification criterion for 19 CNS and PNS syndromes, collectively referred to as Neuropsychiatric SLE (NPSLE) [13]. Despite several efforts to improve the sensitivity and specificity of the SLE criteria, NPSLE diagnosis includes a miscellaneous category of nonspecific neurologic and psychiatric signs. While neurological manifestations have been always grouped together, the criteria for psychiatric disorders have been revised over the years, exhibiting variable prevalence rates [3,14,15].

In this regard, a recent meta-analysis concluded that a high proportion of SLE patients had depressive and anxiety symptoms, with a pooled prevalence of 35% and 25.8%, respectively [15]. However, most of the published studies addressing neuropsychiatric disorders in autoimmune disorders mostly rely on clinical screening tools [14], lacking a comprehensive standardized psychiatric assessment by qualified mental health specialists.

Given that psychiatric disorders have been reported to be among the leading disabling conditions globally [16,17], estimating the true prevalence of these disorders remains necessary to better understand their true impact on patients' quality of life. The aim of this study was to assess the prevalence and clinical correlations of well-defined mood disorders in our cohort of SLE patients.

2. Materials and Methods

2.1. Study Sample

This study utilized a cross-sectional design to assess a sample of 92 patients with systemic lupus erythematosus (SLE) who were actively being followed up at the Autoimmune Diseases Unit at Cruces University Hospital, Spain, the Lupus–Cruces Cohort. This is a well-established cohort, as detailed elsewhere [18]. A cross-sectional study involves data collection at a single point in time, offering a snapshot of the study population at that moment. Unselected consecutive patients attending outpatient clinics between 2017 and 2022 were invited to participate, provided they met the inclusion and exclusion criteria. The inclusion criteria were an age of over 18 years old, a current diagnosis of SLE according to the revised criteria from the ACR/EULAR consensus for the classification of SLE [19], and signing the informed consent form. The exclusion criteria were a history of neurologic damage (including severe head injury, neurodegenerative, vascular or metabolic disorder, and neoplasia); the concurrence of severe or terminal somatic disease; and physical, sensory, or intellectual incapacity impeding the completion of the study protocol. No further criteria related to demographic or clinical characteristics were used, so that the group of study could be considered representative of the whole Lupus–Cruces Cohort. The study was approved by the Basque Ethics Committee (CEI-Euskadi PI2017029, last approval 30 August 2020).

2.2. Psychiatric Assessment

All the participants included in this study were screened by a trained psychiatric specialist using the Semi-Structured Clinical Interview for Axis I DSM-IV Disorders (SCID) [20]. In addition, each participant was screened for major psychiatric disorders according to the 10th Revision of the International Statistical Classification of Diseases and Related Health Problems (ICD-10) [21].

Complementarily, patients were assessed for a broad spectrum of psychiatric symptoms, including depressive and anxious symptomatology, the presence of suicidal ideation, and past traumatic experiences. concluding with the overall global clinical impression using widely utilized psychometric scales in the clinical setting. The scales used are detailed below.

Montgomery–Åsberg Depression Rating Scale (MADRS) [22]: The MADRS is a validated tool of ten items covering various aspects of depression, including affective symptoms (e.g., depressed mood, irritability), somatic symptoms (e.g., sleep disturbances, appetite changes), and cognitive symptoms (e.g., feelings of guilt, suicidal ideation). Each item is rated on a 7-point Likert scale ranging from 0 (no symptoms) to 6 (severe symptomatology). Total scores range from 0 to 60, with higher scores indicating more severe depression.

Hamilton Anxiety Rating Scale (HARS) [22]: The HARS is a clinician-administered widely used instrument for assessing the severity of anxiety. It comprises 14 items that evaluate both psychological (e.g., tension, fear) and somatic (e.g., restlessness, insomnia) manifestations of anxiety. Each item is rated on a 4-point Likert scale ranging from 0 (no symptoms) to 4 (severe symptoms). Total scores range from 0 to 56, with higher scores indicating greater anxiety severity.

Young Mania Rating Scale (YMRS) [23]: The YMRS is a widely used tool designed to assess the severity of manic symptoms in individuals with bipolar disorder. The scale consists of 11 items evaluating core manic symptoms, including elevated mood, increased motor activity, irritability, disruptive behavior, grandiosity, and decreased sleep. Items are rated on either a 4-point or 8-point Likert scale depending on the item. The total scores range from 0 to 60 (or higher depending on the scoring method), with higher scores indicating more severe manic symptoms.

Plutchik Suicide Risk Scale [24]: The Plutchik Suicide Risk Scale is a 15-item self-report measure designed to assess suicide risk. It evaluates various factors associated with suicidal behavior, such as suicidal ideation, previous suicide attempts, and hopelessness. It consists of 15 items that explore various factors related to suicidal ideation, behavior, and intent. Each item is scored as either 0 (no) or 1 (yes), resulting in a total score ranging from 0 to 15. Higher scores indicate an increased risk of suicide.

Traumatic Experiences Screening Questionnaire (ExpTra-S) [25]: The ExpTra-S is a self-report screening tool used to assess exposure to traumatic experiences in individuals. It consists of 18 items rated on a 4-point Likert scale (0 = never to 3 = almost always). The scale covers various types of child abuse (sexual, physical, psychological, and neglect) and includes an open-ended item for other traumatic events. The distress scale, also composed of 18 items rated on a 4-point Likert scale (1 = no distress to 4 = great distress), assesses the emotional impact of these experiences.

Global Clinical Impression Scale (CGI) [26]: The CGI is a clinician-rated instrument used to provide an overall assessment of a patient's clinical status and severity of illness. It consists of two main components: CGI-S (severity) and CGI-I (improvement). The CGI-S is based on the clinician's global impression, using a 7-point scale to rate symptom severity on a scale of 1 (normal) to 7 (extremely ill).

2.3. Clinical Assessment of Lupus Patients

The sociodemographic and clinical characteristics of the study group, including immunomodulatory treatments, were collected for this study. The Systemic Lupus Erythematosus Disease Activity Index (SLEDAI-2K) [27] was used to assess the SLE disease activity. This original SLEDAI was developed in 1985 and later modified to SLEDAI-2K including minor changes [27]. It consists of 24 items comprising 16 clinical (such as rash, arthritis, pleuritis, or psychosis) and 8 laboratory values (including elevated anti-DNA antibodies or hypocomplementemia). Each item has a specific score ranging from 1 to 8, so the global score has a possible maximum score of 105. SLEDAI-2K global scores up to 5 are considered mild activity, 6–12 moderate activity, and >12 severe activity.

Likewise, The Systemic Lupus International Collaborating Clinics/ACR Damage Index (SDI) was used to score the degree of cumulative irreversible damage caused by the disease, therapeutic agents, or concurrent conditions [28,29]. The SDI represents permanent damage, in contrast with SLEDAI-2K, which measures reversible activity. To be counted, items should be present for at least 6 months (with the exception of myocardial infarction and stroke) and need not be attributed to SLE. SDI items are grouped into 12 organ systems: ocular, neuropsychiatric, renal, pulmonary, cardiovascular, peripheral vascular, gastrointestinal, musculoskeletal, skin, endocrine (diabetes), gonadal dysfunction, and malignancy. Notably, the SDI can only be stable or increase over time, with a maximum possible score of 47 points. The SDI has been shown to be a major prognostic predictor in SLE patients [1].

2.4. Data Analysis

Descriptive statistics were calculated for the examined variables. Continuous variables are reported as the mean (standard deviation) for normally distributed data and otherwise as the median (interquartile range). Categorical variables are presented as frequency (percentage). To determine normality, the Shapiro–Wilks test was used. Comparisons between groups were made with Student's t-test in the case of continuous variables following a normal distribution or with the nonparametric Mann–Whitney U test otherwise. The Chi-square test or Fisher's exact test was used for categorical data.

To estimate the associations between the studied variables, Pearson's or Spearman's correlation coefficients were calculated. Multivariate logistic regression models were applied to identify the predictors of affective disorder in patients with SLE. For univariate analysis, clinical variables with $p \leq 0.15$ were used in the final regression model. Collinearity between candidate variables was analyzed with the Spearman correlation and VIF (variance inflation factor) coefficients. The final model calibration was assessed with the Hosmer–Lemeshow goodness-of-fit test ($p > 0.05$).

Finally, the area under the ROC curve (AUC) was calculated for the assessment of model discrimination and diagnostic accuracy. For hypothesis testing, a 95% confidence interval was considered, setting the risk α of 0.05 as the limit of statistical significance. The statistical analysis was performed using IBM SPSS Statistic software (v.21) and R software (v. 4.0.1) [29]. R statistic packages used included compareGroups [30], car [31], ggcorrplot [32], and corrplot [33].

3. Results

The main sociodemographic and clinical characteristics are summarized in Table 1. As expected, a female predominance was observed, accounting for 91% of the sample. Patients were mainly inactive, receiving low-dose prednisone and universal antimalarial therapy, in line with the therapeutic schedules of the Lupus–Cruces cohort [18]. Most patients were in remission, as depicted by a mean (SD) SLEDAI-2K score of 1.59 (2.44). Despite a median disease duration longer than 10 years, the degree of damage accrual was low, with a mean (SD) SDI of 0.33 (0.84), similar to what has been previously reported in our cohort [18]. No significant differences were found in any of the autoimmune clinical manifestations or analytical parameters between the groups (Table 1).

Altogether, the psychopathological assessment revealed that 23 patients (25%) presented a heterogeneous group of clinical syndromes that met the clinical criteria for a psychiatric disorder (Table 2). Additionally, according to the main clinical guidelines, the psychiatric evaluation revealed that nine patients (9.8%) had psychosocial disturbances that could not be classified as mental disorders. In this group of patients, primary support group-related problems and difficulties in managing daily life circumstances were among the main psychosocial difficulties reported.

Among patients who met the diagnostic criteria for a current major psychiatric diagnosis, 15 (16.3% of the cohort) met the ICD-10 criteria for a depressive mood disorder, which was in fact the most common prevalent disorder. According to ICD-10 criteria, only one patient had an in remission organic mood disorder diagnosis.

In contrast, when using the scores obtained on the main clinical scales for the assessment of depression exclusively as diagnostic criteria, and according to the cut-off criteria of the MADRS, as many as 25 patients (27%) met the criteria for depression. Among them, 20 patients (21.7%) met the symptom criteria for "mild depression", 4 patients (4.3%) had "moderate depression", and 1 patient (1.1%) presented "severe depression".

3.1. Autoimmune Clinical Predictors of Presenting a Mood Disorder

Regarding their main clinical characteristics, patients with and without a current mood disorder did not differ significantly in the age at inclusion ($p = 0.995$) or in disease duration ($p = 0.227$). Moreover, as observed in Table 1, patients did not differ on the main clinical variables. No differences were observed among the groups regarding the SLEDAI-2K ($p = 0.995$) and SDI scores ($p = 0.926$); there were no significant differences in current treatment with hydroxychloroquine ($p = 0.16$); immunosuppressive drugs ($p = 0.691$); or in the dose of prednisone, either current ($p = 0.55$) or cumulative ($p = 0.691$). No significant correlations were found between the severity of depression, as measured by the MADRS and the SLEDAI-2K (rho = -0.111, $p = 0.292$) or the SDI scores (rho = -0.043, $p = 0.681$).

3.2. Psychiatric Predictors of Mood Disorder in SLE Patients

Regarding psychopathological assessment, there were significant differences between the groups ($p < 0.001$). Overall, patients with SLE with comorbid major disorder presented a greater percentage of family psychiatric antecedents ($p = 0.003$). Likewise, higher anxiety scores ($p < 0.001$) increased the YMRS and the Plutchik Suicide Risk Scale scores ($p < 0.001$) in SLE patients presenting with a mood disorder. Similarly, greater clinical severity, as measured by the CGI scale, was observed in SLE patients with mood disorders, and a trend toward greater exposure to psychological distress due to childhood traumatic experiences was found.

In the univariate regression, age, ethnicity, the MADRS total score, the HARS total score, the Plutchick Suicide Risk Scale scores, the YMRS scores, the CGI scores, and the reported psychiatric family history had significant associations with presenting a mood disorder. Before adjustment in the multivariate model, ethnicity was removed because its values were not representative. Similarly, the HARS was also removed because it presented a correlation coefficient of 0.83 with MADRS and was related to anxiety, not depression. The remaining variables presented correlation coefficients ≤ 0.60 and appropriate VIF values (<5). As a result, these factors were included as independent variables in the multiple logistic regression model.

Table 1. Sociodemographic and clinical characteristics of the sample included in the analysis.

	Total Sample (n = 92)	Patients without a Mood Disorder (n = 77)	Patients with Mood Disorders (n = 15)	N	p Value
Gender—female	84 (91.3%)	71 (92.2%)	13 (86.7%)	92	0.612
Ethnicity				92	0.053
Caucasian	86 (93.5%)	74 (96.1%)	12 (80%)		
Hispanic	5 (5.4%)	2 (2.6%)	3 (20%)		
Arabic	1 (1.1%)	1 (1.3%)	-		
Age at inclusion, Mean (SD):	44.04 (11.87)	43.23 (11.89)	48.20 (11.23)	92	0.136
Disease duration, Median [25th;75th]:	11.00 [6.00;18.00]	11.00 [6.00;18.00]	9.00 [7.00;21.50]	92	0.966
Main clinical manifestations				92	
Articular	65 (71.4%)	54 (21.1%)	11 (73.3%)		1.000
Cutaneous	46 (50.5%)	40 (52.6%)	6 (40%)		0.410
Serosal	17 (18.7%)	15 (19.7%)	2 (13.3%)		0.728
Hematological	11 (12.1%)	10 (13.2%)	1 (6.7%)		0.684
Renal	19 (20.9%)	14 (18.4%)	5 (33.3%)		0.294
Antiphospholipid syndrome	8 (8.7%)	8 (10.4%)	0 (0%)		0.345
SLEDAI-2K, Mean (SD):	1.59 (2.44)	1.64 (2.60)	1.31 (1.49)	92	0.995
SDI, Mean (SD):	0.33 (0.84)	0.32 (0.84)	0.38 (0.89)	92	0.802
Positive anti-dsDNA	25 (27.2%)	19 (24.7%)	6 (40%)	92	0.224
C3 (mg/dL), Mean (SD):	99.34 (21.31)	98.29 (20.83)	105.07 (25.50)	92	0.397
C4 (mg/dL), Mean (SD):	20.38 (8.13)	20.33 (8.24)	20.64 (7.78)	92	0.721
Anti-ribosomal p positive, N (%)	9 (9.8%)	7 (9.1%)	2 (13.3%)	92	0.637
Prednisone dose (mg/day), Mean (SD):	1.94 (1.94)	1.92 (1.97)	2.03 (1.88)	92	0.553
Cumulative prednisone dose in 1 year (mg), Mean (SD):	671.12 (615.34)	659.61 (626.47)	725.78 (575.24)	92	0.513
Hydroxychloroquine drug therapy (yes), N (%):	90 (97.8%)	77 (100%)	14 (93.3%)	92	0.163
Other immunosuppressive drug therapy (yes), N (%):	34 (36.96%)	26 (33.77%)	8 (53.33%)	92	0.253
Psychiatric family history (yes), N (%)	50 (54.95%)	36 (47.37%)	14 (93.33%)	92	**0.003**
Hamilton Anxiety Rating Scale (HARS), Median [25th;75th]:	2.00 [1.00;6.00]	1.00 [0.00;4.00]	9.00 [6.00;18.50]	92	**<0.001**

Table 1. Cont.

	Total Sample (n = 92)	Patients without a Mood Disorder (n = 77)	Patients with Mood Disorders (n = 15)	N	p Value
Montgomery–Åsberg Depression Rating Scale (MADRS), *Median [25th;75th]*:	2.00 [0.00;7.00]	1.00 [0.00;4.00]	12.00 [8.50;22.50]	92	**<0.001**
Young Mania Rating Scale (YMRS), *Median [25th;75th]*:	0.00 [0.00;0.00]	0.00 [0.00;0.00]	0.00 [0.00;3.00]	92	**<0.001**
Plutchik Suicide Risk Scale, *Median [25th;75th]*:	2.00 [1.00;4.25]	1.00 [1.00;3.00]	5.00 [3.00;7.00]	92	**<0.001**
Global Clinical Impression (CGI), *N (%)*:				91	**<0.001**
1. Normal, not ill	65 (70.65%)	64 (83.12%)	1 (7.14%)		
2. Borderline mental ill	8 (8.70%)	6 (7.79%)	2 (14.29%)		
3. Mildly ill	12 (13.19%)	5 (6.49%)	7 (50.00%)		
4. Moderately ill	5 (5.43%)	2 (2.60%)	3 (21.43%)		
5. Markedly ill	1 (1.09%)	0 (0.00%)	1 (7.14%)		
Traumatic Experiences Screening Questionnaire (ExpTra-S), *Median [25th;75th]*:					
Frequency	0.00 [0.00;2.00]	0.00 [0.00;2.00]	1.00 [0.50;6.00]	87	**0.031**
Distress	0.00 [0.00;3.00]	0.00 [0.00;2.00]	3.00 [1.00;6.00]	87	**0.006**

SD: standard deviation; **SLEDAI-2K**: Systemic Lupus Erythematosus Disease Activity Index; **SDI**: Systemic Lupus International Collaborating Clinics/ACR Damage Index.

Table 2. Prevalence of mental disorders.

Current Psychiatric Diagnoses According to ICD-10 ($n = 32$)	N (%)
Mood disorders	
Major depressive disorder	13 (40.6%)
Persistent depressive disorder	2 (6.3%)
Trauma and Stress-Related Disorders	
Adjustment disorder	5 (15.6%)
Other disorders	
Organic depressive disorder—*in remission*	1 (3.1%)
Generalized anxiety disorder	1 (3.1%)
Eating disorder	1 (3.1%)
Psychosocial conditions not attributable to a mental disorder	
Code Z63. Problems related to primary support group	4 (12.5%)
Code Z73. Problems related to life management difficulty	5 (15.6%)

As shown in Table 3, the final model revealed a statistically significant association between presenting a mood disorder, the MADRS total scores, and the YMRS total scores ($p < 0.001$). The Hosmer–Lemeshow statistic was 6.398 ($p = 0.603$), suggesting a well-calibrated predictive model. These findings suggest that having a mood disorder is associated with greater levels of depressive symptoms and psychiatric disease severity. We further estimated the prediction efficacy of the model by performing an AUC analysis, showing a value of 0.965 (Figure 1). Altogether, these results indicate that the model can precisely detect the presence of a mood disorder in SLE patients.

Table 3. Multiple logistic regression analysis of predictors for mood disorders in SLE patients.

Variables	OR	95% CI	*p*-Value
MADRS total score	1.373	1.180 to 1.679	<0.001
YMRS total score	3.009	1.202 to 10.56	0.022

Abbreviations: OR = odds ratio; **CI** = confidence interval; **MADRS** = Montgomery–Åsberg Depression Rating Scale, **YMRS** = Young Mania Rating Scale.

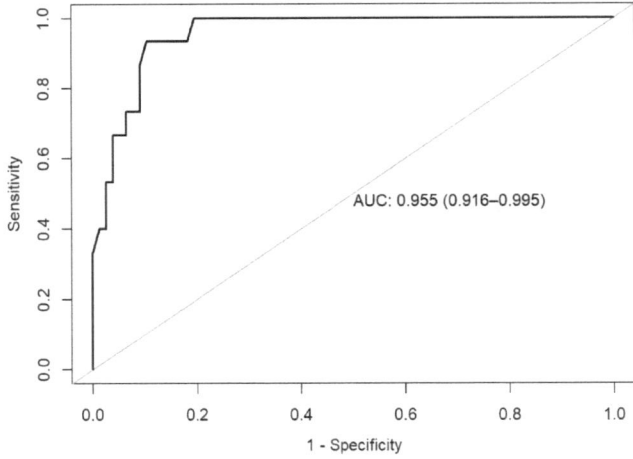

Figure 1. ROC curve. The figure shows the area under the curve (AUC) of the receiver operating characteristic (ROC).

4. Discussion

The aim of this study was to assess the real prevalence of well-characterized mood disorders in a well-defined cohort of SLE patients. Based on our results, patients with SLE showed lower prevalence rates of depressive disorders than those previously reported in the literature. In line with this finding, the prevalence of other psychopathological disturbances, such as anxiety disorders, was also low, with adjustment disorder being the second most common diagnosis. Furthermore, no SLE-related factors appear to influence the presentation of a mood disorder, with psychiatric clinical factors having a significant effect on SLE-depressed patients.

Our findings contrast with previous studies that reported a higher prevalence of psychiatric disorders among patients with lupus [34–37]. Although some studies reported prevalence rates similar to those obtained in our cohort, non-standardized scales were used to support the clinical diagnosis [38]. However, despite this lower prevalence compared to other SLE cohorts, we observed a prevalence of depressive disorders higher than in the general population. According to The Global Health Data Exchange, the overall prevalence of depressive disorders in Spain is 4.13% [39], with variations depending on the methodological aspects of the individual studies [16]. Therefore, it is essential to assess the presence of psychological disturbances in patients with autoimmune diseases through a thorough psychiatric evaluation. Since NPSLE manifestations have a negative impact on the quality of life and day-to-day functional outcomes, the early detection of mental disorders may lead to global improvement in SLE patients [40].

A significant proportion of patients had psychological disturbances that could not be classified as a mental disorder. This classification encompasses a broad spectrum of nonspecific major psychiatric disturbances, which influence health status and attendance to health services. In fact, this reflects the importance of sociocultural circumstances in the emergence and persistence of psychological disturbances. The successful identification and management of these disorders facilitate the adaption of therapeutic interventions based on the individual characteristics of each patient.

It is worth noting that, based on the cut-off criteria of the scores obtained on the MADRS to assess the occurrence of depressive symptoms, approximately 27 percent of our study group would have depression. This fact emphasizes the need for a thorough psychiatric evaluation, which can be supported by clinical screening tools such as the MADRS, among others, for the diagnosis of mental disorders.

We found no correlation between the presence of psychiatric disorders and any of the main autoimmune clinical characteristics of SLE, such as disease duration, disease activity, cumulative disease damage, or immunosuppressive treatment. It is important to note the low prednisone dose and the high use of hydroxychloroquine in both subgroups. The low degree of accrued damage in our cohort has a definite relation with the therapeutic schemes used in our unit [41].

On the other hand, the main psychiatric scales assessed revealed significant differences between groups. Among the main clinical correlators predicting the presentation of a mood disorder, we found global scores such as the MADRS, used to assess depression severity, and the total scores of the Young Mania Rating Scale. Besides that, and despite not being included in the final regression model, the higher overall anxiety scores, the higher scores observed in the Plutchick Risk Suicide Scale, and the greater presence of early traumatic experiences are of clinical significance. On this matter, the impact of early traumatic experiences on the immune system functioning is well established [42,43]. Major pro-inflammatory factors, including IFN-y, Interlucin-6, and TNF-α, among others, have been found to be increased [42]. While research on early traumatic experiences has been replicated in a variety of psychiatric populations, few studies on autoimmune disorders have taken this factor into account.

The main limitations of this study include its limited sample size, particularly in terms of the percentage of SLE patients with mood disorders. Similarly, not all patients in the cohort were evaluated, as only patients who voluntarily agreed to participate in the study were included, all of them in an outpatient clinic setting. Thus, it is possible that some patients presenting with mood disorders have not been effectively assessed. In addition, the large number of patients on hydroxychloroquine and the low current and cumulative dose of prednisone, as well as the low level of activity and damage accrual, as has been shown in our patients in previous studies [41], could have hampered the analysis of the possible predictors of mood disorders. On the other hand, the role of immunosuppressive therapy other than glucocorticoids in the development or protection against mood disorders in SLE patients has not been established [38]. Overall, the availability of a multidisciplinary team for the management of patients with autoimmune diseases should be highlighted as a possible additional explanation for our findings. Patients who show early signs of psychological problems are evaluated jointly by an autoimmune disease team psychiatrist. In this regard, close clinical care and follow-up by a multidisciplinary team can benefit from the early detection of emotional disturbances and prompt rapid therapeutic interventions. This includes a correct diagnosis with the use of a well-accepted and widely standardized semi-structured psychiatric assessment instrument (SCID), which was used in this study in accordance with the ACR guidelines for the assessment of NPSLE [13].

5. Conclusions

In summary, the prevalence of mood disorders in SLE using a comprehensive standardized interview conducted by a trained mental health specialist was lower than previously reported. No associations were found with SLE clinical features, disease activity, damage, or specific therapies. Our results highlight the need for multidisciplinary teamwork for the early diagnosis and therapeutic management of SLE patients with neuropsychiatric disorders.

Author Contributions: R.S. was the principal investigator of this study, contributed to the study design, drafted and reviewed the manuscript, and is the guarantor. G.R.-I. was the co-principal investigator and contributed to the study design. M.R.-B., J.C.-G., J.V., G.R.-I., I.H., J.J.M. and R.S. collected data and reviewed the manuscript. M.R.-B., I.H. and B.S.-Z. performed data analysis and drafted the manuscript. All authors have read and agreed to the published version of the manuscript.

Funding: Funding for this study was supported by the Basque Government via 2016111021 and IT 1512-22 grants.

Institutional Review Board Statement: This study was conducted in accordance with the Declaration of Helsinki, and the protocol was approved by the institutional review board of the Basque Ethics Committee (Code CEIC-Euskadi PI2017029„ last approval 30 August 2020). All patients signed an informed consent form on joining the cohort.

Informed Consent Statement: Written Informed consent was obtained from all subjects involved in the study.

Data Availability Statement: The data that support the findings of this study are available upon request from the corresponding author. The data are not publicly available due to privacy or ethica restrictions.

Conflicts of Interest: J.J. Meana received an unrestricted grant from Janssen-Cilag not related to this research.

References

1. Kaul, A.; Gordon, C.; Crow, M.K.; Touma, Z.; Urowitz, M.B.; van Vollenhoven, R.; Ruiz-Irastorza, G.; Hughes, G. Systemic lupus erythematosus. *Nat. Rev. Dis. Prim.* **2016**, *2*, 16039. [CrossRef] [PubMed]
2. Rees, F.; Doherty, M.; Grainge, M.J.; Lanyon, P.; Zhang, W. The worldwide incidence and prevalence of systemic lupus erythematosus: A systematic review of epidemiological studies. *Rheumatology* **2017**, *56*, 1945–1961. [CrossRef] [PubMed]
3. Schwartz, N.; Stock, A.D.; Putterman, C. Neuropsychiatric lupus: New mechanistic insights and future treatment directions. *Nat. Rev. Rheumatol.* **2019**, *15*, 137–152. [CrossRef] [PubMed]

4. Ugarte-Gil, M.F.; Hanly, J.; Urowitz, M.; Gordon, C.; Bae, S.-C.; Romero-Diaz, J.; Sanchez-Guerrero, J.; Bernatsky, S.; Clarke, A.E.; Wallace, D.J.; et al. Remission and low disease activity (LDA) prevent damage accrual in patients with systemic lupus erythematosus: Results from the Systemic Lupus International Collaborating Clinics (SLICC) inception cohort. *Ann. Rheum. Dis.* **2022**, *81*, 1541–1548. [CrossRef]
5. Mak, A.; Cheung, M.W.-L.; Chiew, H.J.; Liu, Y.; Ho, R.C.-M. Global trend of survival and damage of systemic lupus erythematosus: Meta-analysis and meta-regression of observational studies from the 1950s to 2000s. *Semin. Arthritis Rheum.* **2012**, *41*, 830–839. [CrossRef]
6. Mak, A.; Isenberg, D.A.; Lau, C.-S. Global trends, potential mechanisms and early detection of organ damage in SLE. *Nat. Rev. Rheumatol.* **2012**, *9*, 301–310. [CrossRef]
7. Patten, S.B.; Beck, C.A.; Williams, J.V.; Barbui, C.; Metz, L.M. Major depression in multiple sclerosis. *Neurology* **2003**, *61*, 1524–1527. [CrossRef]
8. Benros, M.E.; Eaton, W.W.; Mortensen, P.B. The epidemiologic evidence linking autoimmune diseases and psychosis. *Biol. Psychiatry* **2014**, *75*, 300–306. [CrossRef]
9. Benros, M.E.; Waltoft, B.L.; Nordentoft, M.; Østergaard, S.D.; Eaton, W.W.; Krogh, J.; Mortensen, P.B. Autoimmune diseases and severe infections as risk factors for mood disorders: A nationwide study. *JAMA Psychiatry* **2013**, *70*, 812–820. [CrossRef] [PubMed]
10. Song, H.; Fang, F.; Tomasson, G.; Arnberg, F.K.; Mataix-Cols, D.; de la Cruz, L.F.; Almqvist, C.; Fall, K.; Valdimarsdóttir, U.A. Association of Stress-Related Disorders With Subsequent Autoimmune Disease. *JAMA* **2018**, *319*, 2388–2400. [CrossRef]
11. Govoni, M.; Hanly, J.G. The management of neuropsychiatric lupus in the 21st century: Still so many unmet needs? *Rheumatology* **2020**, *59*, v52–v62. [CrossRef] [PubMed]
12. Kivity, S.; Agmon-Levin, N.; Zandman-Goddard, G.; Chapman, J.; Shoenfeld, Y. Neuropsychiatric lupus: A mosaic of clinical presentations. *BMC Med.* **2015**, *13*, 43. [CrossRef] [PubMed]
13. The American College of Rheumatology nomenclature and case definitions for neuropsychiatric lupus syndromes. *Arthritis Rheum.* **1999**, *42*, 599–608. [CrossRef]
14. Zhang, L.; Fu, T.; Yin, R.; Zhang, Q.; Shen, B. Prevalence of depression and anxiety in systemic lupus erythematosus: A systematic review and meta-analysis. *BMC Psychiatry* **2017**, *17*, 70. [CrossRef]
15. Moustafa, A.T.; Moazzami, M.; Engel, L.; Bangert, E.; Hassanein, M.; Marzouk, S.; Kravtsenyuk, M.; Fung, W.; Eder, L.; Su, J.; et al. Prevalence and metric of depression and anxiety in systemic lupus erythematosus: A systematic review and meta-analysis. *Semin. Arthritis Rheum.* **2020**, *50*, 84–94. [CrossRef]
16. Vieta, E.; Alonso, J.; Pérez-Sola, V.; Roca, M.; Hernando, T.; Sicras-Mainar, A.; Sicras-Navarro, A.; Herrera, B.; Gabilondo, A. Epidemiology and costs of depressive disorder in Spain: The EPICO study. *Eur. Neuropsychopharmacol.* **2021**, *50*, 93–103. [CrossRef]
17. Santomauro, D.F.; Herrera, A.M.M.; Shadid, J.; Zheng, P.; Ashbaugh, C.; Pigott, D.M.; Abbafati, C.; Adolph, C.; Amlag, J.O.; Aravkin, A.Y.; et al. Global prevalence and burden of depressive and anxiety disorders in 204 countries and territories in 2020 due to the COVID-19 pandemic. *Lancet* **2021**, *398*, 1700–1712. [CrossRef]
18. Ruiz-Arruza, I.; Lozano, J.; Cabezas-Rodriguez, I.; Medina, J.A.; Ugarte, A.; Erdozain, J.G.; Ruiz-Irastorza, G. Restrictive Use of Oral Glucocorticoids in Systemic Lupus Erythematosus and Prevention of Damage Without Worsening Long-Term Disease Control: An Observational Study. *Arthritis Care Res.* **2018**, *70*, 582–591. [CrossRef]
19. Aringer, M.; Costenbader, K.; Daikh, D.; Brinks, R.; Mosca, M.; Ramsey-Goldman, R.; Smolen, J.S.; Wofsy, D.; Boumpas, D.T.; Kamen, D.L.; et al. 2019 European League Against Rheumatism/American College of Rheumatology classification criteria for systemic lupus erythematosus. *Ann. Rheum. Dis.* **2019**, *78*, 1151–1159. [CrossRef]
20. Gorgens, K.A. Structured Clinical Interview For DSM-IV (SCID-I/SCID-II). In *Encyclopedia of Clinical Neuropsychology*; Kreutzer, J.S., DeLuca, J., Caplan, B., Eds.; Springer: New York, NY, USA, 2011. [CrossRef]
21. World Health Organization. *The International Statistical Classification of Diseases and Related Health Problems (ICD-10)*, 10th ed.; World Health Organization: Geneva, Switzerland, 1992.
22. Lobo, A.; Chamorro, L.; Luque, A.; Dal-Ré, R.; Badia, X.; Baró, E.; Grupo de Validación en Español de Escalas Psicométricas (GVEEP). Validación de las versiones en español de la Montgomery-Asberg Depression Rating Scale y la Hamilton Anxiety Rating Scale para la evaluación de la depresión y de la ansiedad [Validation of the Spanish versions of the Montgomery-Asberg depression and Hamilton anxiety rating scales]. *Med. Clin.* **2002**, *118*, 493–499.
23. Colom, F.; Vieta, E.; Martinez-Arán, A.; García, M.; Reinares, M.; Torrent, C.; Goikolea, J.M.; Banús, S.; Salamero, M. Versión española de una escala de evaluación de la manía: Validez y fiabilidad de la Escala de Manía de Young. *Med. Clin.* **2002**, *119*, 366–371. [CrossRef] [PubMed]
24. Rubio, G.; Montero, J.; Jáuregui, J.; Villanueva, R.; Casado, M.A.; Marín, J.; Santo-Domingo, J. Validación de la escala de riesgo suicida de Plutchik en población española. *Arch. Neurobiol.* **1998**, *61*, 143–152.
25. Ordóñez Camblor, N.; Fonseca Pedrero, E.; Paino Piñeiro, M.D.; García Alvarez, L.; Pizarro Ruiz, J.P.; Lemos Giráldez, S. Evaluación de experiencias traumáticas tempranas en adultos. *Papeles Psicol.* **2016**, *37*, 36–44.
26. Busner, J.; Targum, S.D. The clinical global impressions scale: Applying a research tool in clinical practice. *Psychiatry* **2007**, *4*, 28–37. [PubMed]
27. Gladman, D.D.; Ibañez, D.; Urowitz, M.B. Systemic lupus erythematosus disease activity index 2000. *J. Rheumatol.* **2002**, *29*, 288–291.

28. Fortin, P.R.; Abrahamowicz, M.; Clarke, A.E.; Neville, C.; Du Berger, R.; Fraenkel, L.; Liang, M.H. Do lupus disease activity measures detect clinically important change? *J. Rheumatol.* **2000**, *27*, 1421–1428.
29. Gladman, D.D.; Urowitz, M.B.; Goldsmith, C.H.; Fortin, P.; Ginzler, E.; Gordon, C.; Hanly, J.G.; Isenberg, D.A.; Kalunian, K.; Nived, O.; et al. The reliability of the Systemic Lupus International Collaborating Clinics/American College of Rheumatology Damage Index in patients with systemic lupus erythematosus. *Arthritis Rheum.* **1997**, *40*, 809–813. [CrossRef]
30. R Core Team. *R: A Language and Environment for Statistical Computing*; R Foundation for Statistical Computing: Vienna, Austria, 2020; Available online: https://www.R-project.org/ (accessed on 30 November 2023).
31. Subirana, I.; Sanz, H.; Vila, J. Building Bivariate Tables: The compare Groups Package for R. *J. Stat. Softw.* **2014**, *57*, 1–16. [CrossRef]
32. Fox, J.; Weisberg, S. *An R Companion to Applied Regression*, 3rd ed.; SAGE: Los Angeles, CA, USA, 2019.
33. Kassambara, A. Ggcorrplot: Visualization of a Correlation Matrix Using 'Ggplot2'. 2019. Available online: https://CRAN.R-project.org/package=ggcorrplot (accessed on 30 November 2023).
34. Wei, T.; Simko, V. R Package "Corrplot": Visualization of a Correlation Matrix. 2021. Available online: https://github.com/taiyun/corrplot (accessed on 30 November 2023).
35. Brey, R.L.; Holliday, S.L.; Saklad, A.R.; Navarrete, M.G.; Hermosillo–Romo, D.; Stallworth, C.L.; Valdez, C.R.; Escalante, A.; del Rincón, I.; Gronseth, G.; et al. Neuropsychiatric syndromes in lupus: Prevalence using standardized definitions. *Neurology* **2002**, *58*, 1214–1220. [CrossRef]
36. Nery, F.G.; Borba, E.F.; Viana, V.S.; Hatch, J.P.; Soares, J.C.; Bonfá, E.; Neto, F.L. Prevalence of depressive and anxiety disorders in systemic lupus erythematosus and their association with anti-ribosomal P antibodies. *Prog. Neuropsychopharmacol. Biol. Psychiatry* **2008**, *32*, 695–700. [CrossRef]
37. Philip, E.J.; Lindner, H.; Lederman, L. Relationship of illness perceptions with depression among individuals diagnosed with lupus. *Depress. Anxiety* **2009**, *26*, 575–582. [CrossRef] [PubMed]
38. Hanly, J.G.; Su, L.; Urowitz, M.B.; Romero-Diaz, J.; Gordon, C.; Bae, S.; Bernatsky, S.; Clarke, A.E.; Wallace, D.J.; Merrill, J.T.; et al. Mood Disorders in Systemic Lupus Erythematosus: Results From an International Inception Cohort Study. *Arthritis Rheumatol.* **2015**, *67*, 1837–1847. [CrossRef] [PubMed]
39. Global Health Data Exchange (GHDx). Discover the World's Health Data. Prevalence of Depression. 2017. Available online: http://ghdx.healthdata.org/gbd-results-tool (accessed on 30 November 2023).
40. Monahan, R.C.; de Voorde, L.J.J.B.-V.; Steup-Beekman, G.M.; Magro-Checa, C.; Huizinga, T.W.J.; Hoekman, J.; A Kaptein, A. Neuropsychiatric symptoms in systemic lupus erythematosus: Impact on quality of life. *Lupus* **2017**, *26*, 1252–1259. [CrossRef] [PubMed]
41. Ruiz-Irastorza, G.; Ruiz-Estevez, B.; Lazaro, E.; Ruiz-Arruza, I.; Duffau, P.; Martin-Cascon, M.; Richez, C.; Ugarte, A.; Blanco, P. Prolonged remission in SLE is possible by using reduced doses of prednisone: An observational study from the Lupus-Cruces and Lupus-Bordeaux in-ception cohorts. *Autoimmun. Rev.* **2019**, *18*, 102359. [CrossRef] [PubMed]
42. Lord, J.M.; Midwinter, M.J.; Chen, Y.-F.; Belli, A.; Brohi, K.; Kovacs, E.J.; Koenderman, L.; Kubes, P.; Lilford, R.J. The systemic immune response to trauma: An overview of pathophysiology and treatment. *Lancet* **2014**, *384*, 1455–1465. [CrossRef]
43. Elwenspoek, M.M.; Kuehn, A.; Muller, C.P.; Turner, J.D. The effects of early life adversity on the immune system. *Psychoneuroendocrinology* **2017**, *82*, 140–154. [CrossRef]

Disclaimer/Publisher's Note: The statements, opinions and data contained in all publications are solely those of the individual author(s) and contributor(s) and not of MDPI and/or the editor(s). MDPI and/or the editor(s) disclaim responsibility for any injury to people or property resulting from any ideas, methods, instructions or products referred to in the content.

MDPI AG
Grosspeteranlage 5
4052 Basel
Switzerland
Tel.: +41 61 683 77 34

Journal of Clinical Medicine Editorial Office
E-mail: jcm@mdpi.com
www.mdpi.com/journal/jcm

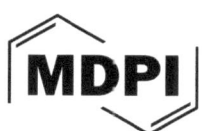

Disclaimer/Publisher's Note: The title and front matter of this reprint are at the discretion of the Guest Editor. The publisher is not responsible for their content or any associated concerns. The statements, opinions and data contained in all individual articles are solely those of the individual Editor and contributors and not of MDPI. MDPI disclaims responsibility for any injury to people or property resulting from any ideas, methods, instructions or products referred to in the content.

www.ingramcontent.com/pod-product-compliance
Lightning Source LLC
LaVergne TN
LVHW072315090526
838202LV00019B/2289